The WASP Textbook on Social Psychiatry

The WASP Textbook on Social Psychiatry

Historical, Developmental, Cultural, and Clinical Perspectives

Edited by

Rama Rao Gogineni,
Andres J. Pumariega,
Roy A. Kallivayalil,
Marianne Kastrup, and
Eugenio M. Rothe

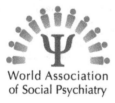

World Association
of Social Psychiatry

OXFORD
UNIVERSITY PRESS

OXFORD
UNIVERSITY PRESS

Oxford University Press is a department of the University of Oxford. It furthers the University's objective of excellence in research, scholarship, and education by publishing worldwide. Oxford is a registered trade mark of Oxford University Press in the UK and certain other countries.

Published in the United States of America by Oxford University Press
198 Madison Avenue, New York, NY 10016, United States of America.

Library of Congress Cataloging-in-Publication Data
Names: Gogineni, Rama Rao, editor. | Pumariega, Andres J., editor. | Kallivayalil, Roy Abraham, editor. | Kastrup, M., editor. | Rothe, Eugenio, editor. | World Association of Social Psychiatry, issuing body.
Title: The WASP textbook on social psychiatry : historical, developmental, cultural, and clinical perspectives / Rama Rao Gogineni, Andres Pumariega, Roy Abraham Kallivayalil, Marianne Kastrup, Eugenio Rothe, editors.
Other titles: Textbook on social psychiatry
Description: New York : Oxford University Press, 2023. |
Includes bibliographical references and index.
Identifiers: LCCN 2022040702 (print) | LCCN 2022040703 (ebook) |
ISBN 9780197521359 (paperback) | ISBN 9780197521373 (epub) | ISBN 9780197521380
Subjects: MESH: Community Psychiatry
Classification: LCC RC455 (print) | LCC RC455 (ebook) | NLM WM 30.61 |
DDC 616.89—dc23/eng/20221209
LC record available at https://lccn.loc.gov/2022040702
LC ebook record available at https://lccn.loc.gov/2022040703

DOI: 10.1093/med/9780197521359.001.0001

This material is not intended to be, and should not be considered, a substitute for medical or other professional advice. Treatment for the conditions described in this material is highly dependent on the individual circumstances. And, while this material is designed to offer accurate information with respect to the subject matter covered and to be current as of the time it was written, research and knowledge about medical and health issues is constantly evolving and dose schedules for medications are being revised continually, with new side effects recognized and accounted for regularly. Readers must therefore always check the product information and clinical procedures with the most up-to-date published product information and data sheets provided by the manufacturers and the most recent codes of conduct and safety regulation. The publisher and the authors make no representations or warranties to readers, express or implied, as to the accuracy or completeness of this material. Without limiting the foregoing, the publisher and the authors make no representations or warranties as to the accuracy or efficacy of the drug dosages mentioned in the material. The authors and the publisher do not accept, and expressly disclaim, any responsibility for any liability, loss, or risk that may be claimed or incurred as a consequence of the use and/or application of any of the contents of this material.

Printed by Marquis Book Printing, Canada

Contents

SECTION 2. DEVELOPMENTAL PERSPECTIVES

SECTION 3. SOCIOCULTURAL PERSPECTIVES

SECTION 4. CLINICAL PERSPECTIVES

SECTION 5. SPECIAL TOPICS

Foreword

Norman Sartorius, MD, PhD, FRCPsych

It is a pleasure and an honor to be invited to write a preface for a book that brought together so many leaders of social psychiatry, covering the entire field of action of social psychiatry with their comprehensive and insightful contributions.

It could be argued that social psychiatry must not exist because its existence means that there can be a psychiatry which is not taking social factors into account. This is not an acceptable conclusion: psychiatry, by definition, must be social. Regrettably, however, much is still done in psychiatry without any consideration of the role of social determinants of mental health and illness, and it is therefore of essential importance to maintain and develop the field of social psychiatry, which must influence the discipline as a whole and ensure that social aspects of psychiatry are receiving the attention they deserve.

The best way to ensure that knowledge about social factors affecting health and the practice of medicine becomes an integral and essential part of the theory and practice of psychiatry is to ensure that social psychiatry is included in undergraduate and postgraduate education of health workers regardless of their field of action. Materials which should be used in this educational effort are not always easy to find, and those which are easy to reach are often inadequate. The 41 chapters of the textbook—authored by more than 50 experts from 13 countries, carefully edited by the five editors—present an invaluable assembly of material which can be used as fundamental teaching aid in the education of different categories of health workers.

The textbook is not only a teaching aid: it is also a thoughtful review of current knowledge which practitioners and researchers in the field of psychiatry will be able to use in their daily work and research.

The timing of the production of this book is also one of its strong points. The continuous growth of comorbidity of mental and physical disorders in today's world, exposed to powerful social trends ranging from globalization to continuously growing commercialization of medicine and dehumanization of social interaction, makes the facts and wisdom contained in the book a wonderful resource for all practitioners of medicine in general and psychiatry in particular who wish to make their work useful to society.

It is for these reasons that I wish to end this Preface by expressing our gratitude to the authors and editors of the *Textbook*. Jointly they have created a most valuable opus which is and will remain a key element in the optimal development of medicine, psychiatry, and social science, and will help all those working in these fields.

Contributors

Abhinav Tando, MD
Associate Professor
Department of Psychiatry
United Institute of Medical Sciences
Allahabad, India

Debasish Basu, MD
Professor and Head
Department of Psychiatry
Postgraduate Institute of Medical
Education and Research
Chandigarh, India

Basie Bostic, BBA
Research Assistant
Austin, TX, USA

Jeff Q. Bostic, MD, EdD
Professor of Clinical Psychiatry
Department of Child Psychiatry
MedStar Georgetown University
Washington, DC, USA

Daniel Buhalo, MD
Psychiatry Resident
Department of Psychiatry
Tower Health Phoenixville Hospital
Phoenixville, PA, USA

Martin-Carrasco, PhD
Medical Director
Department of Psychiatry
Clínica Psiquiátrica Padre Meni
Pamplona (Navarra), ES

Rakesh K. Chadda, MBBS, MD, FAMS, FRCPsych
Professor and Head
Department of Psychiatry, and
Chief, National Drug Dependence
Treatment Centre
All India Institute of Medical Sciences
Ansari Nagar, New Delhi, India

Nidhi Chauhan, MD (Psychiatry), DM (Child & Adolescent Psychiatry)
Assistant Professor
Department of Psychiatry
Postgraduate Institute of Medical
Education and Research
Chandigarh, India

Carl I. Cohen, MD
Distinguished Service Professor
Department of Psychiatry, Division of
Geriatric Psychiatry
SUNY Downstate Health Sciences University
Brooklyn, NY, USA

Doina Cozman, MD, PhD
President of Romanian Association of
Psychiatry and Psychotherapy
Department of Clinical Psychology and
Psychiatry
Iuliu Haţieganu University of Medicine and
Pharmacy
Cluj-Napoca, Romania

Thomas Craig, MD, PhD
Professor Emeritus Social Psychiatry
Health Service and Population Research
King's College London Institute of
Psychiatry, Psychology and Neuroscience
London, UK

Claudia Dima, MD, PhD
Public Health and Management Consultant
National Centre of Evaluation and Health
Promotion
National Institute of Public Health
Bucharest, RO

Vincenzo Di Nicola, MPhil, MD,
DipPsych, PhD, FRCPC, FCAHS,
DLFAPA, DFCPA
Professor
Department of Psychiatry & Addiction
Medicine
Division of Child & Adolescent Psychiatry
University of Montreal
Montreal, QC, Canada

Kyra Doumlele, MD
Resident Physician
Department of Psychiatry
Dartmouth-Hitchcock Medical Center
Lebanon, NH, USA

April Fallon, PhD
Clinical Professor
Department of Psychology
Drexel University College of Medicine and
Fielding Graduate University

Philadelphia and Santa Barbara, PA, USA

Sari Fröjd, PhD (Social Psychiatry)
Docent, University Lecturer
Faculty of Social Sciences, Department of
Health Sciences
Tampere University
Tampere, Finland

Sonu Gaind, MD, FRCP(C), DFAPA
Professor
Department of Psychiatry
University of Toronto
Toronto, ON, Canada

Rachid Bennegadi, MD
Chair of the Transcultural Psychiatry
Section of the World Psychiatric
Association (WPA-TPS)
Director of the Research and Teaching Pole
at Minkowska Centre
Centre Françoise Minkowska
Paris, France

Rama Rao Gogineni, MD
Professor
Department of Psychiatry
Cooper Medical School of Rowan
University
Camden, NJ, USA

Kristine Goins, MD
Child Psychiatrist
Formerly MedStar Georgetown University
Hospital
Division of Child and Adolescent
Psychiatry
Washington, DC, USA

Brian Harlan, MD
Associate Professor
Department of Psychiatry
University of Florida College of Medicine
Gainesville, FL, USA

Gabriel Ivbijaro, MBBS, MMedSci, MA, PhD, FRCGP, FWACPsych, IDFAPA
Professor
Department of Mental Health
NOVA Medical School
Faculdade Ciências Médicas
Lisbon, Portugal

Prasad Joshi, MD, PhD
Child Psychiatrist
Horsham Clinic
Ambler, PA, USA

Roy Abraham Kallivayalil, MD, DPM
Professor and Head
Department of Psychiatry
Pushpagiri Institute of Medical Sciences
Thiruvalla Kerala, India

Olga Karpenko, MD, PhD
Head of Department
Department of Scientific Collaborations
Mental-health Clinic No.1 named after
N.A. Alexeev
Moscow, Russia

Marianne Kastrup, MD, PhD
Specialist in Psychiatry
Chairperson Anti Torture Support
Foundation, Copenhagen Head National
Centre Transcultural Psychiatry,
Copenhagen University Hospital (retired)
Copenhagen, DK

**G. Kostyuk, MD, PhD, Dr Habil.,
Professor of Psychiatry**
Head of Department
Department of Mental Health, Faculty of
Psychology
Lomonosov Moscow State University
Moscow, Russia

Mircea Lazarescu, PhD
Professor and Head
Department of Psychiatry
Eduard Pamfil Psychiatric Clinic
Timisoara, Romania

Fernando Lolas, MD
Professor of Psychiatry and Director,
Center for Bioethics, University of Chile;
Professor and Researcher, Universidad
Central de Chile
Center for Bioethics and Psychiatric Clinic
University of Chile; Central University
of Chile
Santiago de Chile, CL

Maria Ines Lopez-Ibor, PhD, MD
Professor
Legal Medicine, Psychiatry and Pathology
Department, Faculty Medicine
Complutense University
Madrid, ES

Maryssa Lyons, MD
Resident Physician
Department of Psychiatry
Tower Health
Philadelphia, PA, USA

**Savita Malhotra, MD, PhD, FAMS, Hon
Fellow Amer College of Psychiatrists**
Professor of Psychiatry
Former Dean and Head Department of
Psychiatry
Post Graduate Institute of Medical
Education and Research
Chandigarh, India

Shivananda Manohar, DNB, DPM
Assistant Professor
Department of Psychiatry
JSS Academy of Higher Education
Mysuru, India

Angus McLellan, MBChB, MRCPsych
Consultant Psychiatrist
South Oxfordshire Adult Mental
Health Team
Oxford Health NHS Foundation Trust
Oxford, UK

Greeshma Mohan, MA
Psychologist
Schizophrenia Research Foundation
Chennai, India
Andrew Molodynski
Consultant Psychiatrist and Honorary
Senior Lecturer
Oxford Health NHS Foundation Trust and
Oxford University
Oxford, UK

Kishan Nallapula, MBBS
Clinical Assistant Professor
Department of Psychiatry
University of Florida
Gainesville, FL, USA

Kirsti Nurmela, MD
University Instructor
Faculty of Social Sciences
Tampere University Hospital—Tampere
Pirkanmaa, FI, USA

Yoshiro Ono, MD, PhD
Director
Wakayama Prefecture Mental Health and
Welfare Center
Wakayama, JP

R. Padmavati, MD, DPM
Director
Schizophrenia Research Foundation
Chennai, TN, India

Alexandru Paziuc, PhD
Associate Professor
Hospital of Psychiatric Campulung
Moldovenesc
Câmpulung Moldovenesc, RO

Sami Pirkola, PhD
Professor
Social Psychiatry in Health Sciences of
the Tampere University Faculty of Social
Sciences
Helsinki, FI

Basant Pradhan, MD
Associate Professor of Psychiatry &
Pediatrics
Department of Psychiatry & Pediatrics
Cooper Medical School of Rowan
University
Camden, New Jersey, USA

Andres J. Pumariega, MD
Professor and Chief, Division of Child and
Adolescent Psychiatry
Department of Psychiatry
University of Florida
Gainesville, FL, USA

Vijaya Raghavan, MD
Consultant Psychiatrist
Department of Psychiatry
Schizophrenia Research Foundation
Chennai, India

Mariam Rahmani, MD
Clinical Associate Professor
Department of Psychiatry
University of Florida
Gainesville, FL, USA

Suman S. Rao
Researcher
PES College of Pharmacy
Bengaluru, Karnataka, India

T. S. Sathyanarayana Rao
Professor
Department of Psychiatry
JSS Medical College and Hospital
Mysore, Karnataka, India

Eduardo Rodriguez-Yunta, PhD
Coordinator Ethics of Research
Interdisciplinary Center for Studies on
Bioethics
University of Chile
Santiago, CL

Anthony Rostain, MD, MA
Professor and Chair of Psychiatry
Department of Psychiatry and
Behavioral Health
Cooper Medical School of Rowan
University
Camden, NJ, USA

Eugenio Rothe, MD
Professor
Department of Psychiatry
Herbert Wertheim College of Medicine/
Florida International University
Miami, FL, USA

Pedro Ruiz, MD
Clinical Professor of Psychiatry, Baylor
College of Medicine
Past President, World Psychiatric
Association
Past President, American Psychiatric
Association
Houston, Texas

Karim Sedky, MD, MSc, DFAPA
Professor of Psychiatry and Medical
Student Education Director
Department of Psychiatry
Cooper Medical School of Rowan
University
Camden, NJ, USA

Michael Shapiro, MD, DFAPA, DFAACAP
Associate Professor
Division of Child and Adolescent
Psychiatry, Department of Psychiatry
University of Florida
Gainesville, FL, USA

Shridhar Sharma, MD, DPM, FRC Psy
(Lond), FRANZCP, DFAPA, FAMS
Emeritus Professor
Department of Psychiatry
National Academy of Medical Sciences and
Institute of Human Behaviour and Allied
Sciences
New Delhi, India

Angela Shrestha, MD
Director of Psychiatry
Howard Brown Health Center
Chicago, IL, USA

Suzan Song, MD, MPH, PhD
Professor and Director of Global Child and
Family Mental Health
Global Health
Harvard/Boston Children's Hospital
Boston, MA, USA

R. Srinivasa Murthy, MD Psychiatry
Professor of Psychiatry(retd)
Department of Psychiatry
NIMHANS, Bangalore
Bengaluru Urban, India

Nada Stotland, MD, MPH
Professor of Psychiatry
Rush Medical College
Chicago, IL, USA

Jacob Swartz, MD
Inpatient Adolescent Attending
Department of Psychiatry, Child and
Adolescent Division
Medstar Georgetown University Hospital
Washington, DC, AUS

R. Thara, PhD, FRCPsych (hon)
Vice Chairman, and Chair Research
Schizophrenia Research Foundation
(India)
Chennai, India

Kenneth Thompson, MD
Medical Director
Pennsylvania Psychiatric Leadership
Council
Pittsburgh, PA, USA

Joseph E. Thornton, MD
Clinical Associate Professor
Department of Psychiatry
University of Florida College of Medicine
Gainesville, FL, USA

**Lakshmi Venkatraman, MBBS, DPM,
MRCPsych**
Consultant Psychiatrist
General Adult Psychiatry
Schizophrenia Research Foundation
(India)
Chennai, India

Prologue

The Relevance and Need for a Comprehensive Textbook on Social Psychiatry

Roy Abraham Kallivayalil

In every bit of honest writing in the world, there is a base theme. Try to understand men, if you understand each other you will be kind to each other. Knowing a man well never leads to hate and nearly always leads to love.
—John Steinbeck, *Of Mice and Men*

There have been rapid advances in neurosciences today, leading to higher expectations for psychiatry to "cure" mental illnesses. The new psychopharmacological agents were often seen as the answer to many mental illnesses, and breakthroughs were believed to be imminent, which unfortunately has not happened as expected. There seems to be a renewed interest in social psychiatry and its relevance to clinical practice. Times like these, which are unprecedented, further augment the relevance of social psychiatry and the need for a comprehensive book on social psychiatry.

Social psychiatry is that branch of psychiatry concerned with effects of the social environment on the mental health of the individual and with the effects of the mentally ill person on his/her social environment. The multifaceted nature of the word "social" often makes it difficult to encompass what social psychiatry is. Man is a social animal, and social circumstances and society as a whole figure in the pathogenesis of not only mental illness but also physical illness.

The roots of social medicine can be found in the ancient civilizations.[1] Adding a social paradigm to the conceptualization of health made it more holistic and comprehensive. The origin of social medicine can be traced back to ancient Greek, Chinese, and Ayurvedic practices. The World Health Organization (WHO) in its definition of health talks about "a state of complete physical, mental and social well-being and not merely the absence of disease or infirmity."[2] It is important for the modern-day physician to identify and understand the social paradigm of health, and this will go a long way in the curative, preventive, and promotive aspects of managing health. The earliest roots of social medicine can be found in the ancient texts of Ayurveda. The focus of the physician in Ayurveda is on the patient's health, rather than the disease. There is often a stipulated harmonious framework for health and life. There is a greater emphasis on quality of life, rather than just the curative aspect of disease. The treatment approach in Ayurveda is person centered and often takes into consideration the person as a whole. The same would apply to ancient Greek philosophy. Socrates, Plato, Aristotle, and Hippocrates talked about the importance of the social paradigm of health. The concept is summarized in Socrates's quote, "If the whole is not well, it is impossible for the part to be well."[3]

For centuries, psychiatry was known for its treatments aimed at making patients behave in a way acceptable to society, since society generally defined behavioral deviance.[4] Patients were often locked away in distant institutions away from the so-called civilized society. Although there has always been an emphasis on etiology and biological aspects of mental illness, there is an increasing need to focus more on social determinants and consequences of such illnesses, according to the biopsychosocial model. The social aspects remain an essential component in understanding the genesis and management of psychiatric disorders, but are often ignored due to too much emphasis on pharmacological treatments in contemporary psychiatry. A closer look at the research in mental disorders in the past few decades reveals allocation of massive resources toward biological research, whereas hardly any funded research has been carried out into the psychosocial domains, which are important not only in psychiatry, but also in other fields of medicine.[5] The limitations of drug therapy also provide a strong case for investing more to learn about the social domains in the etiopathogenesis of mental illness. There is increasing evidence that social determinants of health play a major role in the genesis of both physical and mental illness.[6] Human beings grow up and develop within society and specific cultures, and their upbringing and learned interactions define their behaviors, which in turn affect brain structures, leading to dysfunctions. Critics of earlier definitions of health by the WHO, which focused on just the "absence of diseases," have argued that this does not include the social domain and individuals' ability to manage their life by fulfilling their potential and obligations with a degree of independence. This becomes very important now, since people are living longer, sometimes with comorbidities. People can be well at times, but can be unwell at other times, sometimes battling several comorbidities. It can be argued that health is a dynamic balance between opportunities and limitations, which is directly affected by social and environmental conditions. In addition, the social domain is highly pertinent in our understanding and management of psychiatric disorders, and can be seen as a crucial etiological factor. Current advances, such as mirror neuron systems, reflect the importance of social cognition that governs human social interactions.

Building on these basic premises, the need arose for a comprehensive textbook in social psychiatry. The World Association of Social Psychiatry (WASP) at its Executive Committee (EC) meeting held at Vienna on April 5, 2018, chaired by Roy Abraham Kallivayalil (WASP president) made a formal decision in this regard and entrusted the preliminary work to Rama Rao Gogineni (past president of American Association of Social Psychiatry [AASP]). Subsequent EC meetings held at Versailles on September 13, 2018, approved the *WASP Textbook on Social Psychiatry*, to be published by Oxford University Press, and the EC meeting held at Versailles on September 12, 2019, appointed Rama Rao Gogineni as the lead editor and Roy Kallivayalil and Marianne Kastrup as editors representing the EC. On October 25, 2019, during the WASP World Congress in Bucharest, Rama Rao Gogineni presented a report on the *WASP Textbook of Social Psychiatry*. This first of its kind textbook focuses on understanding social psychiatry, based on the inputs from stalwarts who have advocated for a paradigm shift from biological reductionism to a more holistic biopsychosocial approach.

The preface of the textbook is written by Norman Sartorius, who has remained an inspiration for all of us to undertake such a challenging task. We start with the history of social psychiatry in Chapter 2, by Roy Kallivayalil, Marianne Kastrup, Rama Rao Gogineni, Vincenzo Di Nicola, and Shridhar Sharma, who take us on a journey of global variations in the practice of social psychiatry. The chapter looks to trace the philosophical origins of social psychiatry and its evolution through the years, dwelling on the dynamic factors that bring about these variations in practice. In Chapter 3, Thomas Craig sheds light upon the dynamic biopsychosocial approach and provides updates to our understanding of this approach. Fernando Lolas and Eduardo Rodriguez, in Chapter 4, then discuss the ethical dimensions of social psychiatry and its ever-increasing relevance in the current times. Chapter 5, by Vincenzo Di Nicola, takes into account these dynamic changes and ethical dimensions of social psychiatry to set a manifesto for the practice of social psychiatry in the 21st century. In Chapter 6, Eugenio Rothe discusses professionalism and social psychiatry. Recommendations for a social psychiatry training curriculum are presented by Eugenio Rothe, Andres Pumariega, and Rama Rao Gogineni in Chapter 7.

To begin Section 2, Developmental Perspectives, Savita Malhotra and Nidhi Chauhan in Chapter 8 share their insights into the developmental perspectives in social psychiatry particularly of relevance to children. Eugenio Rothe then takes the journey further in Chapter 9 by discussing the relevance of social psychiatry during the often tumultuous stages of adolescence and young adulthood. We then delve into the relevance of social psychiatry to issues of aging in Chapter 10 by Carl Cohen and Kyra Doumlele. In Chapter 11, H. Steven Moffic takes us to a discussion of death and dying in the context of social psychiatry. In Chapter 12, Nada Stotland and Angela Shrestha touch upon the relevance of social psychiatry for women. Social psychiatry perspectives for men are discussed by Marianne Kastrup, Kenneth Thompson, and Rama Rao Gogineni in Chapter 13.

In Section 3, Sociocultural Perspectives, Andres Pumariega and Professor Pedro Ruiz (Chapter 14) discuss social psychiatry and culture. María Inés López Ibor and Manuel Martín Carrasco, in Chapter 15, write about the relevance of social psychiatry in the context of religion. Jeff Bostic, Kristine Goins, and Basie Bostic, in Chapter 16, discuss the relevance of music, dance, and the arts in the realm of social psychiatry. In Chapter 17, Jacob Swarz writes about the potential of sports and exercise. The relevance of social psychiatry in sexuality is well described in Chapter 18 by Shivanand Manohar, Abhinav Tandon, Suman S. Rao, and T. S. Sathyanarayana Rao. Marianne Kastrup in Chapter 19 then talks about the relevance of social psychiatry for particularly vulnerable and marginalized sections of society. In Chapter 20, Vincenzo Di Nicola and Suzan Song give us their valuable insights into the relevance of social psychiatry for immigrants, refugees, and displaced populations. Rama Rao Gogineni and Andreas Pumariega, in Chapter 21, discuss in detail the relevance of social determinants like poverty, hunger, and homelessness.

In Section 4, Clinical Perspectives, Basant Pradhan discusses the brain and biology in Chapter 22, thereby looking at the biological underpinnings in social psychiatry. In Chapter 23, Rama Rao Gogineni, Prasad Joshi, and Tony Rostain write on social perspectives in neurodevelopmental disorders. Sami Pirkola, Sari Fröjd, and Kirst Nurmela, in Chapter 24, discuss the relevance of social perspectives in depression and anxiety disorders. In Chapter 25, Maryssa Lyons, Daniel Buhalo, and April Fallon explore traumatic disorders with particular relevance to social psychiatry. In Chapter 26, Lakshmi Venkatraman, Greeshma Mohan, Vijaya Raghavan, Ramachandran Padmavati, and Rangaswamy Thara share their valuable insights into the relevance of social psychiatry in psychotic disorders. Rakesh Chadda and Roy Abraham Kallivayalil, in Chapter 27, discuss substance use disorders in the context of social psychiatry. In Chapter 28, Sonu Gaind takes us to the topic of suicide. We then move on to a discussion of medical illness in psychiatry by Joseph Thornton in Chapter 29, and an exploration of major cognitive disorders by Brian Harlan and Joseph Thornton in Chapter 30. Abram Estafanous and Karim Sedky share their valuable insights on sleep disorders in Chapter 31, and Michael Shapiro discusses child maltreatment in Chapter 32. In Chapter 33, Angus Mclellan and Andrew Molodynski share their insights on prisoners.

In Section 5, we discuss some special topics of contemporary relevance. Social psychiatry has and will have a major role in tackling stigma around mental illness. In Chapter 34, Mariam Rahmani, Gabriel Ivbijaro, and Andres Pumariega discuss this issue. Terrorism and violent conflict and the role of social psychiatry are discussed by Debasish Basu in Chapter 35. In Chapter 36, Eugenio Rothe, Yoshiro Ono, and Andres Pumariega discuss youth violence. Of particular relevance to contemporary times is Chapter 37, by Andres Pumariega, Marianne Kastrup, and R. Srinivasa Murthy, on the COVID-19 pandemic, international response, and the impact of the pandemic on mental mealth. Kishan Nallapula discusses the topic of mental health aspects of information technology in Chapter 38. Olga Karpenko and George Kostyuk, in Chapter 39, write about social psychiatry in Russia. In Chapter 40, Alexandru Pazuic, Doina Cozman, and Mircea Lazarescu discuss education and training in social psychiatry in Romania. Final reflections, in Chapter 41, are presented by Rachid Bennegadi, current president of the WASP.

The biopsychosocial model tries to understand suffering and illness and how they are affected at multiple levels, from the molecular to societal. It values patients' subjective experiences as important for diagnosis, care, and management. Thus, it is a philosophy, on the one hand, while being a practical guide, on the other. The biopsychosocial approach is also providing new directions to global mental health by exploring synergies and opportunities in bridging inequities and inequalities in mental healthcare services worldwide. This book is a product of many like-minded individuals coming together for the cause of social psychiatry. It will give the reader a comprehensive overview of where social psychiatry stands today and the limitless possibilities ahead!

References

1. Rastogi S. Building bridges between Ayurveda and modern science. *Int J Ayurveda Res*. 2010;1(1):41–46.
2. Conference IH. Constitution of the World Health Organization. 1946. *Bull World Health Organ*. 2002;80(12):983.
3. Mezzich JE. Psychiatry for the person: Articulating medicine's science and humanism. *World J Psychiatry*. 2007 Jun;6(2):65.
4. Haack K, Kumbier E. History of social psychiatry. *Curr Opin Psychiatry*. 2012 Nov;25(6):492–496.
5. Khandelwal SK, Chadda RK, Chavan BS. Social psychiatry: Looking at the horizon. *Indian J Soc Psychiatry*. 2016 Jul 1;32(3):179.
6. Marmot M. Social determinants of health inequalities. *Lancet*. 2005 Mar 19;365(9464):1099–1104.

Introduction and Orientation

Introduction and orientation presents a unique aspects on origins and philosophical and academic aspects of social psychiatry. The section focuses on History of Social Psychiatry and Historical Aspects of the WASP, Biopsychosocial Model, Ethical Perspectives, Manifesto for the 21st Century, Professionalism and Developing a Curriculum to Teach Social Psychiatry.

History of Social Psychiatry and Historical Aspects of the World Association of Social Psychiatry

Roy Abraham Kallivayalil, Marianne Kastrup,
Rama Rao Gogineni, Vincenzo Di Nicola, and
Shridhar Sharma

Introduction

Social psychiatry is a discipline that focuses on the social dimension of mental health, mental illness, and mental healthcare. Social psychiatry uses concepts and methods of social sciences, including psychology and anthropology, to investigate social factors influencing and relevant to the occurrence, expression, course, and care of mental disorders. Social psychiatry starts from the position that because humans are social animals, the cause, course, and response to treatment of mental health problems are powerfully determined by the social environment. For example, childhood trauma within the home and bullying at school are associated with both internalizing and externalizing disorders and exert their influence through lifelong impacts on an individual's ability to form supportive relationships with others, their self-esteem, and their resilience in the face of future adversity. Difficulties forming and sustaining personal relationships are intensified by the emergence of illness, consequent social exclusion, and discrimination, that in turn intensify damaging beliefs of low self-worth and rejection. In contrast, we have considerable evidence for the "therapeutic" value of good relationships, notably the role of family and social support in the remarkable resilience shown by those who have come through the most appalling environmental and personal crises. It is therefore surprising that the balance of psychiatric therapeutic effort is stubbornly focused on the individual patient as the problem, with less attention paid to developing and implementing social interventions targeted at the family and the wider social network to prevent and alleviate mental illness.[1]

Social Psychiatry: Origins and Evolution

Reil et al. introduced, in 1803, the word "psychiatry" in Germany. After 100 years, in 1903, the term "social" was first linked to psychiatry, when Ilberg from the Grotschweidnitz asylum in Saxony, Germany, wrote a paper entitled simply "Soziale Psychiatrie."[2] Ilberg[3] defined "social psychiatry" as a theory of the detrimental influences that affected the mental health of the whole population (Gesamtheit) and as a useful means for their prevention. In 1911, Fischer[4] advocated psychiatric care outside the asylums and called this kind of extramural psychiatry "Soziale Psychiatrie." During the same period, Kolb stressed that asylum care and extramural psychiatric care were two inseparable and complementary parts of one single system of mental healthcare. Dr. E. E. Southard of Harvard Medical School, in 1922, taught his students about "social psychiatry," which he termed "an art now during development by which the psychiatrist deals with social problems" and as "that part of the knowledge of psychiatry which has a bearing upon social problems. "[5]

World Wars

The First World War had shaken psychiatry and medicine as a whole, because of the considerable incidence of battle neurosis, or "shell shock," a result of the massive disruptions of war. The Second World War contributed to American and British psychiatry due to social and political complexities and international alliances and brought about major changes in the psychiatric system and ideology. Military psychiatrists came to some important conclusions: that neuropsychiatric problems were more serious than had been previously recognized, that environmental stress was a major contributor to mental maladjustment, and that purposeful human interventions could alter psychological outcomes. Psychiatrists had seen that treating servicemen in the context of their social relationships was essential. With enough supportive forms of psychotherapy, combined with rest, sleep, and food, severely stressed combatants were able to rapidly return to the front.[6]

Social Reforms

The major psychiatric reforms in the second half of the past century were mainly based on concepts and reforms of Swiss, and especially Zurich, psychiatry. Professional associations and expert groups, including the World Health Organization (WHO), stimulated service improvements in the direction of social psychiatry, and promoted education, training, and the professional role of future psychiatrists. Social psychiatry concepts became consolidated over a century ago under the auspices of mental and racial hygiene, but after the Second World War, social psychiatry embraced the concepts of community-based care and deinstitutionalization. And it was not the specific treatments that mattered. William Menninger believed that it was vital to determine the "more serious community-based sources of emotional stress" if effective strategies were to be developed to treat that stress.[6]

After leaving military service, these psychiatrists applied the same notions to civilian care and began to emphasize treatment in a family and community setting, rather than within the state hospital systems exclusively. Cultural factors were found to contribute significant stress and played a central role in mental health and mental illness. These observations led to a dramatic increase in social activism and an optimism that was typical of the times. Prominent psychiatric leaders called upon the mental health professions to deal with "ignorance, superstition, unhealthy cultural patterns, and the rigidities and anxieties of parents, as well as with social conditions which foster the development of neuroses and maladjustments."[6]

Social psychiatry developed from the work of these and other pioneers. Rennie wrote, "Social psychiatry is etiological in its aim, but its point of attack is the whole social framework of contemporary living" and "[t]o include all social, biological, educational, and philosophical considerations which may come to empower psychiatry in its striving towards a society which functions with greater equilibrium and with fewer psychological casualties."[7]

The Principles of Social Psychiatry

1. Human behavior can only be understood in the context of the total social and other energies (including living and inert physical matter) of this universe.
2. A person should always be a subject and never an object of an interpersonal transaction. There is meaningful interrelationship, a relativity, between the behaviors of one individual and all social and mythological institutions and groups.
3. Social problems, including individual, institutional, and group deviant behaviors, cannot be solved without collaboration between all the institutions and disciplines of human knowledge, influence, and action.
4. Values of compassion, caring, and consideration for all human beings are essential to the operations of social psychiatry.
5. Human behavior acquires purpose and meaning about and by adherence to these postulates.[8]

The Contributions of the 1960s and 1970s

The tumultuous 1960s provided an opportunity for the re-evaluation of psychiatry's traditional role. The fundamental health of society was questioned. In the aftermath of two Worlds Wars, genocide, racial discrimination, discrimination against and abuse of women, child abuse, and gross economic inequality became focal points in assessing mental illness. Strident criticisms began in the postwar period and continued through the 1970s, advocating professional responsibility to make visible the hidden moral values in psychiatry and mental health by advocating preventive psychiatry. In 1969, one of the original family therapists, Don Jackson, said, "The important point here is that the behavior which is usually seen as symptomatic in terms of the individual can be seen as adaptive, even appropriate, in terms of the vital system within which the individual operates."[9]

By the turn of the 19th century, the Kraepelinian rather than Meyerian approach to presenting problems was in the ascendancy, expunging both the patient's personal accounts of his or her life and the past and present social circumstances it illuminated. Social psychiatry became marginalized within the medical specialty as biomedical reductionism grew with the "decade of the brain."

Theoretical Foundations

Social psychiatry incorporates evolutionary generalizations, sociocultural evolution, stages of life cycle in the sense of stages from infantile to mature, or creative and productive behavior. And it seeks general laws or principles concerning human history and human psychology in social frameworks. The limited clinical approach of the institution-centered psychiatrist and clinical psychologist has gradually been replaced by a wider, multidimensional, and interdisciplinary method in which clinicians share responsibility with others working in connected social science disciplines, and with socially motivated patients themselves, to understand the total situation of the individual as part of a wider cultural and community setting. This approach, called social psychiatry, has produced not only new community methods, but has resulted in cross-cultural and comparative fields of social psychiatry (or ethnopsychiatry), along with ecological and epidemiological studies of mental health in groups under various conditions of cultural existence. The anthropologist and sociologist, as well as persons working in action programs of health organizations, have founded this field, or sub-field, of general anthropological studies, and have contributed to its scientifically quantified base of knowledge, its reorganization of health practices, and even to fields like therapy and after-care. While cultures are many and diverse, the unity of mankind and the generic similarity of human psychological processes make each of them but a part of a larger dynamic whole. The psychological content of specific cultures, while having overwhelming importance in individual lives, is epiphenomenal and resultant to the conditions under which the culture operates, and certainly but a part of the life of culture in general.

In this chapter we will argue that psychiatrists should be more active in developing and leading interventions that focus on the social and interpersonal networks of their patients, with illustrations from past and ongoing efforts to this end. There is a close link to the structure of society, access to care for all, protection of marginalized segments of society, etc.

Psychological, Social, and Anthropological Underpinnings

Nietzsche's moral framework and "will to power" in modern culture find an expression in social psychology in the focus on social competition, external goods, and the backgrounding of internal goods, skill, and judgments. Freud and Jung postulated man as a complex energy system which maintains itself by means of transactions with the external world. The ultimate purposes of these transactions are individual survival, propagation of the species, and an ongoing evolutionary development.[10] Alfred Adler, Karen Horney, Erich Fromm, and Harry Stack Sullivan incorporated concepts of anthropology and sociology in their explanations of mind.

Sullivan considered an understanding of the course of human development to be essential to understanding individuals. He described seven developmental epochs: infancy, childhood, juvenile, pre-adolescence, early adolescence, late adolescence, and adulthood. Erikson links intergroup violence to the manner in which communities train their members to see themselves and otherness. The result of role learning, or identity formation, is regrettably but typically "pseudospeciation," a tendency to see one's own group as something more than human while denigrating other groups to an inferior position. Erikson proposes to master pseudospeciation through the practice of judiciousness or "mutuality," the psychological equivalent of the political value of tolerance, whose practice he claims to have found demonstrated by Gandhi.

Emile Durkheim believed that the emotional experience of collective effervescence is a necessary condition for generating and maintaining society. Feelings of reverence and obligation create the social bond that holds the individual to society. Overcoming Durkheim's theories suggest several emotions social solidarity, shared symbols, pride shame, might play a role. Durkheim argues that society is defined by groups, not by interactions. For Durkheim, the social causation of emotions appears to consist in linking biologically given emotions to an ever-increasing range of social situations, and in eliciting, intensifying, or suppressing the emotions that have been linked in this way.[11]

Piaget explains that a person's cognitive development influences social development.

Leo Vygotsky asserts, in the social development theory (SDT), that social interaction has a vital role in the cognitive development process, that socialization affects the learning process in an individual, and that consciousness or awareness is the result of socialization. This means that when we talk to our peers or adults, we talk to them for the sake of communication. After we interact with other people, we tend to internalize what we uttered. Social learning theory, developed by Albert Bandura, uses theories of classical and operant conditioning. In this theory, the environment plays a large part in learning. We model the behavior of the people around us, especially if we find these models to be like ourselves or if we want to emulate them. One learns by observing others. A person's mental state is important in the learning process.

Learning doesn't mean there will be a change in behavior. Bandura concluded that children learn aggression, violence, and other social behaviors through observation, learning, or watching the behaviors of others. At the opposite end, kindness and compassion can be imitated as well.[12]

Hinduism encourages people to achieve a certain life purpose, often closely tied to fulfillment in the afterlife. Hindus believe the objective of earthly life is to respect the laws of Dharma and gain benefit in the cycle of life and reincarnation. In the same fashion, religious rites give expression to communal beliefs, and the self-perceived role of everyone becomes a physical manifestation of these beliefs. The five relationships of Confucian philosophy serve as regulating social parameters and determine acceptable individual identities by setting out acceptable behaviors associated with each position in the hierarchy.[13]

World Association of Social Psychiatry (WASP) History

Key Milestones

The World Association of Social Psychiatry (WASP) was founded in 1964 under the leadership of Joshua Bierer of the United Kingdom. The origins of the association lie in the first International Congress of Social Psychiatry in London in 1964 under his leadership. He had championed the importance of social aspects of psychiatry for many years previously, being an early voice calling for the closure of the hospital asylum and for a leading role for patients in the design and running of psychiatric services. He had many achievements to his credit, including founding one of the earliest psychosocial day hospital programs and serving as founding editor of the *International Journal of Social Psychiatry*.[8]

The Early Years, 1969–1976

While Bierer had long championed the benefit of having an international association, the first real step in this direction came at the Second International Congress in 1969. The theme was the "sick society" and hosted such luminaries as Linus Pauling, Julian Huxley, and Walter Schindler. The International Association was launched with Jules Wassermann as president, Henry Mayer as secretary, and M. Hanison as treasurer. A year later, the first congress of the new association was held in Zagreb under the leadership of Vladimir Hudolin, with the active involvement of key scholars from across Europe and the United States. Hudolin was to continue his involvement with the organization over many succeeding years.[8]

In 1972, at the Fourth Congress in Israel on the theme of social change and social psychiatry, the leadership baton was passed from Bierer and Wassermann to Arthur Sacker (US), along with a considerable expansion in members to an executive council representing very broad interests, spanning experts on hospital closure programs, nascent community care, and psychosocial intervention. The Fifth Congress in Athens in 1974 marked auspicious events in Greece and Portugal with the ousting of dictatorial regimes. Vladimir Hudolin was elected to the chair of the association. Initially, it was named the International Congress of Social Psychiatry. From the Sixth Congress, it was named the World Congress of Social Psychiatry.[8]

In 1976, the term "World Congress of Social Psychiatry" was used for the first time at the international congress in Opatija, Croatia, under the theme of "The Future of the Family in a Rapidly Changing World." Further international congresses followed at regular intervals over the subsequent 3 decades, including Lisbon, Portugal (1978); Zagreb, Croatia (1981); Paris, France (1982); Osaka, Japan (1983); Rio de Janeiro, Brazil (1986); Washington, DC, US (1990); New Delhi, India (1992); Hamburg, Germany (1994); Rome, Italy (1995); Vancouver, Canada (1998); Agra, India (2001); Kobe, Japan (2004); Prague, Czech Republic (2007); Marrakech, Morocco (2010); Lisbon, Portugal (2013), and a special congress to mark 50 years of the WASP in London in 2014. The organization has also supported and sponsored many other regional events and international conferences led by member organizations and others closely associated with its broad aims and objectives.

In 2001 the World Association of Social Psychiatry (WASP) was officially launched, with statutes drawn up, and the organization was formally registered as an international association in Paris, France.

WASP in the Past Decade

WASP had a phenomenal growth, especially during the past decade. Some of the major events included the following.

The 20th World Congress of Social Psychiatry, Marrakech, October 23–27, 2010, was organized under the leadership of Driss Moussaoui. Julio Arboleda-Flórez was the Congress president. The theme was "Promoting Integral of Health and Mental Health." The General Assembly elected Driss Moussaoui as president, Tom Craig as president-elect, Roy Abraham Kallivayalil as secretary general, and Michaela Amering as treasurer, and resolved to revise the statutes. The event was a grand success with about 700 delegates participating.[8]

The 21st Congress, Lisbon, was held from June 29 to July 3, 2013. The theme was "The Biopsychosocial Model: The Future of Psychiatry." Organized by Maria Luisa Figueira, the Congress was a big success. The WASP statutes were revised and adopted by the General Assembly at Lisbon. Driss Moussaoui was the Congress president. New office-bearers— Tom Craig as president, Roy Abraham Kallivayalil as president-elect, Rachid Bennegadi as secretary general, and Marianne Kastrup as treasurer—assumed office at Lisbon.[8]

On November 13–15, 2014, the WASP celebrated its Golden Jubilee at an international congress in London under the leadership of Tom Craig, attended by over 1,000 delegates from across the world.[8]

The 22nd WASP Congress, New Delhi, was held from November 30 to December 4, 2016. The Congress theme was "Social Psychiatry in a Rapidly Changing World." Tom Craig was the president of the Congress and it was ably organized under the leadership of Rakesh Chadda. With more than 1,000 delegates attending, it was one of the most successful WASP Congresses to date. The General Assembly elected Roy Kallivayalil as president, Rachid Bennegadi as president-elect, Fernando Lola as secretary-general, and Marianne Kastrup as treasurer.[8]

The 23rd WASP Congress, Bucharest, was held from October 25 to 28, 2019. The theme was "Social Determinants of Health/Mental Health and Access to Care." Nearly 700 delegates from 66 countries participated. There were 441 scientific presentations, including 16 plenary sessions, 53 symposia, 19 workshops, 97 free papers, and 81 e-posters. Roy Abraham Kallivayalil was the Congress president and it was organized under the dynamic leadership of Doina Cozman and Alexander Paziuc. The inauguration and release of the first issue of *World Social Psychiatry*, the official journal of WASP, was one of the highlights of the Congress. Debasish Basu is the founding editor. The Yves Pelicier Prize was awarded to Norman Sartorius, and the Joshua Bierer Lecture was delivered by Daniel David. WASP Honorary Fellowships were presented to 31 eminent persons, and 21 early career psychiatrists across the world received WASP ECP Fellowships. The General Assembly elected Rachid Bennegadi as president, Vincenzo Di Nicola as president-elect, Rakesh Chadda as secretary-general, and Andrew Molodynski as treasurer.[8]

The purpose of the WASP is as follows, and as is defined in the constitution:[8]

- To study the nature of man and his cultures and the prevention and treatment of his vicissitudes and behavioral disorders;
- To promote national and international collaboration among professionals and societies in fields related to social psychiatry;
- To make the knowledge and practice of social psychiatry available to other sciences and to the public; and
- To advance the whole health and well-being of humankind.

World Association of Social Psychiatry Meetings

- I: London, UK, 1964
- II: London, UK, 1969
- III: Zagreb, Yugoslavia, 1970
- IV: Jerusalem, Israel, 1972
- V: Athens, Greece, 1974
- VI: Opatija, Yugoslavia, 1976
- VII: Lisbon, Portugal, 1978
- VIII: Zagreb, Yugoslavia, 1981
- IX: Paris, France, 1982
- X: Osaka, Japan, 1983
- XI: Rio de Janeiro, Brazil, 1986
- XII: Washington, DC, US, 1990
- XIII: New Delhi, India, 1992
- XIV: Hamburg, Germany, 1994
- XV: Rome, Italy, 1995
- XVI: Vancouver, Canada, 1998
- XVII: Agra, India, 2001
- XVIII: Kobe, Japan, 2004
- XIX: Prague, Czech Republic, 2007
- XX: Marrakech, Morocco, 2010
- XXI: Lisbon, Portugal, 2013
- XXII: Delhi, India, 2016
- XXIII: Bucharest, Romania, 2019.[8]

Presidents of World Association of Social Psychiatry

- 1964–1968: Joshua Bierer, United Kingdom
- 1968–1974: Jules H. Masserman, United States

- 1974–1978: Vladimir Hudolin, Croatia, Yugoslavia
- 1978–1983: George Vassiliou, Greece
- 1983–1988: John L. Carleton, United States
- 1988–1992: A. Guilherme Ferreira, Portugal
- 1992–1996: Jorge A. Costa e Silva, Brazil
- 1996–2001: Eliot Sorel, United States
- 2001–2004: Shridhar Sharma, India
- 2004–2007: Tsutomu Sakuta, Japan
- 2007–2010: Julio Arboleda-Flórez, Canada
- 2010–2013: Driss Moussaoui, Morocco
- 2013–2016: Thomas Jamieson-Craig, United Kingdom
- 2016–2019: Roy Abraham Kallivayalil, India
- 2019–2022: Rachid Bennegadi, France.
- 2022– : Vincenzo Di Nicola, Canada.[8]

WASP Member Societies

The organization of member societies within WASP is a relatively new development. Julio Arboleda-Flórez, president at the time, constituted the New Member Societies Committee in 2010, considering the importance of creating interest in new countries to develop their national Social Psychiatry Societies. Roy Abraham Kallivayalil, India, was the chair of this committee.[14]

A workshop on "National Social Psychiatric Societies: Best Practices & Lessons Learned" was held during the WASP Congress in Marrakech, October 2010, in which the following presentations were made:

1. Roy Abraham Kallivayalil (India): "Cultural Perspectives and Networking among National Social Psychiatry Societies"
2. Heinz Katschnig (Austria): "Biological Uniformity and Social Psychiatric Diversity—Implications for Organizing Local and International Associations"
3. Driss Moussaoui: "Moroccan Association of Social Psychiatry"
4. Mizuno Masafumi: "Japanese Society for Social Psychiatry"
5. Harishchandra Gambheera: "Social Psychiatry in Sri Lanka"
6. Andrzej Cechnicki (Poland) / Elmar Spancken: "Polish-German Association for Mental Health"
7. Harry Minhas (Melbourne): "Section of Social and Cultural Psychiatry of the Royal Australian and New Zealand College of Psychiatrists"
8. Habib: "French Association of Social Psychiatry"
9. Yueqin Huang (Beijing): "Social Psychiatry in China"
10. J. K. Trivedi: "Indian Association for Social Psychiatry"

This was the beginning of the organization of WASP into Member Societies.

In the 2016 General Assembly, WASP had the following 19 Member Societies:

1. Austria (Austrian Association of Social Psychiatry)
2. Brazil (Brazilian Association of Social Psychiatry)
3. Chile (Chilean Association of Social Psychiatry)
4. Egypt (PHASE)
5. France (French Association of Social Psychiatry)
6. Germany (German Academy for Psychoanalysis)
7. India (Indian Association for Social Psychiatry)
8. Italy (Italian Association of Social Psychiatry)
9. Japan (Japanese Society for Social Psychiatry)
10. Korea (Korean Association of Social Psychiatry)
11. Madagascar (Société Malgache de Psychiatrie)
12. Morocco (Association Marocaine de Psychiatrie Sociale)
13. Nepal (Nepalese Society of Social Psychiatry)
14. Pakistan (Pakistan Association of Social Psychiatry)
15. Romania (Romanian Society of Social Psychiatry)
16. Sri Lanka (Sri Lanka Association for Social Psychiatry)
17. Sweden (Swedish Social Psychiatric Forum)
18. Switzerland (Swiss Society for Social Psychiatry)
19. United States (American Association for Social Psychiatry).

The 2016–2019 WASP-EC, under the leadership of President Roy Kallivayalil, considered membership development as a priority item, and by the 2019 General Assembly, 8 more Member Societies were added, taking the strength from 19 to 27. This was as significant leap forward in spreading the WASP movement to all parts of the globe. The following were the new Member Societies:[14]

1. Argentina: Argentina branch of WASP; President Alejandra Maddocks
2. Bangladesh: National Society of WASP of Bangladesh; President Mohammod Rabbani
3. Canada: Canadian Association of Social Psychiatry; President Vincenzo Di Nicola
4. Dominican Republic: Dominican Society of Social Psychiatry; President Fernando Sanchez Martinez
5. Finland: Finnish Association of Social Psychiatry; President Sami Pirkola
6. Greece: Society of Preventive Psychiatry; President George Christodoulou
7. Lithuania: Lithuanian Cultural Psychiatry Association; President Palmira Rudalev
8. Serbia: Serbian Association of Social Psychiatry; President: Dusica Lecic-Tosevski.

Some Unique Aspects of Member Societies

Sub-Saharan Africa

Sub-Saharan Africa has 46 countries, with a combined population of 1.1 billion in 2019, speaking several languages and practicing many religions, and a variety of sub-cultures. Extended families are made up of various individuals and families who have shared responsibilities within the community. Most of the countries are affected by globalization and information technology, including social media. The region has 1.4 mental health workers per 100 000 people, compared with a global average of 9.0 per 100 000, and inadequate hospital beds and outpatient facilities. Mental health problems appear to be increasing in importance in Africa.[15]

Asia

Asia has a population of 4.7 billion, dozens of cultures, religions, languages, and ethnic groups. Its highly varied political systems spawn a wide variety of healthcare systems, often based on historical roots and at times colonial heritages. Comparable to Western countries, there is a widespread tendency to stigmatize and discriminate people with mental illness in Asia. Like Africa, Asian countries are also affected by urbanization, globalization, and national and transnational migration, as well as global health crises, and need to incorporate social, cultural contexts into mental healthcare.[2]

Australia and New Zealand and the Pacifics

A population of about 31 million of this region speak English, French, and at least 20 other languages. Diversity enriches the region's languages, arts, music, and lifestyles. At times, however, this same diversity may cause disagreements over issues such as immigration, health benefits, employment, and the effects of colonial rule. The RANZC Section of Social, Cultural and Rehabilitation Psychiatry and the Society for Mental Health Research (https://www.smhr.org.au/) and the Alliance for the Prevention of Mental Disorders (http://www.apmd.org.au/) promote social psychiatry, which includes diverse social and cultural factors impacting recovery from mental illness, quality of life, and reintegration into family and community circles.

Europe

Europe includes 44 countries and a combined population of 743 million, with 24 official languages. Mental disorders are affecting about 25% of the population every year. In all countries, mental health problems are much more prevalent among those who are most deprived. Europe has been very active through its national psychiatric and social psychiatric organizations in promotion of social aspects of psychiatry by publications, meetings, and advocacy.

Latin America

With 23 countries, Latin America is home to a population of more than 652 million. Mental disorders are highly prevalent in Latin American countries, with rates ranging from 11.6% to 20.1%. Most countries of the region have developed national and local initiatives to improve delivery of community-based programs.

Middle East and Northern Africa (MENA)

The Middle East–North Africa region comprises 20 countries and territories, with an estimated population of 315 million, predominantly practicing Islam. The migrant population, mostly within the Gulf nations, practice mostly the religions of their homeland, such as Buddhism and Hinduism among South Asians. The Arab population is plagued by issues that are no different from any other population in the world: depression, anxiety, eating disorders, addiction, suicide, self-mutilation, post-traumatic stress disorders, mood disorders, and so on.

North America

Canada and the United States have a combined population of 597 million. Different racial and ethnic groups of the North American region have contributed to the shaping of cultures in the United States and Canada: Native Americans; European immigrants who brought their Western-oriented traditions, combined with rugged individualism; and the slavery of African peoples all laid the foundations of the North American cultures. Later European, Asian, Latin, and other international immigrants contributed to the diversity of the region. Mental and substance use disorders accounted for 10.5% of the global burden of disease in the Americas.

Concluding Remarks and Recommendations

Social psychiatry is a discipline that focuses on the social dimension of mental health, mental illness, and mental healthcare. In the current atmosphere of COVID-19, social distancing, Black Lives Matter, school closures, and economic hardships, understanding and making use of social constructs and social interventions have risen with proposals for social interventions. In psychiatric and psychological interventions, the importance of social etiology and social interventions has increased significantly. The future of social psychiatry will be shaped by public expectations and the acceptance of community-based services. Today, the practice of social psychiatry is being increasingly influenced by the growth of science and technology, the changing ideology of economics, and the rapid urbanization and migration. Thus, today, social psychiatry has great relevance and a bright future. The new journal of WASP, *World Social Psychiatry*, can play an important role in this through advocacy, research, and dissemination of knowledge. In addition, we must continuously strive to empower our patients, involving them at all levels in decisions about their care and its delivery. As clinicians and teachers, we have the responsibility to spread knowledge of mental health and social psychiatry. The WASP has a very important role to play in this endeavor. It can take the lead role to promote the best mental health practices in the world, growing beyond our organizational activities.

Social psychiatry deals with marginalized populations, inequity in health, institutional racism, sociopolitical issues, and more. We close the chapter with the following statement from WHO:

> Good mental health is integral to human health and well-being. Social, economic, and physical environments shape a person's mental health and many common mental disorders. Risk factors for many common mental disorders are heavily associated with social inequalities, whereby the greater the inequality the higher the inequality in risk. In order to reduce these inequalities and reduce the incidence of mental disorders overall, it is vital that action is taken to improve the conditions of everyday life, beginning before birth and progressing into early childhood, older childhood and adolescence, during family building and working ages, and through to older age. Action throughout these life stages would provide opportunities for both improving population mental health, and for reducing risk of those mental disorders that are associated with social inequalities. As mental disorders affect physical health these actions would also reduce inequalities in physical health and improve health overall. Taking a life-course perspective recognizes that the influences that operate at each stage of life can affect mental health. Populations are made vulnerable by deep-rooted poverty, social inequality and discrimination. . . . Risk and protective factors act at several different levels, including the individual, the family, the community, the structural, and the population levels. A social determinants of health approach requires action across multiple sectors and levels. Empowerment of individuals and communities is at the heart of action on the social determinants.[16]

References

1. Jamieson-Craig T. Social psychiatry in a global perspective 24th European Congress of Psychiatry. *European Psychiatry*. 2016;33S:S8–S11.
2. Shridhar S. Social psychiatry: a global and Indian perspective. *WSP*. 2019;1(1): 39–42.
3. lberg G. Soziale psychiatrie. *Monatsschr Soz Med*. 1903;1:321–329, 393–398.
4. Fischer M. Neue aufgaben der psychiatrie in baden. *Allg Z Psychiatr*. 1912;69:S34–S68.
5. E. E. Southard papers. Center for the History of Medicine, Francis A. Countway Library of Medicine.
6. Uchtenhagen A. Which future for social psychiatry? *Int Rev Psychiatry*. 2008 Dec;20(6):535–539.
7. Rennie T. Social psychiatry: a definition. *Int J Soc Psychiatry*. 2022;1(1):5–13.
8. World Association of Social Psychiatry website. https://www.worldsocpsychiatry.org.
9. Jackson D. The individual and the larger contexts. *Family Process*. 1967 Sept;6(2):139–147.
10. Leiter B. Nietzsche's moral and political philosophy. 2004. https://plato.stanford.edu.
11. Cole NL. Emile Durkheim and his impact on sociology. ThoughtCo. https://www.thoughtco.com 1-29. 2020.
12. Tudge J. Vygotsky, Piaget, and Bandura: perspectives on the relations between the social world and cognitive development. *Human Devel*. 1993 Jan;36(2):61–81.

13. Fernando Tevez Rosales. The role of Eastern religious traditions in society. https://www.methodist.edu.
14. Kallivayalil R. Notes from WASP president's desk, 2021.
15. Sankoh O, Sevalie S, Weston M. Mental health in Africa. *Lancet Glob Health*. 2018 Sep;6(9):e954–e955.
16. World Health Organization and Calouste Gulbenkian Foundation. *Social Determinants of Mental Health*. Geneva: World Health Organization; 2014:43.

3

The Biopsychosocial Model of Health

An Update

Tom K. J. Craig

Background: Engel's Psychosocial Model

The biopsychosocial model of health was first proposed by Roy Grinker[1] in 1964 and was then taken up in a now classic paper by George Engel in 1977.[2] Engel argued that a purely biomedical model provides a very limited understanding of illness. Embracing reductionism and mind-body dualism, the biomedical model regards the complex phenomena of illness as derived from abnormalities at a fundamental molecular level, governed by the basic laws of physics and chemistry. Engel argued that there are several limitations to this reductionist formulation. He pointed out that the presence of a biological abnormality may be a necessary but not sufficient condition for the emergence of illness. Someone may show signs of disease on a laboratory test yet have no symptoms and consider themselves well; another person may be severely incapacitated but show no signs of disease. The boundary between being "well" and "sick" are far from clear, as psychological and social factors play a vital role in determining when and how a person comes to view themselves as sick, whether to seek help, and their response to treatment. He proposed a biopsychosocial model that applied across physical and psychiatric disorders with social and psychological influences linked with each other and with biology as a complex system in which change in one causes change in the other. His paper concludes with the bold assertion that the biopsychosocial model could be "a blueprint for research, a framework for teaching and a design for action in the real world of health care."[2(p135)]

Despite the attraction of the model, there have been compelling critiques claiming that it lacks practically useful specific scientific content and validity. For example, Ghaemi[3,4] argues that the role of the physician has always been to treat disease in the body while also attending to the human being as a person, but beyond this, there is no need for Engel's "psychologised scientism." He makes the point that under the assumptions of the biopsychosocial model, all conditions should benefit from combinations of biological and psychological treatment, but that this is empirically not the case. Using one treatment is often all that is necessary and may even be superior to combined approaches. The model might have been useful in its day for countering extreme biomedical reductionism, but in practice is little more than a compromise to solve ideological conflicts between biology, psychology, and sociology, whose proponents can each turn to the model to claim equal rights for their unique ideology concerning the causes and treatments of illness.[3,4]

A Fresh Look at the Biopsychosocial Model

Ghaemi provides a tough view that, on the face of it, given the notable advance in the understanding of biological mechanisms in disease, is really quite persuasive. But he has in turn been challenged by a recent thoughtful review of the slowly amassing evidence to defend and elaborate Engel's original ideas. In a recent book, Bolton and Gillett[5] draw a distinction between the challenge that the model lacks specific scientific content from that of the validity of an overarching general model that applies across different disorders. In terms of specific scientific content, they point out that in the decades since Engel first advocated the model, new research in biomedicine, psychology, and social epidemiology have clearly shown complex interactions of biological, psychological, and social factors in the cause and course of many medical and psychiatric conditions and in the response to treatment. However, the relevant biopsychosocial interactions are largely specific to particular health conditions and further, to "particular stages of particular health conditions,"[5(p15)] leaving open the question of the validity and use of a general model.

Before turning to review some of the evidence from specific examples, the point is well made that these are not enough to address the validity or even the need for a *general* model. To have broad relevance, such a model should be "a core philosophical and scientific theory of health, disease and healthcare which defines the foundational theoretical constructs—the ontology of the biological, the psychological and the social—and especially the causal relations within and between these domains."[5(p19)] Key to Bolton and Gillet's reformulation is the observation of regulatory mechanisms that operate within and across biological, psychological, and social aspects of health. At the molecular level, the fundamental laws of chemistry and physics are inviolable and cannot be changed by psychosocial factors, but the higher biological functions that are formed by activity at the molecular level are themselves subject to regulatory mechanisms that may be responsive to the psychosocial environment. Events in the social world "get into" the body through cognitive processes that are fully embodied as an aspect of brain function and so are linked to the regulation of many bodily systems (e.g., the HPA axis and the release of stress hormones). Cognition is also the fundamental driver of behaviors to secure what the organism needs for survival (access to natural resources, identification of opportunities and threats, and the knowledge of what to do in response to these). Bolton and Gillet[5] refer to this ability to act in the world as "psychological agency." Agency is first determined biologically but subsequently is shaped throughout childhood and beyond by experience of the "social" world. A reasonably caring and orderly society (including family and wider personal relationships), whose members respect each other's agency and teach the essential skills to get by in life, is necessary for optimal function and even survival. But society also teaches rules (regulatory processes) intended to manage the distribution of resources and to ensure that individuals conform to culturally and agreed-upon behavioral norms. Sometimes these rules are misused, and power is deliberately manipulated to constrain individual agency with harmful effects on the individual's mental and physical health.

The crucial insight is that all three biopsychosocial levels interact, and all involve systems of regulation which direct the *expression* of basic processes (social factors enable and constrain agency, which in turn affects biological systems). For example, epigenetic changes (modification to DNA such as methylation and histone modification) can be brought about by environmental conditions that in turn are governed by psychological and social processes.[6]

Biopsychosocial Specifics: Some Examples with an Emphasis on the Social

An obvious way in which psychosocial factors influence biology is through access to essential resources for survival, including water, nutrients, shelter, and freedom from toxins. As an example, Vitamin B_{12} and folic acid, available through diet, play a fundamental role in neurotransmission and are key methyl donors. Methylation of DNA controls the activation of genes that turn on and off protein synthesis. Vitamin D modulates dopamine and noradrenaline, and a deficiency of the vitamin is thought to be associated with schizophrenia, with neonatal deficiency linked to the disorder in adulthood.[7,8]

The access to essential minerals and food obviously requires agency as defined earlier, but is also clearly socially controlled and far from evenly distributed across society. In 2018, it was estimated by the World Food Programme that around 124 million people in 51 countries were facing crisis levels of food insecurity, with many more people significantly undernourished.[9] Malnutrition may be the result of natural disasters beyond human control, but are also the direct result of social actions implemented without concern for their impact or done for the good of one tribe at the expense of another. The famine associated with Mao Zedong's Great Leap Forward in the late 1950s–early 1960s killed 18 million Chinese, with damaging effects on countless others. Evidence for a lingering impact on mental health includes higher incidence of schizophrenia in the children of mothers who were malnourished in early pregnancy as a result of the famine.[10]

Exposure to environmental toxins is also an issue, particularly for those living near industrial sites. Lead pollution is a familiar example, surprisingly still a problem at population levels, related to contaminated drinking water and the use of leaded paint. The large nuclear plant disasters at Chernobyl and Fukushima had health effects from radiation exposure in the short and long term, raising the incidence of not only cancers but also mental health effects from the horror of the incident itself and from a wide range of social, economic, and public health consequences that followed. At Chernobyl, people lost homes, were forced to move away from family ties, and suffered stigmatization. High levels of anxiety and "medically unexplained" symptoms have been reported.[11]

These environmental examples are extreme, but many other sociopolitical actions have unintended consequences that are harmful to both mind and body. The unequal distribution of wealth across society (personal wealth being prized in most economies) has robust associations with poor mental and physical health. Evidence is consistent, across all the countries that have looked at it, that socioeconomic disadvantage, measured in terms of educational attainment, employment, and material wealth, is associated with poor mental and physical health, and the association is almost certainly causal. It is also apparent that it is not only absolute levels of deprivation that matter, but the extent of the disparity between the richest and poorest in a society that explains differences in health status both within and between countries.[12,13] Take the example of obesity and the downstream health consequences of conditions such as type 2 diabetes, which has now reached epidemic proportions worldwide. Not only are rates rising, but the rise is unequally distributed across social groups so that it is those who are disadvantaged in terms of wealth, education, and occupation, and typically all three together, who are most at risk. A recent analysis of data from 11 Organisation for Economic Co-operation and Development (OECD) countries showed England and the United States to have the highest rates of obesity associated in all 11 countries with large social inequalities, including educational level and economic status.[14]

Similar results are apparent for associations with mental health. Data from 25 years of European population surveys find high rates of common mental disorders such as depression and anxiety linked to material disadvantage, unemployment, and poor education.[15]

The increase in mortality rates for non-Hispanic Americans after 1999 has also been shown to be predominantly among the least educated, the causes of death largely from suicide, drug, and alcohol poisoning—all obviously reflecting rising levels of emotional distress.[16]

As with mental disorders in adulthood, there is an association between social disadvantage and child development that also follows a social gradient. Low educational attainment, living in deprived neighborhoods, and material poverty all associate with worse behavioral and cognitive problems,[17] which of course predispose or extend into adult mental ill health as well. Perhaps the gloomiest observation of all is that social disadvantage present before birth accumulates throughout life and runs, in some cases, across generations. The steepness of this health/inequality gradient varies from country to country and from time to time, suggesting that it can be reduced by addressing the worst of the disparity in power, wealth, and resources and improving the conditions in which people are born, live, are educated, and are employed. These are largely political changes, beyond the reach of an individual health worker perhaps, but not beyond the professional group's power in lobbying for change.

There are, of course, many components to the observed gradient in macro-social factors. People from disadvantaged populations have higher levels of debt, live in poorer housing, often in quite run-down neighborhoods with high levels of crime, high unemployment, and poor working conditions over which they have less control. The impact of this deprivation on childhood development is particularly concerning. Part of the impact is not just material, but also involves how it affects parent-child behavior, and here something can be done that does not rely solely on welfare policies. A study of 19,000 children born in the United Kingdom during 2000–2001 using detailed assessments of the behavior and verbal ability of the children when they were between 3 and 5 years of age showed the expected socioeconomic gradient. Children from the poorest families were more likely to show behavioral problems and lower verbal ability than those from successively higher income families. However, when the data were adjusted for the quality of parenting, this gradient virtually disappeared. When a parent read stories to their child, taught the alphabet, and sang songs together, the disparity gradient was reduced, with the poorest families benefiting the most from these supportive parenting skills.[18]

Macro-social risk is also well established for severe mental illness. Two circumstances are worth a brief mention. First is the very well-established increase in incidence of psychosis in urban settings.[19] Being raised in densely populated urban environments doubles the incidence of psychosis over that of people who grow up in more rural settings, with a dose-response relationship in terms of population density and the length of exposure. Furthermore, changing the exposure by moving from an urban to a rural environment in childhood leads to a reduction in risk. Studies have been careful to control for a range of potential confounders, and the effect is generally now considered as causal.[20] It is, however, not clear what is going on at an individual level that might explain this effect. The risk is greatest among those with a family history of psychosis, suggesting that some psychological or biological mechanism that is relevant to these disorders may be at play. Perhaps heightened vigilance is needed to negotiate the complexity of urban life, or these environments result in persistently higher levels of general arousal. One interesting experiment suggests this may be the case. In this study, healthy volunteers were divided into two groups on the basis of the length of time they had spent living in urban or rural environments, currently and as children. They then took part in an experiment involving a social evaluative stressor (criticism for failures in an arithmetic task) while undergoing a functional magnetic resonance imaging (fMRI) brain scan. During the social stress test, current city living was associated with increased activity in the amygdala, while urban upbringing was associated with increased activity in the anterior cingulate cortex, which is involved in regulating amygdala activity, negative affect, and stress.[21]

The second social circumstance related to the incidence of psychosis is the markedly increased incidence among migrants from many cultures compared to that in the host country, now found in studies carried out in several countries around the world.[22] The relatively increased incidence is seen among first- and second-generation migrants and even among minority groups without recent migration. At least four studies in different countries have shown an association with the ethnic density of the area in which the person lives. Higher rates occur in places where the migrant is in the minority, a member of a socially marginalized group, and perhaps subject to discrimination. In a recent data-linkage study of 203,829 individuals, almost all the variation in the risk of psychosis from urbanicity was explained by individual and school-level markers of social fragmentation. Foreign-born individuals were at higher risk if they attended a school with very few others who were foreign-born, and similar patterns were observed for other measures of social fragmentation and deprivation. In short, it seems that characteristics that mark out an individual as different from most others in their environment increases risk of psychosis.[23]

Getting Under the Skin: From Social to Psychobiological

Social factors can increase the risk of ill health by facilitating exposure to the environmental hazards that are bad for health or by changes to downstream regulatory processes at a psychological and biological level. Examples of the first include economically driven activities, such as the food-industry promotion of low-cost, energy-rich "fast foods" and alcohol and the decline of physical activity in work and leisure that together result in behavior and lifestyle choices that are harmful to health, increasing obesity and the risk of type 2 diabetes and cardiovascular disease.

The effects of chronic stress are possibly the best-known example of the second route linking social factors and ill health. Research into the social causes of common mental disorders of depression and anxiety have clearly established a causal link with stressful experiences, with replicated findings across the depressive spectrum from community cases through hospitalized patients with melancholia.[24,25] Furthermore, the most toxic events are those that involve disruptions in personal relationships, particularly those involving socially excluding experiences of shame and humiliation.[26]

These associations of social experience and depression may also be important for physical disease. Major depression is a bad prognostic factor for coronary heart disease. It is associated in a dose-response relationship with worse health-related quality of life, recurrent cardiac events, and poor physical functioning. Major depression confers a two-fold increase in the risk of incident coronary heart disease over that seen in non-depressed populations.[27,28] Treating depression reduces risk. Similarly, comorbid depression and type 2 diabetes increase disease burden, reduce quality of life, and increase healthcare costs. Associations between the two are bidirectional, with major depression increasing the risk of diabetes, and once established, diabetes increasing the risk of depression. The mechanisms linking the two conditions are likely to be the lifestyle changes noted earlier, as depression increases sedentary behavior and has been linked to "comfort eating" of high-calorie food.[29]

A role for stressful experience has also been documented for schizophrenia and other severe mental illness, with a suggestion that stressors involving intrusion (experiences of a persecutory nature) may have the most powerful effect.[30,31] While an etiological role of stressful events in psychosis is less established than that for depression, there is very consistent evidence that less severe hassles of everyday life can precipitate a relapse of an established disorder. Studies using momentary event sampling methods in which participants make a brief record of thoughts, mood, and current context (where they are, doing what, and with whom) on several occasions throughout a day have shown that people suffering from schizophrenia and their first-degree relatives have a higher level of emotional reactivity to minor hassles of daily living than do healthy controls.[32] Interestingly, sensitivity to stress and enhanced threat anticipation in psychosis have also been shown to be associated with the sense of being an "outsider" and of the environment appearing more personally meaningful (i.e., salient) in first-episode patients but not in healthy controls, these associations being most marked in those who also reported a history of childhood sexual abuse.[33,34]

The quality of parenting in childhood, particularly the damaging experience of childhood maltreatment (i.e., physical or sexual abuse and severe neglect), plays a prominent role in the etiology of many mental disorders,[35] though the effect is rather nonspecific in the sense that the same broad risk is found in several conditions. For depression, early maltreatment appears to exert its effect through an impact on other psychological mediators, such as self-esteem, that extend into adulthood, not only affecting emotional responses to adversity, but even influencing life choices and increasing the likelihood of experiencing one or more interpersonal difficulties and humiliating events mentioned earlier.[36] The experience of childhood maltreatment also has lasting effects on the attachment behaviors that possibly explain some of the less satisfactory partnerships in adulthood.[37]

Of course, not everyone experiencing a stressful event, or exposed to a potentially toxic environment, will go on to develop a disorder. Many explanations are put forward to account for the variation in susceptibility. From a social perspective, support may be key to buffering the impact of stressors, and there is evidence for a heightened vulnerability when expected support is not forthcoming in a crisis.[38] But a clear role for biological vulnerability is also apparent. For example, genetic risk may determine who is susceptible to stressful experiences. The urbanicity risk described earlier is greatest for people who have a family history of psychosis, and there is an increased risk of psychosis in the second-generation offspring of migrants, independent of ethnicity.[39,40]

It is also possible that some stressful experiences have an adverse effect on the brain, thereby raising the risk of disorder. Studies have reported that early childhood maltreatment is linked to structural changes in the corpus callosum, hippocampus, and prefrontal cortex (PFC), and to altered functional activity in the amygdala, PFC, and the striatum, all areas that are involved in processes important for social interaction, including how individuals understand and respond to the social environment. In animal studies, maternal separation increases striatal dopamine release in the separated cub, which is further maintained if the animal is then returned to the group in a subordinate position to other members of its social group. While comparable separation studies are not possible in humans, studies have noted that retrospective reports of poor-quality maternal care in childhood was associated with higher dopamine release in the presence of a social stressor, proving an intriguing suggestion of a mechanism for the observed association of maltreatment and later disorder. However, the changes have also been reported in maltreated people who do not have any disorder, leading one of the reviewers of this literature to conclude that some of the changes may be adaptations that, rather than predicting disorder, are responses to facilitate resilience and survival.[41]

Biopsychosocial Aspects of Treatment and Healthcare

While psychological treatments such as cognitive behavior therapy are effective for some mental disorders, psychosocial interventions seem to be incapable of reversing physical disease once it is established. Bolton and Gillet[5] acknowledge this fact as a serious challenge to the biopsychosocial model. Of course, if there is any biological impact of psychosocial factors, it is likely restricted to organ systems that are controlled or influenced by the central nervous system (CNS), and here there are some signals, especially for mental disorders and in the progression of physical disease. The impact of depression on cardiovascular outcomes is one example where cardiologists are calling for increased screening for and identification of depression, noting that treatments for depression (both pharmacological and psychological) are safe and effective.[28]

The need for approaches that combine all three biopsychosocial components are perhaps most apparent in public health primary prevention programs. For example, there is no doubt that vaccination is effective for many diseases. While the mechanism is entirely biological, the uptake and hence effectiveness at a population level are determined by social and psychological factors. Under the influence of religious and other opinion formers, some people in Pakistan refuse vaccination on the grounds that it is not intended to prevent disease, but is a hostile act of foreign powers aimed to sterilize their children, and many others believe that the vaccine they are offered has been mishandled in some way.[42] Similarly, some people in Europe and North America refuse the measles, mumps, and rubella (MMR) vaccine on the grounds of wholly discredited beliefs that it can cause their children to develop autism. In both examples, change will not occur by simply repeating a biological mantra, but requires social action, including community engagement, close attention to social media to remove misleading information, and involvement of trusted health workers and community leaders in delivering the message.

Public health programs aimed at tacking social exclusion, including that arising from poverty, is another approach that has the potential of a considerable impact on health, though what is possible is clearly determined by wider social and political forces. As is the case with the vaccination program, many potentially beneficial interventions fail because of resistance from the target population or because of the actions of powerful commercial organizations that resist changes that might be economically damaging.

One preventive intervention that shows considerable promise is the promotion of nurturing relationships between parents and their children. There are several well-established programs with evidence of effectiveness, improving parenting skills and the child's behavior at home and at school.[43,44] Aiming these at high-risk groups may be particularly beneficial, as shown in a meta-analysis of parental skills training targeted at mentally ill parents that could reduce the risk of their children developing mental and behavioral disorders by as much as 40%.[45]

Conclusion

Far from being obsolete, the biopsychosocial model of illness continues to be very relevant to healthcare today. As a general model of health and disease, it is a good way of summarizing the aspects of disease that are more than the biology alone, notably the importance of social, lifestyle factors in non-communicable disorders, and moving toward understanding the contribution to disease of disturbance of regulatory processes that are at least partly under the influence of the CNS and thereby psychosocial factors.

References

1. Grinker RR. A struggle for eclecticism. *Am J Psychiatry*. 1964;121:451–457.
2. Engel GL. The need for a new medical model: a challenge for biomedicine. *Science*. 1977;196:129–136.
3. Ghaemi SN. Toward a Hippocratic psychopharmacology. *Can J Psychiatry*. 2008;53:189–196.
4. Ghaemi SN. The rise and fall of the biopsychosocial model. *Br J Psychiatry*. 2009;195:3–4.
5. Bolton D, Gillett G. The Biopsychosocial Model of Health and Disease: new philosophical and scientific developments. *Palgrave Macmillan* ebook. Accessed October 5, 2019. https://doi.org/10.1007/978-3-030-11899-0.
6. McGuinness D, McGlynn LM, Johnson PC, et al. Socio-economic status is associated with epigenetic differences in the pSoBid cohort. *Int J Epidemiology*. 2012;41:151–160.
7. Murri BM, Respino M, Masotti M, et al. Vitamin D and psychosis: mini meta-analysis. *Schizophr Res*. 2013;150(1):l235–1239.
8. McGrath JJ, Eyles DW, Pedersen CB, et al. Neonatal vitamin status and risk of schizophrenia: a population-based case-control study. *Arch Gen Psychiatry*. 2010;67:889–894.
9. Food Security Information Network: global report on food crises. 2018. Accessed October 12, 2019. https://www.wfp.org/publications/global-report-food-crises-2018.
10. Song S, Wang W, Hu P. Famine, death and madness: schizophrenia in early adulthood after pre-natal exposure to the Chinese Forward Famine. *Soc Sci Med*. 2009;68:1315–1321.
11. Bromet EJ, Havenaar JM. Psychological and perceived health effects of the Chernobyl disaster: a 20-year review. *Health Physics*. 2007;93:516–521.
12. Wilkinson R, Pickett K. *The Spirit Level: Why More Equal Societies Almost Always Do Better*. London: Allen Lane; 2009.
13. Marmot M, Bell R. Social inequalities in health: a proper concern of epidemiology. *Ann Epidemiol*. 2016;26:238–240.
14. Devaux M, Sassi F. Social inequalities in obesity and overweight in 11 OECD countries. *Eur J Public Health*. 2013;23:464–469.
15. Fryers T, Melzer D, Jenkins R, Brugha T. The distribution of the common mental disorders: social inequalities in Europe. *Clin Pract Epidemiol Ment Health*. 2005;1:14.
16. Case A, Deaton A. Rising morbidity and mortality in midlife among white non-Hispanic Americans in the 21st century. *Proc Natl Acad Sci USA*. 2015;112:15078–15083.
17. Marryat L, Martin C. Growing up in Scotland: maternal mental health and its impact on child behaviour and development. 2010. Accessed December 31, 2019. http://www.scotland.gov.uk/resource/doc/310448/0097971.pdf
18. Kelly Y, Sacker A, Del Bono E, Francesconi M, Marmot M. What role for the home learning environment and parenting in reducing the socioeconomic gradient in child development? Findings from the Millennium Cohort Study *Arch Dis Child*. 2011;96:832–837.
19. March D, Hatch SL, Morgan C, et al. Psychosis and place. *Epidemiol Rev*. 2008;30:84–100.
20. van Os J, Rutten BP, Poulton R. Gene-environment interactions in schizophrenia: review of epidemiological findings and future directions. *Schizophr Bull*. 2008;34:1066–1082.
21. Lederbogen F, Kirsch P, Haddad L, et al. City living and urban upbringing affect neural social stress processing in humans. *Nature*. 2011;474:498–501.

22. Bourque F, van der Ven E, Malla A. A meta-analysis of the risk for psychotic disorders among first- and second-generation immigrants. *Psychol Med.* 2011;41:987–910.

23. Zammit S, Lewis G, Rasbash J, Dalman C, Gustafsson JE, Allebeck P. Individuals, schools, and neighborhood: a multilevel longitudinal study of variation in incidence of psychotic disorders. *Arch Gen Psychiatry.* 2010;67:914–922.

24. Brown GW, Harris TO. *Social Origins of Depression: A Study of Psychiatric Disorder in Women.* London: Tavistock Press; 1978.

25. Tennant C. Life events and depression: a review of recent findings. *ANZCP.* 2002;36:173–182.

26. Kendler KS, Hettema JM, Butera MA, Gardner CO, Prescott CA. Life event dimensions of loss, humiliation entrapment and danger in the prediction of onsets of major depression and generalized anxiety. *Arch Gen Psychiatry.* 2003;60:789–796.

27. Hare DL Toukhsati SR, Johansson P, Jaarsma T. Depression and cardiovascular disease: a clinical review. *Eur Heart J.* 2014;21:1365–1372.

28. Celano CM, Huffman JC. Depression and cardiac disease: a review. *Cardiol Rev.* 2011;19:130–142.

29. Nouwen A, Adriaanse MC, van Dam K, et al. Longitudinal associations between depression and diabetes complications: a systematic review and meta-analysis. *Diabetic Med.* 2019;36(12):1562–1572. https://doi.org/10.1111/dme.14054.

30. Beards S, Gayer-Anderson C, Borges S, Dewey ME, Fisher HL. Morgan C. Life events and psychosis: a review and meta-analysis. *Schizophr Bull.* 2013;39:740–747.

31. Raune D, Kuipers E, Bebbington P. Stressful and intrusive life events preceding first episode psychosis. *Epidemiol Psychiatr Sci.* 2009;18:221–228.

32. Myin-Germeys I, van Os J, Schwartz JE, Stone AA, Delespaul PA. Emotional reactivity to daily life stress in psychosis. *Arch Gen Psychiatry.* 2001;58:1137–1144.

33. Reininghaus U, Kempton MJ, Valmaggia L, et al. Stress sensitivity, aberrant salience and threat anticipation in early psychosis: an experience sampling study. *Schizophr Bull.* 2016;42:712–722.

34. Reininghaus U, Gayer-Anderson C, Valmaggia L, et al. Psychological processes underlying the association between childhood trauma and psychosis in daily life: an experience sampling study. *Psychol Med.* 2016;46:2799–2813.

35. Morgan C, Fisher H. Environment and schizophrenia: childhood trauma—a critical review. *Schizophr Bull.* 2007;33:3–10.

36. Brown GW, Craig T, Harris TO, Handley RV, Harvey AL. Early maltreatment and adulthood cohabiting partnerships: a life-course study of adult chronic depression. *J Affect Dis.* 2008;110:115–125.

37. Brown GW, Harris TO, Craig TKJ. Exploration of the influence of insecure attachment and parental maltreatment on the incidence and course of adult clinical depression. *Psychol Med.* 2019;49:1025–1032.

38. Brown GW, Andrews B, Harris T, Adler Z, Bridge L. Social support, self-esteem and depression. *Psychol Med.* 1986;16:813–831.

39. van Os J, Hanssen M, Bak M, Bijl, RV, Vollebergh W. Do urbanicity and familial liability co-participate in causing psychosis? *Am J Psychiatry.* 2003;160:477–482.

40. van Os J, Rutten BP, Poulton R. Gene-environment interactions in schizophrenia: review of epidemiological findings and future directions. *Schizophr Bull.* 2008;34:1066–1082.

41. Telcher MH, Samson JA, Anderson CM, Ohashi K. The effects of childhood maltreatment on brain structure, function and connectivity. *Nat Rev Neurosci.* 2016;17:652–666.

42. Ali M, Ahmad N, Khan H, Ali S, Akbar F, Hussain Z. Polio vaccination controversy in Pakistan. *Lancet.* 2019;394:915–916.

43. Webster-Stratton C, Reid MJ, Hammond M. Preventing conduct problems, promoting social competence: a parent and teacher training partnership in Head Start. *J Clin Child Psychol.* 2001;30:283–302.

44. Vreeman RC, Carroll AE. A systematic review of school-based interventions to prevent bullying. *Arch Pediatr Adolesc Med.* 2007;161:78–88.

45. Siegenthaler E, Munder T, Egger M. Effect of preventive interventions in mentally ill parents on the mental health of the offspring: systematic review and meta-analysis. *J Am Acad Child Adolesc Psychiatry.* 2012;51:8–17.

4

Social Psychiatry

Ethical Perspectives

Fernando Lolas and Eduardo Rodríguez

Psychiatry: An Integral View

Ever since psychiatry entered the Western language as a designation for an attitude toward healing, the community of its practitioners has been assimilated into the ethos of the medical profession. Partaking of its values and orientations, it also inherited the orientation of Western medicine toward the causal thinking of the natural-scientific disciplines. Discrepant voices arise from time to time, requesting that it be ascribed either to the sciences of the spirit or to the social sciences. Examples of this tension are the disputes between *Psychiker* and *Somatiker* in 19th-century Germany, the adoption of psychoanalytical insights by different streams of practice, and the famous declaration of Rudolf Virchow, "medicine is a social science."[1]

A heterogeneous community of practice such as psychiatry is characterized by theoretical and methodical pluralisms. This means that different approaches are needed depending upon the definition of the problem at hand. If a problem is defined as psychological, the answer is psychological; if considered a somatic problem, the method is that of the biological sciences. Viktor von Weizsäcker, the founder of anthropological medicine, called this the *Drehtürprinzip*, the principle of the revolving door: one way of looking at the issues precludes or obscures the other.

The basic discipline of psychiatry is a meta-text, composed of different texts not easily compatible with each other.[2] This finds expression in our formulation of the psychophysiological triad, or the incompatible discourses of *illness, disease,* and *sickness,* not easily framed in the traditional ways of conceptualizing psychiatric "disorders." The very idea of assimilating these disorders to disease entities poses two problems: one is the substrate (where the problem lies in the body) and the other is the related issue of causation.

In terms of substrate, the individual is considered the site of disease, except for some proposals to consider the group as susceptible to pathological conditions,[3] a notion repeated from time to time. As for causation, aside from genetics, biological derangements, and unhealthy habits, the emphasis of social psychiatry lies in the cultural, social, and economic factors that may have etiological or pathogenic relevance. It is important to note, however, that meaningful relations between social factors and disease do not always imply causalities that can be removed by the work of medical practitioners. At this interface, the practice of psychiatry reaches the limits of political and social action.

Moral, Ethics, Bioethics

Every human being is born into a moral community. This means that by tradition, custom, and use, certain behaviors and ways of thinking conform to *values*, universals of meaning implying that some attitudes and behaviors are acceptable and others are not. Morality is an implicit standard, and human beings are entities embedded in a world of actions and expectations constructed by previous generations. In this regard, all unreflected morality is imposed on individuals from the outside, rather than arising from their inner feelings.

Ethics, on the other hand, is a linguistic construction (a language game, as Wittgenstein says) designed by individual thinkers who justify why certain actions are permissible and others not. Ethics begins from the inner reflection of persons who orient their lives according to reason, belief, or utility.

In contemporary thinking, stress has been laid upon the way in which ethical convictions are attained, instead of the regulations or abstract theories of practical philosophies. This meta-ethics, procedural in essence, is what we call bioethics, meaning to imply the use of dialogue for formulating moral dilemmas and resolving them. Social institutions have been established in the form of "ethics committees" for regulating the practice of the professions and for conducting research.[4]

Two main traditions can be discerned in Western ethical discourse. Deontological thinking,[5-7] based on the idea of duties imposed by reason (Kantian approach), which limits spontaneous *Neigung* (inclination) and replaces it by *Pflicht* (duty). Duties are to be respected because reason demands it and human nature should obey its dictates (the basic tenet of Western Enlightenment, which defined humans as rational beings).

The other mainstream is teleology, a way of posing and solving moral problems based on the consequences of human actions.[8] Utilitarians believe that any action is ethically justified if its consequences contribute to the welfare of most people or contribute to the common good of society.[9]

It is evident that in common practice individuals make use of these two modes of ethical justification. In ethical decision-making, teleological moments are intertwined with teleological ones.

In the health professions, some particular forms of ethical reflection can be discerned. Virtue ethics[10,11] emphasizes the moral constitution of subjects; it is based upon the notion that good persons perform good actions. Traditionally, the medical profession based its ascendancy and power on the idea that its practitioners are virtuous and their actions directed toward the well-being of the persons they serve. It has been the basis of medical paternalism (beneficence to others without permitting autonomy). "Doctors know best" what is good for people is an idea already present in ancient documents (e.g., the Hippocratic Oath).

Another tradition in the health professions relies on the idea of care. Care ethics is a mixture of compassion, solidarity, and beneficence, and rests on the notion that good intentions produce good results.[12,13]

An additional stream of thought can be found in the idea of casuistry.[14-16] Moral problems are best approached, formulated, and solved by resorting to cases, or previous examples of similar situations; a crucial notion is that of context. Stories, fables, parables, and narratives derive their meaning and usefulness from what is narrated and the context in which it occurs. Circumstance (*circum-stare*), the context, permits an analysis of current situations based on previous instances in which a similar problem arose and was solved.[17]

In essence, the bioethical movement brings to light the idea that *dialogical deliberation* is a key to understanding the dilemmas presented by the practice of the professions, that discourses form the basis of rhetorics aimed at satisfying the expectations and hopes of different social agents and actors (sometimes termed "stakeholders" when a social interest is at issue), and that the main aim of ethics is to harmonize technical expertise with moral justification. Not everything good is also correct. Written regulations, norms, and principles must be balanced against the major interests of all persons and institutions involved. If problems cannot be resolved, they can be dissolved in the common good of a democratic and egalitarian society. Bioethical reasoning is the product of consultation or committee work and serves the needs of communities of practice, which are at the same time interpretive communities that define and legitimize what a "real" problem is. In this regard, a hermeneutic/interpretive/dialogical approach is appropriate.[18]

Bioethical deliberation may be applied in different contexts. *Micro bioethics* refers to the analysis of person-to-person interactions. *Meso bioethics* covers the institutional determinants of moral behavior. *Macro bioethics* refers to the global challenges faced by humanity due to ecological problems, interspecies relations, and global access to the benefits of science and civilization.

Social Psychiatry, Methodical Pluralism, and the Ethical Challenges

Psychiatry may be considered more than a medical specialty. It can be construed as a distinct profession partaking of the ethos of medicine but extending its reach to cultural, biological, and social dimensions of care.[19]

In common parlance, the word "social" is employed for distinguishing between biological and other determinants of behavior. The cultural construction of the individuum as the seat of disorder calls for elaboration on the ethical distinction between individual good and societal welfare. However, all ethical thinking is by definition a social enterprise and is always linked to the actual contexts in which people live. Written codes of conduct are derived from the idea that moral behavior cannot be based solely on personal conviction but the rules must be accessible to anyone. This made the difference between the *ethos* of the medical profession based exclusively on the conscience of practitioners and the fact that professional activities are accountable in light of duties and compromises made public. In this way, activities such as healthcare, research, policymaking, and administration can be monitored by peers, expert opinion, and the public at large. Codes of conduct complement the law, which is the written expression of popular will that orders, permits, and prohibits.

The ethical dimensions of psychiatric practice, when viewed from the perspective of the social, can be analyzed at different levels.[20] *Public health* alludes to the organized efforts of communities to regulate the practice of healthcare. *International health* indicates the need for a comparative analysis of practices and their applicability in different countries or territories. *Global health* emphasizes the ethical need to grant access to the benefits of science and technology to everyone.

Certain inequalities discernible between and within nations can be considered unjust and solvable and thus become inequities that should be removed. From an egalitarian perspective, it is unfair that certain groups are deprived of assistance or denied access to good conditions of life. Many different "gaps" have been identified. The 10/90 gap indicates that 10% of people benefit from the 90% of effort in scientific advances.[21] The treatment gap suggests that not everyone has access to the correct treatment of illness and disease.

To eliminate gaps derived from inequities requires an analysis of their causes. Some of them are structural, based on cultural determinants, since cultures are moral entities with a value architecture sometimes not consciously perceived by their members. Others are individual or contextual determinations due to personal biases. In many cases, the health professions, although conversant with health disparities and inequities, are not in a position to eliminate or correct them. In the long term, what can be achieved through ethical reasoning is to conform to the uses of the communities and provide for the common good of populations, respecting individual dignity. This is particularly true when dealing with phenomena such as stigma and discrimination caused by labels that persons receive: to be a "patient," to be different because of gender or sexual orientation, to belong to an ethnic minority, among others.

Principles in Ethical Reasoning as Applied to Diagnosis, Research, and Healthcare

For practical reasons, the bioethics movement exemplified by the tradition started at Georgetown University adopted an approach based on *principles* when dealing with problems presented by research, healthcare, and policymaking. Despite possible shortcomings and conflicting definitions, the idea that *prima facie* principles can be of help for formulating problems and dilemmas serves well the purpose of finding ways for dealing with them in the context of consultation and committee work. Autonomy, beneficence, nonmaleficence, and justice, as established by the Belmont Report[22] and presented in standard textbooks, permit the identification of moral problems with a clash of principles; autonomy versus beneficence, justice versus autonomy, and so forth. Thus, the deliberation can center around contextual issues justifying the preeminence of one or other principles for adequate decision-making. Cultural and structural factors may influence the relative weight of each principle in concrete cases, with the proviso that a hierarchy of them is not always evident. However, in democratic societies, justice and non-maleficence may rank higher than beneficence and autonomy, particularly when policies affect large populations and a decision must be made between the individual and group welfare.[23]

Principles as concrete deployment and value expression can be expanded. In some traditions and documents, solidarity, reciprocity, and vulnerability may be also construed as useful guidelines for framing discussions and arriving at reasoned (rational) and reasonable decisions.

Methods of Ethical Reasoning Applied to Psychiatric Practice from a Social Perspective

The use of written norms and their interpretation have been the standard practice for posing and analyzing moral quandaries. In Tables 4.1 and 4.2, relevant documents are presented, applicable both to medicine in general and to psychiatry in particular.

The social practice of psychiatry (as opposed to a discipline termed "social psychiatry") is faced with quandaries and dilemmas dictated both by the state of the art (individualistically oriented) and by structural problems originating in the methodical pluralism of the psychiatric practice. It is difficult to understand that "meaningful" connections are not necessarily "causal" connections. Problems derived from structural conditions are understandable, but this does not imply that they can be solved with the aid of the resources available to the psychiatric profession. Poverty, war, and natural disasters are understandably linked to psychiatric ailments, and demonstrations are easily obtained. However, to think of their impact as causes is another matter, since it implies that they can be managed by medical actions.

Ethics Committees in Healthcare Institutions and Bioethical Deliberation

Professionals and patients in healthcare institutions face difficult decisions that require deliberation. Dialogue and deliberation may take place in institutions called ethics committees. Deliberation is a method of reflection and collective analysis for making rational and reasonable decisions based on argumentations by all interested parties. Circumstances, values, and interests are taken into account. The model is based on the following: all arguments must be considered, and participants must be open to modifying their account to achieve a consensus. The ethical committee looks for a consensus, making a hierarchy determining which ethical principles have priority. Bioethical reflection has developed a methodological analysis for the resolution of conflicts and ethical problems related to health.

TABLE 4.1 Main Declarations and Guidelines on Ethics of Healthcare and Research Involving Humans, Especially Mental Health

Declaration	Organization	Purpose	Year
International Code of Medical ethics	World Medical Association	Code of ethics of the medical profession derived from the Declaration of Geneva	1949, 1968, 1983
Belmont Report	US National Commission for the Protection of Human Subjects of Biomedical and Behavioral Research	Basic ethical principles underlying the conduct of biomedical and behavioral research involving human subjects	1976
Declaration of Helsinki	World Medical Association	Statement of ethical principles for medical research involving human subjects	1964, 1975, 1983, 1989, 1996, 2000, 2008, 2013
Declaration of Tokyo	World Medical Association	Statement on torture and cruel, inhuman, or degrading treatment of detainees	1975
Declaration of Hawaii	World Psychiatric Association	Ethical guidelines for the practice of psychiatry	1977, 1983
Principles of medical ethics	United Nations	Code of medical ethics relating to the roles of health personnel in the protection of persons against torture and other cruel, inhuman, or degrading treatment or punishment	1982
International Ethical Guidelines for Health-Related Research Involving Humans	Council for International Organizations of Medical Sciences	International guidance for the application of ethical principles for health research involving humans	1982, 1993, 2002, 2016
Ethical principles for mental health care	United Nations	Principles for the Protection of Persons with Mental Illness and for the Improvement of Mental Health Care	1991
Madrid Declaration	World Psychiatric Association	Ethical guidelines for the practice of psychiatry in specific situations	1996, 1999, 2002
Statement on ethical issues concerning patients with mental illness	World Medical Association	Ethical responsibilities of physicians regarding mental illness	1995, 2006, 2015
Guidelines for good clinical practice	International Council for Harmonization of Technical Requirements for Pharmaceuticals for Human use	Ethical and technical guidelines for clinical trials involving human beings	1996

Edmund Pellegrino[24] considers the following questions as relevant for bioethical deliberation. They need to be adapted when population issues are considered:

- What are the scientific and technical facts? Which alternatives of action do they offer?
- Which ethical problems are raised by each choice?
- Which ethical principles are involved?

TABLE 4.2 Ethical Codes of Psychiatric Associations

Association	Code, Year	Website
American Academy of Child and Adolescent Psychiatry	Code of Ethics, 2014	https://www.aacap.org/App_Themes/AACAP/docs/about_us/transparency_portal/aacap_code_of_ethics_2012.pdf
American Psychiatric Association	The Principles of Medical Ethics with Annotations Especially Applicable to Psychiatry, 1973; most recent revision, 2013	http://www.psychiatry.org/practice/ethics
American Academy of Psychiatry and the Law	Ethics Guidelines for the Practice of Forensic Psychiatry, 2005	https://aapl.org/ethics.htm
United Kingdom Royal College of Psychiatry	Good Psychiatric Practice Code of Ethics, 2014	https://www.rcpsych.ac.uk/docs/default-source/improving-care/better-mh-policy/college-reports/college-report-cr186.pdf?sfvrsn=15f49e84_2
Australian and New Zealand College of Psychiatrists	Code of ethics, 1992; fifth edition, 2018	https://www.ranzcp.org/files/about_us/code-of-ethics.aspx
Institute of Australian Psychiatrists	Ethics Code, 1997	http://iap.org.au/ethics.htm
Japanese Society of Psychiatry and Neurology	Code of Ethics for Psychiatrists, 2015	https://www.jspn.or.jp/uploads/uploads/files/about/Code%20of%20Ethics%20for%20Psychiatrists_2015.pdf
Japanese Psychiatric Nursing Association	Code of Ethical Practice for Psychiatric Nursing, 2020	http://www.jpna.jp/english/pdf/ethicalandfoundations.pdf
College of Psychiatrists of Ireland	Professional Ethics for Psychiatrists, 2019	https://www.irishpsychiatry.ie/wp-content/uploads/2019/05/CPsychI-HRE-Professional-Ethics-for-Psychiatrists-FINAL.pdf
Canadian Medical Association	Code of Ethics Annotated for Psychiatrists, 1978	
Registered Psychiatric Nurses of Canada	Code of Ethics and Standards of Psychiatric Nursing Practice, 2010	https://www.bccnp.ca/Standards/RPN/ProfessionalStandards/Pages/Default.aspx
Indian Psychiatric Society	Code of Ethics, 1989	
Spain Psychiatry Society	Code of Good Practices, 2012	http://www.sepsiq.org/informacion/buenasPracticas

- Who are the patients, and which values do they hold?
- Who is the physician, and which values does he/she hold?
- Are the values of physicians and patients in conflict?
- In which ethical level are the values placed?
- Can the conflict be solved while respecting all moral values of the interested parties?
- Which will be a good moral choice for the specific patient?
- Can the moral process chosen be defended by arguments?
- Can all the necessary steps be defended with rational criteria?

The deliberative method of Diego Gracia[25] serves such purposes. This method consists of three levels, each with steps for reflection, presented here with slight modifications:

Comprehensive Level

This level considers the facts and moral values implied in the problem under analysis in its context. Facts relate to clinical history and technical considerations, and moral values relate to ethical decisions. The following steps are considered:

- The case presented by the person who has the main responsibility for the decision, narrated specifying the facts, biopsychosocial situation, actions, omissions, persons implicated, and opinions or circumstances surrounding the case.
- Discussion of clinical, epidemiological, or political aspects
- Identification of problems both technical and moral.

Analytical Level

Analysis of the bioethical principles implicated in deliberating on circumstances and concrete consequences, determining diverse possible courses of action. The following steps may be considered:

- Specify the relation of dependence between ethical problems and conflicts between them.
- Select a problem for deliberation. The complexity of moral conflict demands that one choose specific problems. Each problem must be solved separately in a sequential manner and not simultaneously.
- Identify the values or ethical principles in conflict. The specific ethical conflict, the principles involved, and their level must be identified, considering the specific circumstances of the case. In the analysis of the conflict between ethical principles, two levels are considered: level I, or universal (two principles: non-maleficence and justice, ethics of minimum); level II, or private (two principles: autonomy and beneficence (ethics of maximum). Level I has preference over level II.
- Identify the extreme courses of action and reflect on the consequences derived from each one.

Decision Level

Decisions must be made with a moral judgment or ethical recommendation. The following steps are suggested:

- A search for intermediate courses
- Analysis of the best course of action
- Final decision
- The confrontation of the decision made with legal accountability, whether the decision would be accepted publicly, and realization if the same decision could be made in the future or under diverse conditions.

Research Ethics Committees in Psychiatry

Research ethics committees bring into discussion and deliberation different social expectations and forms of expertise for studying new ways of approaching mental health issues. Research ethics committees have the following tasks for deliberation:[26] adequate research methodology; adequacy of research team and resources to identify and balance potential benefits and risks, to evaluate social adequacy and protection of vulnerable populations in the study, to evaluate the process of informed consent and the written documents, to evaluate inclusion and exclusion criteria, to evaluate risks for breaks of confidentiality, to prevent the influence in research results of potential conflicts of interest, to prevent any form of discrimination, to evaluate safety procedures, and to monitor research procedures. Among the members of these research ethics committees, apart from a psychiatrist, a lawyer, and an ethicist, it is also important to include members of the community where the study will be taken and representatives of mental health associations, since they may identify specific risks and benefits in the particular context of the study.

In the field of psychiatry, care must be taken in the process of informed consent since generally mental health patients are required to enter into studies. Competency for informed consent must be assessed. The comprehension and voluntary capacities may vary among subjects; some of them will be fully able to participate, others may require an authorized tutor, others may be able to participate only by assent (a way of accepting to participate but requiring the help of a tutor), and for others care may be taken to take informed consent in lucid periods. Specific safeguards for protection must be taken into consideration when carrying out research with mental health disorders since they are a vulnerable population risking social discrimination.

Ethical, Cultural, and Structural Competencies: The Goals of Education

Teaching ethics in the context of a socially responsible practice of psychiatry means not only making students familiar with norms and regulations and inculcating respect for persons, human rights, and duties, but also developing cultural and structural competencies that permit an understanding of conditions relevant to the interpretation and application of the principles. Beneficence, for instance, is a higher-order principle that no professional is obliged to follow if contextual conditions make it impossible to have the means of exercising it.

There has been some discussion about the best way to develop cultural, structural, and moral personal competencies among students and researchers. In addition to standard courses and familiarity with the main ethical documents, students must be exposed to fieldwork to enhance their capacity to experience diversity and confront cultural and structural determinants of health conditions.[27] In the field of psychiatry, in particular, the stigma and discrimination often associated with diagnostic labels must be examined and reflected upon.[28]

Social factors must be taken into account when training future mental healthcare practitioners since mental health differs from other medical fields in that the primary expressions of mental health problems are manifested in social or psychological disequilibriums of multiple causalities, with the alteration of behavior through emotional, cognitive, and perception processes.[29] Part of the disequilibrium may come from neurophysiological malfunctioning and may be treated pharmacologically, but other causes may come from personal relations or lack of adaptation to particular social situations. Community experience and resources in the form of social networks may help to develop ways of diminishing mental health problems[30] by addressing socially the causes that increase these problems. For example, in the mental health field, poverty, unemployment, and the lack of social relations increase the risk of suffering mental disorders.[31] Taking into account social determinants that affect mental health can inform public health measures for preventing disease by identifying social structural changes that may remedy social inequalities.

Furthermore, cultural psychiatric studies may help to understand cultural variabilities relevant for mental health problems, taking into account anthropological, psychological, and sociological factors, including the belief system.[29] Cultural factors may influence the way to envision mental disorders, how to address the symptoms, and how to find ways of adaptation for living with the disorder.[29]

References

1. Lange W. Rudolf Virchow, poverty and global health: From "politics as medicine on a grand scale" to "health in all policies". *Global Health Journal.* 2021;5(3):149–154.
2. Lolas F. The basic discipline of psychiatry as metatext. *Acta Bioethica (Santiago).* 2015;21:61–64.
3. Halliday JL. *Psychosocial Medicine: A Study of the Sick Society.* New York: Norton; 1948.
4. Lolas F. *Bioethics: Moral Dialogue in the Life Sciences.* Santiago: Universitaria; 1999.
5. Kant I. *Groundwork of the Metaphysic of Morals* (1785), HJ Paton, trans. New York: Harper and Row; 1964.
6. Darwall SL, ed. *Deontology.* Malden, MA: Wiley-Blackwell; 2002.
7. Kamm FM. *Intricate Ethics: Rights, Responsibilities, and Permissible Harms.* Oxford: Oxford University Press; 2007.
8. Seidel C. *Consequentialism: New Directions, New Problems.* Oxford: Oxford University Press; 2019.
9. Rachels J. *Elements of Moral Philosophy.* 4th ed. Boston: McGraw-Hill; 2003:96–121.
10. Crisp R, Slote M. *Virtue Ethics.* Oxford Readings in Philosophy. Oxford: Oxford University Press; 1997.
11. Van Zyl L. *Virtue Ethics: A Contemporary Introduction.* London: Routledge; 2018.
12. Gilligan C. *In a Different Voice: Psychological Theory and Women's Development.* Cambridge, MA: Harvard University Press; 1993.
13. Groenhout RE. *Connected Lives: Human Nature and an Ethics of Care.* Lanham, MD: Rowman & Littlefield; 2004.
14. Jonsen AR. Casuistry as methodology in clinical ethics. *Theor Med.* 1986;7:295–307.
15. Jonsen AR, Toulmin S. *The Abuse of Casuistry: A History of Moral Reasoning.* Berkeley: University of California Press; 1988.
16. Arras JD. Getting down to cases: the revival of casuistry in bioethics. *J Med Philos.* 1991;16:29–51.
17. Bloch S, Chodoff P, Green SA, eds. *Psychiatric Ethics.* New York: Oxford University Press; 1999.
18. Lolas F. The hermeneutical dimension of the bioethical enterprise: notes on the dialogical/narrative foundations of bioethics. *Acta Bioethica (Santiago).* 2018;24(2):153–159.
19. Lolas F. Psychiatry: medical specialty or specialized profession? *World Psychiatry.* 2010;9(1):34–35.
20. Lolas F. Social psychiatry: ethical challenges. *World Soc Psychiatry.* 2019;1:33–35.
21. Global Forum for Health Research. 2011. https://sk.sagepub.com/navigator/global-health/n24.xml

22. National Commission for the Protection of Human Subjects of Biomedical and Behavioral Research, Department of Health, Education and Welfare (DHEW). *The Belmont Report*. Washington, DC: United States Government Printing Office; 1978.

23. Beauchamp TL, Childress JL. *Principles of Biomedical Ethics*. New York: Oxford University Press; 1994.

24. Pellegrino ED. The healing relationship: the architectonics of clinical medicine. In: Shelp EE, ed. *The Clinical Encounter: The Moral Fabric of the Patient-Physician Relationship*. Dordrecht: Springer; 1983:153–172.

25. Gracia D. *Procedimientos de Decisión en Ética Clínica* [Decision procedures in clinical ethics]. Madrid: Eudema; 1991.

26. World Health Organization. *Standards and Operational Guidance for Ethics Review of Health-Related Research with Human Participants*. 2011. World Health Organization. Genebra Switzerland. https://apps.who.int/iris/handle/10665/44783

27. Crump JA, Sugarman J, Working Group on Ethics Guidelines for Global Health Training (WEIGHT). Ethics and best practice guidelines for training experiences in global health. *Am J Trop Med*. 2010;83(6):1178–1182.

28. Hatzenbuehler ML, Link BG. Introduction to the special issue on structural stigma and health. *Soc Sci Med*. 2014 Feb;103:1–6. doi:10.1016/j.socscimed.2013.12.017.

29. Kirmayer LJ, Swartz L. Culture and global mental health. In: Patel V, Prince M, Cohen A, Minas H, eds. *Global Mental Health: Principles and Practice*. New York: Oxford University Press; 2013:41–62.

30. Kirmayer LJ, Pedersen D. Toward a new architecture for global mental health. *Transcult Psychiatry*. 2014;51(6):759–776.

31. Patel V, Lund C, Heatherill S, et al. Social determinants of mental disorders. In: Blas E, Sivasankara Kurup A, eds. *Priority Public Health Conditions: From Learning to Action on Social Determinants of Health*. Geneva, Switzerland: World Health Organization; 2009:115–134.

5

"A Person Is a Person Through Other Persons"

A Social Psychiatry Manifesto for the 21st Century

Vincenzo Di Nicola

Introduction: What Is Social Psychiatry?

Social Psychiatry is the science of Anthropos.
—George Vassiliou and Eliot Sorel[a]

As the founder and president of the newly reconstituted Canadian Association of Social Psychiatry (CASP), I immersed myself in the rich history and significant achievements of the World Association of Social Psychiatry (WASP) and encountered a recurrent issue: *What is social psychiatry?* George Vassiliou and Eliot Sorel, two WASP past presidents, defined it as nothing less than the science of Anthropos (humanity). In this article, I address this definitional task by breaking it down into three major questions for social psychiatry and conclude with a call for action, a manifesto for 21st-century social psychiatry:

- What is *social* about psychiatry? I will address definitional problems that arise, such as binary thinking,[1] and the need for a common language.[2]
- What are the *theory* and *practice* of social psychiatry? Issues include social psychiatry's core principles, values, and operational criteria; the social determinants of health[3,4] and

This book chapter is the permitted republication of the article originally published in the journal World Social Psychiatry (published by Wolters Kluwer India Private Limited) under Creative Commons licensing terms. The full citation of the original published source is: Di Nicola V. "A person is a person through other persons": A social psychiatry manifesto for the 21st century. World Soc Psychiatry 2019;1:8–21.

a. From a dialogue between George Vassiliou and Eliot Sorel following the symposium on "The Role of the Psychiatrist in International Conflict Resolution" at the 8th World Congress of Social Psychiatry in Zagreb, Yugoslavia, in 1981.

the Global Mental Health Movement;[5,6] and the need for translational research. This review establishes the *minimal criteria for a coherent theory of social psychiatry* and the view of persons that emerges from such a theory: *the social self*.[7]

- Why has the time come for a *manifesto for social psychiatry*? I will outline the parameters for a theory of social psychiatry, based on both the social self and the social determinants of health, to offer an inclusive social definition of health,[8] concluding with a call for action, a manifesto for 21st-century social psychiatry.

What Is *Social* about Psychiatry?

Jules Masserman,[9(pp211-212)] a founder and early president (1969–1974) of the WASP, affirmed the social nature of psychiatry:

> Humanistic philosophers from Plato and K'ung Fu-Tze (L. *Confucius*) to Émile Durkheim have taught us that an individual's welfare ultimately depends on the merited support of his or her social group, from family and clan to nation. . . .
> We as psychiatrists are . . . called upon in our triune roles as physicians, cultural ombudsmen and philosophic savants to restore our patients' (L. *patient*, sufferer) vitality, social adaptation and relative serenity. In the sense that "social" is derived from L. *socius*, companion, all psychiatry is social.

While Masserman and other social psychiatrists contend that all psychiatry is social,[10,11] the history of psychiatry shows that this must be demonstrated and continually affirmed. At a time when the community psychiatry movement is losing support, with a return to hospital care, and a large burden of psychiatric care shifting to prisons,[12,13] the hard-won knowledge and perspective of social psychiatry must be continually integrated into teaching, research and practice, policymaking, and healthcare planning.

In my view as a social psychiatrist, different approaches such as systemic family therapy and epidemiological studies are tools for investigation based on "*n* greater than 1." They are tools, nonetheless, not ends in themselves. Mara Selvini Palazzoli, a founder of family therapy, stated this presciently: "Family therapy is the starting point for the study of ever wider social units."[14(p241)] Social psychiatry is the ultimate apparatus for the study of the social context of human predicaments, the widest possible context. Understanding humans out of context is not only limited but deeply misleading, as many contend,[11] yielding pseudo-problems and the conundrums that psychiatry and the social sciences have created in their descent into the "spiral staircase of the self," in Montaigne's memorable phrase.

What, then, is *social* about psychiatry as a branch of medicine and a social perspective on health? A corollary is: what are the roots of our concerns as social psychiatrists?

Social Psychiatry—False Friends or an Odd Pair?

In the work of translation, we have the experience of false analogies and ambiguous affinities between languages, what one specialized Italian-English dictionary calls "odd pairs and false friends".[15,-17] This is a metaphor for the state of social psychiatry today, since the two terms, *social* and *psychiatry*, are at times false friends and at others, get along just fine as an odd pair.

If our starting point is Samuel Guze's *Why Psychiatry Is a Branch of Medicine*,[18] *social* is a strong counterpoint to *psychiatry* understood as biomedicine and psychiatric illness as brain disorders, making for a very odd pair. Guze's defense of the medical model in psychiatry now holds sway in North American academic psychiatry to the point that the National Institute of Mental Health (NIMH) established its own Research Domain Criteria (RDoC) based on genomics and neuroscience,[19] airily dismissing a half century of research and refinements into descriptive psychiatric nosography by the American Psychiatric Association's DSM project as a "mere dictionary." The translation of psychiatric illness to disorders of the brain elevates neuroscience to the status of a foundational science. In a parallel shift, academic psychology has now become cognitive neuroscience and evolutionary psychology.[20] This has engendered enthusiastic affirmations such as Eric Kandel's psychiatric extrapolations from his Nobel Prize–winning neuroscience research,[21,22] countered by trenchant criticisms from psychology,[23] philosophy of science,[24] and other branches of medicine.[25] Fernando Lolas,[26] WASP secretary general and an authority on psychiatric ethics, opines that psychiatry should be a specialized profession rather than a branch of medicine.

On the other hand, if we start with Arthur Kleinman's *Social Origins of Distress and Disease*,[27] an essay in medical anthropology that widens our understanding of psychiatry to encompass the personal distress and despair and the social suffering that accompany psychiatric illness, we create false friends, an illusion of harmony within psychiatry as a whole. Kleinman exhorts us to "rethink psychiatry," moving "from cultural category to personal experience."[28] As an authoritative voice for the social sciences in psychiatry, Kleinman poignantly criticizes the pathologization and the medicalization of human suffering, calling for a "rebalancing of academic psychiatry"[29(p421)] to include social, clinical, and community studies within a broader biosocial framework. Yet, the successes of the community mental health movement[30,31] and the creation of research centers for social and cultural psychiatry, along with the inclusion of cultural competence and the cultural formulation in the DSM, have only sharpened the debate. Sartorius and associates[10(pix)] argued that since "all psychiatry is social," it would be "unimaginable that psychiatry could be practiced or that psychiatric research could be conducted without constant reference to social factors and to the social environment." Unimaginable but true! The vaunted biopsychosocial (BPS) approach,[32] offering an integration of three domains, became a convenient cover for psychopharmacology and neuroscience research to appear inclusive, yet in practice, as DSM-IV chairman Allen Frances later observed, BPS became "bio-bio-bio." The social determinants of health,[3,4] based on populational research that is as robust and durable as anything we have in medicine with powerful implications for health and illness, are discounted or ignored. In this environment, to believe that *social* is a descriptor for *psychiatry* today is aspirational. Social sychiatry is, at best, a subfield, like child psychiatry or geriatric psychiatry.

Like other examples of binary opposition, pitting *social* against *psychiatry* can lead to polarization and false divisions. Addressing such conundrums, Wittgenstein[33] dismissed

---

BOX 5.1 Defining Features of Social Psychiatry

Concerned with people in numbers

Studies relationships between mental disorders and sociocultural processes

Responsible to a society or group

Conducts knowledge from clinical psychiatry to strategic points in the sociocultural system to foster reductions in psychiatric disorders

Conducts knowledge from the social sciences into clinical psychiatry

Adapted from Leighton.[36]

---

them as "pseudo-problems" based on linguistic confusions. How can we move beyond unfruitful divisions, whereby practitioners of subspecialties simply agree to disagree, hiving off into their specialized meetings and journals, while psychiatry as a whole lacks coherence and integration?[34,35] To anticipate my conclusion, social psychiatry offers the specialty of psychiatry and all of medicine greater coherence through an integration of the biomedical model with the larger context of the social determinants of health and the relational aspects of all human interactions.

Defining Social Psychiatry

> *Social psychiatry is concerned with the relationships between mental disorder and sociocultural processes.*
> —Alexander Leighton[36]

Leighton[36] was a pioneer of psychiatric epidemiology in Canada whose textbook of social psychiatry offers the defining features of the field (see Box 5.1) with a succinct definition that is both theoretical and pragmatic.

Before going further, let us examine the word *social.* Cultural historians carefully dissect words concerned with the practices and institutions described as "culture" and "society."[37,38,39] Several entries are of interest here: *society, social, societal,* and *sociology,* and related words such as *socialism* and *solidarity.* For our purposes, the lesson is that these terms are plastic and mutable and both *social* and *society,* with roots in the Latin, *socius,* companion, and *societas,* meaning a union for common purpose, association, community, were transformed from relational descriptions of association and sociability to more abstract meanings, clearly signifying a distinction from the individual, as in "man and society" meaning "the individual in society." We may conclude that in the Western cultural lexicon *social* has moved from a relational *description* to a kind of ethical *prescription.*

How Did We Get Here?

How did Western societies move from an ancient worldview where divine forces created and controlled the human world to the contemporary vision of humanity and society following natural laws?

"Man in Nature"—The Age of Reason: From Child of Nature to the Nature of the Child

We can reconstruct a history where we see Western cultures moving from a worldview in which humanity is seen within a divine order of things called the Great Chain of Being (Latin, *scala naturae*), challenged by the Enlightenment and humanism that created natural philosophy and the origins of modern biological sciences.[40,41] The concept of man (which we now call humanity) that emerged in the Enlightenment was "man in nature." And here we see the origins of pedagogy in the work of Jean-Jacques Rousseau, psychology, and the construct of mind in thinking about humans as natural beings.[42,43]

It took a full two centuries before empirical research into what became developmental psychology and developmental psychopathology (child psychiatry) finally studied the adverse events of childhood,[44,45] demonstrating the consequences of childhood trauma.[46] This is the real birth of a socially informed pedagogy, pediatrics, and child psychiatry, and the roots of social psychiatry.

"Man in Society"—19th-Century Social Realism: Society Is Greater than the Sum of Its Parts

With the rise of cities came the study of "man in society" and sociology as a social science. Its founder, Durkheim, studied how society maintained coherence in the face of populational concentration and social dispersion, pioneering methods for studying social currents rather than individuals. He viewed knowledge in social terms and coined the term "collective consciousness." Durkheim channeled 19th-century social and political concerns into a methodology for studying society as greater than the sum of its parts. He is the forefather of social epidemiological research and the social determinants of health and mental health, with a concern for social justice.

"Man Alone"—20th Century: Social Psychiatry in a Time of Loneliness

The 20th century witnessed intense contradictions from the traumas of world wars and genocides to the affirmations of humanistic values in opposition to increasing mechanization and speed leading to isolation and marginalization. Many trends converged to create social psychiatry, which was motivated to bridge the divides in society, in medicine, and in psychiatry. Barely acknowledged in medicine and psychiatry were major trends away from the usual power centers—toward the Global South,[47] toward feminism and postcolonialism, in short, toward a multipolar, pluricultural world which made social psychiatry ever more relevant, and yet the coming Global Mental Health Movement[5,6,13,48,49] would take center stage.

"Liquid Humanity"—21st Century: Humanity Unbound, Social Psychiatry Without Borders

Inheriting the tired term *postmodernism* from the end of the last century, we now seem to be in a *post* era—postmodernism, post everything, including truth. In this spirit, the new century heralds a new era, the Anthropocene, in which human activity dominates the planet. That may be true about the natural environment which we are polluting and destroying,[50,51] but when it comes to the social environment, we are marginalizing our own human capacities in favor of intelligent machines, leading Jaron Lanier,[52] the father of virtual reality, to call his manifesto, *You Are Not a Gadget*.

If some thought leaders in our field worried that the 20th century "lost its mind" (psychologist Cyril Burt)[53] or became "mindless" (child psychiatrist Leon Eisenberg),[54] in the 21st century we may be "losing our humanity" altogether. Rather than the two 20th-century extremes of fulfilling humanity or ending it, there is talk of the *transhuman*, modified by bioengineering and digital technology.[55] The best epithet for our century may be "liquid humanity," a variation of sociologist Zygmunt Bauman's liquid modernity.[56] Rather than overcoming modernity or humanity, it has become liquid. Everything is fluid and subject to change. Never has the Greek philosopher Heraclitus (*ta panta rhei*, "everything flows") seemed so relevant, as we are fast becoming a century of massive, rapid change.[57] And we need a psychiatry adequate to the task of documenting the consequences. There are crises in all three spheres—*the natural environment* (climate change and mental health),[50,51] *the built environment* (homelessness, the housing crisis),[58] and *the social environment* (identity, belonging, migration, massive change).[57,59,60]

If social psychiatry is to become a comprehensive, integrative, transdisciplinary field of medicine and social science, we must now concern ourselves with all three spheres, above all with the social impacts of deteriorations and the challenges in these essential environments. Because of such potential social impacts, it is more artificial than ever to compartmentalize health into separate domains due to their porous borders and reciprocal influences. At the same time, our expertise as social psychiatrists allows us to discern emerging patterns and challenges as we see the social sphere fragmenting into several bubbles. In each bubble, we may perceive a dichotomy or polarization, with both positive and negative impacts.

What Does This Augur for Social Psychiatry?

For social psychiatry to maintain its relevance and affirm the claim that "all psychiatry is social," echoed by both Masserman, a WASP founder,[9] and Sartorius, a WHO leader,[10] we must demonstrate the validity of this general claim in theoretical terms and the specificity of social psychiatry to bolster theory and practice.

Specifically, we must address the binary oppositions not only of psychiatry but of Western and Northern cultural categories. Ciompi[61] urged pluralism as a philosophical foundation for social psychiatry, and Sartorius[62] offered multiple scenarios for the future of psychiatry. We must clarify our principles, values, and operational criteria. We must elucidate a theory of social psychiatry upon which to base a practice of social psychiatry with its integration into teaching, clinical work, research, healthcare planning, and policymaking. And we must set an agenda for social psychiatry in the 21st century.

Binary Oppositions

A simple dichotomy of individual and environment is no longer a sufficient concept in understanding the etiology of mental health and illness.
—Michele S. Trimarchi[63]

In *This Idea Must Die*,[64] a powerful collection of poor theories that block progress, the threads running through many of them are unproductive binary oppositions and false dichotomies. Part of our Western/Northern historical legacy, these include:

- *Nature versus nurture* and its iterations in psychiatry (endogenous vs. exogenous factors, inherited vs. acquired traits);
- *Individual versus collective* (individual versus group therapy, individual versus family therapy, clinical psychiatry versus community psychiatry);
- *Subjectivity versus objectivity*;
- And finally, *social versus biological*.

Investigations into trauma,[1,65] reveal a dichotomy that is built into all discourses about trauma, which expresses itself differently in different fields and times but always founders on the same reductive binary opposition. In trauma studies, I characterize it as the "clinical trauma community" and the "cultural trauma community."[1] This dichotomy defeats all efforts to change the conversation about trauma. Scholars in the humanities, scientists, and clinicians use similar terms, quote the same literature, and yet arrive at radically different understandings and polarizing conclusions, such as whether we should treat or simply witness trauma. That is why we need theory; empirical investigations cannot sort this out. I concluded that psychiatry cannot resolve this dichotomy, which is why I resorted to the conceptual apparatus of philosophy to do so.

Nature versus nurture has been an abiding theme of all thinking about childhood as a model of humanity[42] and investigators and clinicians in all disciplines tend to separate into two camps, with few synthesizers in between.[20,66] In the social sciences, the issue of power has been a dominant theme in the critique of society and the professions, including psychiatry. This includes power issues running through society, including the corrosive myth of racial supremacy. As a social psychiatrist, I believe that power is an illusion and race is a myth. However, as the struggle for power and the discourse on race are social realities, we cannot easily change the subject and need to study how people experience power, race, and stigmatization as social phenomena with complex and profound impacts.

Another issue is to differentiate social psychiatry from its cognate fields: transcultural psychiatry, cultural psychiatry, comparative psychiatry, cross-cultural psychology, medical anthropology, medical sociology, and global mental health. I see them as tessellated fields of study, each tile having its uses and adding its color and shape to form a larger pattern, but as Sartorius[2] observed, if psychiatry is to have credibility, we need to create an accessible and easily understood common vocabulary. Along with promising studies and new ideas and paradigms, we also need to retrench and redefine and then integrate and synthesize.[67]

What may be a solution? I believe the solution lies in interdisciplinary studies and multi-method research programs working toward a transdisciplinary approach—the very pluralism that Ciompi[61] proposed for social psychiatry. We need more integration and synthesis of what is known, with a focus on problems and solutions rather than narrow sectarian interests. The key words here are a pluralistic philosophy that recognizes that different temperaments will lead to different sorts of questions and methodologies,[23,68] while creating integration and syntheses to refresh the language of biomedical and social sciences.[69]

Psychiatry, Fast and Slow

If we cannot defeat binary thinking, let us at least put it to good use as a metaphor. Adapting Nobel Prize–winning psychologist Daniel Kahneman's[70] approach to *thinking, fast and slow*, and my own investigations on *slow thinking* and *slow psychiatry*,[71,72] we can imagine two poles of psychiatry as it is currently constructed: *fast psychiatry* and *slow psychiatry*. This way of looking at modes of thinking, styles of investigation, cuts across many disciplines, as in the celebrated essay by Isaiah Berlin[79] contrasting Russian thinkers Dostoyevsky and Tolstoy, characterized as the deeply burrowing hedgehog and the wide-ranging fox (Table 5.1).

Fast psychiatry yields William James's tough-minded empiricism,[74] converging on solutions,[23] using technocratic algorithms for pragmatic ends,[68] deploying etic or experience-distant approaches with "thin" descriptions,[75] focused on rapid change to gain mastery within a definitive, uniform research paradigm. (*Key words*: fox, empirical, convergent, technocratic, algorithmic, pragmatic impact, rapidity, mastery, paradigmatic/uniform, research.)

TABLE 5.1 Fast Psychiatry and Slow Psychiatry

Fast Psychiatry	Slow Psychiatry
Key words	*Key words*
the wide-ranging fox	the deeply burrowing hedgehog
empirical	rational
convergent	divergent
technocratic	phenomenological
etic, experience-distant	emic, experience-near
thin descriptions	thick descriptions
algorithm	heuristic
pragmatic impact	knowledge accumulation
rapidity	slowness/incrementalism
mastery	comprehension
paradigm/uniform	syntagm/pluralistic
research	investigation

Adapted from Di Nicola.[71,72]

Slow psychiatry offers James's tender-minded rationalism,[74] pursuing divergent questions,[23] deploying phenomenological heuristics to pursue knowledge,[68] using emic or experience-near approaches, incrementally aiming at comprehensive "thick" descriptions[75] and understanding in a syntagmatic (pluralistic) approach to investigations. (*Key words:* hedgehog, rationalistic, divergent, phenomenological, emic/experience-near, heuristic, knowledge accumulation, slowness/incrementalism, comprehension, syntagm/pluralistic, investigation.)

Examples of fast psychiatry include: behavior therapy; cognitive-behavior therapy; brief therapies; solution-focused therapy; psychiatric pharmacotherapy; clinical trials; aspects of psychiatric genetics; and the reductive use of biological psychiatry and neuroscience.

Slow psychiatry includes: psychoanalysis and its derivations; aspects of systemic family therapy (on the more phenomenological side);[17,68] the "narrative turn" in therapy; dialogical methods;[76,77] transcultural psychiatry (both in its original "classical" version at McGill University[78,79] and the "new cross-cultural psychiatry" at Harvard, even more clearly focused on emic, experience-near approaches[80]); epidemiological studies;[81] social determinants of health;[3,4] the human genome project; social neuroscience[82,83] and mirror neurons[84,85] to investigate all forms of imitation from empathy to learning to social skills; and, finally, social psychiatry, thus redefined.

What Is the *Theory* and *Practice* of Social Psychiatry?

Principles, Values, Operational Criteria

Given its role as a bridge between academic disciplines and distinct societies, social psychiatry's *main principles* should include: *transdisciplinarity* and a *multicentric world perspective* (not only Western/Northern). As an ethical matter, our *values* should ensure the *dignity* of all those involved in social psychiatry's activities, and be guided by *beneficence*. Our operational criteria need to balance *coherence*[68] with *theoretical pluralism*,[61,62,86] to conduct *translational research* of social psychiatry's powerful populational studies, in order to provide *ground-level prescriptions* (aimed at prevention, promotion, intervention, and adaptation).

What Is Social Psychiatry?

Here are some ways to imagine social psychiatry's disparate program:

- *An envelope*—a container, a context for human situations, including medical and psychiatric problems;
- *A bridge*—between the natural sciences and the human and social sciences;
- *A map* of human experience based on affectionate bonds and family and social relationships.

Bringing this together, social psychiatry is the widest, broadest envelope for situating human experience, acting as a bridge between fields of expertise and between personal and social or relational being, and thus equipped, offers a comprehensive map of human experiences. Unlike biological psychiatry[18,19] or evolutionary psychology[20,66] which purport to explain human behavior through evolutionary models of brain structures, social psychiatry describes the social context and conditions in which human experiences give rise to psychiatric problems, which I describe as mental, relational, and social problems. I define the difference between *social and relational aspects* as public and private, the difference between living in the same neighborhood (social) and living in the same household (relational). Biological psychiatry and evolutionary psychology face the same paradoxes and blind alleys that behavioral psychology faced: in an effort to circumvent tough questions about consciousness and social relations, they offer somewhat useful tools while explaining too little.

In this sense, social psychiatry as a *map* is also the *territory* of human problems.[87] It doesn't assume, discount, or reduce any other causes or descriptions. And the social determinants of health and mental health are among the most robust and durable findings we have in the human sciences. These are now established insights of social psychiatry.

By describing the environments in which problems arise, social psychiatry in the 21st century offers what phenomenological psychiatry in the 20th century promised but could not deliver: a descriptive nosology of human problems—and key examples are: the social determinants of health, from a populational, epidemiological perspective, and the social context, from the studies of human relations (including attachment theory, family theory, and therapy, and relational aspects of psychotherapy, as well as relational psychology and psychiatry).

The social psychiatry I envision parallels the best intentions of behaviorism in wishing to stay close to observable behavior (without its explanatory overreach in eliminating both mind and brain). My social psychiatry is inspired by such congenial approaches as systems theory, which situates human beings in relational contexts called systems, and attachment theory, which situates human development in the context of parent-child bonds and family-based caregiving. Together, attachment theory and systems theory highlight the crucial, life-defining importance of early childhood growth and lifelong family and social support. Projected onto the larger screen of social psychiatry, these theories become the critical issue of belonging. In a world of complex, competing, and often confusing identities, belonging reminds us that we are first social beings who need to relate to others through family, friendship, and communal relationships.

Social psychiatry has been, since its inception, sometimes an *approach*, closer to an *attitude* in wishing to place psychiatry in a social context, and sometimes a group of *observational studies* about that context—all without a coherent, consensual, and compelling theory. Both ends of this spectrum (an approach, observational studies) lack a comprehensive and compelling theory which marshals the evidence and gives it a coherent theoretical framework. Social psychiatry has often generated a group of powerful observations in search of a theory. Two empirically driven social psychiatry models from the Institute of Psychiatry in London, where I trained, are the Expressed Emotion paradigm[88,89] and the social origins of depression in women;[90] both research models that were initiated by sociologist George Brown.

As a result, social psychiatry has offered important descriptions accompanied by rather anemic explanations and vague, generic prescriptions. The social determinants of health paradigm and the Global Mental Health (GMH) Movement have taken flight and cruising at 35,000 feet gives them a global reach. What are needed now are prescriptions at ground level (Schwab called this "clinical applicability").[91] Competing worldviews of our field show no reticence to make bold claims. Psychopharmacology, biological psychiatry, neuroscience, evolutionary psychology and psychiatry, and others all want to take our place. Social psychiatry needs a comprehensive theory that asserts its powerful observations in a meaningful way while offering ways of bringing together current practices in line with its core principles, values, and operational criteria.

First, however, let me sound a note of caution. While we should harness the power of research methodologies and promising cognate models and allied approaches to social psychiatric questions, we should resist the reduction of social psychiatry to methodologies or cognate allied fields and subdisciplines that produce data. I call these temptations *methodolatry* and *scientism*.[71] Social psychiatry should remain the name of our field and not be subordinated to the limitations imposed by research methodologies or the redefinitions inherent in any kind of reductionism, however seductive their promise may be. As Sartorius recommended, "If psychiatry is to remain a coherent and socially useful discipline it is essential that it redefine its borders."[2(p30)] Lolas[26] weighed in on this issue, arguing for social psychiatry as a specialized profession. If social psychiatry is to have any meaning, it must define and defend its own domain without being sutured to a methodology, model, or practice.

To be specific, social psychiatry cannot be narrowly defined by the social determinants of health, nor can a populational approach alone be our guiding model. Physician-researcher Mukherjee[92] discerned one of the laws of medicine as: *"Normals" teach us rules; "outliers" teach us laws.* The epidemiological approach establishes the denominator of our task as physicians—its social distribution. It teaches us about what is or is not normal in a given population and sets out the parameters of health. Yet it is important to examine outliers—unusual, unrepresentative cases and currents—the numerators that cry out for understanding and intervention. For example, someone had to notice and then describe the first case of anorexia nervosa[93–95] or self-mutilation[96] as an outlier, something that stood apart from the norm. The clinician is also an investigator, attuned to social context to discern patterns and variations.

That said, we may identify allies and partners in our work. Behavioral approaches and relational approaches are natural allies in the clinic. Public health and epidemiology are natural partners for investigation.[96] Attachment theory is a powerful model that has already integrated a wealth of psychosocial observations and clinical knowledge into a coherent theory; we must use it as a model and integrate it into our own expanded model of social psychiatry for a more encompassing theory of belonging. The study of life events, stress, and trauma-related disorders are both the heart of social psychiatry as a map of the territory to be studied and of the problems to be treated.

So, bringing it all together, what is 21st-century social psychiatry?

Minimal Requirements for a Theory of Social Psychiatry

First, we need to articulate requirements for a comprehensive, compelling and consensual theory:

1. We need a *theory of how humans work*—mind, brain, and relations (integrating psychology, neuroscience, and society).
2. We need a *theory of psychiatry as both a branch of medicine and a social science* embracing other pertinent domains as a descriptive "science of Anthropos" that is congruent and theoretically coherent. Part of this theory of social psychiatry is how human problems arise—mentally, relationally, and socially.
3. We need a *model of practice*—i.e., what do social psychiatrists actually do?

What Model of Mind, Self, and Society Emerges from Social Psychiatry?

At issue: the biggest question in the human sciences today is how to conceive of mind.[43,97] The 20th century, from philosophy and psychology to neurology, physiology, and psychiatry, staged endless debates over the concept of mind.[43,98] It opened with two opposing theses: Pavlovian conditioning (based on physiologist Ivan Pavlov's Nobel Prize–winning research) and Freudian psychoanalysis (founded by a neuropathologist), culminating in Watson's behavioral manifesto in academic psychology and a half-century of psychoanalytic predominance in Western psychiatry and mental healthcare. Intriguingly, none of these leaders was a psychiatrist.

We have entertained some false starts on defining mind: just as mind is not reducible to behavior (Chomsky vs. Skinner), the mind is not a computer (Fodor vs. Pinker) and "you are not a gadget" (Lanier vs. Silicon Valley), social psychiatry holds that the mind is not simply the brain (Kagan, Tallis vs. Guze, NIMH). Until we have a consensus on the matter, we should consider competing theories, without accepting reductionist and simplistic claims. Let us accept a levels approach, whereby we name the domains of human activity:[17,68]

- *Biomedical science* (biology and medicine);
- *Cognitive science* (cognitive psychology and neuroscience);
- *Critical thinking* (social science and the humanities);
- *Relational psychology* (from dialogism to social psychology and from relational psychoanalysis to family therapy).

The key feature of such a levels approach is not how each level works as much as what the rules of translation are between levels and how their integration works in reality. What social psychiatry may offer with its encompassing, pluralistic approach is precisely such an integration.

Why the Time Has Come for a *Manifesto for Social Psychiatry*

I will outline the parameters for a theory of social psychiatry, based on both the social self[7,68] and the social determinants of health,[3,4] to offer an inclusive social definition of health,[8] concluding with a call for action, a manifesto for 21st-century social psychiatry.

Why Social Psychiatry Needs a Theory Now

Without theory, blind empiricism produces data without an explanation, observations with no goal. A theory can bring cohesion and coherence to apparently unrelated phenomena and data. Attachment theory, for example, brought together a wide range of clinical observations and studies from psychoanalysis to René Spitz's hospitalism that are given coherence and meaning to create a rich explanatory model. Two great theorists constructed modern psychiatry—Emil Kraepelin with his classification of the psychoses, and Karl Jaspers who brought phenomenology to psychiatry, the greatest coherence brought by a single theorist in the field. Theory brings coherence and meaning to seemingly disparate facts, observations, and studies—what we have called since Jaspers the *clinical phenomenology of psychiatry*.

Social psychiatry has harnessed powerful methodologies from epidemiology and adopted some compelling community and social principles (often in reaction or resistance to institutional psychiatry), yet a comprehensive, compelling, and consensual theory eludes the field. The best we have are statements of social psychiatry's principles and values, thoughtfully expressed. Each of the three definitions cited in this article—Leighton's epidemiological model,[36] Vassiliou's and Sorel's embracing "science of Anthropos," and Ciompi's philosophical pluralism wedded to community psychiatry[61]—brings us closer to a mission statement, but none of them explicitly formulates a theory of social psychiatry.

Practical Implications of Social Psychiatry

Together, three branches of social psychiatry signaled a shift in psychiatry:

- Epidemiological studies, where the shift is away from the individual and the clinic, and *populations* became the *focus* of research;
- Community psychiatry, where the shift is away from the individual in the institution, and the community became the *locus* of intervention;
- Relational therapies (marital, family, and group therapies), where the shift is from the individual to relationships, and relations became the *praxis*, the object of study and intervention.

In contrast to the characterization of Jung's work as "depth psychology," I describe social psychiatry as *a psychiatry of breadth*—expanding the range of observations from the individual to the family and group (relational therapies), to the community (community psychiatry), and to populations (psychiatric epidemiology).

What we need now is translational research to bring these solid findings to the ground level and start converting them to programs for health promotion, illness prevention, and therapeutic interventions, and to harness them to well-established principles of community psychiatry and relational therapies to make these other branches compelling not only as values but backed up by studies demonstrating their utility.

Translational research needs to address four domains: *service* (models of practice), *training and teaching* (bridging all the other domains and transmitting a coherent theory to the field and the next generation), *healthcare planning* (utilitarian questions about efficacy, reliability, and utility), and *values-based medicine* (ethical questions about validity).[95,99]

Qualities of the 21st-Century Social Self—the *Self-in-Relation*

After the atomized individual, alienated by industrial progress in the late 19th century and early 20th century, succumbing to the "lonely crowd" by mid-century,[100] and the "saturated self"[101] by century's end, what kind of self can social psychiatry conjure up in the 21st century? The *social self* that emerges from such studies is: *porous, relational, and quick.*

Porous

"Porosity" is a quality of incompleteness, "a work in progress" and of loosely defined margins.[102] It is closely allied to *liminality* and *threshold persons* described in Victor Turner's anthropology.[103] This is Bauman's "liquid modernity"[56] harking back to the Heraclitan flux. A positive experience of being comfortable with porosity and liminality is "flow," a deep, fluid immersion into activities.[104] *Cognate ideas*: liminality,[103] interdependence,[17] liquid modernity,[56] flow.[104] *Contrasting ideas*: coherence, homeostasis, stability.[68]

Relational

The social self is relational, drawing on Bakhtin's[76,77] *dialogism* and Levinas's *face-to-face encounter.*[105] Relational is more than social, it implies a greater degree of mutual exchange, knowledge, and intimacy. In this view, culture is a border that runs through everything in society.[106] Society is an interface and human relations at their best are face to face. Richard Mollica's[107] groundbreaking work on trauma reminds us that trauma is "a story that must be told" (dialogical) and, I would add, it must be told to another person (face to face) as opposed to being written or deposed as a document. *Cognate ideas:* dialogism, face-to-face encounter, narrative therapy.[76,77,105] *Contrasting ideas*: agency, individuation, solitude.

Quick

This is a quality of the social self inspired by Italo Calvino's reflections on literature,[108] meaning alertness, responsiveness, and economy of expression. Think of the quickness of the fox rather than the velocity of cars as in the "dromology" of Paul Virilio.[109] *Cognate ideas*: adaptability, cleverness. *Contrasting ideas:* lingering, digression, slowness;[72] development; speed/dromology;[109] the deeply burrowing hedgehog and the wide-ranging fox.[73] These contrasts are brought together in the Latin maxim, *Festina lente*, "hasten slowly."

In this new world, where borders are porous and identities are fluid, the quickness and alertness of the fox offer survival skills while the single-mindedness of the hedgehog maintains coherence and stability. Slow thought[72] is a "counter-method" that counsels a strategic pause for reflection before precipitating into action in response to the challenge of rapid change.

A Global Agenda for 21st-Century Social Psychiatry

An agenda that is coherent with a theory of social psychiatry and responsive to its dual clinical and populational mandate needs to be articulated. The agenda of social psychiatry should address three environments or spheres of human activity:

- *Natural environment:* climate change; disaster psychiatry ;
- *Built environment:* homelessness; crowding; worker safety; child labor and exploitation;
- *Social environment:* rapid, massive change; social class, culture change; the Global South; global epistemologies; migration and borders; stigmatization; crime and violence; mass murder and suicide.

The *Still* Hidden Injuries of Class

Despite *social class* having been set aside for theoretical reasons, the rise of cultural psychiatry with its emphasis on culture as a primary focus means that the "hidden injuries of class"[110] have become invisible to academics. In fact, these injuries are still present yet hiding in plain sight. We have become inured to their presence, especially in mid- to large cities, where, sadly, we can ignore poverty, homelessness, and urban violence through social segregation. The discourse of social class has been essentially replaced by issues related to culture such as migration and racism. This means that social psychiatry for a time was eclipsed by cultural psychiatry. We must reopen the discussion about social segregation and health care equity, as the WHO CSDH recommends.[3]

Rapid, Massive Change

These are two different issues: radical change and the acceleration of everything. Social psychiatry is uniquely positioned to take stock of rapid and massive cultural and social change.[42,93,94] The debate on migration and borders in many countries has become polarized. Accusations of racism and xenophobia on one side and fear of lawlessness and loss of sovereignty on the other abound. These are the wrong questions which generate wrong answers. In another era, people studied history to understand cycles and social changes in order to cope with the massive disruptions associated with disasters and wars. From this, they created strategies to deal with them. Most societies deal with rapid, massive change with difficulty, and this may be exploited for short-term gains or planned wisely to deal with its implications and opportunities. For example, many complex economies now require a highly skilled workforce which their home populations cannot sustain; hence immigration is not only desirable but necessary to maintain their levels of economic productivity and social stability.

That said, rapid social change may generate many adaptational problems.[57,111] In the early literature of transcultural psychiatry, much attention was given to Culture-Bound Syndromes, but I have argued for the study of Culture-*Change* Syndromes, notably among youth, in whom rates of selective mutism and anorexia nervosa are greatly elevated in first-generation immigrants.[42,93,94,112] My clinical practice as a child psychiatrist demonstrates that these problems are still treated as passing phases or transitional problems (e.g., adjustment disorders) rather than serious mental health issues that can become chronic.[42]

Psychiatric Problems Are Socially Constructed

Human problems, including psychiatric disorders, broadly conceived, are richly contextual in which even genetics (via epigenetics) are now known to be socially situated. This means that the cross-cultural distribution and historical evolution of psychiatric disorders not only reflect dominant models of mind, self, and society, but are constantly changing. Across cultures and over time, psychiatric disorders are themselves porous, under construction, and are not easily codified.[42,93,94] The complex evolutionary basis and neurophysiological substrates teach us that mind and brain reflect the plasticity of adaptation and the porosity of human identity. Social neuroscience is a bridge between brain and mind and not a reductive science.[82–85]

A priority should be integrating descriptive populational studies with ground-level prescriptions through translational research. The social determinants of health, the ACE Study, and key ideas such as the social gradient of health and treatment gaps identified by the GMH Movement should serve as blueprints for wise and responsive healthcare planning and practice.

Moving Beyond Binary Oppositions

Above all, social psychiatry needs to:

- Create a synthesis of populational research with ground-level programs;
- Move beyond dichotomies such as personal/social and individual/group;
- Accept that domains of inquiry reflect different temperaments among the investigators, addressing different sorts of hypotheses;[23,68]
- Acknowledge that we need both phenomenological and technocratic approaches, divergent and convergent methods, to properly define and thereby solve social problems. Nowhere is this clearer than in the emerging fields of transgender health,[113–115] part of whose message is to move beyond binary identities.

The Global South and Southern Epistemologies

In order to be inclusive and responsive to social realities in different societies around the world, we need to move beyond Western and Northern epistemologies to embrace the Global South[47] and "southern epistemologies."[116]

Migration and Borders

The global flow of migrants and refugees is an international problem that must be recognized as a global, transnational priority.[117] As Thomas Nail[59,60] argues in his work, there are two implications. First, global migration is not a mere uptick or a passing crisis to be imagined as an exception, it is rather the rule in human history. Human history is the history of our migrations. Second, such a perspective implies that we need to rethink everything, from what Nail calls *kinopolitics*—a politics based on movement and migration, which challenges current notions of borders and sovereignty, to *kinopsychology*—the psychology of migrants and refugees, which challenges our conceptual models of human behavior.[112]

Social Psychiatry's Public Works: Health Promotion, Human Rights, Destigmatization

The foci of social psychiatry's public works projects are health promotion, human rights, and combating stigmatization of psychiatric illness[11,118–120] and the traumatic consequences of disaster, war, and conflict.[121] An emerging allied field is disaster psychiatry.[122]

The Language of Social Psychiatry

Finally, a new model requires a refreshed vocabulary.[68,69] After centuries of situating human beings in a social context and more than a half century of WASP, social psychiatry is now in a position to develop its own lexicon of keywords.[2] Social psychiatry has numerous "plastic words"[38] that are polysemic and whose professional meanings are at odds with general usage. Life events, stress, and trauma are three examples. These terms have expanded to mean almost anything and researchers have had to coin more specific notions with stricter criteria to represent their impacts on health, e.g., "complex PTSD" to differentiate serious cases from the now generic "trauma".[1]

Social self: The self is best imagined as a *social self*, a *self-in-relation*. In this view, the concept of "self-esteem" is understood as *social esteem*.

Relational disorders: Many human problems have their roots in social contexts, starting with attachment and family process, which are *relational processes*. Renewed attention must be given to *relational disorders* understood through relational psychology and social psychiatry with an emphasis on relational interventions and therapies.

Psychiatric problems: The problems we treat are *psychiatric problems*, which include problems with many complex causes, from more genetically loaded ones such as bipolar disorder to brain, behavioral, emotional, cognitive, and relational disorders. All of these exist in evolving social contexts which are often determinant of the expression of symptoms. Many thoughtful psychiatrists would add ethical, moral, and spiritual domains to this enlarged vision of psychiatry.[26,68,123] "Mental illness" focuses exclusively on the mind and was first challenged by behaviorists, who eschewed any reference to mental processes and consciousness, and now many neuroscientists, for whom mind equals brain.

Patients: Our concerns are with preventing disease, attenuating illness, and improving the social health of *patients*, an ancient term that speaks to suffering, as Masserman observed.[9] Calling them "clients" and "consumers" implies a commercial exchange, not a medical or therapeutic relationship. When addressing "*n* greater than 1," especially outside the clinic, we should refer to the appropriate relational or social group, e.g., *family, community, culture,* and *society.* In policy and healthcare planning, the term *population* is appropriate but more distancing.

Psychiatry: Our field is *psychiatry,* not "mental health" which conflates the nuances among *disease, illness, health,* and *well-being.* Above all, I am arguing for an enlarged vision of medicine to include psychosocial and sociocultural perspectives in the integrated view of human health we call social psychiatry.

Health is first social: Sartorius[2(pp31–32)] affirmed that health is "a dimension of human existence which remains present in disease and in spite of impairments which diseases may cause."[124(p194)] Lewis[124,125] concurred: "Health is a single concept: it is not possible to set up essentially different criteria for physical and mental health." Instead, health may be fruitfully imagined as a series of contextual envelopes—physical, mental, relational, and social—the largest, broadest, and most encompassing of which is social.[8] Just as we can recast self-esteem as social esteem, we can understand the social self in illness and health through its social contexts. Today, understanding the social determinants of health leads us to formulate health as first social—where identity is porous and plural, expression is dialogic in face-to-face encounters, and community action is relational and social.[8]

Conclusion: From Society to Self—"A Person Is a Person Through Other Persons"

Being is always "being with," "I" is not prior to "we," and existence is essentially co-existence.
—Jean-Luc Nancy[126]

Social psychiatry upends much of the Western tradition that reasons from self to society. Employing other strands in the Western tradition and supported by much wisdom and cultural traditions in other societies,[30,127–131] Social psychiatry reasons from *society to self.* We are born with the capacity—properly nurtured—to become fully human, as we construct that notion in different places and different times. Social psychiatry focuses on attachment, on the caregiver bond, and lifelong social relations to create a sense of self and of belonging in the human community. Self emerges from social relationships and this *social self* is most properly seen as a *self-in-relation.* The "self-made man" is a myth that found its avatar in the work of Ayn Rand where the heroic individual is responsible to no one. In the solipsistic Randian universe, social relations count for nothing, only the endless affirmations of the heroic self.[132]

Because of the binary thinking built into our now globally dominant Western/Northern culture,[133–135] we cannot take the social for granted in psychiatry. In fact, bringing the two words together in the field of social psychiatry makes for an odd pair which demands explanations and a theory. Social psychiatry, thus redefined, is not only a context for understanding the self and its relations, but offers two critical things for medicine and society. It is an embracing definition of *health as first social* that enriches and expands the field of biomedicine, and a *theory of humans as social beings*, with diverse methodologies and observational studies that follow from it, as well as the practices it inspires. Out of all my training, research, teaching, and practice over more than four decades, it is social psychiatry that encompasses and unites them as an abiding concern and a guide for practice.

In the end, we must find ways of continually suturing the individual to the society and for society to respond to the individual's uniqueness. So while the social is our heuristic, our path forward, social psychiatry must try to bypass the binary opposition between the individual and the community, as William James so wisely put it:[b]

> *The community stagnates without the impulse of the individual.*
> *The impulse dies away without the sympathy of the community.*

In Africa's Ubuntu philosophy, personhood is not innate but acquired through experience, as the Zulu saying, *Umuntu ngumuntu ngabantu*, captures it—"A person is a person through other persons."[136] This is the slogan for a manifesto of social psychiatry that reaches for more than a methodology to a social theory of human being, the science of Anthropos.

Acknowledgments

This chapter first appeared as an invited review article in the inaugural issue of the WASP journal, *World Social Psychiatry*, and appears here with the kind permission of the publisher, Wolters Kluwer, and Editor-in-Chief, Debasish Basu.[137] It was accompanied by the invited commentaries of three distinguished social psychiatrists—Norman Sartorius, Eliot Sorel, and Thomas Jamieson-Craig—to which I had the pleasure to reply and expand my original manifesto.[138-141]

I am grateful for dialogues with the WASP past presidents Eliot Sorel (1996–2001) on the history and definition of social psychiatry, Guilherme Ferreira (1988–1992) on the history of the WASP, and Rachid Bennegadi (2019–2022) on information technology, as well as with Jack Drescher on transgender health and Lise Van Susteren on climate change and mental health.

Dedicated to Giambattista Vico (1668–1744), the father of *constructivist epistemology* which sees knowledge as a social construction rather than a discovery of the natural world— *Verum esse ipsum factum*, "What is true is precisely what is made."

References

1. Di Nicola V. Two trauma communities: a philosophical archaeology of cultural and clinical trauma theories. In: Capretto PT, Boynton E, eds. *Trauma and Transcendence: Limits in Theory and Prospects in Thinking.* New York: Fordham University Press; 2018:17–52.
2. Sartorius N. Challenges to psychiatry of the next century. *Soc Psychiatry.* 1994;1:30–32.

---

b.   Source: Plaque at the entrance of William James Hall at Harvard University.

3. CSDH. Closing the gap in a generation: health equity through action on the social determinants of health. Final report of the Commission on Social Determinants of Health. Geneva, Switzerland: World Health Organization; 2008.

4. Satcher D, Okafor M, Nottingham JH. The social determinants of mental health. In: Sorel E, ed. *21st Century Global Mental Health*. Burlington, MA: Jones & Bartlett Learning; 2012:73–94.

5. Patel V, Prince M. Global mental health: a new mental health field comes of age. *JAMA*. 2010 May 19;303(19):1976–1977.

6. Cohen A, Patel V, Minas H. A very brief history of global mental health. In: Patel V, Minas H, Cohen A, Prince MJ, eds. *Global Mental Health: Principles and Practice*. Oxford: Oxford University Press; 2013:3–26.

7. Carrithers M. An alternative social history of the self. In: Carrithers M, Collins S, Lukes S, eds. *The Category of the Person: Anthropology, Philosophy, History*. Cambridge, UK: Cambridge University Press; 1985:234–256.

8. Di Nicola V. Family, psychosocial, and cultural determinants of health. In: Sorel E, ed. *21st Century Global Mental Health*. Burlington, MA: Jones & Bartlett Learning; 2012:119–150.

9. Masserman JH. Social psychiatry: individual to global. In: Varma VK, Kulhara P, Masserman CM, Malhotra A, Malik SC, eds. *Social Psychiatry: A Global Perspective*. Delhi: Macmillan India; 1998:211–216.

10. Sartorius N, Gaebel W, López-Ibor JJ, Maj M, eds. *Psychiatry in Society*. Chichester, UK: John Wiley & Sons; 2002.

11. Ventriglio A, Gupta S, Bhugra D. Why do we need a social psychiatry? *Br J Psychiatry*. 2016;209:1–2.

12. Beynon J, Drew N. Information sheet: mental health and prisons. WHO/ICRC [Internet]. 2005 [cited 2019 Jun 1]. Available from: https://www.who.int/mental_health/policy/mh_in_prison.pdf.

13. Kleinman A. Global mental health: a failure of humanity. *Lancet*. 2009;374(9690):603–604.

14. Selvini Palazzoli M. *Self-starvation: From Individual to Family Therapy in the Treatment of Anorexia Nervosa*. Pomerans AJ, translator. London: Chaucer; 1974.

15. Browne V, Mendes E, Natali G. *Odd Pairs and False Friends: Dizionario di false analogie e ambigue affinita fra inglese e italiano* (English and Italian edition). Modena: Zanichelli Editore; 1987.

16. Di Nicola VF. Beyond Babel: family therapy as cultural translation. *Int J Fam Psychiatry*. 1986;7(2):179–191.

17. Di Nicola VF. *A Stranger in the Family: Culture, Families, and Therapy*. New York and London: W. W. Norton; 1997.

18. Guze S. *Why Psychiatry Is a Branch of Medicine*. Oxford: Oxford University Press; 1992.

19. Insel TR, Landis SC. Twenty-five years of progress: the view from NIMH and NINDS. *Neuron*. 2013;80(3):561–567.

20. Pinker S. *The Blank Slate: The Modern Denial of Human Nature*. New York: Penguin Press; 2003.

21. Kandel ER. *Psychiatry, Psychoanalysis, and the New Biology of Mind*. New York: American Psychiatric Publishing; 2005.

22. Kandel ER. *The Disordered Mind: What Unusual Brains Tell Us About Ourselves*. New York: Farrar, Straus and Giroux; 2018.

23. Kagan J. *An Argument for Mind*. New Haven, CT: Yale University Press; 2000.

24. Fodor J. *The Mind Doesn't Work That Way: The Scope and Limits of Computational Psychology*. Cambridge, MA: MIT Press; 2000.

25. Tallis R. *Aping Mankind: Neuromania, Darwinitis, and the Misrepresentation of Humanity*. London: Acumen/Routledge; 2014.

26. Lolas F. Psychiatry: medical specialty or specialized profession? *World Psychiatry*. 2010;9(1):34–35.

27. Kleinman A. *Social Origins of Distress and Disease: Depression, Neurasthenia, and Pain in Modern China*. New Haven, CT: Yale University Press; 1986.

28. Kleinman A. *Rethinking Psychiatry: From Cultural Category to Personal Experience*. New York: Free Press; 1991.

29. Kleinman AM. Rebalancing academic psychiatry: why it needs to happen—and soon. *Br J Psychiatry*. 2012;201(6):421–422.

30. Barreto A, Grandesso, M. Community therapy: a participatory response to psychic misery. *Int J Narr Ther Comm Work*. 2010;4:33–41.

31. Basaglia F. *Psychiatry Inside Out: Selected Writings of Franco Basaglia*. Scheper-Hughes N, Lovell AM, eds. Lovell AM, Shtob T, trans. New York: Columbia University Press; 1987.

32. Ghaemi SN. *The Rise and Fall of the Biopsychosocial Model: Reconciling Art and Science in Psychiatry*. Baltimore, MD: Johns Hopkins University Press; 2009.

33. Wittgenstein L. *Philosophical Investigations*. Anscombe, GEM, trans. London: MacMillan; 1953.

34. Di Nicola V, Stoyanov, DS. *Psychiatry in Crisis: At the Crossroads of Social Science, the Humanities, and Neuroscience*. New York: Springer International; 2021.

35. Katschnig, H. Are psychiatrists an endangered species? Observations on internal and external challenges to the profession. *World Psychiatry*. 2010;9(1):21–28.

36. Leighton AH. *An Introduction to Social Psychiatry*. Springfield, IL: Charles C. Thomas; 1960.

37. Cassin B, ed. *Dictionary of Untranslatables: A Philosophical Lexicon*. Randall S, Hubert C, Mehlman J, Stein S, Syrotinski M, trans., Apter E, Lezra J, Wood M, trans. eds. Princeton, NJ: Princeton University Press; 2014.

38. Poerksen U. *Plastic Words: The Tyranny of a Modular Language*. Mason J, Cayley D, trans. University Park: Pennsylvania University Press; 1995.

39. Williams R. *Keywords: A Vocabulary of Culture and Society*. London: Flamingo/Fontana Paperbacks; 1984.

40. Arieti S. Vico and modern psychiatry. *Soc Res*. 1976;43:739–752.

41. Lollini M. On becoming human: the "Verum Factum" principle and Giambattista Vico's humanism [Internet]. *MLN*. 2012;127(1):S21–S31 [cited 2019 Jun 1]. Available from: http://www.jstor.org/stable/41415841.

42. Di Nicola VF. De l'enfant sauvage à l'enfant fou: a prospectus for transcultural child psychiatry. In: Grizenko N, L Sayegh L, P Migneault P, eds. *Transcultural Issues in Child Psychiatry*. Montréal, QC: Éditions Douglas; 1992:7–53.

43. Makari G. *Soul Machine: The Invention of the Modern Mind*. New York: W. W. Norton; 2015.

44. Chapman DP, Dube SR, Anda RF. Adverse childhood events as risk factors for negative mental health outcomes. *Psychiat Annals*. 2007;37(5):359–364.

45. Felitti VJ, Anda RF. The relationship of adverse childhood experiences to adult medical disease, psychiatric disorders and sexual behavior: implications for health care. In: Lanius RA, Vermetten E, Pain C, eds. *The Impact of Early Trauma on Health and Disease: The Hidden Epidemic*. Cambridge, UK: Cambridge University Press; 2010:77–87.

46. Di Nicola V. Family, psychosocial, and cultural determinants of health. In: Sorel E, ed. *21st Century Global Mental Health*. Burlington, MA: Jones & Bartlett Learning, 2012:119–150.

47. Di Nicola V. The Global South: an emergent epistemology for social psychiatry. *World Soc Psychiatry*. 2020;2:20–26.

48. Prince M, Patel V, Saxena S, et al. No health without mental health. *Lancet*. 2007;370(9590):859–877.

49. Sorel E, ed. *21st Century Global Mental Health*. Burlington, MA: Jones & Bartlett Learning; 2012.

50. Clayton S, Manning CM, Hodge C. *Beyond Storms and Droughts: The Psychological Impacts of Climate Change*. Washington, DC: American Psychological Association and ecoAmerica; 2014.

51. Watts N, Adger WN, Agnolucci P, et al. Health and climate change: policy responses to protect public health. *Lancet*. 2015;386:1861–1914.

52. Lanier J. *You Are Not a Gadget: A Manifesto*. New York: Vintage Books; 2010.

53. Burt C. The concept of consciousness. *Br J Psychol*. 1962;53(3):229–242.

54. Eisenberg L. Mindlessness and brainlessness. *Br J Psychiatry*. 1986;148(5):497–508.

55. Carvalko J. *The Techno-Human Shell—A Jump in the Evolutionary Gap*. Mechanicsburg, PA: Sunbury Press; 2012.

56. Bauman Z. *Liquid Modernity*. Cambridge, UK: Polity Press; 2000.

57. Mau B. *The Institute Without Boundaries: Massive Change*. London: Phaedon Press; 2004.

58. Kovess V. The homeless mentally ill. In: Sartorius N, Gaebel W, López-Ibor, JJ, Maj M, eds. *Psychiatry in Society*. Chichester, UK: John Wiley & Sons; 2002:221–240.

59. Nail T. *The Figure of the Migrant*. Stanford, CA: Stanford University Press; 2015.

60. Nail T. *Theory of the Border*. Oxford: Oxford University Press; 2016.

61. Ciompi L. The philosophy of social psychiatry. *J World Assoc Soc Psychiatry*. 1995 Jan–Feb;2:22–27.

62. Sartorius N. More than one scenario exists for the future of psychiatry. *Lancet Psychiatry*. 2017 Oct;4(10):738–739.

63. Trimarchi MS. Foreword. In: Price RK, Shea BM, Mookherjee HN, eds. *Social Psychiatry Across Cultures: Studies from North America, Asia, Europe, and Africa*. New York: Plenum Press; 1995:vii–viii.

64. Brockman J, ed. *This Idea Must Die: Scientific Theories That Are Blocking Progress*. New York: HarperPerennial; 2015.

65. Leys R. *Trauma: A Genealogy*. Chicago: University of Chicago Press; 2000.

66. Tooby J, Cosmides L. Conceptual foundations of evolutionary psychology. In: Buss DM, ed. *The Handbook of Evolutionary Psychology*. Hoboken, NJ: Wiley; 2005:5–67.

67. Eisenberg L. The impact of sociocultural and economic changes on psychiatry. In: Sartorius N, Gaebel W, López-Ibor JJ, Maj M, eds. *Psychiatry in Society*. Chichester, UK: John Wiley & Sons; 2002:1–14.

68. Di Nicola V. *Letters to a Young Therapist: Relational Practices for the Coming Community*. New York and Dresden: Atropos Press; 2011.

69. Di Nicola VF. The postmodern language of therapy: at the nexus of culture and therapy. *J Syst Ther*. 1993;12(1):49–62.

70. Kahneman D. *Thinking, Fast and Slow*. New York: Farrar, Straus and Giroux; 2011.

71. Di Nicola V. Badiou, the event, and psychiatry, Part 1: trauma and event. Online blog of the American Philosophical Association [Internet]. 2017 Nov 23 [cited 2019 Jun 1]. Available from: https://blog.apaonline.org/2017/11/23/badiou-the-event-and-psychiatry-part-1-trauma-and-event/.

72. Di Nicola V. Take your time: the seven pillars of a slow thought manifesto. *Aeon Magazine* [Internet]. 2018 Feb 27 [cited 2019 Jun 1]. Available from: https://aeon.co/essays/take-your-time-the-seven-pillars-of-a-slow-thought-manifesto.

73. Berlin I. The hedgehog and the fox. In: Berlin I, *Russian Thinkers*. Hardy H, Kelly A, eds., Kelly A, introduction. New York: Penguin; 1979:22–81.

74. James W. *Pragmatism*. New York: Dover; 1995.

75. Geertz C. Thick description: toward an interpretive theory of culture. In: Geertz C, *The Interpretation of Cultures: Selected Essays*. New York: Basic Books; 1973:3–30.

76. Bakhtin MM. *The Dialogic Imagination: Four Essays by M.M. Bakhtin*. Holquist M, ed., Emerson C, Holquist M, trans. Austin: University of Texas Press; 1981.

77. Salgado J, Gonçalves M. The dialogical self: social, personal, and (un)conscious. In: Vaalsiner J, Rosa A, eds. *The Cambridge Handbook of Sociocultural Psychology*. Cambridge, UK: Cambridge University Press; 2007:608–621.

78. Prince R. Mental health workers should be trained at home: some implications of transcultural psychiatric research. *African J Psychiatry*. 1972;2:277–282.

79. Murphy, HBM. *Comparative Psychiatry: The International and Intercultural Distribution of Mental Illness*. Berlin: Springer-Verlag; 1982.

80. Kleinman AM. Depression, somatization and the "new cross-cultural psychiatry." *Soc Sci Med*. 1977 Jan;11(1):3–10.

81. Marmot M. The health gap: the challenge of an unequal world. *Lancet*. 2015;386(10011):2442–2444.

82. Cacioppo JT. Social neuroscience: understanding the pieces fosters understanding the whole and vice versa. *Am Psychol*. 2002;57(11):819–831.

83. Cacioppo JT, Berntson G. *Social Neuroscience: Key Readings*. New York: Psychology Press; 2005.

84. Gallese V. Mirror neurons and the social nature of language: the neural exploitation hypothesis. *Soc Neurosci*. 2008;3:317–333.

85. Gallese V. Bodily selves in relation: embodied simulation as second-person perspective on intersubjectivity. *Phil Trans Roy Soc*. 2014;B.369(1644). https://doi.org/10.1098/rstb.2013.0177

86. Rakoff V. The necessity for multiple models in family therapy. *J Fam Ther*. 1984;6:199–210.

87. Korzybski A. *Science and Sanity: An Introduction to Non-Aristotelian Systems and General Semantics*. Fort Worth, TX: International Non-Aristotelian Library; 1933.

88. Leff J, Vaughan C. *Expressed Emotion in Families: Its Significance for Mental Illness*. New York: Guilford Press; 1985.

89. Di Nicola VF. Expressed emotion and schizophrenia in North India: an essay-review. *Transcult Psychiatr Res Rev.* 1988;25(3):205–217.

90. Brown GW, Harris T. *Social Origins of Depression: A Study of Psychiatric Disorder in Women.* New York: Free Press; 1978.

91. Schwab JJ. Social psychiatry: a reappraisal. *J World Assoc Soc Psychiatry.* 1995 Jan–Feb;2:16–21.

92. Mukherjee S. *The Laws of Medicine: Field Notes from an Uncertain Science.* New York: TED Books/Simon & Schuster; 2015.

93. Di Nicola VF. Overview: anorexia multiforme: self-starvation in historical and cultural context. I: Self-starvation as a historical chameleon. *Transcult Psychiatr Res Rev.* 1990;27(3):165–196.

94. Di Nicola VF. Overview: anorexia multiforme: self-starvation in historical and cultural context. II: Anorexia nervosa as a culture-reactive syndrome. *Transcult Psychiatr Res Rev.* 1990;27(4):245–286.

95. Di Nicola V. Antonella—"A stranger in the family": a case study of eating disorders across cultures. In: Stoyanov DS, Van Staden CW, Stanghellini G, Wong GM, Fulford KWM, eds. *International Perspectives in Values-Based Mental Health Practice: Case Studies and Commentaries.* New York: Springer International; 2021:27–35.

96. Bhugra D, Till A. Public mental health is about social psychiatry. *Int J Soc Psychiatry.* 2013 Mar;59(2):105–106.

97. Restak RM. *Mind: The Big Questions Series.* London: Quercus Editions; 2012.

98. Ryle G. *The Concept of Mind.* New York: Viking Penguin; 1966.

99. Fulford KWM. Editorial: values-based practice: a new partner to evidence-based practice and a first for psychiatry? *Mens Sana Monographs.* 2008;6(1):10–21.

100. Riesman D, Glazer N, Denney R. *The Lonely Crowd: A Study of the Changing American Character.* New Haven, CT: Yale University Press; 1963.

101. Gergen KJ. *The Saturated Self: Dilemmas of Identity in Contemporary Life.* New York: Basic Books; 1991.

102. Benjamin W, Lacis A. Naples. In: Benjamin W. *Reflections: Essays, Aphorisms, Autobiographical Writings.* Jephcott E, ed., Demetz P, introduction, Wieseltier L, preface. New York: Schocken Books; 2007:163–173.

103. Turner V. *The Ritual Process: Structure and Anti-Structure.* Ithaca, NY: Cornell University Press; 1969.

104. Csíkszentmihályi M. *Flow: The Psychology of Optimal Experience.* New York: Harper & Row; 1990.

105. Levinas E. *Entre Nous: Thinking-of-the-Other.* Smith MB, Harshav, B, trans. New York: Columbia University Press; 1998.

106. Matusov E, Smith M, Albuquerque Candela M, et al. "Culture has no internal territory": culture as dialogue. In: Valsiner J, Rosa A, eds. *The Cambridge Handbook of Sociocultural Psychology.* Cambridge, UK: Cambridge University Press; 2007:460–483.

107. Mollica RF. *Healing Invisible Wounds: Paths to Hope and Recovery in a Violent World.* Orlando, FL: Harcourt; 2006.

108. Calvino I. *Six Memos for the Next Millenium: The Charles Eliot Norton Lectures 1985–86.* Cambridge, MA: Harvard University Press; 1988.

109. Virilio P. *Speed and Politics.* Polizzotti M, trans. Los Angeles: Semio-text(e); 2016.

110. Sennett R, Cobb J. *The Hidden Injuries of Class.* Reissued. New York: W. W. Norton; 1993.

111. Rutz W. Social psychiatry and public mental health: present situation and future objectives. Time for rethinking and renaissance? *Acta Psychiatr Scand Suppl.* 2006;429:95–100.

112. Nail T. *Theory of the Border.* Oxford University Press; 2016.

113. Drescher J. Queer diagnoses: parallels and contrasts in the history of homosexuality, gender variance, and the Diagnostic and Statistical Manual (DSM). *Arch Sexual Behav.* 2010;39:427–460.

114. Leibowitz S, de Vries A. Gender dysphoria in adolescence. *Int Rev Psychiatry.* 2016;28(1):21–35.

115. Reed GM, Drescher J, Krueger RB, et al. Revising the ICD-10 Mental and Behavioural Disorders classification of sexuality and gender identity based on current scientific evidence, best clinical practices, and human rights considerations. *World Psychiatry.* 2016;15:205–221.

116. Santos, B de Sousa. *Epistemologies of the South: Justice Against Epistemicide.* New York: Routledge; 2016.

117. Grinberg L, Grinberg R. *Psychoanalytic Perspectives on Migration and Exile.* Kernberg O, foreword, Festinger N, trans. New Haven, CT: Yale University Press; 1989.

118. Arboleda-Flórez J, Sartorius N, eds. *Understanding the Stigma of Mental Illness: Theory and Interventions*. Chichester, UK: John Wiley & Sons; 2008.

119. Arboleda-Flórez J, Stuart, H. Human rights, stigma, mental health policy, and the media. In: Sorel E, ed. *21st Century Global Mental Health*. Burlington, MA: Jones & Bartlett Learning; 2012:329–347.

120. Cuenca O. Mass media and psychiatry. In: Sartorius N, Gaebel W, López-Ibor J, Maj M, eds. *Psychiatry in Society*. Chichester, UK: John Wiley & Sons; 2002:263–279.

121. Dyer AR, Bhadra S. Global disasters, war, conflict, and complex emergencies: caring for special populations. In: Sorel E, ed. *21st Century Global Mental Health*. Burlington, MA: Jones & Bartlett Learning; 2012:171–208.

122. Stoddard FJ Jr, Pandya A, Katz CL. *Disaster Psychiatry: Readiness, Evaluation, and Treatment*. Washington, DC: American Psychiatric Association; 2011.

123. Okasha A. The new ethical context of psychiatry. In: Sartorius N, Gaebel W, López-Ibor JJ, Maj M, eds. *Psychiatry in Society*. Chichester, UK: John Wiley & Sons; 2002:101–130.

124. Lewis A. Health as a social concept. In: *The State of Psychiatry: Essays and Addresses*. New York: Science House; 1967:179–194.

125. Lewis A. Social psychiatry. In: *Inquiries in Psychiatry: Clinical and Social Investigations*. New York: Science House; 1967:251–269.

126. Nancy J-L. *Being Singular Plural*. Richardson RD, O'Bourne AE, eds. Stanford, CA: Stanford University Press; 2000.

127. Kallivayalil RA. Lessons in social psychiatry at unexpected times! *Indian J Soc Psychiatry*. 2018;34:263–264.

128. Price RK, Shea BM, Mookherjee HN, eds. *Social Psychiatry Across Cultures: Studies from North America, Asia, Europe, and Africa*. New York: Plenum Press; 1995.

129. Sorel E, ed. *Family, Culture, and Psychobiology*. Brooklyn, NY: Legas; 1990.

130. Sorel E, ed. *Social Psychiatry in the 20th Century: Selected Proceedings of the XII World Congress of Social Psychiatry*. Brooklyn, NY: Legas; 1993.

131. Varma VK, Kulhara P, Masserman CM, Malhotra A, Malik SC, eds. *Social Psychiatry: A Global Perspective*. Delhi: Macmillan India; 1998.

132. Cleary SC. Philosophy shrugged: ignoring Ayn Rand won't make her go away. *Aeon Magazine* [Internet]. 2018 June 22 [cited 2019 Jun 1]. Available from: https://aeon.co/ideas/philosophy-shrugged-ignoring-ayn-rand-wont-make-her-go-away.

133. Watters E. *Crazy like Us: The Globalization of the American Psyche*. New York: Free Press; 2010.

134. Mills C. *Decolonizing Global Mental Health: The Psychiatrization of the Majority World*. London: Routledge; 2013.

135. Mills C. From "invisible problem" to global priority: the inclusion of mental health in the sustainable development goals. *Dev Change*. 2018;49(3):843–866.

136. Birhane A. Descartes was wrong: "a person is a person through other persons." *Aeon Magazine* [Internet]. 2017 Apr 7 [cited 2019 May 1]. Available from: https://aeon.co/ideas/descartes-was-wrong-a-person-is-a-person-through-other-persons?utm_source=Aeon+Newsletter&utm_campaign=bcaa6b60e4-EMAIL_CAMPAIGN_2019_03_14_05_59&utm_medium=email&utm_term=0_411a82e59d-bcaa6b60e4-70338641.

137. Di Nicola V. "A person is a person through other persons": A social psychiatry manifesto for the 21st century. *World Soc Psychiatry*. 2019;1:8–21.

138. Sartorius N. Medicine is medicine through its disciplines. *World Soc Psychiatry*. 2019;1:22.

139. Sorel E. The social brain: Wired to connect and belong. *World Soc Psychiatry*. 2019;1:23–24.

140. Craig TK. The importance of the social in psychiatry. *World Soc Psychiatry*. 2019;1:25–26.

141. Di Nicola V. "There is no such thing as society": The pervasive myth of the atomistic individual in psychology and psychiatry. *World Soc Psychiatry*. 2021;3:60–64.

6

The Importance of Medical Professionalism in Social Psychiatry

Eugenio M. Rothe

Introduction

In the late 19th century, Sigmund Freud began to develop the techniques of psychoanalysis, which served as a foundation to all the other psychotherapeutic modalities. Psychoanalytic psychotherapy and all its offshoots were grounded in an approach to the patient that focused almost exclusively on the individual, and the root of this sprung from the fact that most of Freud's patients were members of the upper classes of Viennese society, had significant ego strengths, and their problems were mostly intra-psychic.[1] In contrast, many of the patients who are seen by psychiatrists and residents today also suffer from problems that are extra-psychic, such as poverty, social and political oppression, and abuses of power in relationships that threaten to overwhelm their coping capacities. This called for a new theoretical model that would allow for a better understanding and more effective treatment of these patients. So in the second part of the 20th century, psychiatrists began to focus on the environment and the social surroundings and how these impacted the mental health of the individual, which led to the emergence of the Community Psychiatry Movement; some of these psychiatrists began to define themselves as *social psychiatrists*. The writings of Harry Stack Sullivan, Karen Horney, Erik Erikson, Lev Vigotsky, and later Gerald Kaplan, Robert Coles, and Arthur Kleinman, followed by the empirical studies of Albert Bandura, August Hollingshead, Lloyd Rogler, Frederick Redlich, E. J. Anthony, Bertram Cohler, and others, brought even more into focus the interconnectedness of the individual's mental health with the human and material environment. The anthropologist Margaret Mead, her husband Gregory Bateson, and other psychiatrists such as Salvador Minuchin and Murray Bowen who pioneered the Family Therapy Movement, also brought attention to the importance of the individual within the family context.[2] In addition, the sociologist Oscar Lewis published the controversial document titled *The Culture of Poverty*[3] in which he argued that in order to adapt to their environment, people who live in poverty for long periods of time develop a series of coping mechanisms that become engrained and paralyzing and that affect the individual, the family, the slum community, and the community in relation to society. All of these writings led Jules Masserman[4] and others to contend that *all psychiatry is social*. So understanding and treating patients from this biopsychosocial perspective calls for physicians with high levels of empathy and professionalism. *Medical professionalism* includes having a scientific and technical knowledge base, skills and altruism, with an emphasis on the public good, always upholding the primacy of patient welfare, and advocating for justice in healthcare.[5]

The Crisis of American Medical Professionalism

Since the 1960s American medicine has become dominated by for-profit third-party insurance providers that often deny needed medical services to the patient and limit the earnings of the doctor with the purpose of maximizing their financial profits. Only the very poor, the elderly, the military, and prisoners in the United States are eligible for government subsidized universal healthcare. In addition, the legal profession has accosted those practicing medicine with litigious malpractice lawsuits where the bounty collected by the lawyers and victims often reaches millions of dollars. This has caused physicians to sometimes view the patient as a potential aggressor and forces physicians to purchase expensive malpractice insurance policies and to practice *defensive medicine*. As a result of all of this, the public perception of prestige, authority, and respect that had been previously accorded to physicians has suffered a decline. Some argue that this current culture of medicine in the United States is hostile to altruism, compassion, integrity, fidelity, self-effacement, and other qualities traditionally associated with being a physician; also, that hospital culture and the narratives that support it often embody a set of professional qualities that are diametrically opposed to virtues that are explicitly taught as constituting a good doctor.[6,7,8] Studies in the United States have demonstrated that the erosion of altruism and ethical values in medicine begins in medical school with a traumatic de-idealization and loss of the heroic-idealized image of the doctor,[9] and that for many students, medical school is a "de-humanizing experience."[10] Collier[11] found that 61% of students reported becoming "more cynical" during medical school, and Hojat et al.[12] argued that some of the reasons that account for this include: (1) lack of positive role models, (2) vulgar language by attending physicians, (3) extreme fatigue and sleep deprivation, (4) harassment and belittlement by faculty, (5) and students being encouraged to maintain emotional distance. Other studies found that students who demonstrated poor professionalism in medical school were 9 times more likely to be cited by their State Medical Boards for disciplining actions, in particular for negligence and substance abuse[13,14] and that as a physician matures, it becomes more difficult to teach values of professionalism, which suggests that medical professionalism should be taught early in the medical school curriculum.[15]

The Healing Effect of the Doctor-Patient Relationship

The main goal of being a physician is to "uphold the primacy of the patient" (altruism) and that a good-quality interaction and maintenance of the patient-doctor relationship is the core mission of the medical profession;[16] thus the new concept of medical professionalism recognizes that all healthcare occurs reciprocally, that emotions and affect are important parts of all human interactions, and that it is important to recognize the personhood and humanity of all the participants. The curative effect of the doctor-patient relationship was evaluated in a meta-analysis of 25 randomized controlled trials. In this study the doctor-patient relationship showed an independent (statistically significant) positive effect over outcome that improved patient treatment adherence, patient satisfaction, decreased the risk of malpractice lawsuits, enhanced physician and staff morale, and generated an enhancement of the prestige of the profession. These authors also highlight the fact that the placebo effect may be as high as 30%, which also plays a part in a positive doctor-patient relationship.[17] The doctor-patient relationship is enhanced when the patient perceives that the doctor has empathy and understands the plight of the patient. So in the United States[18] and elsewhere,[19] there is an increasing recognition that empathy is one of the most desirable qualities in a physician, and that professionalism and etiquette enhance the quality of the patient-doctor interaction.[20] Professionalism is now considered to be one of the most important aspects of medical training and has become one of the core competencies of the American Association of Medical Colleges[21] necessary for graduation from American medical schools; professionalism in medical education is supported by most medical-specialty associations.[22]

Professionalism, Empathy, and the Process of Self-reflection

Empathy, *the capacity to understand what another being is going through*, is an important developmental leap in human evolution and the foundation of morality. Empathy is one of the most desirable qualities in a physician.[23,24] There is an element of empathy that is innate, but empathy can also be learned. *Vicarious empathy* refers to the person's immediate-natural response to an emotionally laden event and is considered to be an automatic response, like a reflex reaction. The intensity of vicarious empathy can vary in each person according to the individual's temperament, culture, and life experience. In contrast, *cognitive empathy* involves qualities of the former, but it differs in that in requires cognitive processing; in other words, it involves self-reflection. This second type of empathy is a cognitive skill that can be taught and reliably assessed.[12] In order for cognitive empathy to occur, the particular experience needs to be understood, processed, and talked about. The process of self-reflection involves active listening and creating a narrative of the experience. The patient-physician interaction will affect both parties in all spheres: physical, emotional-psychological, and spiritual, but detachment by the doctor decreases self-reflection and cognitive empathy.

The exercise of self-reflection begins by asking three fundamental questions: (1) *What are we reflecting about?* (2) *How?* (What style or method are we using?); and (3) *Why are we reflecting?* This process involves returning to the experience, evaluating the patient's and the doctor's feelings and the feelings that emerge from the interaction between both, creating a narrative of the experience, and re-evaluating the experience in its entire dimension in order to improve and grow from it.[25] The exercise of self-reflection that is involved in the doctor-patient relationship is very similar to that of psychodynamic psychotherapy, since it involves analyzing emotion, affect, transference and countertransference, and the interpersonal dimension of the experience,[26] and creating a narrative, which will allow the doctor to attain an understanding and a degree of mastery over the experience.[27] So applying the necessary medical-technical skills in order to help the patient is essential, but the process will be incomplete if the physician does not involve in self-reflection.

Defining Professionalism across Cultures

Despite over 20 years of intense scrutiny of the medical literature, there is still a lack of consensus as to what defines professionalism.[28] Remen and Rabow[29] prefer the term *professional formation*. Swick[30] lists nine qualities that he considers essential for medical professionalism: (1) physicians must subordinate their own interests to the interests of others; (2) physicians must adhere to high ethical and moral standards; (3) physicians must respond to societal needs, and their behaviors must reflect a social contract with the communities served; (4) physicians must exemplify core humanistic values, including honesty and integrity, caring and compassion, altruism and empathy, respect for others, and trustworthiness; (5) physicians must exercise accountability for themselves and for their colleagues; (6) physicians must demonstrate a continuing commitment to excellence; (7) physicians must exhibit a commitment to scholarship and to advancing their field; (8) physicians must be prepared to deal with high levels of complexity and uncertainty; and (9) physicians must reflect carefully upon their actions and decisions. Hafferty[31(p21)] adds that medical professionalism is "something that resides in the interface between the possession of specialized knowledge and a commitment to use that knowledge for the betterment of others," and other authors argue that professionalism should be *narrative based* as opposed to *rule based*, since rules vary with different patient settings and circumstances.[32,33] Medical professionalism is context-specific, but most literature on professionalism stems from Western countries. There is no single framework of professionalism that can be globally acknowledged. A culture-oriented concept of professionalism is necessary to understand what the profession is dedicated to, and to incorporate the concept into the medical students' and physicians' professional identity formation. The concepts of professionalism that were articulated by the American Board of Medical Specialties[34] do not always reflect the traditions of cultures other than those in the West. These differences with other cultures are rooted in societal core values, community needs, and the particular reality of the culture in question. In an attempt to better understand this gap, Chandralitake et al.[19] interviewed a total of 584 medical practitioners, representing the United Kingdom, Europe, North America, and Asia, about which attributes they considered essential to medical professionalism. The participants listed a total of 46 different attributes which varied in importance according to the physicians' culture of origin, underscoring the importance of cultural differences in this aspect of the practice of medicine. In addition, Al-Rumayyana et al.[35] studied the similarities and differences between the Western concepts of medical professionalism with those of other cultures. These authors concluded that in most cases the basic concepts of ethics, altruism, and benevolence were held in common by all cultures, but they noted certain cultural differences. In the *Chinese Model*, which is based on the Confucian tradition, there is an emphasis on a dignified persona and a collective community approach. The Chinese integrated four additional qualities of professionalism: *teamwork, health promotion, self-management*, and *economics*. The *Arabian Model* represents the blend of culture, traditions, beliefs, and behaviors that are being practiced by nations in the Middle East where Arabic is the official language and Islam is the religion of the majority. In addition to the traditional values of medical professionalism, in the Arabian context *Allah* (God) plays an important role in the daily life and rituals of the people. Belief in Allah includes attributes of *self-accountability* and *self-motivation* and the reward for upholding these professional values is received directly from Allah, not from people or from the patient. The *Japanese Model* also overlaps with the traditional Western attributes of professionalism, but its values derive from the concept of *bushido*, a value system that means "the way of the warrior," and includes *rectitude, honesty, benevolence, politeness, courage, honor*, and *loyalty*. Benevolence, the third virtue, combines the concepts of love, sympathy, and pity and is valued as the highest attribute of the human soul. The Japanese concept of medical professionalism adds the concept of *loyalty* to the interests and needs of the group, such as hospital staff and family, and it places the needs of the group above individual interests and needs. Understanding cultural differences seems particularly relevant given the rapid demographic changes that are taking place in the United States, which is rapidly becoming a predominantly multicultural society.[2]

The Need for Medical Professionalism in Social Psychiatry

Medical professionalism proposes that medicine is the reciprocal relationship between the doctor and patient and recognizes of the feelings and the humanity of the participants. In their award-winning course for teaching medical professionalism,[36] Rothe and Bonnin[22] outline six basic concepts that can be taught and learned in order to educate medical students, residents, and physicians so that they can develop and acquire the qualities needed for medical professionalism. These concepts overlap with the needs and goals of social psychiatry and include the following:

The Dyadic Quality of the Doctor-Patient Relationship

The medical encounter, like all human interactions, is unavoidably laden with emotions, and rather than viewing them as something to be overcome, the emotional responses of the physician and of the patient should be analyzed and understood. Even early in their careers, medical students have strong emotional responses to their patients. The British pediatrician-psychoanalyst Donald W. Winnicott[37] was one of the first to recognize and legitimize the intersubjective quality of the doctor-patient relationship and that this relationship can be analyzed for information about the patient and about the physician, and that a better understanding of these psychodynamic factors can help to cement the *therapeutic alliance*, whereby patient and doctor establish a rational agreement or contract to support the treatment goals.[38] In turn, social psychiatry postulates that the circuits of the mind extend beyond the brain to include our interactions with others, which take place through mental processes that are intrinsically social and that take place through bodily and verbal communication.[39] This eco-social view of mind, brain, and culture takes into account that the doctor should consider persons in the social role of patients as partners in the process of healing and curing, while respecting privacy and confidentiality.[40]

Self-awareness

Bringing to consciousness negative and positive feelings in the doctor-patient relationship is not always an easy task, and resistance usually occurs because we want to avoid, rather than confront, an aspect of ourselves. So, self-awareness is the key to utilizing these feelings and reactions to improve the patient-physician relationship, because bringing these emotional responses to consciousness allows us to harvest the wealth of clinical information that they contain.[41] The attempts to address this issue by developing the qualities of medical professionalism are evidenced by the call to action that has taken place in medical schools in the United States[42] and abroad.[19,35] In turn, the efforts of social psychiatry have moved in the direction of developing an integrative theory and practical tools to better understand, assess, and intervene in the social-ecological cultural systems that constitute our essence as biopsychosocial entities. Practicing medicine includes developing narrative capacities, skills, practices, and a fund of knowledge that contribute to our understanding of the causes, course, and outcomes of psychopathology, as well as the processes of coping, resilience, healing, and recovery. Culturally responsive medical care seeks to integrate the knowledge of the individual's life-world, family, and community as the sources from which the person will cope, adapt, heal, and recover,[39] and a realization that knowledge about oneself and about others is obtained by different means and approaches, and that human groups differ in their realization of self-awareness.[40]

Understanding Transference and Countertransference

Transference is the phenomenon whereby we unconsciously transfer feelings and attitudes from a person or situation in the past onto a person or situation in the present; *countertransference* in this case refers to the reciprocal process in the doctor toward the patient. Heimann[43] was one of the first to point out that analysis of transference and countertransference could provide diagnostic information about both of the participants and that in spite of the importance of these insights, the natural tendency had been to suppress, rather than to analyze the significance of these feelings. In turn, social psychiatry postulates that, like the understanding of transference and countertransference, our brains are designed to acquire culture in order to be able to navigate a social world, find support from others, and cooperate to construct our own eco-social niche; social psychiatry seeks to analyze and understand these variables. The circuits of the mind extend out into the world, through our tools, discourse, practices, and institutions that enable cooperation. They allow us to construct identities, to form groups and communities to which to belong, and to position ourselves within and against social constraints.[39] Like transference and countertransference, social psychiatry also highlights the need to understand that societies and individuals within those societies may have different beliefs, customs, and traditions through which their particular society conceptualizes well-being, illness, sickness, and disease.[40]

Understanding the Importance of Narratives

The effective practice of medicine requires *narrative competence*, that is, the ability to acknowledge, absorb, interpret, and act on the stories and plights of others. As the physician listens to the patient, he or she follows the narrative thread of the story, imagines the biological, familial, cultural, and existential situation of the teller, recognizes the multiple and often contradictory meanings of the words used and the events described, and in some way enters into and is moved by the narrative world of the patient as the patient asks: "What is wrong with me?" or "Why did this happen to me?" and "What will become of me?" Asking these questions provides a rich, deep, and resonant comprehension of a person's situation as it unfolds in time. The complexity of the story is told not only in words, but also in gestures and silences, and is burdened not only with the objective information about the illness, but also with the fears, hopes, and implications associated with it.[27] In turn, social psychiatry also postulates that the human brain is a story machine, weaving webs of meaning through language, imagery, and performance, and that these memories, identities, and actions are organized in terms of narratives that locate us in space and time.[39] Both medical professionalism and social psychiatry agree in that culturally responsive care seeks to integrate the knowledge of the individual's life-world, their family, and community, and that narrative capacities, skills, practices, and specific content all contribute to a better understanding of the causes, course, and outcomes of psychopathology, as well as to processes of coping, resilience, healing, and recovery.

Understanding Conflict Resolution

Conflict has also long been identified as a critical component of professional development, and is found as a dominant element in some measures of medical professionalism. Medical students, residents, and practicing physicians are often placed in conflictual situations where their ethical and professional values are faced off against loyalty toward the group, or against the unspoken rules of the institutional culture, and going against these rules threatens their place and belonging in the group, or may result in retaliation by members of the group. Many of the ethical and professional conflicts of medical students and physicians are *context-dependent* and cannot be accurately addressed by applying universal, unbending rules. So for doctors and medical students, the capacity for self-reflection, understanding of transference and countertransference issues, and narrative knowledge can prove to be invaluable tools when facing complex ethical and professional dilemmas.[22] In turn, social psychiatry is grounded on the commitment to help victims of the devastating effects of structural violence, social inequality, discrimination, and racism, recognizing that these factors play a key role as determinants of health;[39] in addition to a strong advocacy attitude toward inequalities, inequities, and suffering, irrespective of geographical determinants, race, religion, or ethnicity.[40]

Understanding Cultural Issues

Medical professionalism is context-specific, but most literature on professionalism stems from Western countries. There is no single framework of professionalism that can be globally acknowledged. A culture-oriented concept of professionalism is necessary to understand what the profession is dedicated to and to incorporate the concept into the physicians' professional identity formation. These differences with other cultures are rooted in societal core values, community needs, and the particular reality of the culture in question. Empathy, humility, curiosity, and respect are necessary on the part of the physician in any attempt at understanding these differences.[22] In turn, social psychiatry is grounded in the recognition that we are fundamentally cultural beings and that our brains are designed to acquire culture to navigate a social world, because mental processes are intrinsically social and provide us with the tools, discourse, practices, and institutions that enable cooperation, and that this opens the door to a creative engagement with human diversity in all its forms.[39]

Conclusions and Future Directions

The principles of medical professionalism and of social psychiatry aim at attaining the necessary scientific and technical knowledge base, skills, and altruism for a practice of the medical profession that emphasizes the public good, always upholding the primacy of patient welfare and advocating for justice in healthcare. These principles are the best suited to provide the most compassionate and effective healthcare to patients in changing world communities which are rapidly becoming multicultural and globalized.[2]

References

1. Kanzer M, Glenn J. *Freud and His Patients*. New York/London, NJ: Jason Aronson; 1993:3–23.
2. Rothe EM, Pumariega AJ. *Immigration, Cultural Identity and Mental Health: Psychosocial Implications of the Reshaping of America*. Oxford: Oxford University Press; 2020.
3. Lewis O. Culture of poverty. In: Moynihan DP, ed. *On Understanding Poverty: Perspectives from the Social Sciences*. New York: Basic Books; 1969: 187–220.
4. Masserman JH. Social psychiatry: I]individual to global. In: Varma VK, Kulhara P, Masserman CM, Malhotra A, Malik SC, eds. *Social Psychiatry: A Global Perspective*. Delhi: Macmillan India; 1998:211–216.
5. Bhugra D., Till A. Public mental health is about social psychiatry. *Int J Soc Psychiatry*. 2013;59(2):105–106.
6. Cruess RL, Cruess SR. Expectations and obligations: professionalism and medicine's social contract with society. *Perspect Biol Med*. 2008;51:579–598.
7. Cruess SR, Cruess RL, Steinert Y. Linking the teaching of professionalism to the social contract: a call for cultural humility. *Med Teach*. 2010;31:357–360.
8. Starr P. *The Social Transformation of American Medicine*. New York: Basic Books; 1982.

9. Kay J. (1990). Traumatic de-idealization and future of medicine. *JAMA*. 1990;263:572–573.

10. Edwards MT, Zimet CN. (1976). Problems and concerns among medical students. *J Med Educ*. 1976;51:619–625.

11. Collier R. (2012). Professionalism: can it be taught? *Can Med Assoc J*. 2012;184(11):1234–1236.

12. Hojat M, Vergare MJ, Maxwell K, et al. The devil is in the third year: A longitudinal study of erosion in empathy in medical school. *Acad Med*. 2009;84:1182–1191. http://www.ama-assn.org/delivering-care/ama-code-medical-ethics.

13. Papadakis MA, Hodgson CS, Teherani A, Kohatsu ND. (2004). Unprofessional behavior in medical school is associated with subsequent disciplinary action by a state medical board. *Acad Med*. 2004;79:244–249.

14. Papadakis MA, Banach MA, Knettler TR, et al. (2005). Disciplinary action by medical boards and prior behavior in medical school. *N Engl J Med*. 2005;353:25:2673–2682.

15. Goldie J, Dowie A, Cotton P, Morrison J. Teaching professionalism in the early years of a medical curriculum: a qualitative study. *Med Educ*. 2007;41:610–617.

16. Shapiro J. (2008). Walking a mile in their patients' shoes: empathy and othering in medical students' education. *Philos Ethics Humanit Med*. 2008;3:1–11.

17. DeBlasi Z, Harkness E, Ernst E, Gorgiou A, Kleijnen J. Influence of context effects on health outcomes: a systematic review. *Lancet*, 2001;357:757–762.

18. Newton BW, Barber L, Clardy J, Cleveland E. Is there hardening of the heart during medical school? *Acad Med*. 2008;83:244–249.

19. Chandratilake M, McAleer S, Gibson J. Cultural similarities and differences in medical professionalism: a multi-region study. *Med Educ*. 2012;46:257–266.

20. Kahn MW. Etiquette-based medicine. *N Eng J Med*. 2008;358:1988–1989.

21. American Association of Medical Colleges. *Core Entrustable Professional Activities for Entering Residency: Curriculum Developers Guide*. 2014. www.mededportal.org/icollaborative/resource/887.

22. Rothe EM, Bonnin R. Utilizing psychodynamic principles to teach professionalism to medical students through an innovative curriculum. *Psychodyn Psychiatry*. 2020;48(4):477–497. doi:10.1521/pdps.2020.48.4.477.

23. Spiro HM. What is empathy and can it be taught? *Ann Inter Med*. 1992;116:843–846.

24. Spiro HM. The practice of empathy. *Acad Med*. 2009;84(9):1177–1179.

25. Cruess SR, Cruess RL. The cognitive base of professionalism. In: Cruess RL, Cruess SR, Steinert Y, eds. *Teaching Medical Professionalism*. New York: Cambridge University Press; 2009:7–31.

26. Hughes P, Kerr I. Transference and countertransference in communication between doctor and patient. *Adv Psychiatr Treat*. 2000;6:57–64.

27. Charon R. Narrative medicine a model for empathy, reflection, profession, and trust *JAMA*. 2001 Oct 17;286(15):1897–1902.

28. Birden H, Glass N, Wilson I, Harrison M, Usherwood T, Nass D. Defining professionalism in medical education: a systematic review. *Med Teach*. 2014;36:47–61.

29. Remen RN, Rabow MW. The healers art: professionalism, service and mission. *Med Educ*. 2005 Nov;39:1167–1168. PMID: 1626843,

30. Swick HM. (2000) Toward a normative definition of medical professionalism. *Acad Med*. 2000 June;75(6):612–616.

31. Hafferty FW. Professionalism and the socialization of medical students. In: Cruess RL, Cruess SR, Steinert Y, eds. *Teaching Medical Professionalism*. New York: Cambridge University Press; 2009:53–73.

32. Coulehan J. Today's professionalism: engaging the mind but not the heart. *Acad Med*. 2005;80:890–898.

33. Verkerk MA, de Bree MJ, Mourits MJE. Reflective professionalism: Interpreting CanMEDS' "professionalism." *J Med Ethics*. 2007;33:663–666.

34. American Board of Medical Specialties. *Definition of Professionalism*, July 16, 2017. http://www.abms.org/media/84742/abms-definition-of-medical-professionalism.pdf.

35. Al-Rumayyana A, Van Mook WK, Magzoubd ME, et al. Medical professionalism frameworks across non-Western cultures: a narrative overview. *Med Teach*. 2017;39(S1):S8–S14.

36. Alpha Omega Alpha Honor Medical Society Edward B. Harris Medical Professionalism Award, 2018. http://alphaomegaalpha.org/news_2018_professionalism.html.

37. Winnicott DW. Hate in the counter-transference. *Int J Psychoanal.* 1949;30:69–74.

38. Greenson RR. *The Technique and Practice of Psychoanalysis.* London: Hogarth Press; 1985.

39. Kirmayer LJ. Toward an ecosocial psychiatry. *WSP.* 2019 Sept–Dec;1(1):30–32.

40. Lolas F. Social psychiatry: the ethical challenges. *WSP.* 2019 Sept–Dec;1(1):33–35.

41. Zinn WM. Doctors have feelings too. *JAMA.* 1988;259:3296–3298.

42. Inui TS. *A Flag in the Wind: Educating for Professionalism in Medicine.* Washington, DC: Association of American Medical Colleges; 2003.

43. Heimann P. On countertransference. *Int J Psychoanal.* 1950;11:81–84.

7

Developing a Curriculum to Teach Social Psychiatry

Eugenio M. Rothe, Andres J. Pumariega, and Rama Rao Gogineni

Introduction

In addition to the mental health problems that afflict the psychiatric population around the world, most patients seen by psychiatrists and residents today also suffer from problems that are extra-psychic, such as poverty, stigma, marginalization, social and political oppression, and abuses of power in relationships that threaten to overwhelm their coping capacities.[1,2] The majority of psychiatry residency-training programs in the United States and other countries are located in public hospitals that provide care for underprivileged patients and expose residents to ancillary services associated with social and community psychiatry, such as community mental health centers, day hospitals, community residencies, addiction treatment clinics, assisted living facilities, school consultation programs, family-based community clinics, prison programs, and homeless shelters. Yet, few residency programs provide a formal curriculum of social psychiatry that teaches residents about the social determinants of health and the evidence-based treatment approaches to treat the particular problems that afflict these populations. In many cases, residents learn the principles of social psychiatry by "doing" in their daily contact with these patients, and the experiences are incorporated at a "gut level" without a formal methodological discussion of the principles of this therapeutic perspective.

Social psychiatrists aim to understand their patients in the context of the society in which they were raised and the larger social order of which they are a part. For this biopsychosocial understanding of the patient, it is also important to incorporate knowledge about history, sociology, social anthropology, and other allied disciplines.[2] This chapter will present suggestions about how a social psychiatry curriculum should be taught and incorporated at a residency level, will review the existing residency-training programs in the United States that offer such curricula, will present a list of contents that should be included in a formal social psychiatry curriculum, and will suggest possible models for how they can be taught.

Social Psychiatry: Historical Perspective

Residents should be taught that social psychiatry is a paradigm that combines medical training with the perspectives of social anthropology, social psychology, cultural psychiatry, sociology, and other disciplines relating to the human condition and to mental distress and disorder. The discipline of social psychiatry emerged in the 20th century, placing its main focus on the person's social milieu and economic circumstances. Social psychiatry has been associated with highlighting the effect of socioeconomic factors on mental illness and issues that are pertinent to the current realities of the 21st century,[3,4,5] such as the weight of stigma on patients who suffer from mental illness and on their families, as well as problems that result from poverty, wars, natural disasters, social and political oppression, and the massive human migrations that often follow these crises.[6] In 1965, sociologist Oscar Lewis[7] published the controversial document titled "The Culture of Poverty," in which he argued that in order to adapt to their environment, people who live in poverty for long periods of time develop a series of coping mechanisms that become engrained and paralyzing and that affect the individual, the family, the community, and the community in relation to society. For these populations, social psychiatry provides a deeper understanding of their surrounding circumstances, which in turn leads to more holistic and effective therapeutic approaches. Social psychiatry was the dominant form of psychiatry for the second half of the 20th century, but has sometimes been less visible than biological psychiatry.[4] Some of the pioneers who brought attention to social psychiatry in the past century included Karen Horney, Erik Erikson, Harry Stack Sullivan, August Hollingshead, Frederick Redlich, Alexander H. Leighton, and Lloyd Rogler. In the field of child and adolescent psychiatry, Robert Coles, William Rutter, E. James Anthony, and Bertram Cohler opened new windows into the social circumstances that molded the lives of children. More recently, the work of Arthur Kleinman[2] and others have continued to expand the field. Social psychiatry was instrumental in the development of therapeutic communities and the social treatments for chronic schizophrenia focusing on the treatment of the socially disadvantaged and on vulnerable populations. Studies demonstrating the efficacy of social psychiatry approaches in these populations have been replicated in many countries around the world, and the social inclusion of people with mental health problems continues to be a major focus of modern social psychiatry.[8] On the world stage, pioneers such as Abraham Halpern, John Mack, and Robert J. Lifton have also highlighted the role of social psychiatry in protecting patients from political oppression.[9] Social psychiatrists strive to pay close attention to their patients' cultural milieus and to their "idioms of distress," which are the characteristic way in which members of different cultures describe what is wrong, and which may differ from the expressions found in mainstream American culture.[10] In addition, they also try to listen closely to the metaphors or therapeutic stories contained in their patient's "life-meaning stories," which often reveal past traumatic experiences that explain treatment resistance and can help avoid treatment failures. So, as long as human beings continue to be human, there will continue to be social psychiatry.

Existing Teaching, Mentoring Social Psychiatry Programs in the United States

The authors were able to identify the following structured training modules in social psychiatry in North American psychiatry residency-training programs:

1. *The McGill University Division of Social and Transcultural Psychiatry*[11] is a network of scholars and clinicians within the Faculty of Medicine, McGill University, devoted to promoting research, training, and consultation in social and cultural psychiatry. The broad themes of research and training conducted by members of the Division include: social psychiatry teaching and training in psychiatric epidemiology, social determinants of mental health, community mental health, psychiatry in primary care, evaluation of mental health services, and global mental health. Cultural psychiatry focuses on the mental health of indigenous peoples, immigrant and refugee mental health, ethno-psychology and ethno-psychiatry, indigenous healing systems, responding to diversity in mental healthcare, and anthropology of psychiatry. The Division is home to several programs related to social and cultural psychiatry:

2. *New York University (NYU) Langone Department of Psychiatry*[12] offers a residency curriculum in cultural, structural, and global mental health. The curriculum exposes the trainee to cross-cultural psychiatry and the social determinants of health, both nationally and internationally. The trainee also learns ways in which physicians can intervene by collaborating with community organizations, non-health institutions such as schools and correctional facilities, and policymakers. This helps practitioners to recognize that the primary drivers of socioeconomic, ethnic, and racial inequalities in mental health are socially based, such as housing, education, employment, and exposure to violence. The program provides lectures and invited speakers, and offers electives to learn about various aspects of social psychiatry. Much of curriculum is taught in the third and fourth year of training.

3. *Columbia University Program in Global Mental Health and Social Change,*[13] established in 2009, serves as a conduit for implementation-based training and research in global mental health delivery, linked to expanding programmatic work at *Partners in Health* global sites. The program seeks to bring together students, scholars, researchers, educators, and healthcare practitioners to address the global burden of mental disorders, and to develop best-practice models for global mental health delivery and implementation science.

4. *University of Washington (UW)*[14] in Seattle provides psychiatric services in rural areas and roll-out models of collaborative care tracks in community and public psychiatry,

works closely with family physicians, provides the opportunity for rural psychiatry electives, and provides tele-psychiatry and health services development. The program is strongly focused on identifying and addressing mental health disparities with a large lesbian, gay, bisexual, and transgender (LGBT) community, and a strong LGBT mental health movement in the State of Washington.

5. *University of California, San Francisco (UCSF)*,[15] has program of community engagement initiatives and a track record in public and community psychiatry with inpatient teams divided by patient ethnicity. In addition to developing strong cultural competence, there are opportunities to develop interests in women's health, HIV psychiatry, and LGBT mental health through an array of clinical services and more outpatient focus than many residency programs.

6. *University of California, San Diego (UCSD), Department of Psychiatry*[16] offers a community psychiatry fellowship and a number of public psychiatry fellowships covering addictions, HIV, eating disorders, stress reduction, and a combined psychiatry–family medicine residency-training program with a student-run clinic that provides treatment to the medically underserved, including a burgeoning homeless population, and promotes non-hospital residential alternatives for psychotic crises.

7. *Cambridge Health Alliance/Harvard University*[17] has an enduring commitment to social justice, activism, health disparities, and a promotion of cross-cultural and LGBT health. It offers a diverse array of clinical services and community-based rotations, as well as opportunities to obtain a master's degree in Public Health or a master's degree in Public Health (MPH) Administration (MPA) at Harvard University. The faculty has included such pioneers as Arthur Kleinman, Robert Coles, John Mack, Bessel Van der Kolk, Edward Khantzian, and Margarita Alegria.

8. *University of Pennsylvania (UPenn)*[18] provides training leading to bioethics, community psychiatry, and cultural psychiatry certificates involving mental health services research, health disparities, and health policy. There is also a community psychiatry track allowing for creation of a more social- and community-based training for those who are interested.

9. *New Haven Connecticut Mental Health Center/Yale University (CMHC)*[19] offers an array of recovery-oriented services for the chronically mentally ill, and fellowships in public psychiatry, addictions, and forensic and social psychiatry didactics in the curriculum. Residents can take various elective courses in social and community psychiatry, and the West Haven Veterans Administration Hospital, which is one of the rotations, also offers a wealth of recovery and social services.

10. *The European Congress of Social Psychiatry*[20] organizes programs to promote greater understanding of the interactions between individuals and their physical and human environment (including their society and culture), and the impact of these interactions on the clinical expression and the treatment of mental and behavioral problems and disorders, and their prevention. The Congress also promotes mental health through education of health workers, policymakers, and decision-makers and the community at large, and promotes research that can facilitate the understanding of the interaction between social factors, psychological functioning, and mental health or illness.

In this process the Congress organizes several programs for early career psychiatrists. Similar programs are organized across the globe in several national social psychiatry organizations.

Proposed Social Psychiatry Didactic Curriculum

Anthropology and Cultural Studies

A social psychiatric didactic curriculum should begin by focusing on studies of human evolutionary theory and the history of the origins of culture, and the functions of cultures and sub-cultures in human development. Definitions of race and ethnicity and how these interact with the concept of culture, with a focus on the cultural manifestations of medical and mental illness, should be explored. The curriculum should include the origins and the pioneers of social psychiatry, with their respective contributions and the concepts of culturally competent clinical practice, with the introduction of the concept of cultural humility, as well as the practice parameters for cultural competence. In addition, an introduction to the new field of global social psychiatry should be provided.

Sociology

The field of sociology is of utmost importance to the understanding of social psychiatry and contributes a rich literature on socioeconomic differences, differences related to levels of education, social marginalization, stigma, access to care, and the social determinants of health. There should also be an emphasis placed on medical ethics as it relates to access to care for the different world populations.[2,21]

Human Developmental Studies

Human developmental concepts are fundamental to the understanding of social psychiatry, including neurological, cognitive, and psychosocial development, focusing on the cultural influences and differences among the diverse world populations.[22,23]

Economics

Social psychiatry places great importance on the influence of economics on human behavior. Understanding concepts of economic theory, economic models, macroeconomics, labor economics, the impact of poverty, and the modern realities of health economics, which includes the funding for public and private healthcare systems, healthcare benefits, and access to medical and psychiatric care, is fundamental to better understand the concept of social psychiatry.

Political Sciences

How countries and populations are governed is fundamental to understanding health policies and the psychological adaption of its citizens to a particular society. It is important to touch upon theories of government, the differences in the structure of governments, the civil liberties allowed or restricted by governments, and how these governments structure health policy.[1]

Behavioral Epidemiology

Knowledge of behavioral epidemiology is key to understanding the prevalence of mental illness and addictions in particular populations, the risk factors and protective factors, ethnic and racial disparities, social determinants of health, and the effects of violence and trauma in the different members and generations of a population.[1,3,5]

Preventive Social Psychiatry

Theories of prevention, including the levels of prevention (primary, secondary, and tertiary) and the knowledge about model programs for adults and children, the elderly, and addiction prevention programs, are an integral part of the practice of social psychiatry.

Community Mental Health and Addiction

Community mental health is at the heart of social psychiatry, so it is important to learn about the beginnings of the community mental health movement, and it is fundamental to understand the principles of community-based systems of care, and model clinical programs for adults, children, family, the elderly, the chronic mentally ill, and addictions, and the state and local levels of care.[24,25,26]

Mental Health and the Judicial System

A great number of mentally ill persons are currently confined to jails and prisons, which serve as a receptacles that substitute broken or nonexistent services for these populations. Knowledge of the functioning of family courts, drug diversion courts, domestic violence courts, juvenile delinquency programs, and diversions programs, as well as penal psychiatry and social reintegration programs, is also a fundamental part of social psychiatry.[27]

Immigration Studies

The United States is, and has been throughout its modern history, a country of immigrants. In the past three decades the world has been changed by large displacements of populations, due to wars, political turmoil, and socioeconomic factors, and the globalization of the world economy and the improvements in communication and transportation technologies have made many world populations more racially and ethnically diverse. An understanding of the intervening factors and the trauma that results from these population displacements, many of whose members are refugees, and the changes that these individuals bring to the receiving the communities, as well as the effects on those compatriots who are left behind, is fundamental to the practice of social psychiatry.[6,9,28]

Suggested Learning Objectives in a Social Psychiatry Core Curriculum

1. *Proficiency in knowledge in the above-mentioned areas*;
2. *Skills domain*: social-case documentation; social methods in psychiatric research; therapeutic aspects with family, larger social groups, community psychiatry and rehabilitation;

3. *Skills domain*: social case-taking; social methods in psychiatric research; therapeutic aspects with family, larger social groups, community psychiatry and rehabilitation;
4. *Effective (attitudinal) domain*: appreciating the social context of mental health and illness; social and structural determinants of mental health; being able to see and understand the "broader picture" through empathy and social cognition.

Other Methods of Teaching and Training

1. *Group work* (workshops, projects, brainstorming sessions);
2. *Field visits*: to courts, community mental health centers, prisons, Head Start and other children's programs, nursing homes, halfway houses, diversion programs, and other community programs in the area;
3. *Assessment in training and continuing professional development*;
4. *Formative*: learning during the course;
5. *Summative*: at the end of the course, for certification purposes (several residency programs already offer fellowships in community psychiatry and specialization of care with particular ethnic and social groups).

Developing and establishing a formal curriculum to teach social psychiatry at a residency level help to cement the principle and to convey the message to the psychiatrists of the future and to other health professionals[29] that *all psychiatry is social.*[24]

Conclusions

1. Social psychiatry emerged in the 20th century, focusing on the person's social milieu and economic circumstances.
2. In the United States and around the globe, few residency programs provide a formal curriculum of social psychiatry and the evidence-based social treatment approaches to treat the afflicted populations.
3. Many North American psychiatry training programs incorporate social psychiatry into their general psychiatry curriculum of a combined program of global, community, cultural, and family psychiatry.
4. A social psychiatry curriculum may focus in didactics on anthropological, developmental, social, economic, political, community, and preventive aspects.
5. In addition to didactics, exposure to social, community, religious, and cultural aspects of society will enhance learning and mentalization.
6. By encouraging a separate identity in the didactic curriculum, the "social" aspect of psychology and treatments can be enhanced, providing a holistic approach for the understanding and treatment of human mental suffering

Editors' note: This chapter is predominantly written with references and knowledge based on North American universities. But we feel and hope that the observations apply universally to the rest of the globe.

Other Resources

MULTIMEDIA

World Association of Social Psychiatry https://www.worldsocpsychiatry.org
Websites of all the national social psychiatry organizations, APA website, and websites of all the programs mentioned in this chapter.

TEXTBOOKS

Bhugra D, Craig T, Moussaoui D, eds. *Oxford Textbook of Social Psychiatry*. Oxford: Oxford University Press; 2022.
Chadda R, et al., eds. *Social Psychiatry: Principles and Clinical Perspectives*. Jaypee Brothers. 2019.
4. Principles of Social Psychiatry, 2nd edition Craig Morgan (Editor), Dinesh Bhugra (Editor), Wiley.
Stylianidis S, ed. *Social and Community Psychiatry: Towards a Critical, Patient-Oriented Approach*. (eBook). Springer International Publishing; 2016. doi:10.1007/978-3-319-28616.

JOURNALS

Frontiers in Psychiatry, https://www.frontiersin.org/journals/psychiatry.
Indian Journal of Social Psychiatry, https://www.indjsp.org.
International Journal of Social Psychiatry: SAGE Journals, https://journals.sagepub.com.
World Social Psychiatry. http://www.waspsocialpsychiatry.com, official journal of the World Association of Social Psychiatry (WASP), Wolters Kluwer.

References

1. Dohrenwend BP, Levav I, Shrout PE, et al. Socioeconomic status and psychiatric disorders: the causation-selection issue. *Science*. 1992;255:946–952.
2. Kleinman A. *Rethinking Psychiatry: From Cultural Category to Personal Experience*. New York: Free Press; 1991.
3. Alegria M, Vallas M, Pumariega AJ. Racial and ethnic disparities in pediatric mental health. *Child Adolesc Psychiatr Clin N Am*. 2010;19(4):759–774. doi:10.1016/j.chc.2010.07.001.
4. De Nicola V. A person is a person through other persons: a social psychiatry manifesto for the 21st century. *WSP*. 2019 Sep–Dec;1(1):8–21.
5. Kastrup MC. Inequity in mental health: an issue of increasing public health concern. *WSP*. 2019 Sep–Dec;1(1):36–38.
6. Rothe EM, Pumariega AJ, Gogeneni RR. The current refugee problem around the world: implications for social psychiatry. *WSP*. 2019 Sep–Dec;1(1):50–52.
7. Lewis O. Culture of poverty. In: Moynihan DP, ed. *On Understanding Poverty: Perspectives from the Social Sciences*. New York: Basic Books; 1969:187–220.
8. Bhugra D, Till A. Public mental health is about social psychiatry. *Int J Soc Psychiatry*. 2013;59:105–106.
9. Lifton RJ. *Witness to an Extreme Century: A Memoir*. New York: Free Press; 2011.
10. Kaiser BN, Weaver LJ. Culture-bound syndromes, idioms of distress, and cultural concepts of distress: new directions for an old concept in psychological anthropology. *Transcult Psychiatry*. 2013 Aug;56(4):589–598. doi:10.1177/1363461519862708.
11. The McGill University Division of Social and Transcultural Psychiatry (2021). Department of Psychiatry, Global Mental Health Program, Culture, Mind and Brain Program (1A). https://www.mcgill.ca/tcpsych/
12. New York University (NYU) Langone Department of Psychiatry (2021). Cultural, Structural, and Global Mental Health Curriculum. https://med.nyu.edu/departments-institutes/psychiatry/education/residency-programs/psychiatry-residency-curriculum/curriculum-cultural-structural-global-mental-health.
13. Columbia University Program in Global Mental Health and Social Change (2021). https://www.cugmhp.org/.

14. University of Washington Integrated Care Training Program (2021). http://ictp.uw.edu/.
15. University of California, San Francisco Department of Psychiatry Community Engagement Initiatives (2021). https://psych.ucsf.edu/engagement.
16. University of California, San Diego (2021). https://medschool.ucsd.edu/som/psychiatry/education/Programs/Pages/default.aspx.
17. Cambridge Health Alliance/Harvard University (2021). https://www.challiance.org/academics/psychiatry/adult-psychiatry-residency.
18. University of Pennsylvania (2021). https://www.med.upenn.edu/psychres/.
19. New Haven Connecticut Mental Health Center/Yale University (2021). https://medicine.yale.edu/psychiatry/care/cmhc/?locationId=405.
20. European Congress of Social Psychiatry (2021). http://www.esspsy.org/.
21. Rutz WA. Need to rethink social psychiatry. *Int J Public Health.* 2007;52(3):137–139. doi:10.1007/s00038-007-7024-7.
22. Rothe EM, Pumariega AJ. Culture, identity and psycho-social development. In: *Immigration, Cultural Identity and Mental Health: Psychosocial Implications of the Reshaping of America.* Oxford: Oxford University Press; 2020.
23. Pumariega AJ, Joshi S-V. Culture and development. *Child Adolesc Psychiatr Clin N Am.* 2010;19(4):661–680.
24. Masserman JH. Social psychiatry: individual to global. In: Varma VK, Kulhara P, Masserman CM, Malhotra A, Malik SC, eds. *Social Psychiatry: A Global Perspective.* Delhi: Macmillan India; 1998:211–216.
25. Kovess V. The homeless mentally ill. In: Sartorius N, Gaebel W, López-Ibor JJ, Maj M, eds. *Psychiatry in Society.* Chichester, UK: John Wiley and Sons; 2002:221–240.
26. Hawkley LC, Cacioppo JT. Loneliness matters: a theoretical and empirical review of consequences and mechanisms. *Ann Behav Med.* 2010;40:218–227.
27. Mentally Ill Persons in Corrections (2021). *National Institute of Mental Health.* https://nicic.gov/projects/mentally-ill-persons-in-corrections.
28. Rothe EM, Pumariega AJ. *Immigration, Cultural Identity and Mental Health: Psychosocial Implications of the Reshaping of America.* Oxford: Oxford University Press; 2020.
29. Uchtenhagen A. Which future for social psychiatry? *Int Rev Psychiatry.* 2008 Dec;20(6):535–539. doi:10.1080/09540260802565471.

Developmental Perspectives

On developmental perspectives presents various aspects of developmental psychiatry and psychology. Focusses on social developmental aspects of Children, Adolescents, Men, Women, Aging and dying and death.

8

Social Psychiatry

Children

Savita Malhotra and Nidhi Chauhan

Introduction

A holistic understanding of mental health and illness requires equal attention to neurobiological as well as sociopsychological and cultural factors. The past five decades of research have seen a burgeoning of neurobiology to such an extent that socio-psychological underpinnings of mental disorders almost receded to the background. Current teaching and research are heavily loaded in favor of neurobiology, and the new generation of psychiatry trainees often neither address nor incorporate the role of socio-psychological factors in their formulation and treatments while treating mental disorders. In this chapter, effort is made to focus on the sociocultural aspects of human development as well as mental health and disease.

Social psychiatry is a branch of psychiatry that considers social determinants of mental health (such as culture, socioeconomic status [SES], psychosocial stressors) and which has a public health perspective and strives for social justice. It focuses on the interpersonal and cultural context of mental disorder and mental well-being and incorporates knowledge from disciplines of social and cultural anthropology; social psychology; cultural psychiatry; sociology; socioeconomic factors; life events; and community aspects of mental illness. Social psychiatry addresses the broader domains of health promotion, prevention, and social policy.

Social factors refer to the environment where an individual lives, grows up, and learns; all these factors influence development at different levels, interacting and moderating one another based on the interactions among its various members, living conditions, relationship between parents and with parents, peers, neighborhood, and educational and sociopolitical context.[1] These factors have the potential to be modified to provide nurturing environmental ingredients for the developing brain and individual.

Now considering social psychiatry as applied to children, it is that component of psychiatry which strives to understand the development of the brain and its vicissitudes in the context of the social environment, and to address social determinants of childhood mental disorders; and that forays into sociocultural aspects of treatments and preventive and promotive strategies, as well as social policy and legislation.

Children are our most valuable natural resources and thus it becomes imperative on everyone's part to care for them and provide them with the most fulfilling and enriching ingredients, enabling them to become the best of what each can be. About one-fourth of the world's population is under 15 years of age, comprising a significant proportion of the total population. When an appropriate, rich, and nurturing environment is provided to developing children, it can enable them to become physically and mentally healthy youth.

Social Factors and Brain Development

Human development is a complex, multifactorial, multifaceted process. There is ample literature emphasizing the fact that development of any living being depends on genetic endowment and socio-environmental conditions which work in sync with each other, interacting with each other and moderating each other's effects—children are no exception to that. Childhood refers to the developmental period between prenatal period to around 8 years of age, and social factors begin to influence the development of living being as early as the prenatal period.[1] When it comes to measuring the development of a child, four domains are important:—cognitive, motor (gross motor and fine motor), speech and language, and the socio-emotional domain—which all have a bearing on future learning, academic achievement, social relationships, employment, and community participation. Development in each specific domain is affected by a multitude of biological, psychological, and social factors acting in unison and altering/modifying the outcome. The early years of life mark a rapid development especially of the central nervous system and the developing brain's ability for neuro-genesis/synapto-genesis and neuronal plasticity. It is this critical phase of development in which the brain can be sculpted or molded according to the environment in which the child is growing. Equally important is the life course perspective, which needs to be acknowledged while talking about development, as genes influence behavior and experiences and vice versa. However, this chapter is about social factors affecting development and here, we shall briefly discuss the various social factors that have an impact on the physical, cognitive, socio-emotional, and mental development of children.

Social factors play an important role starting from conception, pregnancy, postnatal period, early childhood, adolescence, and adulthood. Some social factors may have a causative role in the genesis of physical and mental health problems, for example, maternal health (physical and mental) pre-conception and during pregnancy, safe delivery practices, immunization, early feeding practices; whereas others, like family environment (marital discord, parental substance abuse, interparental violence), neighborhood, living conditions,

sanitation, etc., may act as both causative as well as maintaining factors. It is equally important to mention that not every child has a poorer outcome following exposure to adversities
(which include social pathologies like abuse, war, migration, natural calamities); there are
children who thrive despite these adversities, partly due to presence of some support in
the family or neighborhood and partly because of the innate resilience factors with which
a person is endowed. The following are brief descriptions of various factors affecting child
development—ways in which they are favorable and ways in which they have a deleterious
effect on child development.

Preconception to Birth

Social factors begin to play a role as early as the pre-conception period, with a focus on the
maternal life style factors; for example, maternal nutrition determines birth weight, general
fetal well-being, and health outcomes during childhood and later in life. Poor maternal nutrition is associated with poverty, illiteracy, unemployment, lack of prenatal education, lack
of or non- implementation of governmental policies regarding care and nutrition of pregnant females, safe and hygienic delivery practices, etc.;[2] all these factors contribute to higher
infant mortality and child mortality rates, especially in developing countries. Maternal
smoking, maternal alcohol consumption, exposure to environmental toxins, obesity, and
stress are other factors affecting optimal child development. Dietary deficiency of essential fatty acids in pregnant females adversely affects physical and brain development of the
fetus.[3] Thus, a healthy mother is an essential prerequisite for healthy child development.

At birth, a newborn has millions of neurons still to form meaningful connections
among each other, and this entirely depends on the environmental stimulation provided in
all sensory and developmental processes (i.e., visual, auditory, olfactory, tactile, gustatory,
emotional, verbal, physical), along with biological factors playing a part during the critical periods of development. Any adverse exposure during such period hampers cognitive,
socio-emotional, and physical development and may lead to delays and deviances in development. The early life experiences impact later health and achievements through three key
mechanisms. The first, "biological embedding," is the effect of interaction among various biological, psychological, and social factors which influence not only lifelong health but also
physiological responses seen in neuroendocrine, immune systems of the body.[3] Second is
the toxic stress due to the cumulative effect of adverse life experiences; and the third mechanism is an increase in risk over time, that is, exposure to adverse experience once in early
life increases the probability of similar exposures later in life.[4]

Attachment and Bonding

Attachment refers to the bond of trust, a sense of safety and security, and prompt and appropriate response between infant and caregiver. High levels of trust ensure "secure attachment," which in turn increases successful attempts at exploration of the environment,
fostering mastery, competence and self-confidence.[5] Breastfeeding is another activity
fostering attachment between infant and mother, apart from providing essential nutrients
required for physical and cognitive development. The type of attachment (secure, resistant,
avoidant, disorganized) determines how a child would experience the world and even the

same experience; children with different attachment styles experience even the same environment differently. Secure attachment with a warm, loving, and trusted caregiver ensures emotional well-being, not only during childhood but also during adolescence and adulthood. For working parents, the level of support provided by the government (in terms of parental leave schemes like maternity and paternity leave) and work shift flexibility are important determining factors for the time spent with the newborn and consequently the type of attachment formed with the primary caregiver.[6]

Parenting Style

The varying levels of warmth expressed and control exercised to handle children determine the type of parenting, for example, authoritative (high on control and warmth); authoritarian (high control and low warmth); permissive (high warmth and low control); and neglecting-uninvolved (low both on control and warmth). Consequent to weak and disrupted attachment, parenting is often negligent and inadequate, resulting in adverse health and developmental outcomes for young children. Authoritative parenting is associated with fewer behavior problems in children, better adjustment with peers, good academic achievement, and good socio-emotional competence. Parenting practices are not always influenced by the financial conditions of the family, and both positive and negative parenting may be found at varying levels of SES.[7] At the same time it is seen that low SES, unemployment, and poor parental mental health may impede positive parenting practices. Until a few years back, parenting was seen generally irrespective of either parent, but recently the focus has shifted to the particular parent (i.e., mother or father) given the recent change and shift in parental roles (working mothers, caregiver role of fathers, etc.). Key components of parenting which influence development are availability/accessibility (i.e., for how long the parent is available, even if not interacting), engagement/interaction (i.e., spending quality time doing various activities with children), responsibility in managing child's activities, and arranging for resources.[8] Another important aspect is "co-parenting" (i.e., the extent and ease with which parents work together to rear a child), this being distinct from marital relationship quality and parenting style.

Sibling Issues

Most children gain skills and competencies, as well as maladaptive behaviors, through social learning. Siblings in the family offer this window whereby a young child can learn specific communication patterns and social skills through interaction with them, while at the same time practicing what they have learned from their parents or from significant others around them. When there are older siblings, the young child may either be allowed to explore the world around them or may be restricted, depending upon the demeanor and attitude of the older siblings, acting as gatekeepers, teachers, or mentors for the young child.[9] The siblings' relationship and interaction pattern with their parents also has an indirect influence on development. The processes thus are not direct and are affected by the birth order of the sibling and the young child. In the face of marital discord in the family, a supportive relationship with a sibling can work as a buffer against adjustment problems and behavioral difficulties.[10]

Thus, given the role that a family plays in child development, as highlighted earlier, it can be said that the family regulates the majority of child-environment interactions and helps to shape children's adaptation. Family is the first and the foremost arena within which the child experiences and experiments with expressions and control of emotions and impulses; learns norms and morality; accepts and is exposed to graded responsibility for self and others in the filial group and the larger society; develops social bonds and relationships. Most of the young children's cognitive, emotional, and social repertoire stems directly from the experience they have had within the framework of the family. Family plays a key part in the process of shaping and guiding children's development and thus contributes to overall child mental health.

Social Factors and Functioning

Various social factors act singly or in unison to affect a child's cognitive, emotional, social, and moral functioning. Most factors act parallel to each other in determining a child's development and functioning. A brief account of various social factors affecting child's functioning is given below.

Parental Education

The presence of a supportive environment for early learning paves the way for later learning and development, as development and learning go hand in hand. The learning of new skills fosters future autonomy and competence in children. If parents are educated, it is likely that children will also be sent to school and efforts will be made for providing children with a better education. The mother's education is directly linked to her children's education and well -being.

Parental Health (Physical and Mental Disorders)

Chronic and severe disorders in parents have a negative influence on child development and are known to be predictors of disturbances in the healthy development of children and later functioning gains.[11] Parental physical and mental disorders, especially in maternal health, have a strong influence on child development and functioning. Infants as young as few months old demonstrate the deleterious effects of parental depression, especially maternal depression, with deficits observable in social engagement and interaction and object recognition. Physiological changes like increased heart rate and high cortisol levels are also seen in infants of depressed mothers compared to infants of mentally healthy mothers.[12] Deficits in cognitive development, speech and language development, and age-appropriate social skills, as well as an increase in problem behaviors, are also reported to be higher in children reared by mothers who are depressed in conjunction with not being able to provide positive and responsive child-rearing.[13] The academic attainment scores and cognitive development were lower in children with parents having more severe psychological problems compared to those with parents having lesser psychological problems.[14] The family's financial condition is reported to be an important mediator while studying parental mental health disorders and child's development. Although either parent's mental health problem had a deleterious effect on development, the mother's mental health issues were more strongly associated with developmental problems in boys than girls, emphasizing that boys need an emotionally healthy and sensitive caregiver for optimal development. Whereas maternal mental health issues had a direct bearing on the child's development, the father's mental health issues were mediated through socioeconomic adversity.[14] Thus, paternal and maternal mental health problems impact child development, albeit through different pathways.

Sexually transmitted diseases (e.g., AIDS) in the adult population affect the younger population in many ways. In addition to acquiring the disease through direct transmission from mother to offspring, in many situations the children have to take on adult roles, for example as caregivers for ailing parents, in early employment to support the family financially, and/or looking after younger siblings in place of parents. As a result, children may have to forgo schooling early and also become vulnerable to a plethora of physical and psychological issues.[15] This results in altered development and functioning of children later in adulthood.

Marital Discord

The child's ability to solve problem situations and have adequate coping ability is influenced significantly by the quality of functioning of the marital dyad (i.e., child's parents). The interpersonal relation between parents has a strong influence on the development of emotional security, emotional regulation, and the familial internal representations within the family, as well as the future socio-emotional functioning of the child. What is important for the general well-being of children is the quality of relationships and experiences children have with their parents and significant others. Problems in marital dyad adjustment can lead to impaired parent-child interaction, negative parenting behaviors, or scapegoating of the child, all of which have a deleterious effect on the child's development. It is generally seen that conflicts between parents arising because of children are more harmful for the child's development compared to conflicts involving other issues. Greater feelings of shame, embarrassment, and self-blame are seen in such children. Resolution of the conflict has a positive effect on child's overall adjustment. Cold, detached, and hostile couples impact children's development most negatively. Arguments, quarrels, and conflicts which are resolved positively are better than unresolved conflicts between parents.[16] It is seen that a moderate degree of conflict, expressed positively in the background of a warm and supportive family, enables children to learn and imbibe skills required for the adequate resolution of conflicts and disagreements.[10]

Single Parenthood, Parental Separation/Divorce

There is enough literature emphasizing the positive developmental outcomes of children living with both biological parents, especially in stable parental unions, by spending more time with each other and greater time for interaction while living together.

Cultural Beliefs and Attitudes

There is a huge difference in the way beliefs and behavior are shaped by and in different cultures. The entire process of development, especially during early childhood, also entails that culture is imbibed and internalized as one grows. Through the process of neurogenesis and synaptic plasticity, a series of adaptations result, bringing about evolutionary change in the structure and functions of the brain, crucial for survival of the human being. From as early as birth, infants are beginning to be conditioned to learn the art of meeting external demands, assuming socially adjusted and accepted roles, and accepting the limitations of reality despite strong inner strivings. Stress and conflicts arise as a result of these unfulfilled strivings, and incomplete resolution of these conflicts result in discontent in life, ready to evolve or progress into a disease or aggression. However, if the environment provided to a developing brain and a child is safe, nurturing, repetitive, predictable, and appropriate to the developmental level of the child, development proceeds optimally. On the other hand, a rapidly changing environment and chaotic experiences become overwhelming and prevent the optimal development of children.[17]

According to the ancient Indian philosophy given in the Rig Veda, man has an average life span of 100 years, which is divided into four periods of 25 years each. The first 25 years are designated as the period of *brahamcharya*, which is a period of learning (which makes sense as we know that the brain development is complete only by 25 years of age), during which the child is put through a formal and rigorous education for life and also for different professions, under the conditions of austerity and celibacy. This ideology is reflected in the way children are brought up and treated. They are handled in an authoritative manner, inculcating respect for age and social hierarchy, and are encouraged to live a simple and sober life devoid of luxuries or material pleasures. They are not praised lest they become vain. However, with the increasing influence of Westernization and globalization, this pattern is changing rapidly. Formal authority of family and society over individuals is getting diluted; children are exposed prematurely to the adult world without imbibing or learning the basic values of life that would enable them to evaluate and discriminate between right and wrong.[18]

Cultural factors determine the attitude toward childbirth, child-rearing, and further development. Mothers talk differently to their newborns across different cultures. Mothers in Germany focus on the infant's needs and wishes, whereas African mothers focus on social contexts. Early exposure and interaction help in forming self-image and self-identity. Parenting is also influenced by culture, for example in the ways parents respond and interact with children, who then learn various sociocultural ways and taboos.

Chinese parents are more authoritative and demand obedience from their children, whereas Chinese people who migrated to America tend to follow American culture, and as a result, children follow parental demands less frequently. People in Australia are of the view that newborn children are "passive absorbers of content" and their lives should be "simplified and uncluttered by influences."[19(pp7-8)] Such beliefs influence the attitude of individuals and society toward child-rearing practices on one hand, and governmental investments for healthy children on the other hand. Similarly, childcare and early education are considered to be personal obligations in Australia, rather than a public responsibility; therefore there is minimal support for high-quality early education.[20] Newborns in Bhutan are not given lactation immediately after birth; rather, they are given water/butter as pre-lacteal feed within 24 hours of birth, thus delaying lactation and milk let-down reflex, leading to lactation failure.[21] Also, it is commonly believed in Bhutan that newborns take around 3–4 weeks to have vision and are not able to see at birth. As a result, caregivers do not communicate with the newborn and expose them to under-stimulation, resulting in delayed development of skills. The practice of keeping the newborns wrapped tightly in cloth prevents human touch by the infant, and such infants are unable to move their limbs. Also, it is a common belief in Bhutan that talking to newborns (who do not speak at all) is a sin, thus preventing the stimulation required to develop speech and language.

Social Factors and Mental Illness

The social causation theory posits an inverse relationship between socioeconomic class and rates of mental disorders. On one hand, adverse psychosocial circumstances may precipitate mental illness, and on the other hand, persistent mental illness has a downward trajectory in terms of social status and socioeconomic condition. As highlighted earlier, most factors act in unison with the earlier mentioned social factors affecting development and achievement of optimal functioning in various domains, and the factors enumerated below add on to the already acquired inadequacies.

Socioeconomic Status

In social science literature, SES is understood as the socioeconomic class of an individual/group. It encompasses two different but interrelated aspects: social aspect and economic aspect.[22] Financially disadvantaged families display a gradient effect on the brain development, physical and psychological health, and academic attainments during adulthood.[1,23]

Socioeconomic class also influences language acquisition during early development mainly because of low knowledge and skills of caregivers, in addition to impediments in providing nutrition, safe housing, and good-quality childcare.[3] Despite low SES, adequate family social support, high maternal education, and positive maternal mental health mediated children's IQ scores and development, whereas low SES combined with poor parental mental health and a stressful environment resulted in impaired parent-child interaction, dampening the learning experiences at home.[3] The multiple needs of a family expose them to additional stressors like unstable housing, homelessness, and social isolation, thus negatively affecting child development and health. Thus, family environment may act as a buffer or may exacerbate the deleterious effects of financial disadvantage on the cognitive abilities of children.[24] Low SES has an indirect effect on the stress levels experienced by children and the other family members and consequently on the immune response to stress, making them vulnerable to a number of mental and physical health conditions.[22] Socioeconomic class of the neighborhood is associated with child injury rates and, along with family socioeconomic class, is seen to be related to various physical and mental health conditions, including depressive disorders, anxiety disorders, and disruptive behavioral disorders.[25]

Gender

Inequality with respect to gender starts at home, as early as an infant is born. In some parts of the world, the birth of a boy is rejoiced, while the birth of a girl is still condemned—to the extent that even in the 21st century, we hear/read about female feticide and reports of termination of pregnancy on conceiving a female fetus. As the girl child grows, clear bias and partiality are observed favoring boys. The social framework in most communities promotes female involvement in taking up the entire responsibility of household chores, leaving out on school and forced labor. As a result of their mothers working as household help, many young girls have to drop out of school; according to UNICEF,[26] 1 in every 5 girls is not able to complete primary education. Poorly educated females are not able to achieve their full potential. Thus, gender has important implications with respect to accessibility to power for implementing household and caretaking, as well as schooling decisions for children. In many areas there is a clear bias toward male children and thus they are preferred over females who may be denied adequate food, education, essential health services, and leisure activities. Low educational attainment and poor decision-making skills affect child development adversely.[26]

Overall, there are many societal changes which have taken place, for example, an increase in the number of nuclear families; smaller extended families with fewer cousins, uncles, and aunts; increasing maternal age of first childbirth; increasing number of couples who do not want to have children; increased number of both parents working, with longer work shifts and increasing dependence on hired caregivers to raise children. As a result, the environment in which children are being born and brought up has also seen a rapid shift and has a definite impact on the way children are reared and consequently their overall development and physical and mental health.[4] Children learn not only language and pre-academic skills from significant others in their environment, but also socio-emotional skills. Also, it is imperative for adults to reinforce positive meaningful participation of children in daily activities; their opinions must be heard, which goes a long way in developing self-efficacy, competence, and pro-social adjustments.

Neighborhood Physical and Social Environment

The availability of parks and green spaces, and the level of exposure to environmental toxins (ingested and/or inhaled), toxic waste, poor water quality, overcrowding, and excessive noise have a significant impact on the health and overall development of young bodies and minds.[27] Family functioning and child development are also influenced by the type and quality of social environment available, that is, the level of social support, cohesion among members of the community, safety and security (i.e., level of crime rate in the area) for children. These factors influence child development indirectly by having an impact on family practices and the psychological health of family members. For example, if the outside environment is not considered safe for the child, the family may limit the opportunity for physical activity outside home (e.g., in playgrounds), limiting a child's exposure to social experiences—and is correctly referred to as the "domino effect." A cohesive neighborhood may lessen the anxiety faced by family members when it comes to the safety of children in close vicinity.[28] Neighborhood also determines school readiness, which is stronger for children who have had more social interactions. Rural lives in developing countries, on the other hand, have been posited to bring about a sense of belonging, fostering socio-emotional development and healthy child development, even in adverse circumstances.[3] "Relational community" refers to individuals, groups of people, and organizations who are connected to each other based on commonalities, rather than place of origin or place of residing. These influence child development through the monitoring of children in the community, positive/negative role modeling of individuals in the community, type and quality of social ties, and also help in disseminating information and awareness regarding child-rearing practices, gender roles, and child development.[1] Whereas low- and middle-income countries witness an intergenerational transmission of low SES, with poverty affecting adult attainments and productivity, even the developed countries report adverse developmental outcomes as one goes down the SES spectrum, as around one-fourth of individuals have attained adulthood without having exposure to adequate literacy and numeracy skills. "Social capital" refers to inflow of information into the community and the shared norms and values within the community, which either facilitate or constrain the activities and interaction of the people living in a community. The parental social network is one determinant of possible social exposure and style of social interaction that a child may acquire depending upon the level of exposure to social interactions among adults as well as children and the particular ways of interacting with each other. Positive and supportive social networks favor positive parent-child relationships, both within and outside the family.[29]

Special Circumstances

Social factors which operate at a wider perspective and affect child development may be considered as special circumstances in which a child is forced to grow and develop.

Migration

Parents migrating to geographically and culturally different areas face significant stress while making adjustments in new areas of habitation. Positive relationships foster healthier child development. Migration to areas with a higher concentration of immigrants is a positive predictor of better adjustment of the family and lesser emotional and behavioral problems in children, whereas with immigration to pockets of sparse population of immigrants the opposite is true.[30] It is mostly seen that migrant populations with low SES usually have to take up menial jobs to earn their livelihood; as a result, caregivers have to take their children along with them, exposing them to unsafe conditions, or they are left at home under the care of younger siblings.

Child Abuse

Abuse in any form (physical, emotional, sexual, neglect) is detrimental for the general well-being and development of children.[4] Childhood maltreatment (in the form of physical abuse and neglect, emotional abuse and neglect, sexual abuse) and parental interpersonal violence leading to all forms of abuse act as potent stressors for children by hampering the formation of healthy and emotionally satisfying attachments bonds with their caregivers.[31] The relation of the timing of exposure to abuse (during which developmental period) to the extent of deleterious effects on development is not very well studied, but it appears that the younger the child, the more deleterious effect it has, given the fact that the brain of a very young child is in a stage where molding (due to neurogenesis and synaptic plasticity) takes place depending upon environmental inputs.[31] Apart from being a victim of abuse, these children become more vulnerable to contracting sexually transmitted diseases, anxiety and depressive disorders, substance use, risk-taking behavior, difficulty forming and maintaining relationships, and externalizing behavior, with long-term consequences for health and life achievements. Low IQ scores, academic underachievement, impaired cognitive functioning, and reading and writing deficits are other long-term consequences of abuse. Direct injury to the brain due to head trauma resulting from physical abuse may be one pathway of adverse effects of abuse on development, while stress due to other forms of abuse may be the other mechanism of the same. Additionally, abuse hampers the formation of warm and loving parent-child relationships; psychological issues resulting due to abuse also add to the cognitive deficits and social skill deficits. Abuse victims also may become abusers later in life.[32]

Natural Calamities

Natural disasters like volcano eruptions, hurricanes, floods, and droughts open a wide window for the adversities that children might experience, ranging from serious physical injuries, being orphaned, homelessness, damaged infrastructure, lost income and unemployment in the family, increased demands for basic amenities, mental health consequences, abuse, exploitation, and child trafficking. Around 90% of disease borne by children globally in the near future is attributed to climate change.[33] Many children suffer from anxiety, depression, and most commonly post-traumatic stress disorder symptoms, which tend to persist over years. The experience of these adversities by children is compounded by the low socioeconomic condition experienced by many families. These children are most in need for intervention and require parental support and societal support. Schools can prepare children for these calamities, and overall, a public health approach is required for this preparedness.

The United Nations Children's Fund (UNICEF) takes the lead in providing care to children affected by calamities and war, by offering treatment, psychological aid (counseling), creating "child-friendly" spaces, and protecting children and women from violence and exploitation.

Social Policies and Intervention Strategies

Healthcare Services

Accessibility to various health-related and other services is a challenge to individuals from disadvantaged families; common reasons being percolation of lesser services in such communities, minimal awareness of governmental schemes to members of disadvantaged communities, making less utilization of available resources, and the inability of those in maximum need to access such services.[34] The "when" and "how" of service delivery process seems to be important if disadvantaged families are to be taken care of. A comprehensive, multilevel, multi-sectoral approach is needed to target all factors related to child, family, community, and society for the healthy development of children. Certain policies focusing on early child development (e.g., positive parenting practices, positive learning experiences) prepare young children for entry to formal schooling. Early education programs and care programs also ease the transition from kindergarten to formal school level. A child-care program developed in India, SEWA (Self-Employed Women's Association), is one such program, which takes care of the developmental needs of children and the socioeconomic needs of working mothers. Cognitive, social, and emotional development is ensured by engaging the children in age-appropriate learning activities; the program also offers the advantage of ensuring education of the eldest child, especially the eldest daughter, who otherwise would have had to take up the role of caregiver for the younger siblings.[35]

Policies

Nearly half a century has passed since the acknowledgment of the need for national-level policy in child and adolescent mental health. As the adult or the general mental health policies often lack the developmental framework, there is need for specific policy for child and adolescent mental health. Low-resource countries should be equally active and innovative in formulating specific national-level child mental health policies and programs.[36]

Policies formulated at the national and international level are important factors for child development. The fact remains that child development is better in developed countries compared to developing countries, but at the same time there is another fact: countries giving priority to children in social policies fare better in terms of developmental outcomes. While framing child welfare policies, countries should take into account 5 domains: income and tax benefits, employment; maternity and paternity leaves; maternal employment and issues thereof; early childhood education and early childcare programs; prevention and interventions of teen pregnancy.[37] A public health approach is most suited for healthy development of all children at all ages.

Malhotra,[38(p12)] while highlighting ethnocentrism in child mental health, states:

> there is strong merit in studying traditional, indigenous and alternative systems of health care which most countries have. Unfortunately very little scientific research has been done in the developing countries and these studies have been relegated to obscurity due to the export of modern western thinking that has pervaded the whole world. There is a rich body of knowledge and wisdom that exists in ancient texts in countries like India, China and Japan. There is a huge resource that already exists in terms of the number of people who practice or advocate it and the population that believes in it and follows it. These should be tested for efficacy and potential benefits. The vast potential of culture-specific traditional medicines should be incorporated into health care systems.

Conclusion

The seeds of lifelong determinants of health are sowed during early child development. An adequate and appropriate nurturing environment can be provided by and within the family; warm and caring caregivers determine children's outcomes. Adverse experiences have a multiplicative effect on physical, cognitive, and physiological development. There is a complex interplay of social factors operating at different levels of aggregation in a culture-specific context. Irrespective of geographical distribution and specific cultural practices, it is seen that adequate maternal care during pregnancy, nutrition, stimulation, healthy family environment, safe vicinity, and care are necessary for the optimal development of young children. Policies should aim at providing young children with an environment where exploration is encouraged, basic skills are strengthened and mentored, development is monitored and rejoiced, newer skills are taught and mentored, a safe and secure environment, free from abuse, punishments, and bullying, is made available, and a rich and stimulating atmosphere is provided. Only then can healthier adults develop, who would then contribute toward better socioeconomic development of the nation. Before embarking upon the policies to be initiated for better development of children, it would be prudent to take into account the social conditions of the community where interventions are to be targeted, understanding the cultural context of the area, involving natives as well as immigrants and minority sections of the society, with community awareness targeting local leaders who may be helpful in disseminating information about various policies and schemes and also have a bearing on motivating people. Finally, a program should always be in place to monitor the implementation and growth of all such activities and programs.

References

1. Irwin LG, Siddiqi A, Hertzman C. *Early Child Development: A Powerful Equalizer, Final Report.* WHO Commission on the Social Determinants of Health. World Health Organization, Vancouver; 2007:1–67. https://apps.who.int/iris/handle/10665/69729
2. Karp RJ, Cheng C, Meyers AF. The appearance of discretionary income: influence on the prevalence of under- and over-nutrition. *Int J Equity Health.* 2005;4:10.
3. Maggi S, Irwin LJ, Siddiqi A, Hertzman C. The social determinants of early child development: an overview. *J Paediatr Child Health.* 2010;46:627–635.
4. Moore TG, McDonald M, Carlon L, O'Rourke K. Early childhood development and the social determinants of health inequities. *Health Promot Int.* 2015;30(S2):ii102–ii115.
5. Hertzman C. The case for an early childhood development strategy. *ISUMA.* 2000;1:11–18.
6. O'Brien M. Fathers, parental leave policies, and infant quality of life: international perspectives and policy impact. *Ann Am Acad Pol Soc Sci.* 2009;624:190–213.
7. Chao RK, Willms JD. The effects of parenting practices on children's outcomes. In: Willms JD, ed. *Vulnerable Children.* Edmonton: University of Alberta Press; 2002:149–166.
8. Carlson MJ, Magnuson KA. Low income fathers' influence on children. *Annals, AAPSS.* 2011;635:95–116.
9. Volling BL, McElwain NL, Miller AL. Emotion regulation in context: the jealousy complex between young siblings and its relations with child and family characteristics. *Child Dev.* 2002;73:581–600.
10. Parke RD. Development in the family. *Annu Rev Psychol.* 2004;55:365–399.
11. NICHD Early Child Care Network. Early child care and children's development prior to school entry: results from the NICHD study of early child care. *Am Educ Res J.* 2002;39:133–164.
12. Field T. Infants of depressed mothers. *Infant Behav Dev.* 1995;18:1–13.

13. Cogill SR, Caplan HL, Alexandra H, Robson KM, Kumar R. Impact of maternal postnatal depression on cognitive development of young children. *BMJ*. 1986;292:1165–1172.

14. Mensah FK, Kiernan KE. Parents' mental health and children's cognitive and social development: families in England in the Millennium Cohort Study. *Soc Psychiat Epidemiol*. 2010;45:1023–1035.

15. Richter L, Foster G. *Strengthening Systems to Support Children's Healthy Development in Communities Affected by HIV/AIDS*. Geneva: Department of Child and Adolescent Health and Development, World Health Organization; 2006.

16. Lamb ME. Mothers, fathers, families, and circumstances: factors affecting children's adjustment. *Appl Dev Sci*. 2012;16(2):98–111.

17. Malhotra S, Kumar D. Family issues in child mental health: a cross-cultural perspective. In: Taylor E, et al., eds. *Mental Health and Illness of Children and Adolescents. Book Series "Mental Health and Illness Worldwide"*. https://doi.org/10.1007/978-981-10-0753-8_20-1. Springer Nature Singapore; 2020:1–20.

18. Malhotra S. Challenges for providing mental health services for children and adolescents in India. In: Young JG, Ferrari P, eds. *Designing Mental Health Services and Systems for Children and Adolescents: A Shrewd Investment*. Philadelphia, USA: Brunner/Mazel; 1998:324–325.

19. Kendall-Taylor N, Lindland E. *Modernity, Morals and More Information: Mapping the Gaps Between Expert and Public Understandings of Early Child Development in Australia*. Washington, DC: FrameWorks Institute; 2013:7–8.

20. Fenech M. Quality early childhood education for my child or for all children? Parents as activists for equitable, high quality early childhood education in Australia. *Austral J Early Child*. 2013;38:92–98.

21. Armstrong J, Reilly JJ. Breastfeeding and lowering the risk of childhood obesity. *Lancet*. 2002;359:2003–2004.

22. Webb S, Janus M, Duku E, et al. Neighbourhood socioeconomic status indices and early childhood development. *SSM Popul Health*. 2017;3:48–56.

23. Duncan GJ, Kalil A, Ziol-Guest KM. Early childhood poverty and adult achievement, employment and health. *Fam Matters*. 2013;93:27–35.

24. Brooks-Gunn J, Berlin LJ, Fuligni AS. Early childhood intervention programs: what about the family? In: Shonkoff JP, Meisels SJ, eds. *Handbook of Early Childhood Intervention*. 2nd ed. New York: Cambridge University Press; 2000:549–588.

25. Brownell MD, Derksen SA, Jutte DP, Roos NP, Ekuma O, Yallop L. Socio-economic inequities in children's injury rates: has the gradient changed over time? *Can J Public Health*. 2010;101:S28–S31.

26. UNICEF. *State of the world's children 2007: women and children: the double dividend of gender equality*. New York, USA; 2007:68–86.

27. Sandercock G, Angus C, Barton J. Physical activity levels of children living in different built environments. *Prev Med*. 2010;50:193–198.

28. Sampson RJ, Raudenbush SW, Earls F. Neighbourhoods and violent crime: a multilevel study of collective efficacy. *Science*. 1997;77:918–924.

29. Cochran M, Niego S. Parenting and social networks. In: Bornstein MH, ed. *Handbook of Parenting: Social Conditions and Applied Parenting*. Washington, DC: Lawrence Erlbaum Associates Publishers; 2002:123–148.

30. Clark KD, Oosthuizen J, Beerenfels S, Rowell AM. Making the best of the early years: the Tambellup way. *Rural Remote Health*. 2010;10(3):1407.

31. Enlow MB, Egeland B, Blood EA, Wright RO, Wright RJ. Interpersonal trauma exposure and cognitive development in children to age 8 years: a longitudinal study. *J Epidemiol Commun Health*. 2012;66:1005–1010.

32. Cashmore J, Shackel R. The long-term effects of child sexual abuse. CFCA Paper No. 11. Melbourne, Victoria: Child Family Community Australia Information Exchange, Australian Institute of Family Studies; 2013. Retrieved from: http://www.aifs.gov.au/cfca/pubs/papers /a143161 /index.html.

33. Dyregrove A, Yule W, Olff M. Children and natural disasters. *Eur J Psychotraumatol*. 2018;9:1–3.

34. Leurer MD. Perceived barriers to program participation experienced by disadvantaged families. *Int J Health Promot Educ*. 2011;49:53–59.

35. Dayal M. *Towards Securer Lives: SEWA's Social-Security Programme*. Delhi: Ravi Dayal; 2001.

36. Malhotra S, Padhy SK. Challenges in providing child and adolescent psychiatric services in low re-source countries. *Child Adolesc Psychiatric Clin N Amer.* 2015;24;777–797.

37. Hertzman C. Framework for the social determinants of early child development. In: Tremblay RE, Boivin M, Peters RV, eds. *Encyclopedia on Early Childhood Development.* Canada: University of British Columbia; 2010:1–8.

38. Malhotra S. Socio-cultural diversity and ethnocentrism in child mental health. In: Young JG, Ferrari P, Malhotra S, Tyano S, Caffo E, eds. *Brain, Culture and Development: Tradition and Innovation in Child and Adolescent Mental Health.* New Delhi: Macmillan India; 2003:3–13.

9

The Place of Adolescence in Social Psychiatry

Eugenio M. Rothe

The Invention of Adolescence

Adolescence is defined as the developmental transition between childhood and adulthood. It is the period from puberty until the attainment of adult status, and it is characterized, among other things, by the appearance of sexual reproductive capacity. The completion of adolescence and entry into adulthood vary from culture to culture and are subject to a number of different variables. From a historical perspective, pubescent boys and girls were considered adults in many societies prior to the 1800s, and even today, this continues to be the case in non-affluent and predominantly agricultural societies. Before the common era, pubescent boys usually learned their father's trade or went into the army; girls stayed at home and were taught by their mothers. This undefined period of time usually ended in marriage, and both sexes were expected to follow strict cultural norms. Between the fifth and sixteenth centuries of the common era in Europe, girls were considered adults after the age of 14 and could marry, inherit, and bear children. However, in some countries boys did not reach legal adulthood until the age of 21. In the year 1350 the Black Plague killed half of the population in Europe, which significantly reduced the workforce; to fill this gap many countries in Europe resorted to child labor, and children 7 years and older were often sent away to work for others or to learn a trade as an apprentice. However, in wealthy families, pubertal boys continued their studies, sometimes until early adulthood. In the 1500s to 1700s in Europe, if the children were not able to work in the family farm or if the child was not the oldest or first-born, they were often sent away to work for someone else after the age of 9; most youth moved straight from childhood into adulthood, and many young people emigrated to America in search of new opportunities. In the 1700s the German writer Johann Wolfgang Von Goethe formed a part of the *Sturm und Drang* (German for

Storm and Stress) literary movement, which emerged as a counter-movement to the extreme rationality imposed by the Enlightenment and which encouraged the free expression of emotion. He published a novel titled *The Sorrows of Young Werther*,[1] in which the adolescent protagonist commits suicide after he discovers that his love is already engaged to another man, thus highlighting the impulsivity and passion attributed to adolescence. In the 1800s the Industrial Revolution increased the use of child labor, which triggered a series of social reforms in Europe and the United States, but by the 1890s in the United States only 6% of 14- to 17-year-olds were in school. The modern concept of adolescence in the United States was invented by the psychologist G. Stanley Hall (1844–1924) at Clark University in Massachusetts. At the time, the influence of Protestant clergymen in a predominantly rural nation dictated the Puritan moral tone of the country, and these clergymen advocated for a period between 14 and 25 years of age in which young men were still not ready to marry and assume patriarchal roles in a family. Young men were instead encouraged to learn a trade or profession, develop their moral characters, avoid sex, and learn self-control. Young women were encouraged to be selective about the company they kept, to cultivate religion, and to avoid reading romantic novels.[2] In contrast, G. Stanley Hall, who was influenced by the theories of Charles Darwin, saw the stage of adolescence as parallel to the history of mankind, in which humans move from a period of primitivism and savagery to a more civilized and mature stage of development, and he considered it to be an intermediate stage prior to reaching full maturity and civility. He saw adolescent development as a series of contradictory tendencies that oscillated between impulsivity and euphoria, to lethargy and depressive gloom, and where the higher qualities of altruism and idealism alternated with vanity, selfishness, and conceit. He recognized that adolescents possessed great curiosity, were extremely sensitive to rejection, depended on the approval of their peers, and that their actions oscillated between acts of tenderness, and callousness and cruelty. Hall saw human development as a constantly evolving unfinished product.

Identity Formation in Adolescence

Erik Erkison (1902–1994) theorized that the principal task of the adolescent stage of development is a consolidation of a stable sense of personal identity and avoidance of the opposite result, which he defined as role-diffusion, although the details of this may vary from culture to culture. Failure to complete a consolidation of a stable sense of personal identity would lead to alienation and confusion. According to Erikson, the adolescent must confront him- or herself with the following questions: *Who am I? Where am I going?* and *Who will I become?* The answers to these questions must be acquired through sustained individual efforts, separating from the identity of the parents, and facing change in the present and uncertainty in the future. Adolescents search for affirmation by their peer group. and once the personal identity is established, then the adolescent can move on to find intimacy or to face isolation in interpersonal relationships.[3,4,5] In addition to Erikson's two-pole conceptualization of the psychosocial tasks of adolescence of *identity vs. role-diffusion*, James Marcia[6,7] proposed two other important dimensions in adolescent development: (1)

exploration: actively questioning and weighing various identity alternatives before deciding which values, beliefs, and goals to pursue; and (2) *commitment*: making identity choices and engaging in activities to implement them.[8] Marcia classified this psychological process as having four possible distinct stages:

1. *Identity diffused or identity confused*: these are individuals who have not yet experienced an identity crisis, nor made any commitment to a vocation or set of beliefs.
2. *Foreclosure*: individuals who have not experienced crisis, but have made commitments; however, these commitments are not the result of the individual's own searching and exploring, but they are handed to the adolescent, ready-made, by others, frequently the parents.
3. *Moratorium*: this stage describes individuals who are in an acute state of crisis. They are exploring and actively searching for alternatives and struggling to find their identity, but have not yet made any commitment or have only developed very temporary kinds of commitment.
4. *Achievement of identity*: In this final, culminating stage, individuals have experienced crises but have resolved them on their own terms, and as a result of the resolution of the crisis have made a personal commitment to an occupation, a religious belief, a personal value system, and have resolved their attitude toward sexuality.

According to Marcia, the *moratorium* is the hallmark of adolescent psychological development, and he found that almost 30% of American college students were in this stage. In many developing countries, adolescents do not have the luxury of negotiating these stages, and instead are thrust into adult roles by financial necessity. The anthropologist Margaret Mead (1901–1978) also emphasized the importance of the *moratorium* stage of adolescence as a time to experiment and explore different options and concluded that it was much more difficult to complete the psychological journey of adolescence in developed countries than in primitive societies.[9] The American educator Robert Havighurst (1900–1991) summarized what he considered be the developmental tasks that needed to be completed by the end of adolescence: (1) accepting one's physique and accepting a masculine or feminine role; (2) new relations with age-mates of both sexes; (3) emotional independence of parents and other adults; (4) achieving assurance of economic independence; (5) selecting and preparing for an occupation; (6) developing intellectual skills and concepts necessary for civic competence; (7) desiring and achieving socially responsible behavior; (8) preparing for marriage and family life; (9) building conscious values in harmony with an adequate scientific world-picture).[10] The Swiss psychologist Jean Piaget (1896–1980) mapped the intellectual capabilities of adolescence as the stage of *formal operations*, in which the adolescent can temporarily leave behind the objective world and enter *the world of ideas*. Now, in addition to concrete events, adolescents can also carry out symbolic operations in the mind, putting forth their own propositions and trying to prove or disprove their own hypotheses.[11] Finally, Kurt Lewin (1890–1947) who began his work at the University of Berlin, was one of the first scientists to describe the stage of adolescence as a result of a combination of social and biological influences, which at the time were considered to be contradictory.[12]

Emerging Adulthood: The Unexplored Continent

For most people living in industrialized societies, *emerging adulthood* has become a newly conceptualized developmental stage that begins in the late teens and continues through the twenties, with a focus on the ages 18–25. This stage is neither adolescence, nor adulthood, and in most industrialized societies marriage and parenthood are now delayed until the mid-twenties or late twenties. For most people, this becomes a period of exploration and an opportunity to further the individual's levels of education or to obtain valuable professional experience in order to become more competitive in the workplace. This is also a time in which various forms of interpersonal exploration take place in order to consider new possibilities in work, love, and worldviews, and by the end of this period, most people have made life choices that have enduring ramifications.[13] One particular area that defines emerging adulthood is *residential status*. In many industrialized societies, adolescents now leave the parental home by age 18 or 19 and in the United States about a third of these adolescents go to college. The residential arrangements at this age are diverse; some individuals live in dorms, share apartments, or cohabitate with a romantic partner. This period of semi-autonomy often is punctuated by varying degrees of financial dependence on the parents. Also, there are frequent changes that take place during this period, such as graduating from college, starting a full-time or part-time job, progressing to graduate education, and relocating geographically and changing residential arrangements. In the United States about 32% of people in their twenties have completed a college education, and in the course of these years these emerging adults do not see themselves as adolescents, but many of them also do not see themselves entirely as adults. Emerging adulthood is most likely to be found in countries that are highly industrialized or postindustrial. Such countries require a high level of education and training for entry into the information-based professions that are the most prestigious and lucrative, so many of their young people remain in school into their early twenties and mid-twenties. Marriage and parenthood are typically postponed until well after schooling has ended. In contrast, young people in rural areas of developing countries often receive minimal schooling, marry early, and have little choice of occupations except agricultural work. However, it should also be noted that emerging adulthood is likely to become more pervasive worldwide in the decades to come, with the increasing globalization of the world economy. As developing countries are becoming more integrated into a global economy, there is an increasing number of higher-paying jobs in these countries, jobs that require young people to obtain higher education. At the same time, as technology becomes increasingly available in developing countries, particularly in agriculture, the labor of young people is becoming less and less necessary for family survival, making it possible for many of them to attend school instead. Also, members of minority groups in industrialized countries may be less likely to experience ages 18–25 as a period of independent exploration of possible life directions, since in most industrialized countries opportunities tend to be less widely available in minority cultures than in the majority culture. However, social class may be more important than ethnicity, with young people in the middle class or above having more opportunities for the explorations of emerging adulthood than young people who are working class or below, regardless of their ethnicity. In many countries there is still no name to define this period of development that is located chronologically between adolescence and adulthood, and we continue to know very little about those individuals between 18 and 25 who are not in college; this is due to the fact that studying these young people is difficult, because they are scattered in the workplace and are not available in the confines of an institutional setting. However, there are three objective criteria that appear to clearly define the transition of emerging adulthood into full-fledged adulthood in most cultures: (1) accepting responsibility for one's self; (2) making independent decisions; and (3) becoming financially independent.[13]

The Effects of Poverty on Adolescence

Numerous studies reveal adverse cognitive, socio-emotional, and health consequences of childhood poverty.[14,15] It is safe to assume that when children grow up in poverty and face a plethora of chronic, uncontrollable stressors across multiple life domains, they may also become more helpless, persisting less when confronted with difficult, challenging situations.[16] However, very little empirical work has been done in trying to separate the effects of poverty alone, from the effects of the chaotic social circumstances that often accompany poverty, and how these two variables may function independently to affect adolescent outcomes. It is possible that the fact that these two variables are often lumped together may account for some of the heterogeneity in the research findings that explore the effects of poverty on adverse adolescent outcomes. A third variable is that of *adolescent task-persistence* in the face of adverse life circumstances. Adolescents who persist in the face of difficult challenges tend to achieve positive outcomes, but low-income children who also live in more chaotic households might persist less in the face of difficult challenges, because of the added burden of living in highly unpredictable and unstructured environments. Several studies have identified the relationship of chaos, independently from poverty on adverse child and adolescent outcomes,[17,18] and other previously mentioned studies have shown that when there is a combination of low *socioeconomic status* (SES) and chaos, all groups do poorly. Chaotic home environments include crowding, noise, family instability, and sudden geographic mobility, along with fewer structured activities and routines. which interfere with the development of competency or the belief that one can control and regulate one's environment. The inability to sustain daily predictable activities and routines, so necessary in the process of normal child and adolescent development, undermines a sense of order, continuity, and purpose in life and thus interferes with the child's ability to manage his or her own behaviors. In order to be effective, these activities must occur regularly, over a long period of time, and become progressively more complex as the child matures; chaotic circumstances can undermine these processes. In addition, parents in chaotic home environments are often less responsive to their child's need for attention, are less confident about their parental abilities, and provide positive reinforcement to their children very randomly.[17,18] In essence, in spite of the fact that the existing studies of poverty and chaos, and how they are able to produce adverse outcomes by undermining *adolescent task-persistence*, demonstrate that poverty and chaos function independently, the reality is that poverty and chaos, more often than not, tend to occur together.[15]

Adolescents in Developing Countries

The world population today is counted around 6.7 billion, and more than 1.5 billion people of the world's population are between the ages of 10 and 24 years. About 70% of the young people live in developing countries where social, economic, and health challenges are greater than those in the industrialized countries.[19] The newer generations face different challenges due to globalization, including increasing urbanization, electronic communications, AIDS, and massive migrations due to war and poverty. These challenges impact the physical, psychological, and social landscape of the adolescent period of development. Even though the transition from childhood to adulthood is universal in nature, the experiences of adolescence are by no means universal, given that every society varies in the role definitions and expectations for its young people, including gender expectations and sexual behavior. For many young people in developing countries, the dilemma of their transitory life stage is further complicated by the clashes between the many forces of Westernization and the stricter traditional values of their societies, which have an impact on their dreams, aspirations, interests in participation in the political and social lives of their societies, and the overall quality of their lives.[20] Puberty triggers emotional, cognitive, and behavioral changes in young people, and influences their relationships with others, including parents and peers. Adolescence and youth periods have been considered to be the healthiest period of a person's life due to low mortality rates; however, the changes in recent trends have given rise to concerns. One shortcoming of the adolescent health research studies in developing countries is its primary preoccupation with health problems and the very limited focus on the normal developmental issues of adolescence.

Traditionally, in Western societies, the leading health challenges of young people are sexual and reproductive health issues, accidental and intentional injuries, mental health problems, substance use and abuse, and eating disorders.[21] However, youth age 14 to adulthood in developing countries present a different picture. A recent comprehensive analysis of population health data by Patton et al.[22] clearly shows that young people in developing countries have mortality rates 2.4 times higher than in developed countries. Strikingly, almost two-thirds (1.67 million) of the global deaths among young people occurred in just two areas of the developing world, Sub-Saharan Africa and Southeast Asia, whereas only 42% of young people live in these areas; and the relative risk for death among young people is higher in Africa than in any other region, which is nearly 7 times higher than in high-income countries. Causes of death vary significantly between the regions of the world. The commonest causes of mortality among young people in several developing regions are largely preventable. Communicable diseases and pregnancy-related conditions are the leading causes of mortality among young females, ages 15–24 years, in Sub-Saharan Africa, while in Southeast Asia injury, followed by communicable diseases, has the highest contribution in this age bracket. Violence perpetrated by family members contributes substantially to the high rate of injury among females in Southeast Asia. Among the males, injury and communicable diseases are the leading causes of death in both Sub-Saharan Africa and Southeast Asia. HIV/AIDS, tuberculosis, and lower respiratory tract infections are the leading communicable diseases in the two regions.[20,22] Mortality risk in developing countries compared with developed (high-income) countries was higher for females than for males; a major reason for this pattern is the low mortality figure for young females in high-income countries, unlike the situation in many developing countries, where maternal mortality and AIDS shorten the life span of many young females.[22] More than three-quarters of young people (ages 15–24 years) living with HIV in Sub-Saharan Africa are females.[23] Sub-Saharan Africa, with about 12% of the world's population, accounts for approximately two-thirds of people living with HIV, and in parts of Africa and the Caribbean, young women (ages 15–24) are up to 6 times more likely to be infected than young men of similar ages. HIV transmission in Sub-Saharan Africa is mainly through heterosexual intercourse, and high prevalence of risky sexual behavior among young people contributes substantially to the epidemic. Also, age-mixing, resulting from sexual relationships between young girls and much older men, and sexual coercion, which are both gender-mediated, also contribute to the high HIV infection level in Sub-Saharan Africa, in addition to predisposing biological factors. In Asia, which is the region with the second-highest figure of people living with HIV, nearly half of the adult population living with HIV are under the age of 25 years, most of them males, and injecting drug use contributes substantially to the picture of HIV epidemics in Asia. Latin America and the Caribbean has the second-highest HIV prevalence rate among young people ages 15–24 years after Sub-Saharan Africa, and risky sexual behavior is a major factor in the transmission.[24] As children grow into adolescence and young adulthood, gender role differentials widen between males and females because typically, adolescent males increasingly experience privileges reserved for men in their society. These include increased autonomy, mobility, and access to developmental and economic opportunities. In contrast, adolescent females encounter more restricted mobility, reduced interaction with the opposite sex, and more limited social interaction network, and comparatively less developmental opportunities compared to their male counterparts. Traditionally, societies ascribe youth sexuality-related roles and define the boundaries of acceptable sexual behavior for males and females. Deviations from these roles are often not tolerated and attract sanctions, particularly in the case of female offenders. This pattern is still evident in many societies in developing countries. In many developing countries, society seriously frowns at premarital and extramarital behavior among females, but the same society would often condone such behaviors from young males as an expression of their masculinity. Similarly, the notion of male aggressiveness and female submissiveness as part of gender identity also contributes to poor sexual negotiations skills on the part of females and risky sexual and violence-related behavior among males. This contributes to incidences of sexual coercion, gender-based violence, HIV and other sexually transmitted infections, and unintended and unwanted pregnancies.[20] Schooling represents an important source of change and improved youth outcomes in the developing countries, since a higher proportion of young people in this generation, compared to other generations, are enrolled in school. These changes are particularly notable in Sub-Saharan Africa, with a dramatic narrowing of the gender gap across the continent. Schooling has led to delayed marriage and childbearing among young people, and opportunities for males and females to enhance their intellectual capabilities and increase their potentials to better compete for good employment. Thus, school prepares young people for productive adulthood, and has potential to contribute substantially to the adolescent transition process. It also provides an enlarged opportunity for peer-relationships, social interaction, and opportunity to bond with selected adults in form of teachers and other school staff, leading to *school connectedness*, a feeling that someone in a young person's school cares about his or her well-being. These are important developmental relationships that are associated with youth resiliency and are negatively associated with poor school performance, school dropout, early sexual initiation, risky sexual activity, violence, and substance use.[25] In many developing countries that prescribe expulsion for pregnant schoolgirls, many pregnant schoolgirls who desire to finish school are likely to resort to abortion. Unfortunately, such abortions in developing countries are often carried out in medically unsuitable environments and are handled by non-medically qualified individuals, which puts young women at risk. Yet schools also provide increased opportunity for young people, both males and females, to access essential health-related information, education, and skills that can enhance their health and well-being.[20]

The Neurobiology of Adolescence

A detailed explanation of the neurobiology of adolescence is beyond the scope of this chapter, which focuses more on the social psychiatry aspects of this stage of development. However, it is important to mention that adolescence is a time of dramatic changes, including rapid physical growth, the onset of sexual maturation, the activation of new drives and motivations, and a wide array of social and affective changes and challenges. Two of these motivational changes include: (1) *increases in sensation-seeking* (motivational tendency to want to experience high-intensity, exciting experiences), and (2) *stronger natural interest in, and pursuit of, contact with peers and potential romantic partners*. These motivational changes promote exploration of social experiences, development of skills and knowledge relevant to taking on adult social roles, individuation from family, and establishment of an individual identity, all of which represent core developmental tasks during this period in the life span. The pubertal rise in reproductive hormones activates increasing motivations to attract friends, to attain social status, and more generally, in their natural tendencies to pay more attention to, care about, and react to peer, romantic, and sexual contexts. Brain development is highly sensitive to hormone influence perinatally and again during puberty, which brings about a sharp increase in reproductive hormones and represents a reactivation of specific neuroendocrine axes that were also active in infancy.[26] Another feature that explains behavior in adolescence is related to the notion that immature neuronal processing in the prefrontal cortex and other cortical and subcortical regions, along with their interaction, leads to behavior that is biased toward risk, reward, and emotional reactivity. Recent work on the development of inhibitory interneuron circuits and their changing interaction with neuromodulatory systems during adolescence may also shed light on why illnesses like schizophrenia typically manifest at this time. A better understanding of the neurobiological changes that take place in this stage of development may lead to the development of preventive interventions for other problems common to adolescents, such as depression and substance abuse.[27] The dopamine-modulated neurobehavioral system that underlies incentive-driven behavior undergoes important changes during adolescence and has been thoroughly described, but has not been carefully considered from a developmental perspective. Studies showing differences in the hedonic value of sucrose solutions in the brains of adults versus adolescents reveal marked differences in brain functioning during these periods of life. Some studies show that adolescents, compared to adults, experience more negative affect and depressed mood, and may feel less pleasure from stimuli of low or moderate incentive value; therefore they seek stimuli of greater hedonic intensity to satisfy a deficiency in their experience of reward. Adolescents and adults may also differ in the way they integrate emotional information in decisions: adolescents may be less adept at interpreting or integrating relevant emotional content, or less effective at forming such associations. All of these changes also confer positive evolutionary advantages as the adolescent moves to explore new social environments, acquiring relevant knowledge and skills and moving toward increasing independence.[28]

Social Consequences of Rejection and Ostracism in Adolescence

The social brain is defined as the network of brain regions responsible for social cognition, which enables us to recognize others, and to evaluate our own and others' mental states, their intentions, desires, beliefs, feelings, enduring dispositions, and actions. Many different brain regions are involved in social cognition—including medial prefrontal cortex (mPFC), anterior cingulate cortex (ACC), inferior frontal gyrus, posterior superior temporal sulcus (pSTS), temporo-parietal junction (TPJ), the amygdala, and anterior insula— as well as the attribution of mental states to oneself and to others. This ability is known as *mentalizing* or *theory of mind*, which enables us to understand other people's behavior and actions in terms of underlying mental states such as intentions, desires, and beliefs.[29] There is considerable overlap between these social brain regions and regions that are still developing structurally in adolescence. Adolescence is a time during which peers, rather than parents, become influential in shaping social behavior. Functional magnetic resonance imaging (fMRI) studies have demonstrated how in early adolescence the areas of the brain involved in self-awareness and mentalizing become progressively more activated, and youth at this age become increasingly self-conscious and more aware of, and concerned with, others' opinions and social functions. It appears that adolescents use different cognitive strategies than adults to perform social cognition tasks and that structures in the brain continue to mature and become activated in the transition from adolescence to adulthood. So, as peer relationships become more important in adolescence, the potential negative consequences of rejection or victimization by peers increase. *Relational aggression* in adolescence can occur in various forms, such as socially excluding the victim using the "silent treatment," or by spreading rumors about the victim. Victims of relational aggression often have social-psychological adjustment problems, including low self-esteem, depression, and rage. Studies have demonstrated that adolescents ages 13–17 reported that peer evaluations were more important in determining their sense of personal self-worth than did younger children. Peer rejection was commonly viewed as an indication of their "unworthiness" as an individual; this peer effect on self-evaluation was most apparent in girls ages 13–15, and sensitivity to rejection appears to decline in late adolescence.[29] Williams[30,31] explains that ostracism (which derives from the word *oyster*) threatens four fundamental psychological needs: (1) *self-esteem*, (2) *belonging*, (3) *control*, and (4) *sense of meaningful existence*; and that adolescent girls at this age are the most vulnerable. So hypersensitivity to social rejection during adolescence can be explained by the neurobiological changes that take place at this stage of development.[29]

Adolescents and the Media

The current generation of adolescents are growing up in a media-saturated world and social-media use is currently one of the most popular leisure activities, but it is currently unclear how social media influences the maturational trajectories of brain regions involved in social interactions. As discussed earlier, adolescents are highly sensitive to acceptance and rejection, and this plays out clearly in their interaction with social media. Adolescents can access social media though a variety of different platforms (mobile or computer devices), for different activities (interacting with real-life friends, meeting others based on shared interests, chatting, mailing, sharing or creating pictures, videos, blogging, dating, playing games, and gambling). Facebook is one of the most popular social media among 13–17-year-old adolescents in the United States. However, to date, there is no consensus among researchers regarding the definition of *problematic social-media use*. Some studies on adolescents who overuse social media have demonstrated academic difficulties and problems in interpersonal relationships, which in turn are also correlated to depression. Also, some studies have revealed patterns of addictive behavior with respect to the amount of time spent on media devices, and irritability and anxiety when use of media is denied.[32]

In a sample of Spanish adolescents with *problematic social-media use,* empirical measures demonstrated that adolescents who engaged with social media while performing other activities, such as homework (multi-tasking) made more mistakes (dys-executive problems) in everyday life and had worse cognitive functioning in the components related with working memory, processing speed, and lower academic achievement in language and math.[33] *Social media aggression and victimization* among adolescents have also been another point of concern. In a study addressing these issues, adolescents who reported experiencing social-media aggression and victimization were rated by their parents as more maladjusted, and the parents were frequently unaware that their children were being bullied, or were bullying others, on social media. In these studies, media aggression and victimization were found to be highly correlated with oppositional defiant disorder in the aggressors and depression in the victims. In addition, youth with a diagnosis of attention deficit hyperactivity disorder (ADHD) were often not aware that their communications victimized others. However, what is still unclear is how media influences the maturational trajectories of brain regions involved in social interactions.[34]

The Need for a Worldwide Adolescent Mental Health Policy

Children and adolescents, by and large, have no voice, no political or economic influence, and often abrogated rights, so in 1977 the World Health Organization (WHO) recommended that every country throughout the world should have a National Plan for Child Mental Health.[35] Child and adolescent mental health policy in developing and developed countries is essential for the rational development of systems of care for children. The current science base related to child and adolescent mental disorders is not widely appreciated. Consequently, inappropriate strategies derived only from adult experience often find their way into regulations impacting children. Shatkin and Belfer[36] conducted a study to identify all existing national mental health policies worldwide in which no country was excluded, and the only limitation was that of an inability to find an identifiable policy through the means described. Soon after this study was published, the WHO published a second document to serve as a guide to help nations strategize for the development of mental health legislation, policies, and action plans. This document is titled *Mental Health Policy and Service Guidance Package, World Health Organization, Child and Adolescent Mental Health Policies and Plans.*[37] Currently there are very few countries for which one is able to identify a clearly enumerated child and adolescent mental health policy of any sort. Fourteen countries worldwide were found to have policies both prior to 1990 and since 1990. Nineteen countries lacked an identifiable policy prior to 1990 but developed one sometime after 1990. Of the 191 countries recognized by the United Nations, only 35 countries were found to have identifiable mental health policies that might impact children and adolescents, 11 of which are European. Considering that there are 191 member countries of the WHO, only 7% of countries worldwide (14 of 191) were found to have a clearly articulated child and adolescent mental health policy. Finally, it is rare to find health policy of any sort that integrates publicly and privately supported programming. There are many reasons for the fact that child and adolescent mental health has been left behind in the arena of health policy: (1) the relatively new development of this field of knowledge; (2) the lack of appreciation of a developmental perspective related to mental disorders; (3) stigma; (4) a fragmented advocacy constituency; (5) the reluctance of professionals to engage in debates over policy; and (6) there is no single study or consistent set of independent studies on the epidemiology of child and adolescent disorders in the past 20 years that can be identified as definitive or relevant across societies. The recent delineation of *cultural epidemiology*,[38] combining classical epidemiology with the information derived from cultural anthropological study, offers a unifying approach that may advance the understanding of child and adolescent disorders as seen in developing countries and inform our understanding in clinical settings worldwide. Two of the most important barriers in developing mental healthcare for children and adolescents worldwide include financial constraints and lack of trained professionals. In addition, the move toward *privatization* of mental healthcare constitutes a disturbing trend in many countries. This appears to be a progressive modernization trend, but in resource-poor countries the move away from state-subsidized care toward private care leaves many without any care at all. Also, governments that adopt *managed-care* algorithms often do not understand the many negative consequences that have been seen in the Western Hemisphere countries over time. Managed care is too often focused on cost saving and not on a more altruistic mission of improving the appropriateness and quality of care.[36] The lack of trained child and adolescent psychiatrists in many countries around the world leaves the primary care provider, possessing inconsistent degrees of expertise, as the central figure in the provision of child and adolescent mental health. Special populations of repatriated child soldiers and the growing numbers of child and adolescent refugees and street children that abound in large urban areas around the world are a vivid reminder of the many children who have been deprived of an environment that could support healthy development and the need for a worldwide health policy for children and adolescents. Of even more concern in countries around the world are the increasing immigrant populations. These present with child and adolescent mental health problems that are a direct extension of the traumatic experiences in their home countries, or are related to the difficult task of making an adjustment to a new country. Understanding and treating these contemporary psychological problems are essential if one has an international perspective. They represent some of the many challenges that lay ahead that can be better understood when addressed through the lens of *social psychiatry.*

References

1. Goethe JW. *The Sorrows of Young Werther* [1774]. Boylan RD, trans. Demetra Publishing, Bulgaria; 2018. www.digireads.com.
2. Kett JF. Reflections on the history of adolescence in America. *Hist Fam.* 2003;8:355–373.
3. Erikson EH. *Identity and the Life Cycle: Selected Papers.* Psychological Issues Monograph Series I, No. 1. New York: International Universities Press; 1959.
4. Erikson EH. *The Challenge of Youth.* Garden City, NY: Anchor Books; 1965.
5. Erikson EH. *Identity: Youth and Crisis.* New York: W. W. Norton; 1968.
6. Marcia JE. Development and validation of ego identity status. *J Pers Soc Psychol.* 1966;3:551–558.
7. Marcia JE. Ego identity status: relationship to change in self-esteem, general adjustment and authoritarianism. *J Pers.* 1967;35:118–133.
8. Crocetti, E. Identity formation in adolescence: the dynamics of forming and consolidating identity commitments. *Child Dev Perspect.* 2017;11(2):145–150.
9. Mead M. *Coming of Age in Samoa.* New York: Harper Collins; 2001.
10. Havighurst R. *Adolescent Character and Personality.* New York: Wiley and Sons; 1949.
11. Singer DG, Revenson TA. *A Piaget Primer: How the Child Thinks.* Rev. ed. New York: Penguin Books;1996.
12. Lewin K. *Resolving Social Conflicts in Field Theory and Social Science.* Washington, DC: American Psychological Association; 1997.
13. Arnett JJ. Emerging adulthood: a theory of development from the late teens to the twenties. *Am Psychol.* 2000;55(5):469–480.
14. Blair C, Raver CC. Child development in the context of adversity. *Am Psychol.* 2012;67:309–318.
15. Fuller-Rowell TE, Evans GW, Paul E, Curtis DS. The role of poverty and chaos in the development of task persistence among adolescents. *J Res Adolesc.* 2014;25: 4, 606–613.
16. Peterson C, Maier R, Seligman MEP. *Learned Helplessness.* New York: Oxford University Press; 1993.
17. Ackerman BP, Brown ED. Physical and psychosocial turmoil in the home and cognitive development. In: Evans GW, Wachs TD, eds. *Chaos and Children's Development: Levels of Analysis and Mechanisms.* Washington, DC: American Psychological Association; 2010:35–48.

18. Fiese BH, Winter MA. The dynamics of family chaos and its relation to children's socio-emotional well-being. In Evans GW, Wachs TD, eds. *Chaos and Children's Development: Levels of Analysis and Mechanisms*. Washington, DC: American Psychological Association; 2010:49–66.

19. United Nations. *Young People*. 2009. Available at: www.icpd2015.org/assets/pdf/Young%20People.

20. Fatusi AO, Hindin MJ. Adolescents and youth in developing countries: Health and development issues in context. *J Adolesc*. 2010;33:499–508.

21. World Health Organization. *Growing in Confidence: Programming for Adolescent Health and Development*. Geneva: WHO; 2002. WHO/FCH/CAH/02.13.

22. Patton GC, Coffey C, Sawyer SM, et al. Global patterns of mortality in young people: a systematic analysis of population health data. *Lancet*, 2009;374:881–892.

23. Santosa RF. Young people, sexual and reproductive health and HIV. *Bull WHO*. 2009;87:877–879.

24. United Nations Population Fund (UNFPA). HIV/AIDS: what does gender have to do with it? Chapter 13. *State of the World Population*. 2005. Available at: http://www.unfpa.org/swp/2005/english/ch4/chap4_page1.htm.

25. Hewett PC, Lloyd CB. Progress towards "education for all": trends and current challenges for sub-Saharan Africa. In Lloyd CB, Behrman J, Stromquist NP, Cohen B, eds. *The Changing Transitions to Adulthood in Developing Countries: Selected Studies*. Washington, DC: National Academies Press; 2005:84–117.

26. Forbes EE, Dahl RE. Pubertal development and behavior: hormonal activation of social and motivational tendencies. *Brain Cogn*. 2010;72: 66–72.

27. Blakemore SJ. The social brain in adolescence. *Nature Rev Neurosci*. 2008 Apr;9:267–276.

28. Wahlstrom D, Collins P, White T, Luciana M. Developmental changes in dopamine neurotransmission in adolescence: behavioral implications and issues in assessment. *Brain Cogn*. 2010;72:146–159.

29. Sebastian C, Viding E, Kipling D, Williams KD, Blakemore SJ. Social brain development and the affective consequences of ostracism in adolescence. *Brain Cogn*. 2010;72:134–145.

30. Williams KD. *Ostracism: The Power of Silence*. New York: Guilford Press; 2001.

31. Williams KD. Ostracism. *Ann Rev Psychol*. 2007;58:425–452.

32. BaÂnyai F, ZsilaA Â, KiraÂly O, et al. Problematic social media use: results from a large-scale nationally representative adolescent sample. *PLoS ONE* 2017;12(1):e0169839. doi: 10.1371/journal.pone.0169839. eCollection 2017.

33. Martín-Perpiñá MM, Viñas Poch F, Malo-Cerrato S. *Psicothema*, 2019;31(1):81–87. doi: 10.7334/psicothema2018.178.

34. Barry CT, Briggs SM, Sidoti CL. Adolescent and parent reports of aggression and victimization on social media: associations with psychosocial adjustment. *J Child Fam Studies*. 2019;28:2286–2296.

35. World Health: the magazine of the World Health Organization: November 1977: Traditional Medicine. 5 June 1977 Publication; https://www.who.int/publications/i/item/WH-1977

36. Shatkin JP, Belfer ML. The global absence of child and adolescent mental health policy. *Child Adolesc Mental Health*. 2004;9(3):104–108.

37. World Health Organization. *Mental Health Policy and Service Guidance Package, World Health Organization, Child and Adolescent Mental Health Policies and Plans*. 2005. https://www.who.int/mental_health/policy/Childado_mh_module.pdf.

38. Weiss, MG. Cultural epidemiology: an introduction and overview. *Anthropol Med*. 2001;8: 1, 5–30.

10

Social Psychiatry

Aging

Carl I. Cohen and Kyra Doumlele

What Is Old Age?

It is apropos to begin a chapter on social psychiatry and aging by pointing out how the definition of aging is largely socially determined. In Western countries, the demarcation of "elderly" at age 65 largely arose in the 20th century because of its association with government retirement age pensions that often began at that age. This age was a political decision, not based on any biological criteria. In the literature, demarcations for older adults may be 65, 60 (e.g., World Health Organization studies) and even 50 or 55 (e.g., for persons with schizophrenia who seem to have accelerated aging and higher mortality rates). Although some gerontologists have proposed ages based on physical decline and physiological changes—e.g., age 75—there is no consensus on what these criteria would entail and how they might apply across societies.[1]

The Grey Tsunami

The world population of elderly adults is increasing dramatically. Between 2015 and 2050, the global population aged 60 and over will more than double, from about 900 million people (12% of all people) to about 2 billion people (22%).[2] In 2020, in Western Europe, the United States, and Japan, the percentage of persons age 60 and over represented between one-quarter to one-third of the population. Although the percentages are lower in India and China, the absolute number of elders is growing most dramatically in these countries. Likewise, in other developing countries in Asia, Africa, and Latin America, increased longevity and lower fertility rates are producing populations with proportionately more elderly persons. Thus, the classic population pyramid of a small number of older adults resting atop a wide base of middle-age and younger adults has now been reconfigured so that it looks more like a rectangle. This is troubling since it makes it more difficult for the base to provide support for their elders at the top. The potential impact on societies and the well-being of older adults is enormous.

Political Economy and Aging

Link and Phelan have described underlying social factors ("fundamental causes") that account for many of the health conditions that arise in people.[3] Understanding mental distress in older adults requires an appreciation of the impact of late capitalism on aging populations. Specifically, three trends—globalization of markets, urbanization, and migration (internal and external)—have dramatically altered the life situations of aging individuals.[1] For example, in recent decades, agriculture can no longer support families in developing countries, and younger persons have moved to cities within the same country or have migrated abroad. More than 2% of the world's population lives in countries that were not their birthplace. There is also internal migration in developed countries. Thus, in the United States, persons 65 and over represent proportionately more of the population in rural versus urban areas (18% versus 13%). Elders who were traditionally revered and valued because they owned the land, were sources of traditional knowledge, controlled various resources, and assisted with respect to shelter and grandchild care, have lost their esteemed roles. Moreover, they are often left behind in rural areas with minimal support. Paradoxically, this rapid modernization has had a profound effect on several Eastern countries that have a strong collectivist and Confucian influence of filial piety; recent studies have found more negative views about older adults in many of these countries versus several Western countries that have much a more individualistic focus.[4] It should be underscored that the impact of these changes is differentially influenced by social class and gender. Moreover, it has been observed that these transformations may historically follow a J-shaped curve: in the early phases of social change the occupational and economic status of older persons may decline, but with advanced stages, they may rise relative to younger groups.[4]

In developing countries, many older persons have also been part of the global urban migration, arriving at a younger age and growing older in their new city. Others arrive later in life, often to assist their children in household duties and childcare. For example, in the United States, about 60% of immigrants aged 65 and older entered the country more than 40 years ago and have aged in place; about 10% had been in the country fewer than 10 years and have left their lifelong social connections to join their family in a country where they are unfamiliar with the culture and language.[4] These dramatic and deep-seated social changes can have a marked influence on the psychological well-being of older adults.

In classic Marxist theory, older adults in market societies are generally viewed as "surplus labor." That is, because of their lack of robustness versus younger persons, they are less able to find work. With no source of income, and if they have not accumulated enough savings, they must be cared for by family or by society. Most societies have created a "moral economy" in which persons who are not productive are cared for by society. In developed countries, a variety of government safety net programs have been created to care for elders.

However, as the number of retirees has increased dramatically in recent years, many countries are finding it more difficult to support these programs.

In developing countries, the burden for caring for the elderly falls upon the family. Nevertheless, as noted above, the shrinking base of younger citizens makes it more difficult to care for the aging population in both the developed and developing worlds. In the developed world, some of the proportionate decline in native workers has been augmented by immigration. However, increasingly, this has been met by political resistance in the host countries. While migration may diminish the number of younger persons in their country of origin, this may be offset by money that migrants send to their families in their homeland.

Social and Social Psychological Theories of Aging

Social and psychological theories can enhance our appreciation of various issues of aging, as well as provide theoretical underpinnings to gerontological research. Social theories on aging can be categorized as micro level or macro level, with the former focusing on the individual and the latter on the impact of social structures. The micro-level theories favor a normative perspective—i.e., focus on basic properties of individuals or their social interactions—whereas the macro-level theories tend to be interpretive, i.e., understanding how broader social and cultural forces shape human behavior.[5] Each of these theories has provided models for predicting well-being in later life. A major weakness of these theories, especially on the microlevel, has been their bias toward Western cultures and norms.

Social and Social Psychological Theories of Aging	
Micro Level	**Description**
Disengagement Theory[6]	Withdrawal of the individual from previous roles and activities is natural and protective. In this theory, the older individual and society are mutual participants in this process of disengagement.
Activity Theory[7]	Society imposes withdrawal on older adults, and those who can maintain or replace the activities and social connections of middle age are most likely to find fulfillment.
Continuity Theory[8]	Individuals adapt to aging by attempting to maintain continuity with past life experiences in terms of their inner psychological characteristics and outer social circumstances
Exchange Theory[9]	The degree of engagement in old age is the result of a specific exchange relationship between an individual or group of individuals and the society. Because power resources decline with increased age, older persons become increasingly unable to enter balanced exchange relations with other groups.
Selective Optimization Theory[10]	Successful aging occurs when resilience and adaptation allow the older individual to counterweigh an increasingly negative balance between gains and losses. Through optimization, these remaining skills are utilized disproportionately to compensate for deficits in other areas.
Personality Theory[11]	Successful aging is contingent on outer and inner factors. The outer factors are composed of transitional life events, e.g., marriage, that, when they occur outside of usual time frames, (e.g., early widowhood), can have negative psychological effects. Inner factors, specifically personality type, determine ability to cope with the adaptations necessary for successful aging.

Social and Social Psychological Theories of Aging	
Macro Level	**Description**
Socio-Environmental Theory of Aging[12]	Aging involves the interplay of individual resources (e.g., social capital) and their environment (e.g., community characteristics). The role of the individual within their immediate social environment and the status of this community within the greater society influence the outcomes of the older adult.
Modernization Theory[13]	As societies modernize—transitioning from farm and craft production within families to an industrial mode of production outside the home—the status of older people tends to diminish.
Subculture of Aging[14]	A subculture of older persons forms through a combination of social exclusion and shared experiences and interests. Older adults who fail to find their new role within this subculture risk isolation.
Political Economy of Old Age[15]	Refers to how the economy and government reciprocally interact and affect the distribution of social goods. It can provide a framework for examining the larger social context of problems of later life, and it can be used as a method for analyzing the structural social conditions that affect the socioeconomic determinants of the aging experience in various societies.
Critical Gerontology[16]	Its main goal is to identify wider societal influences on the problems that are examined in aging research, to explore how theorizing is done, and to analyze the consequences of different patterns of research and theory building. It is especially useful in showing how cultural categories enter the field of gerontological research.
Age Stratification Perspective[17]	Members of society may be stratified by age, just as they are stratified by race, class, and gender. Thus, different age groups will have varying access to social resources such as political and economic power, and in some societies, older adults may be discriminated against.

Mental Health Outcomes

Successful Aging

Outcomes with respect to psychiatric status in later life have been examined on a continuum from the degree of psychopathology on one side (see below) to a positive mental health perspective on the other. The latter seeks to describe and explain the factors that contribute to success in the aging process. Rowe and Kahn defined successful aging as "freedom from disability and high cognitive, physical, and social functioning."[18(pp143-149)] Depp and Jeste built upon this definition and worked toward systematically standardizing an optimal definition and measurement of so-called successful aging based on its use as a variable in existing literature.[19] They found that most studies defined this conceptually as an absence of physical disability/physical performance and, to a lesser extent, an absence of cognitive impairment. They also acknowledged that older adults themselves report specific variables to be important for successful aging, including resilience and positive spirituality.

Social Factors and Mental Disorders in Older Adults

Design Issues

In looking at psychopathology and associated social variables, it is important to recognize that these variables are often proximal to the more distal ("fundamental") causes. Thus, gender is associated with higher rates of depression and anxiety in older persons, but it is critical to know whether there are any distal social factors that make women more prone to these disorders. Of course, it may be solely a biological phenomenon, although this is unlikely unless proven otherwise. Moreover, a critical assessment of the validity of the effect of social variables on psychiatric illness in older adults necessitates a consideration of methodological issues that affect findings. Among the methodological concerns that need to be considered are the following:

1. Clinical data may be biased by including only persons who have access to care, which in turn is determined by social class, education, gender, and various cultural factors.
2. Many studies are derived from clinical samples so that they may not be representative of the entire population.
3. Psychiatric symptoms may be expressed differently across cultures and may not be identified as psychiatric symptoms by commonly used assessment instruments.
4. Causal inferences are limited by cross-sectional rather than prospective data.
5. Sample sizes may not have sufficient power to identify significant social variables.
6. Confounding variables such as education and social class may not be adequately controlled.
7. Models may examine variables additively but do not account for interactive or mutually transforming (dialectical) relationships
8. Qualitative data are lacking so that social variables are not fully examined subjectively or contextually.

Specific Disorders

In this section, we examine sociodemographic and other social factors associated with the most common disorders found in later life. Whenever possible, we have included comprehensive reviews, meta-analyses, cross-national studies, or big data community studies. We have focused on general community studies since rates are much higher in clinical populations (e.g., medically ill) or institutionalized settings such as nursing homes.[20] Furthermore, we have focused on studies from the past decade, but the paucity of studies necessitated including some older publications.

Depression

Does Depression Differ by Age?

There have been several cross-national community studies of major depressive disorders. The WHO World Mental Health Survey of 18 countries found 12-month prevalence rates of DSM-IV major depressive disorder (MDD) of 2.6% and 7.5% in developed and developing countries, respectively.[21] In developed countries, the elderly group had significantly lower rates of MDD than the younger group (range: 5.1% to 7.0%), whereas there were no significant differences in the developing countries, with the rates of MDD in the younger group ranging from 5.3% to 6.8%. In virtually all the developed countries, elderly persons had the lowest rates of major depressive episodes; this varied in developing countries, and in the Ukraine elderly adults had the highest rate (13%). An expanded version of this study was published in 2015 that examined 24 countries and again found elderly adults had about half the rates of MDD for lifetime and 12-month prevalence; rates of comorbid anxiety with the MDD were also lower in the oldest age group.[22] Older adults in both developing and developed countries had longer episodes of MDD than younger persons, but were found to have less clinically severe episodes in the developed but not in the developing countries.[21] Haigh and colleagues concluded that findings from a systematic review of more recent longitudinal studies support the notion that depression in older adulthood is associated with a worse course trajectory than in younger persons—likely moderated by depression severity, number of previous episodes, and medical comorbidity.[23] Although data are somewhat unreliable, Fiske and coauthors estimated that about half of geriatric major depression arises in old age.[24]

While there were significant differences in MDD by age, the differences in depressive symptoms by age are less consistent. Some studies demonstrate an inverse relationship, and others a U-shaped relationship between depressive symptoms and increasing age.[25-27] Beekman and coauthors' review of the worldwide prevalence rates of depression in older adults (age 55+) found prevalence rates varied when assessing for the presence of any clinically significant depressive symptoms, ranging from 2.4% in Japan to 35% in China.[28] Prevalence rates were more consistent, however, when studies specifically assessed for MDD. The prevalence of MDD ranged from 0.4% in Japan to 10.2% in Australia; the latter was the only study that reported a prevalence rate above 5%.

Do Depression and Suicidality Differ by Geographic Area?

Although there are cross-national differences, and the prevalence rates of MDD differ by as much as 10-fold, they are in a relatively narrow band. Kessler and colleagues' cross-national study found a prevalence range of between 1.0% and 6.0%, if the outlier Ukraine (13%) was excluded.[21] Likewise, Beekman and coauthors' cross-national review found a range of 0.4% to 5%, if Australia (10%) was excluded.[28]

A meta-analysis by Purtle and colleagues found that depression prevalence was significantly higher among older urban residents in 10 studies and significantly higher among rural residents in 3 studies (all 3 conducted in China), and there were no differences in 5 studies.[29] The associations between urban-rural residence and depression generally remained significant after adjusting for covariates, although several recent studies in China found no differences after controlling for socioeconomic status. In developed countries, the odds of depression were significantly higher among urban than rural residents (pooled OR = 1.44). However, in developing countries, this association was not observed (pooled OR = 0.91).

Shah examined the WHO's 1-year average of suicide rates for persons aged 65+ and found that there were wide cross-national variations in elderly suicide rates.[30] Elderly suicide rates were the lowest in Caribbean and Arabic/Islamic countries, and the highest in Central and Eastern European countries emerging from the former Soviet Union, some Asian, and some Western European countries. In Western countries suicide rates increased with age, at least until age 75, whereas the trend is more variable in developing countries. Globally, suicide rates among men are greater than among women, but there are some notable exceptions; for example, in China, rates among older women may exceed those among men.[31] Within countries, there are also marked differences in suicide rates.[32] For example, in the United States, suicide rates for African Americans and Latino American elders are lower than for Whites, whereas rates among Japanese, Chinese, and Korean American elders are comparable to those for Whites.

What Social Variables Are Associated with Depression?

There have been several extensive reviews that have looked at social variables associated with depression. [28,33,34] A limitation of these reviews was that most articles came from Western European countries and North America. Some recent articles from China have helped supplement these findings.[35-37] It should be underscored that there has been considerable inconsistency with respect to the strength of the associations between various social variables and depression in older adults. The most consistent findings in the literature are that higher rates of depressive symptoms and clinical depression are associated with women, negative stressful events, low income, lower education, being unmarried, widowhood (especially for men), lower quality of life, living in institutions, smaller social networks, low perceived social support, and loneliness. Clearly, there is some overlap among these variables, and their associations with depression might be further attenuated if confounding variables had been controlled for in all studies.

The literature is sparse with respect to mental disorders in older immigrants. In one of the more comprehensive studies, Aichberger and co-investigators studied persons age 50 years and older in 11 European countries and found that first-generation migrants in Northern and Western Europe had higher rates of depression than did their indigenous age peers.[38] Although migrants in Southern Europe had higher rates of depression, these rates did not differ significantly from those of their indigenous age peers. Greater age, lower income, female gender, and physical illness contributed to depression. Van der Wurff and associates postulated that depression risk for immigrants likely depends on the interplay of ethnicity, social class, and health factors.[39]

Anxiety Disorders

Do Anxiety Disorders Differ by Age?

There have been only a few cross-national assessments of anxiety disorders so that comparisons are more difficult. A recent study of 5 European countries and Israel of persons aged 65 and over found a 12-month mean prevalence of any anxiety disorder of 17.2%.[40] This exceeded the 11.6% prevalence rate for depression in that study.[41] The investigators found that compared to persons in the age 65–70 age range, persons age 75+ and age 80+ showed a decrease in anxiety disorders by over 40% and 47%, respectively. In an American study using National Comorbidity Survey Replication data[42] and in a Chilean study,[43] 12-month prevalence rates of anxiety in elderly persons were less than half of those of their younger counterparts. Unlike the European study, the American and Chilean data showed that there was little change in anxiety prevalence rates with increasing age after 65.[43,44] Anxiety often begins early in life, but roughly one-quarter of persons reported an onset of anxiety disorder after age 50.[45]

Do Anxiety Disorders Differ by Geographic Area?

In two cross-national studies of anxiety in older adults there were narrow bands of prevalence—14.4% (Italy) to 20.8% (United Kingdom) in the European study[40] cited above and 0.1% (rural China) to 9.6% (urban Peru) in a study of seven Asian and Latin American countries,[46] although there were considerable differences in the ranges between the two studies. Of note, the prevalence rate for the large American study described above was much closer to the rates found in the latter. The differences between studies may reflect varying methods of assessment as well as reporting issues.

There has been considerable variation in the frequency of the subtypes of anxiety disorders in geriatric samples, with the highest rates for agoraphobia (4.9%) in the European study,[40] specific phobia (4.7%) in the American study,[42] and generalized anxiety disorder (7.3%) in a Dutch study.[47] Here again, the differences in prevalence rates most likely reflect differences in the instruments used and diagnostic criteria.

With respect to urban/rural differences, the Asian/Latin American study[46] found that living in an urban setting was associated with twice the risk of having an anxiety disorder. A review by Vink and coworkers found only two studies examining urban versus rural residence in anxiety (both in the Netherlands) in elderly people, and neither found it to be significant.[34]

What Social Variables Are Associated with Anxiety Disorders?

As with depression, all social risk variables show inconsistencies.[34,40,45,47] Somewhat less is known about anxiety than depression since there have been fewer studies in older adults. Female gender and low social support are most consistently associated with anxiety disorders. There have been a few studies that have found anxiety disorders to be linked to lower quality of life, stressful life events, lower education and poverty. Marital status has not been found to be associated with anxiety disorders.

Dementia

How Does Age Affect Dementia Prevalence?

Dementias (also known as "major neurocognitive disorders") are diseases associated with advancing age. The prevalence of dementia (mild-moderate-severe) in age groups of 5-year differences is similar worldwide, starting from 1950, and that this will be the case until 2050:[48] 1% in age group 60–64 years; 1.5% in 65–69 years; 3% in 70–74 years; 6% in 75–79 years; 13% in 80–84 years; 24% in 85–89 years; 34% in 90–94 years; and 45% in 95 years. There are approximately 55 million persons worldwide with dementia,[49] and about half live in Asia, and nearly three-fifths reside in low- and middle-income countries.[50] The proportion in middle- and low-income countries is expected to rise to 70% by 2050.[51]

Does Dementia Differ by Geographic Area?

Wimo and colleagues estimated the worldwide prevalence of dementia (age 65+) at 6.1%, with prevalence rates of 7.2% in developed countries and 5.4% in developing countries.[52] The rates ranged from 4.7% (Melanesia) to 7.9% (North America and Northern Europe). More recently, Prince and coauthors reported a range of 2% to 4% for Sub-Saharan Africa to 8.5% for Latin America (age 60+).[51] Most countries fell within a narrow band of 5% to 7%.

More than two decades ago, Keefover and co-investigators described mixed findings regarding urban-rural differences in dementia: roughly one-third of studies showed no differences, one-third had lower rates in urban areas, and one-third had lower rates in rural areas.[53] In 2012, a large review by Russ and coauthors found that rural living is associated significantly with an increased risk of Alzheimer's disease but not dementia in general; however, the fact that few studies have been conducted in resource-poor countries limited the generalizability of these results.[54] More recently, a large-scale survey by Weden and colleagues in the United States found that after adjusting for sociodemographic and health factors there remained persistent rural disadvantages for developing dementia (OR = 1.79).[55] Likewise, recent European studies in Spain, Portugal, and Ireland have reported a higher prevalence of cognitive impairment and dementia in rural than in urban areas due, at least in part, to differences in the sociodemographic composition of the populations by age and education,[56] whereas two American studies found no difference.[57,58]

What Social Variables Are Associated with Dementia?

There are many inconsistencies in the literature, but there is modestly strong evidence that women are at greater risk for Alzheimer's disease as well as dementia in general, disproportionate to their over-representation in the aging population, and have higher rates even at the same age;[59–62] however, some studies, such as one in rural Greece, found no gender differences.[63] Higher prevalence rates in women may reflect their lower education levels in many countries, the fact that men die earlier from cardiovascular disease so that the surviving men may be healthier, possible interactive effects with estrogen, and genetic risk factors such as *APOE4* having a stronger effect in women.[59] Lower educational levels are frequently reported as associated with higher rates of dementia, and may be independent of low socioeconomic status, which is also a risk factor.[59,60,64,65] Several writers have identified diminished social participation or loneliness as associated with higher rates of dementia and as a possible risk factor, although this has not been a consistent finding in the literature.[66,67] There have been compelling findings of ethnic differences in the rates of dementia in various countries. For example, Hamid and colleagues noted that there are ethnic differences in dementia rates in Singapore (Malays and Indians have higher rates than Chinese), Malaysia (Bumiputera and Malays have higher rates than Chinese and Indians), and in the United States (African Americans and Hispanics have higher rates than Whites).[60] However, these differences have been thought to reflect educational and social class differences, and the associated risks of unhealthy lifestyles and social stress.[60,68] Indeed, Yaffe and associates found that Black/White differences in dementia risk were eliminated after controlling for differences in participants' characteristics, in particular socioeconomic status.[68]

Schizophrenia and Psychoses

How Does Age Affect the Incidence and Prevalence of Psychotic Symptoms and Disorders?

Psychoses is either primary (caused by a psychiatric disorder) or secondary (due to a medical or neurological disorder). About three-fifths of psychotic disorders in later life are due to a secondary condition, most commonly dementia.[69] In this section, we have limited our discussion to psychotic persons without dementia, although study designs have varied in how they excluded such disorders. The prevalence of psychotic symptoms in non-demented older adults has been estimated to be between 1% and 13.4%.[70] The median prevalence in these studies was 3%. One study from Western Europe found increasing prevalence of psychotic symptoms with advancing age, so that rates were under 2% in persons aged 65–74, but 4% and 7% in those aged 85–94 and 95–104, respectively.[71] Using a large national data set in the United States, Cohen and Marino found lower rates of psychotic symptoms in persons aged 65 and over, but these differences became nonsignificant after controlling for other variables.[72] It was not possible in this study to determine if symptom prevalence increased in the very old. A recent literature survey found that the prevalence of non-affective psychotic disorders (NAP) in older adults ranged between 0.1% and 4.7%, and the median prevalence was 1.2%.[70] The majority of studies find schizophrenia to be the most common NAP disorder. A large-scale review by Jongsma and coworkers reported the incidence of NAP to be about 8 times higher in those under 60 versus those in the 60–64 age group (persons over 65 were not included).[73] Notably, the National Comorbidity Survey-Replication included elderly adults and found prevalence of NAP to be about 3 to 4 times higher in those under 60 versus those age 60 and over.[74] On the other hand, Stafford and colleagues' literature review found evidence that the prevalence of NAP may rise after age 65, although there was considerable variation across studies.[75]

Older adults with schizophrenia can be divided into two groups: early onset (typically defined as prior to age 40 or 45) and late onset, which begins after these age cutoffs. Approximately 20%–25% of patients with schizophrenia have an onset of the disorder after age 40.[76] A Dutch case-register of persons with schizophrenia aged 60 and over found that 64% had early-onset schizophrenia, suggesting that the loss of early-onset individuals (to death or recovery) may be compensated for by the influx of cases with a later onset.[77] Stafford and coworkers found that disproportionately more elderly persons are diagnosed with NAP than schizophrenia, which they thought might be due to the elders' more atypical presentations of psychotic symptoms in the context of medical illness and disability.[75]

Are There Geographical Differences in the Prevalence of Schizophrenia?

To our knowledge there are no cross-national epidemiological studies of older adults with schizophrenia or psychotic disorders or any comparisons between urban and rural elders with these disorders. Saha and colleagues conducted a comprehensive cross-national review of the prevalence of schizophrenia in broad-age-range samples from 46 countries.[78] They found that prevalence rates were lower in the least-developed countries versus emerging and developed nations. Moreover, they found no urban, rural, or mixed site differences. It is not known whether older adults would follow the same patterns.

What Social Variables Are Associated with Psychotic Disorders?

Compared to older adults with early-onset schizophrenia, persons with the late-onset disorder are more likely to be married, to have successful work histories, and to be female. Strikingly, the incident rate of schizophrenia for men is about 1.4 times that of women in younger samples,[79] whereas women may comprise up to 66%–87% of patients with onset after the age of 40–50 years.[80] Stafford and co-investigators found that rates of NAP are also higher among older women, although this was not found as consistently as with late-onset schizophrenia.[75] The reasons for incident differences in gender are not entirely clear. It is postulated that estrogen plays a protective role in the development of schizophrenia due to its mild antidopaminergic effects, and its decline during menopause unmasks some women's inherent vulnerability to schizophrenia (this is known as the "estrogen theory").[81,82] However, the estrogen theory does not provide an explanation for males who develop late-onset schizophrenia or for women who despite having the benefit of estrogen develop schizophrenia before the age of 40. It is also possible that men develop biological and/or psychosocial protection against schizophrenia as they grow older. Other social factors found to be associated with late-onset schizophrenia include social isolation and lower educational and occupational levels than their age peers, although these differences have been less consistently replicated.[70,75]

There have been two longitudinal studies of outcome (clinical remission) among persons aged 55 and over with schizophrenia. With respect to social indicators, a study in New York City of community-dwelling elders found that higher levels of community integration and having more entitlements were associated with higher rates of remission on 52-month follow-up.[83] A study in the Netherlands derived from catchment-area data found that higher remission after 5 years was associated with having a partner.[84] Age and gender were not significant in either study.

There are compelling data showing higher rates of schizophrenia among immigrants versus people in the host population or in the immigrants' country of origin.[78] However, there are little data specific to older adults. With respect to psychotic symptoms, a study in New York City of non-demented persons aged 55+ examined ethnic differences and included two immigrant groups among Black participants.[85] The authors found very high levels of paranoid ideation or psychotic symptoms among Blacks, particularly among persons born in the Caribbean. The investigators found that Blacks were more than twice as likely as Whites to experience paranoid ideation(21% versus 9%). Within the Black population, there were appreciable but statistically nonsignificant differences in the rates of expression of paranoid ideation or psychotic symptoms among U.S.-born Blacks (18%), French Caribbean Blacks (38%), and English Caribbean Blacks (18%).

Mental Illness Paradox

It is apparent from the findings for depression, anxiety, and schizophrenia/psychotic disorders presented above that, in general, older adults have lower incidence and prevalence of formal disorders, despite increased stressors such as medical comorbidity and disability, social isolation, and bereavement. [86] (The age differences for symptom levels may not be as compelling.) This phenomenon has been described as the aging "paradox."[86] This observation appears to be true in both Western societies and non-Western societies, and is found in both cross-sectional and longitudinal studies spanning at least a quarter century. There are several potential explanations for this paradox, including study design issues such as recall of symptoms, attribution of psychiatric symptoms to somatic conditions, generational and cultural differences in discussing mental illness, and the exclusion of institutionalized adults. [87] These concerns notwithstanding, a study in the United States found that emotional well-being rises for older adults in the general population after age 50.[88] Embedded in the construct of enhanced emotional well-being is the older adult's affinity toward positive rather than negative information (cognitive "positivity effect"). That is, versus younger persons, older adults recall past events more favorably, give more positive ratings to negative events, focus more on things that will yield greater well-being, and view social networks more favorably.[88]

Summary

1. The aging process is a biological phenomenon that is affected by social factors. How we define "old age" is mostly socially determined.
2. The world's elderly population will double between 2015 and 2050 to 2 billion persons, or about one-fifth of all people. This is troubling because there will be proportionately fewer younger persons available to fund governmental programs or provide personal care for aging adults. The potential impact on societies and the well-being of older adults is enormous.
3. Understanding the causes of mental distress in older adults requires an appreciation of the effects of late capitalism, especially with respect to globalization of markets, urbanization, and mass migration (internal and external).
4. Social and social psychological theories of aging can enhance our appreciation of aging in a society. Micro-level theories focus on properties of individuals and their social interactions, whereas macro-level theories focus on broader social and cultural forces that shape behavior.
5. With respect to specific psychiatric disorders, worldwide studies have generally found lower incidence and prevalence rates of formal psychiatric disorder in older persons (excluding dementia), although age differences in psychiatric symptoms have been found

less consistently. Thus, rates of psychiatric disorders are lower in the context of seemingly more challenges and stressors with advanced age. This "mental illness paradox" may be the result of an increased cognitive positivity with age, although study design issues may also play a role.

6. A variety of social variables have been found to affect rates of psychiatric disorders, but there are many inconsistencies that may reflect methodological differences across investigations.

References

1. Cohen CI, Elmouchtari M, Ahmed I. Working with elderly persons across cultures. In: Bhugra D, Bhui K, eds. *Transcultural Psychiatry*. 2nd ed. London: Cambridge; 2018:552–569.

2. World Health Organization. *Ageing and Health*. 2018. https://www.who.int/news-room/fact-sheets/detail/ageing-and-health

3. Link BG, Phelan J. Social conditions as fundamental causes of disease. *J Health Soc Behav*. 1995(Extra Issue):80–94.

4. Cohen CI, Lo P, Nzodom C, Sahlu S. Migration, acculturation, and mental health. In: Llorente M, ed. *Culture, Heritage, and Diversity in Older Adult Mental Health Care*. Washington, DC: American Psychiatric Publishing; 2019:53–80.

5. Marshall VW. Analyzing social theories of aging. In: Bengston VL, Schiae KW, eds. *Handbook of Theories of Aging*. New York: Springer; 1999:434–458.

6. Cumming E, Henry W. *Growing Old*. New York: Basic Books; 1961.

7. Havighurst RJ, Neugarten BL, Tobin SS. Disengagement and patterns of aging. In: Neugarten BL, ed. *Middle Age and Aging*. Chicago: University of Chicago Press; 1968:67–71.

8. Atchley RC. A continuity theory of normal aging. *Gerontologist*. 1989;29(2):183–190.

9. Dowd JJ. Aging as exchange: a preface to theory. *J Gerontol*. 1975;30(5):584–594.

10. Baltes PB, Baltes MM. Psychological perspectives on successful aging: the model of selective optimization with compensation. In: Baltes PB, Baltes MM, eds. *Successful Aging: Perspectives from the Behavioral Sciences*. New York: Cambridge University Press; 1990:1–34.

11. Neugarten BL. Adult personality: toward a psychology of the life cycle. In: Neugarten BL, ed. *Middle Age and Aging: A Reader in Social Psychology*. Chicago: University of Chicago Press; 1968:137–147.

12. Gubrium JF. Toward a socio-environmental theory of aging. *Gerontologist*. 1972;12(3,Part 1):281–284.

13. Cowgill DO, Holmes LD. *Aging and Modernization*. New York: Appleton Century Crofts; 1972.

14. Rose AM. The subculture of the aging: a topic for sociological research. *Gerontologist*. 1962;2(3):123–127.

15. Quadagno J, Reid J. The political economy perspective in aging. In: Vern L, Bengston VL, Warner Schaie W, eds. *Handbook of Theories of Aging*. New York: Springer; 1999:344–358.

16. Luborsky M, Sankar A. Extending the critical gerontology perspective: cultural dimensions. Introduction. *Gerontologist*. 1993;33:440–444.

17. Riley MW, Johnson M, Foner A. *Aging and Society: A Sociology of Age Stratification*. Vol. 3. New York: Russell Sage Foundation; 1972.

18. Rowe JW, Kahn RL. Human aging: usual and successful. *Science*. 1987;237(4811):143–149.

19. Depp CA, Jeste DV. Definitions and predictors of successful aging: a comprehensive review of larger quantitative studies. *Am J Geriatr Psychiatry*. 2006;14(1):6–20.

20. Bryant C, Jackson H, Ames D. The prevalence of anxiety in older adults: methodological issues and a review of the literature. *J Affect Disord*. 2008;109(3):233–250.

21. Kessler RC, Birnbaum HG, Shahly V, et al. Age differences in the prevalence and co-morbidity of DSM-IV major depressive episodes: results from the WHO World Mental Health Survey Initiative. *Depress Anxiety*. 2010 Apr;27(4):351–364.

22. Kessler RC, Sampson NA, Berglund P, et al. Anxious and non-anxious major depressive disorder in the World Health Organization World Mental Health Surveys. *Epidemiol Psychiatr Sci*. 2015;24(3):210–226.

23. Haigh EAP, Bogucki OE, Sigmon ST, Blazer DG. Depression among older adults: a 20-year update on five common myths and misconceptions. *Am J Geriatr Psychiatry*. 2018;26(1):107–122.

24. Fiske A, Wetherell JL, Gatz M. Depression in older adults. *Annu Rev Clin Psychol*. 2009;5:363–389.

25. Kessler RC, Birnbaum H, Bromet E, Hwang I, Sampson N, Shahly V. Age differences in major depression: results from the National Comorbidity Survey Replication (NCS-R). *Psychol Med*. 2010;40(2):225–237.

26. Pan A, Franco OH, Wang YF, Yu ZJ, Ye XW, Lin X. Prevalence and geographic disparity of depressive symptoms among middle-aged and elderly in China. *J Affect Disord*. 2008;105(1–3):167–175.

27. Yunming L, Changsheng C, Haibo T, et al. Prevalence and risk factors for depression in older people in Xi'an China: a community-based study. *Int J Geriatr Psychiatry*. 2012;27(1):31–39.

28. Beekman AT, Copeland JR, Prince MJ. Review of community prevalence of depression in later life. *Br J Psychiatry*. 1999;174:307–311.

29. Purtle J, Nelson KL, Yang Y, Langellier B, Stankov I, Diez Roux AV. Urban–rural differences in older adult depression: a systematic review and meta-analysis of comparative studies. *Am J Prev Med*. 2019;56(4):603–613.

30. Shah A, Bhandarkar R, Bhatia G. The relationship between general population suicide rates and mental health funding, service provision and national policy: a cross-national study. *Int J Soc Psychiatry*. 2010;56(4):448–453.

31. Li GH, Baker SP. A comparison of injury death rates in China and the United States, 1986. *Am J Public Health*. 1991;81(5):605–609.

32. Sakauye K. Ethnocultural aspects of aging in mental health. In: Sadavoy J, Jarvik LF, Grossberg GT, Meyers BS, eds. *Comprehensive Textbook of Geriatric Psychiatry*. 3rd ed. New York: W. W. Norton; 2004:225–250.

33. Djernes JK. Prevalence and predictors of depression in populations of elderly: a review. *Acta Psychiatr Scand*. 2006;113(5):372–387.

34. Vink D, Aartsen MJ, Schoevers RA. Risk factors for anxiety and depression in the elderly: a review. *J Affect Disord*. 2008;106(1–2):29–44.

35. Wang Z, Yang H, Guo Z, Liu B, Geng S. Socio-demographic characteristics and co-occurrence of depressive symptoms with chronic diseases among older adults in China: the China longitudinal ageing social survey. *BMC Psychiatry*. 2019;19(1):310.

36. Liu Q, Cai H, Yang LH, et al. Depressive symptoms and their association with social determinants and chronic diseases in middle-aged and elderly Chinese people. *Sci Rep*. 2018 Mar 1;8(1):3841.

37. Gao S, Jin Y, Unverzagt FW, et al. Correlates of depressive symptoms in rural elderly Chinese. *Int J Geriatr Psychiatry*. 2009;24(12):1358–1366.

38. Aichberger MC, Schouler-Ocak M, Mundt A, et al. Depression in middle-aged and older first generation migrants in Europe: results from the Survey of Health, Ageing and Retirement in Europe (SHARE). *Eur Psychiatry*. 2010;25(8):468–475.

39. van der Wurff FB, Beekman AT, Dijkshoorn H, et al. Prevalence and risk-factors for depression in elderly Turkish and Moroccan migrants in the Netherlands. *J Affect Disord*. 2004;83(1):33–41.

40. Canuto A, Weber K, Baertschi M, et al. Anxiety disorders in old age: psychiatric comorbidities, quality of life, and prevalence according to age, gender, and country. *Am J Geriatr Psychiatry*. 2018;26(2):174–185.

41. Andreas S, Schulz H, Volkert J, et al. Prevalence of mental disorders in elderly people: The European MentDis_ICF65+ study. *Br J Psychiatry*. 2017;210(2):125–131.

42. Gum AM, King-Kallimanis B, Kohn R. Prevalence of mood, anxiety, and substance-abuse disorders for older Americans in the national comorbidity survey-replication. *Am J Geriatr Psychiatry*. 2009;17(9):769–781.

43. Kohn R, Vicente B, Saldivia S, Rioseco P, Torres S. Psychiatric epidemiology of the elderly population in Chile. *Am J Geriatr Psychiatry*. 2008;16(12):1020–1028.

44. Byers AL, Yaffe K, Covinsky KE, Friedman MB, Bruce ML. High occurrence of mood and anxiety disorders among older adults: The National Comorbidity Survey Replication. *Arch Gen Psychiatry*. 2010;67(5):489–496.

45. Zhang X, Norton J, Carriere I, Ritchie K, Chaudieu I, Ancelin ML. Generalized anxiety in community-dwelling elderly: prevalence and clinical characteristics. *J Affect Disord*. 2015;172:24–29.

46. Prina AM, Ferri CP, Guerra M, Brayne C, Prince M. Prevalence of anxiety and its correlates among older adults in Latin America, India and China: cross-cultural study. *Br J Psychiatry.* 2011;199(6):485–491.

47. Beekman AT, Bremmer MA, Deeg DJ, et al. Anxiety disorders in later life: a report from the Longitudinal Aging Study Amsterdam. *Int J Geriatr Psychiatry.* 1998;13(10):717–726.

48. Fratiglioni L, Rocca WA. Epidemiology of dementia. In: Boller F, Cappa SF, eds. *Handbook of Neuropsychology.* 2nd ed. Amsterdam: Elsevier; 2001:193–215.

49. World Health Organization. *Dementia Fact Sheet.* September 20, 2022. https://www.who.int/newsroom/fact-sheets/detail/dementia

50. Prince MJ. Wimo A, Guerchet M, Ali G-C, Wu YT, Prina M. *World Alzheimer Report 2015: The Global Impact of Dementia: an Analysis of Prevalence, Incidence, Cost and Trends.* London: Alzheimer's Disease International; August 2015.

51. Prince M, Bryce R, Albanese E, Wimo A, Ribeiro W, Ferri CP. The global prevalence of dementia: a systematic review and metaanalysis. *Alzheimers Dement.* 2013;9(1):63–75.e62.

52. Wimo A, Winblad B, Aguero-Torres H, von Strauss E. The magnitude of dementia occurrence in the world. *Alzheimer Dis Assoc Disord.* 2003;17(2):63–67.

53. Keefover RW, Rankin ED, Keyl PM, Wells JC, Martin J, Shaw J. Dementing illnesses in rural populations: the need for research and challenges confronting investigators. *J Rural Health.* 1996;12(3):178–187.

54. Russ T, Murianni L, Icaza G, Slachevsky A, Starr J. Geographical variation in dementia mortality in Italy, New Zealand, and Chile: the impact of latitude, vitamin D, and air pollution. *Dement Geriatr Cogn Disord.* 2016;42(1–2):31–41.

55. Weden MM, Shih RA, Kabeto MU, Langa KM. Secular trends in dementia and cognitive impairment of U.S. rural and urban older adults. *Am J Prev Med.* 2018;54(2):164–172.

56. Cassarino M, Setti A. Environment as 'brain training': a review of geographical and physical environmental influences on cognitive ageing. *Ageing Res Rev.* 2015;23(Pt B):167–182.

57. Abner EL, Jicha GA, Christian WJ, Schreurs BG. Rural-urban differences in alzheimer's disease and related disorders diagnostic prevalence in Kentucky and West Virginia. *J Rural Health.* 2016;32(3):314–320.

58. Mattos MK, Snitz BE, Lingler JH, Burke LE, Novosel LM, Sereika SM. Older rural- and urban-dwelling Appalachian adults with mild cognitive impairment. *J Rural Health.* 2017;33(2):208–216.

59. Alzheimer's Association. 2019 Alzheimer's disease facts and figures. *Alzheimers Dement.* 2019;15(3):321–387.

60. Hamid TA, Krishnaswamy S, Abdullah SS, Momtaz YA. Sociodemographic risk factors and correlates of dementia in older Malaysians. *Dement Geriatr Cogn Disord.* 2010;30(6):533–539.

61. Azad NA, Al Bugami M, Loy-English I. Gender differences in dementia risk factors. *Gend Med.* 2007;4(2):120–129.

62. Mathuranath PS, Cherian PJ, Mathew R, et al. Dementia in Kerala, South India: prevalence and influence of age, education and gender. *Int J Geriatr Psychiatry.* 2010;25(3):290–297.

63. Jelastopulu E, Giourou E, Argyropoulos K, Kariori E, Moratis E, Metousi A, Kyriopoulos J. Demographic and clinical characteristics of patients with dementia in Greece. *Adv Psychiatry.* 2014;2014:1–7.

64. Jones IR. Social class, dementia and the fourth age. *Sociol Health Illn.* 2017;39(2):303–317.

65. Ngandu T, von Strauss E, Helkala EL, et al. Education and dementia: what lies behind the association? *Neurology.* 2007;69(14):1442–1450.

66. Kuiper JS, Zuidersma M, Oude Voshaar RC, et al. Social relationships and risk of dementia: A systematic review and meta-analysis of longitudinal cohort studies. *Ageing Res Rev.* 2015;22:39–57.

67. Sutin AR, Stephan Y, Luchetti M, Terracciano A. Loneliness and risk of dementia. *J Gerontol B Psychol Sci Soc Sci.* 2020;75(7):1414–1422.

68. Yaffe K, Falvey C, Harris TB, et al. Effect of socioeconomic disparities on incidence of dementia among biracial older adults: prospective study. *BMJ.* 2013 Dec 19;347:f7051.

69. Reinhardt MM, Cohen CI. Late-life psychosis: diagnosis and treatment. *Curr Psychiatry Rep.* 2015;17(2):1.

70. Sigstrom R, Gustafson D. Epidemiology of psychotic disorders: methodological issues and empirical findings. In: Cohen CI, Meesters PD, eds. *Schizophrenia and Psychoses in Later Life: New Perspectives on Treatment, Research, and Policy.* Cambridge: Cambridge University Press; 2019:1–12.

71. Ostling S, Backman K, Waern M, et al. Paranoid symptoms and hallucinations among the older people in Western Europe. *Int J Geriatr Psychiatry*. 2013;28(6):573–579.

72. Cohen CI, Marino L. Racial and ethnic differences in the prevalence of psychotic symptoms in the general population. *Psychiatr Serv*. 2013;64(11):1103–1109.

73. Jongsma HE, Turner C, Kirkbride JB, Jones PB. International incidence of psychotic disorders, 2002–17: a systematic review and meta-analysis. *Lancet Public Health*. 2019;4(5):e229–e244.

74. Kessler RC, Birnbaum H, Demler O, et al. The prevalence and correlates of nonaffective psychosis in the National Comorbidity Survey Replication (NCS-R). *Biol Psychiatry*. 2005;58(8):668–676.

75. Stafford J, Howard R, Kirkbride JB. The incidence of very late-onset psychotic disorders: a systematic review and meta-analysis, 1960–2016. *Psychol Med*. 2018;48(11):1775–1786.

76. Howard R, Rabins PV, Seeman MV, Jeste DV. Late-onset schizophrenia and very-late-onset schizophrenia-like psychosis: an international consensus. *Am J Psychiatry*. 2000;157(2):172–178.

77. Meesters PD, de Haan L, Comijs HC, et al. Schizophrenia spectrum disorders in later life: prevalence and distribution of age at onset and sex in a dutch catchment area. *Am J Geriatr Psychiatry*. 2012;20(1):18–28.

78. Saha S, Chant D, Welham J, McGrath J. A systematic review of the prevalence of schizophrenia. *PLoS Med*. 2005;2(5):e141.

79. Abel KM, Drake R, Goldstein JM. Sex differences in schizophrenia. *Int Rev Psychiatry*. 2010;22(5):417–428.

80. Howard R, Jeste D. Late onset schizophrenia. In: Weinberger DR, Harrison PJ, eds. *Schizophrenia*. Chichester, West Sussex: Wiley Blackwell; 2011:47–61.

81. Seeman MV, Lang M. The role of estrogens in schizophrenia gender differences. *Schizophr Bull*. 1990;16(2):185–194.

82. Li R, Ma X, Wang G, Yang J, Wang C. Why sex differences in schizophrenia? *J Transl Neurosci (Beijing)*. 2016;1(1):37–42.

83. Cohen CI, Iqbal M. Longitudinal study of remission among older adults with schizophrenia spectrum disorder. *Am J Geriatr Psychiatry*. 2014;22(5):450–458.

84. Lange SMM, Meesters PD, Stek ML, Wunderink L, Penninx B, Rhebergen D. Course and predictors of symptomatic remission in late-life schizophrenia: a 5-year follow-up study in a Dutch psychiatric catchment area. *Schizophr Res*. 2019;209:179–184.

85. Cohen CI, Magai C, Yaffee R, Walcott-Brown L. Racial differences in paranoid ideation and psychoses in an older urban population. *Am J Psychiatry*. 2004;161(5):864–871.

86. Thomas ML, Kaufmann CN, Palmer BW, et al. Paradoxical Trend for Improvement in Mental Health With Aging. *J Clin Psychiatry*. 2016;77(08):e1019–e1025.

87. Gurian BS, Miner JH. Clinical presentation of anxiety in the elderly. In: Salzman C, Lebowitz BD, eds. *Anxiety in the Elderly: Treatment and Research*. New York: Springer; 1991:31–44.

88. Stone AA, Schwartz JE, Broderick JE, Deaton A. A snapshot of the age distribution of psychological well-being in the United States. *Proc Natl Acad Sci USA*. 2010;107(22):9985–9990.

11

Social Psychiatry

Death and Dying

H. Steven Moffic

Introduction

Since we are all dying and will die, though pending the immortality projects, death and dying are a ubiquitous experience. Of course, at its essence, this process is a biological one, as everyone's body currently ages over time, although modern medicine can replace or temporarily slow down some of those changes.

As in our field's biopsychosocial model, the psychology part of death and dying is of obvious importance. We each have our own individual psychological reaction to our death and dying. Virtually all patients have had experiences of the deaths of people and/or pets. How they have processed that should be part of any assessment. What tends to be lost with these powerful processes and preoccupations are the social aspects. These social aspects include the variations in how a society and loved ones view death and dying, all the way to societal options for burial and the disposal of the body.

Certainly, some of these social factors become part and parcel of virtually every clinical encounter. At the very least, we are taught to access suicide risk in every patient, both at the beginning and periodically. That is one way a person can control the timing of their own death. Related to that is an assessment of whether a patient is homicidal, and thereby at risk for causing someone else to die. Ethical and legal standards have developed to guide clinicians as to what to do when they judge a patient to be of suicidal or homicidal risk. An important one is that confidentiality should be broken if the clinician deems that someone's life is at risk, either generally the patient or a homicidal target.

Social psychiatric issues in suicide and homicide also extend beyond the individual patient to larger societal events. What about Japanese kamikaze pilots in World War II who would kill themselves for their country in order to help defeat the enemy as they purposely crashed into warships? Or, currently, those who are usually called suicide bombers? These are terrorists who choose to die as they kill others, most commonly currently in the case of Islamic terrorists. Actually, as a social psychiatrist, I think that the terminology is misleading, as these are clearly homicidal bombers or pilots, as the killing of others is the primary psychological and practical goal.

In regard to death and dying, another social psychiatric problem in addition to individual psychopathology is domestic violence, which is a major cause of death, especially toward women. Social policies, such as how and when to use restraining orders, require both social psychological as well as individual psychological expertise.

Society also has had a new social issue in what has at times been called physician-assisted suicide. Perhaps that is the wrong terminology, too. Better may be "physician-assisted death," as most of these patients have never been suicidal before their terminal and often painful illness. That this is a controversial and conflicting issue is reflected in its approval in some states and some countries, but not others to date. Moreover, some psychiatrists feel it is ethically acceptable, and others do not. Psychiatrists are also concerned that a couple of European countries have included unremitting psychiatric illness that is psychologically painful.

Often ignored, but of potential importance, is how any society and person should best think about death and dying. Is it more beneficial to not think of death and dying, or to more constantly think about it? Or, is it best to do so intermittently? Many religions have set up rituals to address those questions.

My Social Psychiatric Experience with Death and Dying

As a clinical psychiatrist, these patient considerations became a typical topic to cover, although I never encountered any evaluation form that specified "Death and Dying" as a topic to be covered for every patient. Even if an evaluation form has "Suicide" and "Homicide" as required topics to cover and document, death and dying cover more than that. Given that death and dying will be of personal interest to our own lives, any countertransference concerns must be monitored and assessed in these considerations.

Indeed, our mainstream American society has been thought to traditionally deny death.[1] Overcoming some of that denial, Kubler-Ross helped society appreciate the common stages of grieving.[2] Now there is a movement to make that denial a reality in stopping the death process, which made the cover of *Time Magazine*.[3]

As a social psychiatrist and part of my community, I have been asked to comment on death and dying to the public. For example, I was asked to write a column in our local Jewish monthly publication, the *Wisconsin Jewish Chronicle*,[4] on death and dying as it relates to our annual holiday of Yom Kippur, when we are supposed to be assessed as to whether God will put us in next year's "Book of Life." Part of that consideration is the recommendation to ask for forgiveness from those you may have harmed, inadvertently or not, as well as to dedicate oneself to "returning" to your better self. Since this process happens yearly, by itself it precipitates at least a yearly personal processing of death and dying. The limited data available suggest that intermittent thinking about one's death is the healthiest frequency.

Another example was a talk with staff at our local synagogue who were becoming overwhelmed with their reactions to so many congregants dying whom they knew. It felt like there was not enough time to mourn, or even enough knowledge about how to mourn. Should they develop some mourning rituals? Yes, I said. Should crying in grief be supported at work? Yes, I said. Should the whole congregations have a reminder session on death and dying? Yes, I recommended.

I've also spoken several times to our Young at Hearts group, which is a group of elders that meets monthly to discuss matters of interest. Topics I've covered with them include loneliness, how to age well (and thereby die well), and their fear about dying. It is clear that the social connections with other congregants is significant in their lives and the clergy important when contemplating death.

One earlier time when clinical psychiatry was infused into our whole congregation was during one of our annual Yom Kippur study sessions. A teenage girl in our congregation had recently committed suicide. Many were shocked. To help the community mourn and to prevent another tragedy, we set up a study session, and I was to talk about suicide and its prevention from a psychiatric perspective. However, I took the paradoxical stance of deciding to talk about my one patient who had committed suicide. I thought that might relieve some of the guilt that family and friends felt. I assumed that they must have felt some responsibility for the suicide.

As I started to speak, and having given many public speeches without a hitch, I started to tear up, then cry. And cry. I looked for my wife in the audience for help, but I couldn't locate her. Suddenly, I heard a whisper from up front to the right of me: "Slow down, relax." That helped. I regained control and continued my speech as planned. Afterward, I looked to see who did that. It was someone I didn't know. To my astonishment, it was the father of the girl who committed suicide! I then realized that I had never mourned, not even cried, about the suicide of an elderly patient over 40 years ago. I finally cried and mourned my unresolved hidden grief. I occasionally had been told over the years that I had a "rescue fantasy." If that was true, perhaps that suicide had caused some countertransference issues and a reaction formation to avoid that again by being overzealous in helping.

Surely, that was a personal lesson for me and the public. Indeed it was I, not the father, who felt guilty and had unresolved countertransference issues. It also led to a community decision to set up ongoing programs to prevent suicides in our youth, as well as support for the parents and loved ones of suicidal teens. The outcomes have been positively dramatic. For me, I can now talk about my patient who committed suicide without crying.

Some of these social psychiatric experiences of mine suggest the many opportunities available to social psychiatrists in regard to death and dying. There are other kinds of dying that seem to proverbially shake our communities. One recent example is the national—and even international—response to the sudden death of the basketball star Kobe Bryant. The impact seemed to be related not only to the memories of his basketball stardom, but perhaps even more so, to what his life outside of basketball meant to people. His public life included redemption for past mistakes. After an apparent extramarital affair, he returned to a lasting marriage with his wife. More than that, coming from a culture of concern for single mothers and missing fathers, he devoted himself to his daughters, one of whom died with him. Social psychiatry can surely help assess how best society can mourn their public figures successfully.

Virtually all religions have grieving rituals to help people start grieving the loss of loved ones that have stood the test of time. Even medicine has adapted what was thought to be a model of the typical process of grieving: denial, bargaining, anger, depression, acceptance.[2] On occasion, the target of the grieving can be a beloved public figure like Kobe Bryant, but in general this refers to family and friends who are loved ones. This can even include the unborn, as in pregnancy miscarriages.

However, general workplace policies and procedures to help grieving employees are few and far between. That includes psychiatric workplaces. Occasionally, workplaces allow "mental health" days, but the vagueness and various reasons to take them may not focus enough on the death of loved ones. Social psychiatry would recommend general policies that would allow enough time off to begin the normal grieving process. Without that, workplace productivity is likely to suffer if the grieving process doesn't go well.

On occasion, someone on a psychiatry clinic's staff will die. Such workplaces should provide a model for how to process the loss, including a mourning service, counseling availability, and time off.

Worst of all may be having a staff member commit suicide. That happened in one of the clinics I led. It was apparently a decision by a staff member to avoid the prolonged suffering of AIDS before adequate treatment became available. Staff noticed some withdrawal by this employee, but when he wasn't heard from over a couple of days, a staff member and I went to his home. She was a friend and had a key. We found him in bed, dead from a bullet, with dried blood surrounding his body.

By the time of this traumatic discovery, there was still a significant amount of fears about AIDS and contracting it, especially in exposure to blood. We had to be careful about our own risks, yet not overly frightened. Some of that epidemic fear rose again with the Ebola epidemic, during which I criticized the lack of quarantining a physician returning from the front lines in Africa, escalating public fear in New York.[5] Now, as of this writing with the spread of COVID-19, even though quarantining is more widespread, some have slipped through. Two of the leading Chinese doctors working to control the epidemic contacted the virus and died. Social psychiatrists can play a role in addressing how such social anxiety can be managed as well as possible, as well the actual cases of infection, as we await better prevention and treatment recommendations.

Though less risky in regard to likely death nowadays, contracting the flu is a yearly risk. Since about half of American adults don't get the flu vaccine, there must be certain cognitive distortions that need correction, and the messaging about the flu shot more psychologically sophisticated and convincing.

A different kind of epidemic has been the opioid crisis, with the vector not being a virus, but an actual medication that can—and should—be used therapeutically. A different sort of psychological contagion is present here, which should come into the wheelhouse of social psychiatry knowledge as far as prevention and treatment.[6]

After recommending enough time off for any who needed it, we had a service to celebrate the staff member who committed suicide. Any patients he worked with were invited. Periodically, ever since, we have looked upon that service as a healing one. And when some of us gather again over 30 years later, we still bring it up to further process.

We can contribute to successful social grieving of the public, patients, and public figures. And there is much more that we can contribute.

The Role of Social Psychiatry and Psychiatrists in Hastening Death

Whatever terminology is used, it is clear that there is a role for social psychiatrists in what has been called physician-assisted suicide or physician-assisted death, or other related terminology, such as "death with dignity," given the disparities in states that have approved such procedures versus those that haven't, as well as similar disparities in Europe and around the world. It is clear that social values about life, death, pain, and dying play a role.

Psychiatrists and some psychiatric organizations, though not the American Association for Social Psychiatry, have been part of this discussion.[7] In general, psychiatrists have tended to not support such endeavors, in the sense that the role of physicians is not to cause death. Yet, even in the best of palliative care and hospice, an alternative ethical case can be made in terms of the relief of suffering and patient autonomy. In the United States, the cost of medical care is another important social value. It is known that end-of-life medical care takes up a significant percentage of healthcare dollars, which of course can be shaved by assisting death for patients with chronic and costly illness.

In those locales where the process is legal, clinical psychiatrists also have a role in assessing whether any clinical depression, or another psychiatric disorder, is responsible for the request and is treatable. Here, society needs not only our clinical expertise, but also our assessment of how the needs of society dovetail with that.

There are important cultural and social values to keep in mind regarding any of the newer services devoted to dying, including palliative care and physician-assisted death.[8] It is crucial to assess the values of the patient and family. Some cultural groups, such as African Americans, may tend to be less accepting of advance directives or any attempt to shorten life, given their historical experience in America with dying early, producing some distrust of mainstream medicine.

The Role of Social Psychiatry and Psychiatrists in Prolonging Death

On the list-serve of members of the American Psychiatric Association, around the turn of the New Year and the annual election of officers, there was a robust discussion about the role of psychiatric and other physicians in hastening death. At the same time, in society there is now a movement to prolong life, if not prevent death. Google is one of the companies that is working on that.

As a crude experiment, I asked the same members on the list-serve for opinions on how psychiatrists might contribute to this societal endeavor. There were no responses. Yet, this brings up many social psychological conundrums. Is such an endeavor just another way to deny death and dying? What would life and society be like to know that one would never die? Would this help to relieve the loneliness epidemic of old age if losses of life were eliminated? Do we have adequate resources to take care of an increasingly aging population? Is there a role for social psychiatry in this particular social issue?

The Role of Social Psychiatry and Psychiatrists in Disaster

From the time of the Coconut Grove Fire in 1942, psychiatrists have played a robust role in the recovery process from acute disasters.[9] Lindemann, who studied this disaster, isolated the new psychiatric management strategies for grief reactions. He also added educational efforts, despite resistance from the medical establishment.[10] Indeed, new ideas for the benefit of society are often met with resistance, the kind of resistance that social psychiatrists should know how to overcome. Lindemann did so with patience, data, and reframing change. Unfortunately, he had to add his own rare cancer in the 1970s, when he had a chance to test his own theories on confronting death for himself.[11]

Now we know, as Lindemann's ideas became accepted and extended, how and when to provide psychological services to assess, prevent, and treat possible post-traumatic stress disorder, such as following the events of 9/11. When there are deaths, we can provide grief counseling and possible medication for loved ones.

Usually, those disasters are sudden and destructive, from such causes as hurricanes, earthquakes, wildfires, and other natural disasters. There are also man-made disasters like war, terrorist attacks, and mass shootings. Trauma, death, and dying are all common.

Societies have learned to use social psychiatric principles to prepare for such disasters. Usually, there are teams of mental healthcare professionals trained and ready to attend to the disasters quickly.

However, currently, we are experiencing another kind of disaster: the chronic, slow-moving disaster of climate change, which is changing the very environment that we have adjusted to, and changing it usually for the worse. This requires something different from psychiatrists and social psychiatry. It requires societal secondary preventive endeavors, which translate into addressing and reducing the psychological processes that contribute to the human behavior that is playing a major factor in climate change.

We know that social contagion contributes to thought leaders and respected citizens being able to influence others, so overt and conscientious environmental leaders from local blocks to our national government are needed. Social psychiatry can point out the social psychiatric problems that are arising, ranging from climate refugees to solastalgia to increased anxiety in children. Dying and death are among the outcomes of concern.

Conclusions and Recommendations

Death and dying have not been a typical focus of attention for social psychiatry and social psychiatrists. The last major comprehensive text on social psychiatry, published to begin the decade of the teens, did not have a chapter devoted to death and dying.[12] However, there is much reason that it should be covered, especially as society develops new methods to both hasten and prolong death. Our social psychiatrists and related mental healthcare disciplines have expertise in the social relationship aspect of our biopsychosocial model of medicine.[13] Without that, we tend to only focus on biological processes and the individual patient, yet we know that social processes have enormous influence on living and dying mentally well, or not. Indeed, the general neglect of the social aspects of the biopsychosocial model calls for this decade of the 2020s to be the "decade of the social" in psychiatry.[14] We'll see if this 20/20 vision comes to pass.

In this particular review of death and dying from the social psychiatric perspective, here are some preliminary recommendations.

1. *Countertransference.* As was seen in my own example of unresolved grief, all psychiatrists have their own experiences and attitudes toward death, which need to be understood and appreciated in order to avoid inadvertently influencing the patient for the clinicians' own reasons.
2. *Mourning.* Organized social psychiatry and social psychiatrists should help to develop principles of public mourning of public figures and celebrations, geared to particularly cultural and social values as well as principles of grieving normally.
3. *Hastening death.* Organized social psychiatry and social psychiatrists should be part of the various societal debates about physician-assisted death that go beyond the clinical assessment of individual patients and the ethical values of individual patient care.
4. *Extending life and stopping death.* Organized social psychiatry and social psychiatrists should begin to weigh in on psychological benefits and harm from the societal endeavors to prolong life and even end death as we know it.
5. *Epidemics.* Organized social psychiatry and social psychiatrists have particular expertise in addressing dangerous epidemics of any source, whether viral or another kind of vector, to help establish—locally, nationally, and internationally—the reasonable and right amount of fear as attempts to reduce death and dying are in process.
6. *Disasters.* Social psychiatry and psychiatrists have long played a role in recovery from acute disasters, but now need to expand into the slowly developing, chronic disasters such as those from climate instability.
7. *Documenting patient perspectives.* Social psychiatry and social psychiatrists should advocate for any patient evaluation to include an item that will document how the patient views their own death and dying, knowing full well that such an item will need to be addressed and documented periodically.
8. *Relationships with other professions.* Organized social psychiatry and social psychiatrists should endeavor to develop relationships with other professionals who commonly address death and dying, especially clergy, family physicians, and oncologists.

9. *Dealing with denial.* As in the case of Lindemann and his ideas about how to deal with disasters, society, like individual patients, will often be initially resistant to new ideas, so social psychiatrists need to be patient and apply their knowledge about overcoming resistance.

10. *The future.* Escalating social challenges, including that of death and dying, calls for an increase of attention to the social aspects of the biopsychosocial model of medicine and psychiatry.

From the standpoint of death and dying, social psychiatry has probably just scratched the surface of what we can contribute.

Editor's Comments

In this comprehensive review on death and dying, Dr. Steve Moffic writes on this complex topic by using examples from his own experiences and clinical work. He covers a vast number of issues related to death and the influence on our professional life and draws the line from the individual patient to society at large. Domestic violence, terrorism, suicide bombers, kamikaze pilots, grieving rituals, fear of dying, death of public figures, the role of religion, and the COVID-19 pandemic are all topics that are touched upon and linked to the role of social psychiatrists.

One particular important aspect is suicide and how suicidal acts among our patients affect—even torment—us as psychiatrists.

Dr. Moffic also shares with us some of the ethical dilemmas related both to physician-assisted death and prolonging life, which is a topic of increasing relevance and concern in many countries. But he further discusses the role of psychiatrists in dealing with disasters and their traumatic after-effects.

As a conclusion, the author lists 10 recommendations in dealing with death and dying. He points out that organized psychiatry and social psychiatrists do play an important role and that we should be aware of our responsibilities in addressing epidemics and severe disasters. We should also take a stand when it comes to prolonging life or assisting death, as well as developing ways to help human beings in mourning their loved ones.

References

1. Becker E. *The Denial of Death.* New York: Free Press; 1997.
2. Kulber-Ross E. *On Death and Dying.* New York: Scriber Classics; 1997.
3. *Time Magazine.* Can Google solve death. Cover story; September 30, 2013.
4. Moffic HS. Dr. Moffic's ABCs of aging well (Jewishly). *The Wisconsin Jewish Chronicle.* October 7, 2019.
5. Moffic HS. The Ebola patient in New York. *New York Times,* letter to the editor. October 24, 2014.
6. Dasgupta N, Beletsky L, Ciccarone D. Opioid crisis: no easy fix to its social and economic determinants. *Am J Public Health.* 2018;108(2):182–186.
7. Conrad, Oh, Canada! Your New Law Will Provide, Not Prevent, Suicide for Some Psychiatric Patients, Psychiatric Times June 1, 2021. https://www.psychiatrictimes.com
8. Appelbaum P. Physician-assisted death in psychiatry. *World Psychiatry.* 2018;17(2):145–146.

9. Searlight HR, Gafford J. Cultural diversity and end of life: issues and guidelines for family physicians. *Am Fam Physician*. 2005;71(3):515–522.
10. Lindemann E. Symptomalogy and management of acute grief. *Psychiatry Online*. 2006 Apr. https://doi.org/10.1176/ajp.101.2.141.
11. Satin DG. Erich Lindemann: the humanist and the era of community mental health. *Proc Am Philos Soc*. 1982;126(4):327–346.
12. Lindemann E. *Beyond Grief: Studies in Crisis Intervention*. New York: Arsonson; 1979.
13. Morgan C, Bhugra D, eds. *Principles of Social Psychiatry*. New York: Wiley; 2010.
14. Give J. How death imitates life: cultural influences on conceptions of death and dying. *Culture and Human Development: Adulthood and Old Age*. 2014;6(2):1–20. https://doi.org/10.9707/2307-0919.1120.

Social Psychiatry

Women's Issues

Nada L. Stotland and Angela Devi Shrestha

Introduction

Social psychiatry is the psychiatry that recognizes that humans are utterly, inescapably social beings—that it makes no sense to diagnose and treat a person without understanding, and sometimes addressing and intervening in, the person's social circumstances and interpersonal relationships.

Social psychiatry should encompass all societies; each has unique attitudes and practices, specifically, in regard to gender roles. Generalizations can be inaccurate and misleading. However, it is not possible for any chapter to cover all societies. The authors of this chapter, while diverse in family origins, are American, write in English, and live and work in a largely Western world. We will do our best to recognize and address issues that differentiate Western from other worldviews and practices.

What is a woman? According to the World Health Organization, gender refers to socially constructed characteristics of women and men.[1] These vary from society to society and can be changed. Most people are born either male or female and are taught cultural gender norms associated with men and women. However, when individuals do not fall within binary sex categories or established gender norms, they often face stigma, discrimination, and social exclusion—all of which adversely affect mental health.[2] It is important to pause and consider the complexity of gender when writing a chapter on those who identify as women.

We note that several other categorizations in this volume are also scrutinized and disputed. The concept of race as a biological given is scientifically questionable but socially persistent and powerful. What identifies a population as "marginalized"? How does the definition of "poverty" vary with social circumstances? We will try to acknowledge these context-dependent, fluid boundaries.

So, considering the shifting definition of the very concept of womanhood, we will offer observations and clinical suggestions. After a brief look at the history of women in society and its impact on their mental health and psychopathology, we will look at women as reproductive beings, as family members, as workers, and as members of society at large, offering some case vignettes to illustrate salient issues. Lastly, we will consider current social conflicts and circumstances critically affecting the well-being, psychopathology, psychiatric treatment of women and offer suggestions for educational, advocacy, policy, organizational, and clinical applications.

History

The history of women in society is one of nearly universal exclusion from positions of power and subjection to oppression and abuse. Why is that? Some might cite that men are, on average, physically larger and stronger than women, or that women bear and nurture helpless children, limiting their availability for other roles. Some trace women's secondary role to the prehistoric shift from hunter-gatherer to agrarian societies, when men's roles as hunters diminished and they assumed control over farming.[3] The notion of "seed" is common to both agriculture and reproduction. When the seed is considered the essence of life, the fertile, life-giving soil or uterus becomes a mere vessel. The cloaks of science and religion have been, and continue to be, used to veil the systematic, emphatic confinement of women to domestic tasks. The menstrual cycle is associated with pollution in many societies, and menstruation and childbearing are said to weaken women not only in the body, but in the brain. In many cultures, women's attempts to demonstrate strength or to advocate for themselves have been and continue to be construed as psychopathology. The pervasiveness of the oppression of women in many societies is such that perpetrators of physical and sexual violence escape any consequence—and women kill themselves out of desperation.

Psychiatry, as both a medical specialty and a product of the societies in which it is practiced, has historically participated in and promulgated these views. Ancient physicians blamed women's psychiatric symptoms on the wandering womb: hysteria. Sigmund Freud, in the treatment of the patient he called "Dora," blamed her symptoms on the unconscious repression of sexual desire and did not consider the role of attempted seduction of this very young woman by an older man. Similarly, contemporary psychiatry is undoubtedly culpable of errors in theory we have yet to understand. The role of social psychiatry is to critically examine all aspects that affect a woman's mental health in order to prevent these misunderstandings and subsequent mismanagement, where at all possible.

Woman as a Reproductive Being

Women experience menarche, menstruation, pregnancy, childbirth, lactation, and menopause. These phenomena result in hormonal changes. The psychiatrist as scientist and clinician walks a fine line between recognizing the influences of sex hormones and reproductive events on one hand, and the danger of seeing them as defining and incapacitating on the other. If, as social psychiatrists, we see disease as a social construct, by according formal status to personal symptoms and social disability, we recognize diseases as conditions with social repercussions. It is important to note that masculinizing hormones are virtually never considered pathogenic, although testosterone is a factor in far more dangerous behaviors, and social consequences, than any feminizing hormone.

While in many indigenous cultures around the world, menstruation is seen as sacred and powerful,[4] there are many more where it is considered impure. One example is the tradition of *chhaupadi* in western Nepal, where menstruating women are isolated from their family, homes, schools, and temples, and even touching a menstruating woman is thought to cause illness.[5] These women are exiled to menstrual huts, which often pose multiple health and safety risks.[6]

As long as menstruation is seen as something to be hidden, this normal function is associated with shame. Only recently has there been a healthy change in the Western world, with open referral to periods on prime-time national television and unveiled advertisements for menstrual hygiene products. In many societies, menarche limits the accepted behaviors of a girl. She must renounce activities such as sports, stay close to home, and prepare for marriage.

Vignette

Maria G was a woman of color working as a surgical nurse. She endured racial discrimination at work. She was regularly assigned as the operating room nurse for a male surgeon who regularly yelled, used obscenities, and threw surgical instruments during the course of surgical procedures. One day, during one of his tantrums, Maria declared, "This behavior is inappropriate and intolerable." The surgeon replied, "I guess it's Maria's time of the month." This surgeon was highly valued by the hospital because of the income he generated. Maria knew that her behavior was completely justified. She knew that it had nothing to do with her menstrual cycle but felt pressured to stay silent in order to keep her job.

The association of average menstrual cycles with negative changes in mood, irritability, thinking, and behavior continues unabated. Premenstrual dysphoric disorder has now been enshrined in the *Diagnostic and Statistical Manual of Mental Disorders* (DSM) of the American Psychiatric Association. The methodological challenge in studying the impact of the menstrual cycle is social. Everybody believes there are negative effects. Given the social mandate for women to be pleasant and compliant, and the social taboos against mental illness, the menstrual cycle can be blamed for perfectly justifiable anger that is otherwise suppressed and for frank psychopathology such as clinical depression. Of women who seek care for premenstrual symptoms, many, when asked to prospectively chart their mood on calendars separate from those used to track their menstrual cycles, will discover their symptoms are not related to menstruation.[7] What many may call premenstrual syndrome (PMS), upon careful interview, is often found to stem from mood changes that result from gender-based violence, as well as other psychiatric disorders, including posttraumatic stress disorder.[8]

With menarche comes fertility. A woman's ability to control her fertility is essential to her well-being: to be educated, to find work commensurate with her preferences and abilities, and to provide adequate and satisfying care for children and other dependents. Men's desire for children, and children they can feel assured are genetically theirs, leads to social preoccupation with virginity and to limitations on women's freedom to move about in the world outside the home.

Societies generally regard menarche, under normal circumstances, as the time of onset of sexual desire and sexual desirability. Societies tend to consider men's sexual desires both comparatively uncontrollable and desirable, while women who openly manifest sexual desire are viewed as immoral. Sexual mistreatment by men is often blamed on the failure of women to dress modestly and restrict their lives to "safe" places. A recent study indicates that, for many women, first sexual intercourse is non-consensual.[9] Since many married women are physically and financially vulnerable, they often have little or no control over sexual intercourse in marriage.

Vignette

Surinder, a married 22-year-old woman in Delhi, India, called a psychiatrist's office begging for an emergency appointment. Her first pregnancy had just been diagnosed. When her mother-in-law received the very welcome news, she announced that Surinder must undergo testing to determine fetal sex at the first opportunity. If the fetus was female, the family would insist Surinder have an abortion. They would resort to force if necessary. Surinder's husband would have accepted a daughter but was unable or unwilling to overrule his mother. Surinder was in a state of panic. In addition to treatment of her psychiatric symptoms, she asked that the psychiatrist intervene in the conflict.

So, with fertility comes reproductive injustice. Before modern reproductive science, and still in places where that science is not understood or accepted, women were and are blamed for infertility and other real or perceived reproductive failures, such as the failure to deliver male children. Despite vulnerability to unwanted and/or unprotected intercourse, they are also blamed for sexually transmitted diseases, including HIV, and for unplanned or unwanted pregnancies. Women's control of their fertility may be the single most important factor in the well-being of families and society in general. The control of women's reproductive functions by others is a central factor in their oppression. When China sought to curtail population growth, women's menstrual cycles were officially monitored, and women were subjected to involuntary abortions and sterilizations.[10] In India, a similar effort was focused on vasectomy in men.[11] In Poland, as this is written, the government proposes forbidding unmarried women to use their own frozen embryos. The custom of child marriage is still widely practiced throughout the globe, subjecting girls to both sexual trauma and serious obstetrical complications.

Sexual access to unwilling women and girls is regarded societally as an entitlement in a wide range of situations. Some fathers, other relatives, and family friends sexually abuse female children. The reluctance of families and societies to acknowledge this exploitation, sometimes blaming and punishing the victim, exacerbates the traumatic impact. Women can be subject to rape for purposes of revenge and subjugation, by invading armies or extremist religious sects. Rape is a major factor in the incidence of post-traumatic stress disorder. Throughout history, some men have considered themselves entitled to the exploitation of slaves, servants, students, and workers. Sexual acts with those in positions of power may even be seen as normal steps toward progress in school or career. The women involved face a lifetime of uncertainty, with a variety of psychopathological effects, about their own ability and culpability.

All of the contexts in which women engage in sexual intercourse, willingly or not, entail the possibility of conception in women of reproductive age. Effective contraception is a personal and social necessity, but often is unavailable because of legality, availability, cost, or other realities of women's lives. "Morning-after" hormonal contraception can reduce the incidence of unwanted pregnancy, but availability is limited. Some religious extremists insist that it is a form of abortion, and many women are not aware that it exists or are unable to obtain it during the window of effectiveness.

Abortion has been a means of fertility control in all or most societies throughout recorded history. It has been practiced at comparable rates whether allowed or forbidden.[12] Where it is forbidden, it is performed unsafely and results in significant morbidity and mortality In 2022, The Supreme Court of the United States, in the Dobbs decision, overturned the 50 year old Roe v Wade ruling making access to abortion a constitutional right and leaving abortion law to be decided by each of the 50 states. State laws, which may change at any time, range from total bans to total access. Some laws include ambiguous exceptions for maternal health or life, leading to consternation among patients and clinicians at risk of arrest and imprisonment, and life-threatening delays in the care of women experiencing miscarriages, ectopic pregnancies and other complications. We can anticipate years of litigation over proposed bans on interstate travel for abortions and the provision of abortion medications by mail or personal delivery. Some laws forbid the mere discussion of abortion; psychiatrists practicing in those states have to decide between obeying the law and their professional obligation to do what is best for their patients. Under the guise of religious liberty, healthcare providers are allowed to limit access to contraception and other women's health care due to their personal religious and "conscientious" objections.[14] Many state laws privilege the legal rights of the fetus over those of the mother. This takes us back to a woman as no more than a vessel.

There are several implications for social psychiatry. There is a great deal of misinformation about abortion, including the belief that abortion causes psychiatric symptoms or disorders. Abortion providers are required by law to pass on this misinformation to patients in several American states. The fact is that abortion, in and of itself, does not cause psychiatric illness.[15] Psychiatrists need to supply accurate information to patients and society at large. There is considerable social stigma, as well as religious disapproval of abortion, which patients who have had or are contemplating abortion have to work through.

There is a tragic disconnect between the incidence of abortion—about one-third of women in the United States—and the willingness of the public to allow abortion restrictions.[16] That is, women who oppose abortion, and who support elected leaders who vote to impose restrictions on it, have abortions when their pregnancies threaten their own well-being or that of their families. The religious affiliations of women who have abortions are in the same proportions as those of the general population. This is an example of an exquisite interplay of social and psychological factors.

Pregnancy and childbirth are usually regarded as biological and psychological experiences, but they are social experiences as well. Society will judge the appropriateness or acceptability of a pregnancy. Pregnancy outside a socially sanctioned relationship or circumstance can lead to severe approbation and exclusion, raising terrifying concerns about one's own survival and the fate of one's coming child.

The advent of reproductive technologies has complicated the social aspects of pregnancy. Women who wish to delay pregnancy beyond the age when fertility declines can have their eggs extracted and frozen for future use. Women can be impregnated and bear children after menopause. Technology enables many infertile couples to have children. The ability to overstimulate ovulation hormonally and then harvest eggs also allows for those eggs to be donated or sold to others. Eggs from women of particular ethnicities or accomplishments fetch premium prices. Finally, women can volunteer, or more often be paid, to gestate fetuses at the behest of couples who cannot or choose not to do so, known as surrogacy. There are cases in which the birth mother subsequently refuses to relinquish the baby, and others in which the intended parents refuse to accept it. The effect of these arrangements on the existing children of surrogates is unknown and unaddressed. Although women who agree to serve as surrogates are said to do so because they enjoy pregnancy and the prospect of bringing joy to the prospective parents, the risk of exploitation is clear. In fact, some surrogates are recruited among poor women outside the United States. All of these arrangements create social pressures and uncertainties.

Postpartum depression appears to occur worldwide and has gained recognition, acceptance, and treatment approaches. Nevertheless, in social terms, it poses a particular challenge. Having a baby is supposed to be one of the most joyful experiences in a woman's life. Women are aware of this expectation, and many women are frustrated in their attempts to achieve it. When instead they experience depression, they, their friends, and relatives may consider them ungrateful rather than ill. Next, many women are geographically distant from family support. Lastly, in the United States especially, there is neither sufficient maternity leave, financial support, nor childcare to support new mothers. There are also few hospitals able to psychiatrically admit and care for postpartum women together with their babies. One bright light for social psychiatry is the effectiveness of peer and group support for postpartum depression.

Menopause could be said to be just as much a social as a hormonal function. In Western societies, menopause is socially pathologized through medicalization, with expectations not only of debilitating physical symptoms, but of cognitive decline and negative moods and behaviors.[17] In many Eastern societies, aging accords women increased status and relief from domestic responsibilities. In the West, aging women are the witches of folklore and the critical and demanding mothers and mothers-in-law of comedy, and menopause means aging. There are compelling evolutionary reasons for women to live beyond their reproductive years; they need years after having children to care for those children, and grandmothers offer grandchildren measurable advantages. Some women grieve when their children leave home, and some women are abandoned by their partners in favor of younger partners. On the other hand, many women thrive, with or without partners and children.

Women in the Family

In many societies, a female newborn is viewed as a liability, or, perhaps worse, an asset to be sold or traded. When Chinese couples were restricted to one child, many female fetuses were aborted, and female newborns abandoned.[18] In India, pregnant women are sometimes forced by their husbands' families to undergo prenatal gender testing and to abort female fetuses. In some societies, girls' fathers choose their husbands and marry them off so young that they experience serious obstetrical complications. In some societies, male members of the family may punish any daughter's behavior or circumstance perceived to stain the family honor by murdering her. Husbands' families dissatisfied with brides may disfigure or murder them. They will not be welcomed back by their families of origin.

Motherhood is the basis of the social relationship. Motherhood is a primal psychological and social experience. Motherhood changes a woman's social status, social opportunities, and social regard. It can expand or narrow her social contacts and activities. Social mores have changed, making it more acceptable for unmarried women to have and raise children. In much of the Western world, the average age of marriage has risen, and the rate of marriage has fallen. The decision to have children and the decision to marry are separate. The entrance of most mothers into the paid workforce, because of increased opportunities for women as well as financial need, this is a major social revolution.

The birth of a child puts major strains on a relationship: strains that neither member has anticipated. For centuries, women were expected to devote all their time and energy to caring for the house and family. Those responsibilities are little diminished when women are employed. For poor women, this is understood as a necessary burden. Mothers with successful careers may be characterized to "have it all," while a more accurate description may be that they do it all.

The entrance of vast numbers of women into the paid workforce also means that many of them have very different lives than their own mothers. The maternal wisdom of the past may not be applicable in the family of the present. Grandmothers and grandmothers-in-law may be jealous of modern women's opportunities. They may be fearful that the children of employed mothers will be neglected. Employed grandmothers are less likely to reside close to their grandchildren and are less available to help care for them than in the past.

While women have been, and continue to be, oppressed and limited within families, it is also within families that women play the most powerful roles and derive much life satisfaction. Traditionally, in many societies, men bear the primary responsibility for providing financial support for their families. In many, men also are responsible for discipline: making and enforcing rules. Most, if not all, other family functions are served by women. Women are responsible for the family's health and healthcare, for their diets, for the activities of young children and the studies of older children. Women assemble the family for daily, weekly, and holiday meals; make arrangements for meetings with friends;

follow neighborhood and subcultural developments with impacts on the family. Women teach and advise younger women, particularly their daughters, on household management and child-rearing.

Nearly everywhere, women are paid less than men for the same jobs. Employed women remain responsible and uncompensated for most domestic tasks. Even when men assume some of the physical tasks, they are largely oblivious to the many managerial tasks: planning the meals, seeing that dental and medical care is scheduled, knowing children's school and other schedules.

The family is also the place where women are most at risk of psychological abuse and physical violence. The abuse of women in the family is tolerated in many societies worldwide. Psychiatry, in the past, played an unfortunate role by labeling women who tolerated pain as masochistic. It is still difficult for many to understand the realities and dynamics that keep women in abusive relationships: financial need, damaged self-esteem, social stigma, hope of redemption, and fear of mayhem and murder. Women seeking psychiatric care may not reveal, or even recognize, that their symptoms are the result of abuse. Every clinician must be alert for that possibility. Seeking psychiatric care and receiving psychiatric diagnoses can alleviate damaging consequences but can also put these women at increased risk of abuse and of losing custody of their children to their abusers.

Women in School and Workplace

All over the world, women have entered educational programs, jobs, and careers denied to them for centuries. This has largely been a boon to their well-being, but there are both backlash and ongoing limitations. Societies, or countries, vary in terms of their concern about population. Women who pursue education and careers enjoy their freedom and postpone or limit their childbearing.[19] China, once so desperate to limit population, is now faced with a population of women who wish to have just one child, and more aging citizens than young ones to earn and care for them.

Programs providing training and small amounts of capital to women in impoverished villages have received considerable attention. While they may have improved the lives of those women and their families—the women generally prioritize spending on their children's education—they do not address the poverty and lack of opportunity in those societies.

Women's entry into some careers may be met with considerable resistance, varying from mistrust to outright harassment. They may also experience "imposter syndrome"—imagining that they are unqualified.[20] In schools there have always been and continue to be male teachers who take advantage of the trust, ambition, and vulnerabilities of female students; teachers who have lower expectations of women; and teachers who deny female students the opportunities they offer men. Women discriminated against, harassed, and abused in the workplace—including those in the military and in medicine—have little protection or recourse.[21] These are realities. These problems at the lower levels, as well as outright discrimination at the upper levels, result in the major underrepresentation of women at leadership levels in nearly all fields, including government. Some countries have addressed gender inequality by legislating mandatory quotas for elected and other leadership roles. Others have active programs to recruit and train more women in scientific, technical, and medical careers.

Women in Society: Current Challenges and Crises

The media have reported that there is a global war on women.[22] Women constitute the majority of the poor. Women's heart attacks are more likely than men's to be unrecognized and untreated. Women's rights, in ascendance in a few places, are under attack in others. Fundamentalist expressions of religion are used as a major tool in restricting women's roles and rights. It would appear to a non-expert that the scriptures on which the fundamentalists rely seldom spell out the rules they espouse. Does the Qur'an require women to cover every part of their bodies but their eyes when they leave home, or to be stoned to death if accused of adultery? Did Jesus condemn lesbians to an eternity in hell? Restrictions and punishments appear to reflect a passion to return to an imaginary golden time. This view appears to be incompatible with scientific and other advancement, which in turn leaves people unemployed, frustrated, humiliated, and angry. Women's lives may be the one thing that men can control.

Vignette

Violet B, a married woman with a one-year-old and a newborn, was brought to the Emergency Room by family in a decompensated state of anxiety. There had been a huge blizzard just as her second baby was being born, and she had been shut in with the babies for many days. In treatment, she exhibited signs and symptoms of borderline personality disorder: dissociative episodes, dramatic mood shifts, regressive behaviors. After years of weekly psychotherapy, she finally recognized and communicated the fact that she had been abused since birth and had been, and was continuing to be, physically and psychologically abused by her husband. He justified his behavior on the basis of the teachings of their Evangelical church. The correct diagnosis was post-traumatic stress disorder. Her signs and symptoms improved; she divorced her husband; and she successfully completed nurses' training and worked as an excellent nurse.

In most countries, some part of the population is considered to be a minority and is discriminated against for racial, religious, or cultural reasons. Women members of minorities bear a double burden. While minority women must face discrimination by the majority population, they often are also discriminated against by minority men. The flagrant abuse and mass incarceration of Black men in American society has left many Black women alone with the burden of rearing their children and grandchildren. This has given rise to the myth of the strong, indomitable Black woman.[23] In circumstances where Black men may discriminate against or even cause physical harm to their female counterparts, Black women often also feel it their responsibility to protect Black men from further societal injustice by staying silent.[24] The stress of managing conflicts such as these contributes to depression and anxiety in Black women.[25]

The influence of attitudes toward women, race, and politics can come together in the courtroom. One example is the astonishingly lenient sentence of 6 months given to a male university student in California who was convicted of rape. The victim was subjected to sexist questioning by the defense attorney. The man's father and the judge were preoccupied by the potential negative impact of the rape and punishment on the assailant's life. The victim, whose identity had been confidential, later wrote a memoir, revealing that she was Chinese American and that the failure to treat her fairly and to take the impact of the assault on her simply echoed the treatment she had perceived all her life.[26]

We are said to be living in the #MeToo era. Several powerful and prominent men have lost their positions after being accused of harassing and abusing women over many years. Their accusers report relief at having finally been believed and seeing their abusers held to justice. However, #MeToo is far from a resolution of women's challenges. The number of men who have suffered deserved consequences is vanishingly small. There is no evidence that the masses of abused women are safer or better off than they were before #MeToo. There has been, at best, lip service and mandated employee harassment seminars without measurable outcomes.

There is concern that #MeToo has exacerbated a tendency for women to be seen as helpless, vulnerable victims. Women who question #MeToo and men accused without proof of sexual misbehavior have been reviled and ejected from college campuses by angry students and fearful administrators. Many women who report abuse have been terrorized by online attacks. Men are complaining that they cannot mentor or collaborate with women for fear of being accused of sexual misbehavior.[27] Have most women's lives in society been improved?

Not all women are pleased about changing gender roles. Their positions as wives and their primacy as mothers have been the major source of status, self-regard, and gratification. They tend to see feminism—the belief and practice of gender equality—as a diminishment of these cherished values and a rejection of femininity.

One positive social effect of #MeToo is the emergence of mutual support among women victims. Women are more likely than men to have close friendships in which they express intimate concerns and feelings. The realities of women's lives today leave little time or energy for getting together to exchange experiences, commiserate about hardships, and share coping ideas. The internet is a significant resource. Groups of women in particular professions, stages of motherhood, or any other common factor, have gathered electronically. Sisterhood can be a powerful force.

Clinical and and Social Applications

- Take nothing for granted. It is tempting to assume that persons with similar circumstances or backgrounds to one's own are similar to oneself.

- Work with medical students, residents, and physicians in all patient-care specialties to insist that psychological and social factors be made a part of every diagnostic and treatment-planning process.
- Remember that physicians are reluctant to seek patient information that will make patients emotionally expressive or that will make it clear that patients need services that the clinician cannot provide.
- Patients often need to form a trusting relationship with a clinician before revealing that they are victims of abuse. Although social psychiatrists appropriately may find it important to see patients along with their loved ones, the presence of the abuser, who may seem benign, will prevent the victim from reporting the abuse. A woman and her children in an abusive relationship can be in a life-or-death situation.
- Take note of patients' dependent-care obligations when making a treatment plan. Women will sacrifice their own healthcare before jeopardizing the well-being of their children. The fate of children removed from their families for protection is problematic; there are few institutions and foster families able to substitute for parents and address children's reactions to separation. Parenting support can be crucial for the well-being of patients who are mothers and for their children.
- Helping patients who report workplace harassment, discrimination, and/or abuse is a complicated process. The psychiatrist must validate the patient's feelings and observations while considering the patient's possible contributions to the difficult situation. Sometimes a patient needs help coping with the realities of a situation that she cannot afford to leave. At other times, a patient needs help to realize that she is not as helpless as she feels and to mobilize to obtain relief and redress.
- There is a similar challenge with regard to hormonal influences on mood and behavior. Some women appear to be more sensitive to hormonal changes than others. Premenstrual symptoms and menopausal hot flashes are unpleasant, but they are very rarely incapacitating. Given the stigma against mental illness, and the widespread belief that women's hormones cause problems with mood and behavior, it is tempting for women to attribute psychiatric symptoms to hormones. There must be a careful exploration of the patient's social circumstances.
- Be prepared to talk with patients about their religious affiliations and beliefs. Sometimes harmful attitudes of a given religious organization do not genuinely reflect the scriptures of their religion. Religious beliefs and institutions can also be crucial psychosocial supports.
- Every physician should be an advocate for health-promoting social policies. Few have or take the time and have the expertise to be effective advocates. Social psychiatrists have a particular expertise and obligation to serve as advocates.

Areas for Further Research

Women constitute half the world's population. Although there are powerful social forces limiting their influence and power, it is also true that women are too often complicit in the social mores and rules that work against their own well-being. We need to understand the mechanisms that deter them from advocating for themselves and their daughters. A specific example is the split between the frequency of abortion and the failure of women to mobilize against abortion limitations.

Another area for study is backlash. Is there more to the global and local wars on women than men's fears of losing control of the family, the workplace, or the government? The literature on the unconscious fears of men is very old. What makes women so terrifying to men?

Lastly, how can we incorporate the impact of social realities into the practice of medicine, and psychiatry in particular? An exclusive biomedical model leaves gaping holes in treatment and minimal attention to prevention.

Concluding Remarks

This chapter documents the oppression of women throughout history and throughout the world. This social reality inevitably results in anxiety, depression, trauma responses such as post-traumatic stress disorder, and suicide. The field of psychiatry has generally focused on the individual patient. By utilizing the principles of social psychiatry, we have the opportunity to contextualize women's psychiatric conditions: in the classroom, the hospital ward, the clinic, and in outreach to policymakers, as well as in individual treatment.

References

1. World Health Organization. Gender and genetics. https://www.who.int/genomics/gender/en/ Website. Accessed August 8, 2020.
2. World Health Organization. Gender mainstreaming for health managers: a practical approach. *WHO*. 2011. https://www-who-int.proxy.cc.uic.edu/gender-equity-rights/knowledge/health_managers_guide/en/. Accessed August 5, 2020.
3. McElvaine RS. Perspective: the ancient metaphor that created modern sexism. *Washington Post*. October 17, 2018. Available from: https://www.washingtonpost.com/outlook/2018/10/17/ancient-metaphor-that-created-modern-sexism/. Accessed August 5, 2020.
4. Miles T. Review of Cherokee women: gender and culture change, 1700–1835. *J Soc History*. 2000;33(4):1022–1024.
5. Ranabhat C, Kim CB, Choi EH, Aryal A, Park MB, Doh YA. Chhaupadi culture and reproductive health of women in Nepal. *Asia Pac J Public Health*. 2015;27(7):785–795. doi: 10.1177/1010539515602743.
6. Amatya P, Ghimire S, Callahan KE, Baral BK, Poudel KC. Practice and lived experience of menstrual exiles (chhaupadi) among adolescent girls in far-western Nepal. *PLoS One*. 2018;13(12):e0208260. doi: 10.1371/journal.pone.0208260.
7. Walker A. Theory and methodology in premenstrual syndrome research. *Soc Sci Med*. 1995;41(6):793–800. doi: 027795369500046A [pii].
8. Ussher JM, Perz J. PMS as a process of negotiation: women's experience and management of premenstrual distress. *Psychol Health*. 2013;28(8):909–927. doi: 10.1080/08870446.2013.765004.
9. Hawks L, Woolhandler S, Himmelstein DU, Bor DH, Gaffney A, McCormick D. Association Between Forced Sexual Initiation and Health Outcomes Among US Women. *JAMA Intern Med*. 2019;179(11):1551–1558. doi: 10.1001/jamainternmed.2019.3500
10. Hu H. Family planning law and China's birth control situation. *China Daily*. October 18, 2002. Available from: http://www.china.org.cn/english/2002/Oct/46138.htm.

11. Biswas S. India's dark history of sterilisation. *BBC News.* November 14, 2014. Available from: https://www.bbc.com/news/world-asia-india-30040790. Accessed August 5, 2020.

12. Stotland NL. Reproductive rights and women's mental health. *Psychiatr Clin North Am.* 2017;40(2):335–350. doi: S0193-953X(17)30013-8 [pii].

13. Nash E. Abortion rights in peril—what clinicians need to know. *N Engl J Med.* 2019;381(6):497–499. https://doi-org.proxy.cc.uic.edu/10.1056/NEJMp1906972. Accessed August 5, 2020. doi: 10.1056/NEJMp1906972.

14. Bronstein JM. Radical changes for reproductive health care—proposed regulations for title X. *N Engl J Med.* 2018;379(8):706–708. doi: 10.1056/NEJMp1807125.

15. Gold LH. Abortion and suicide. *Am J Psychiatry.* 2018;175(9):813–814. doi: 10.1176/appi.ajp.2018.18050513.

16. Jones RK, Jerman J. Abortion incidence and service availability in the United States, 2014. *Perspect Sex Reprod Health.* 2017;49(1):17–27. doi: 10.1363/psrh.12015.

17. Meyer VF. The medicalization of menopause: critique and consequences. *Int J Health Serv.* 2001;31(4):769–792. doi: 10.2190/M77D-YV2Y-D5NU-FXNW.

18. Johansson S, Nygren O. The missing girls of China: A new demographic account. *Popul Dev Rev.* 1991;17(1):35–51.

19. Cain Miller C. The costs of motherhood are rising, and catching women off guard. *New York Times.* August 17, 2018. Available from: https://www.nytimes.com/2018/08/17/upshot/motherhood-rising-costs-surprise.html.

20. Mullangi S, Jagsi R. Imposter syndrome: treat the cause, not the symptom. *JAMA.* 2019;322(5):403–404. https://jamanetwork-com.proxy.cc.uic.edu/journals/jama/fullarticle/2740724. Accessed August 5, 2020. doi: 10.1001/jama.2019.9788.

21. Fairchild AL, Holyfield LJ, Byington CL. National academies of sciences, engineering, and medicine report on sexual harassment: making the case for fundamental institutional change. *JAMA.* 2018;320(9):873–874. https://jamanetwork-com.proxy.cc.uic.edu/journals/jama/fullarticle/2697842. Accessed August 5, 2020. doi: 10.1001/jama.2018.10840.

22. Beinart P. The new authoritarians are waging war on women. *The Atlantic.* January/February 2019. Available from: https://www.theatlantic.com/magazine/archive/2019/01/authoritarian-sexism-trump-duterte/576382/.

23. Bennet J. The pressure of being a "strong black woman" often leads to depression. *Ebony.* May 28, 2019. Retrieved from: https://www.ebony.com/the-pressure-of-being-a-strong-black-woman-often-leads-to-depression/

24. Lacey KK, Parnell R, Mouzon DM, et al. The mental health of US Black women: the roles of social context and severe intimate partner violence. *BMJ Open.* 2015;5:e008415. doi: 10.1136/bmjopen-2015-008415

25. Abrams JA, Hill A, Maxwell M. Underneath the mask of the strong black woman schema: disentangling influences of strength and self-silencing on depressive symptoms among U.S. black women. *Sex Roles.* 2019;80(9–10):517–526. doi: 10.1007/s11199-018-0956-y.

26. Miller C. *Know My Name.* New York: Viking; 2019.

27. Byerley JS. Mentoring in the era of #MeToo. *JAMA.* 2018;319(12):1199–1200. https://jamanetwork-com.proxy.cc.uic.edu/journals/jama/fullarticle/2676115. Accessed August 5, 2020. doi: 10.1001/jama.2018.2128.

13

Men Under Stress

Evolutionary, Sociocultural, and Clinical Perspectives on Masculinity and Mental Health

Marianne Kastrup, Kenneth Thompson, and
Rama Rao Gogineni

Introduction: The Male Health Crisis

We live today in a world that no longer sees human beings as divided into two sexes—male and female—and that now includes a more diversified complexity, as individuals may no longer identify with being either male or female. Sexual preferences are not set in stone and can change over time, often depending on the immediate situation the individual is in. This has been described as fluidity. Four different types of sexual fluidity are identified: (1) fluidity as overall erotic responsiveness to one's less-preferred gender, (2) fluidity as situational variability in erotic responsiveness to one's less-preferred gender, (3) fluidity as discrepancy between the gender patterning of sexual attractions and the gender patterning of sexual partnering, and (4) fluidity as instability in day-to-day attractions over time. Another related concept, erotic plasticity, is defined as change in people's sexual expression—that is, attitudes, preferences, and behavior. In other words, someone's sexual response can fluctuate depending on their surrounding environment.

And yet we still present statistics as divided into males and females. Globally, male life expectancy, at 68 years, lags 5 years behind female life expectancy. There is not a single country in which male life expectancy exceeds female. Overall, the gap between the sexes has widened since 1970 and will continue to widen. By 2030, male life expectancy is expected to be 7 years shorter than female life expectancy. Men have a more than 40% probability of dying between the ages of 50 and 74, while for women the probability is less than 30%.[1]

Of 67 risk factors and risk-factor clusters identified in the Global Burden of Disease (GBD) 2010 study, 60 were responsible for more male than female deaths and the top 10 risk factors were all more common in men. In 2010, three times as many men as women died because of tobacco use. 3.14 million men died due to alcohol-related issues, compared with 1.72 million women. Almost 1 million more men than women died from dietary risk factors, such as low fruit and vegetable intake and eating too much processed meat.[1] Almost 90% of deaths attributable to occupational risk factors in 2010 were male. About 1.25 million people die each year as a result of road traffic accidents; some three-quarters (73%) are men.[1]

With respect to mental health. we see in many countries a high incidence of male suicide, in particular in middle-aged single men, and severe alcohol abuse is very prevalent. Further, male depression is frequently manifest in forms that are poorly recognized and consequently inadequately treated. Similarly, many men may not know how to manage psychological stress, and a high proportion of men in Western societies have acquired psychological coping strategies that are dysfunctional. As a result, men underutilize mental health services, with negative implications for clinical outcome.[2] But men are still more present in the workplace, have the primary responsibility of being the principal financial provider, and face shame if they fail in this task.

In the light of the above health issues, the Global Action on Men's Health (GAMH)— that represents a wide range of men's health and related organizations with a focus on public health and the social determinants of health—aims to improve health and well-being in men and boys irrespective of background and encourages health practitioners to pay attention to the specific needs of males in service delivery, health promotion, and clinical practice.

Taking a social psychiatric perspective, the chapter will provide an overview of the historical dimension of male supremacy, mental distress in men, and the frequency and manifestations of the most common mental disorders in males. Finally, the utilization of mental health services will be discussed, and recommendations will be provided on how to satisfy the needs of the male population suffering from mental illness.

The Paradox of Power and Powerlessness
Evolution, Sociology, and History

Men are seen in a traditional sense to have "power" in relation to women. There is some truth to this belief. It is also true that relative to some men with more power, many men are subservient, exploited, oppressed, and excluded, usually based on class, race/ethnicity/ tribe, religion, sexual orientation, age, geography, etc. The men with all the power rule a very tight hierarchy to their advantage. One of the key elements of their power is the ability to establish and maintain the hierarchy that keeps them in power, pitting some against the other. This is what Wilkerson calls "caste"-based hierarchy, rather than gender-based hierarchy. This hierarchy of power can be detrimental to many, including men themselves.

Biologically, men in general are larger and are built stronger than women. Unlike the theory of brute strength, the reasons are based on evolutionary need for propagation of the species. Sexual dimorphism between males and females of a species is common in most species, but men and women are more physically similar than we are different. Nonetheless, there are a few key distinctions in our physiques. Some of them are designed to suit each sex for the role it plays in reproduction, while others exist to help us tell each other apart and to aid in our mutual attraction. Women have breasts which give them ability to feed their children. Men have deeper voices than women. Women have evolved to seek out men who have all the indicators of fitness and health; studies have shown time and time again that women tend to be more attracted to men with lower-pitched voices. They are looking for a mate with whom to produce healthy offspring. The more testosterone a man has, the stronger his brow, cheekbones, and jaw line. Meanwhile, the more estrogen a woman has, the wider her face, the fuller her lips, and the higher her eyebrows. In short, sex hormones control the divergence of male and female facial features. Women found men with facial hair more attractive than men without it, and thus were more likely to mate with bearded men. This attraction could arise because beards not only signal high testosterone levels, they also signify sexual maturity (in much the same way as breasts on women), as well as possibly signifying dominance by increasing the perceived size of a man's jaw. Also to some degree this may have been a factor in the survival of the species in earlier societies, where a predominating role of males contributed to the development of the patriarchy that has manifested itself in the economic, political, legal, and social organization of most cultures. The patriarchal system contributed to an ideology of seeing males as inherently superior and thereby justifies the dominance of males in all areas of society.

It is a matter of debate when and how patriarchy developed. Some find that is it linked with the domestication, others that it is related to when the concept of fatherhood took root. Whatever the causes of its development, patriarchy has taken shape according to the culture where it is practiced, and today we still find that most contemporary societies are for all practical reasons patriarchal even though this may not explicitly be reflected in their laws and national policies.[3] A very important explanation for the origin of patriarchy was given by Frederick Engels in 1884 in his book *The Origins of the Family, Private Property and the State*. At the stage when private property arose in tsociety, men wanted to retain power and property and pass it on to their own children. According to Engels, it was in this period that both patriarchy and monogamy for women were established. According the first tools of production, and if they were to M. Mies,[4] women were the first producers of life, of social production, of also the first to initiate social relations, why were they unable to prevent the establishment of a hierarchical and exploitative relationship between the sexes? She answers this by saying that male supremacy, far from being a consequence of men's superior economic contribution, was a result of the development and control of destructive tools through which they controlled women, nature, and other men. According to Lerner, patriarchy was not one event, but a process developing over a period of almost 2500 years (from approximately 3100 BC to 600 BC), and several factors and forces were responsible for the establishment of male supremacy as we see it today. However, there are several ways to consider the dominance of patriarchy. From a biological perspective, it has been argued[5] that males have developed to be more aggressive in order to get access to territories, resources, and mates. From a sociological perspective, patriarchy can be seen as a construction that through time has been passed from generation to generation, favoring male dominance, and that patriarchy developed due to historic rather than biological conditions.

Culture and Cross-Cultural Variations

According to Edwards,[6] we have seen a three-phase model of masculinity studies. The first wave, from the 1970s, focused on demonstrating the socially constructed nature of masculinity and its reliance on socialization. In the 1980s, the second wave reacted against the fact that Black, working-class, and gay men were seen as subordinated to the hegemonic White, Western, middle-class, heterosexual men, and dealt with power and its polyvalent meanings. The third wave is influenced by the advent of post-structural theory in questions of normativity. The growing development of studies of non-Western masculinities has yet to develop analyses of race, ethnicity, and masculinity.[6] Edwards's study describes college men engaged in a process of gender identity development that centered on a complex interaction between them as individuals and society's expectations of them as men. Over time, they were socialized into and then internalized dominant society's increasingly complex expectations of them as men. These men spent their lives wearing a mask and performing these expectations, which was a struggle because it did not reflect their true selves. This performance had consequences for women, for other men, and for the participants themselves. Each of the men had begun to remove the mask and transcend society's expectations of them in certain situations or under certain circumstances. They described critical influences and critical events that helped them to begin transcending these external expectations of them as men.

In recent years we see an increasing interest in whether there is a link between violence and Muslim men. It is a belief that in the Qur'an certain characteristics are seen as prescribing masculinity: submissiveness, altruism, righteousness, steadfastness, and combativeness—however, they are not only overlapping but also contradictory, depending on the institutional context in which the people are acting, as well as their religious status.[7] The United Nations reports that globally, the absolute number of war deaths has been declining since 1946. And yet, conflict and violence are currently on the rise, with many conflicts today waged between non-state actors, such as political militias, criminals, and international terrorist groups. In 2016, more countries experienced violent conflict than at any point in almost 30 years. But today, crime kills far more people than armed conflicts. In 2017, almost half a million people across the world were killed in homicides, far surpassing the 89,000 killed in active armed conflicts and the attacks. Countries in the Americas have the worst homicide rates by a wide margin, accounting for 37% of the global total in a region that accounts for only 13% of the world's population. Political instability engenders organized crime, including targeted attacks against police, women, journalists, and migrants. Meanwhile, political violence no longer affects only low-income states. In the past 15 years, more than half of the world's population has lived in direct contact or proximity to significant political violence. For women and girls, the home remains the most dangerous place. Some 58% of female homicides were carried out by intimate partners or family members in 2017, up from 47% in 2012. Women bear the heaviest burden of lethal victimization, often because of misogynistic beliefs, inequality, and dependency, which persist globally, especially in low-income countries. While terrorism remains widespread, its impact has been waning in recent years. Globally, the number of deaths attributed to terrorism. More than 99% of all terrorist-related deaths occur in countries involved in a violent conflict or with high levels of political terror. Most deadly attacks take place in the Middle East, North Africa, and Sub-Saharan Africa, with Afghanistan, Iraq, Nigeria, Somalia, and Syria bearing the heaviest burden.

Recent research interest in Muslim men has mainly focused on youthful masculinities[8] and accounts showing how problematizing ideas about Muslim masculinities have become commonplace, and describing Muslim men as self-interested defenders and chief beneficiaries of a deeply patriarchal, oppressive culture with a focus on abusive, exploitative familial gender relations, arising from culturally situated unequal power relations and leading to deviant cultural practices.[8] But research in the United Kingdom following a child sexual exploitation crisis suggests the emergence of new masculine subject positions that are adjusting to a changing gender order and raising important questions about the extent to which Muslim men's involvement in caring facilitates greater gender equality.

Studies of male samples from five Asian countries showed that the majority of men considered "having a good job" (20.3%), "being seen as a man of honor" (15.6%) and "being in control of his own life" (14.6%) as the most important attributes.[9] The relative importance differed across countries but did not vary with age.

Men and Changes in Family Structure

Over the past decades, huge changes have taken place in family patterns in most parts of the world, with a decrease in fertility, later marital age, women being employed outside the home, and divorce becoming very common, to mention a few. Family life is changing in the United States and most of the world. Two-parent households are on the decline as divorce, remarriage, and cohabitation are on the rise. And families are smaller now, both due to the growth of single-parent households and the drop in fertility. Single motherhood is on rise. Less than half (46%) are living in two-parent families in the United States. The declining share of children living in what is often deemed a "traditional" family has been largely supplanted by the rising shares of children living with single or cohabiting parents. Non-marital cohabitation and divorce, along with the prevalence of remarriage and non-marital coupling in the United States, make for family structures that in many cases continue to evolve throughout a child's life. An additional 15% of children are living with two parents, at least one of whom has been married before. The share of children living without either parent stands at 5%; most of these children are being raised by grandparents. There are significant variations in racial and ethnic makeup in the incidence of family structure. In 2000, one-third of births occurred to unmarried women. One in five children born within a marriage will experience the breakup of that marriage by age 9. In 2014, just 11% of women with a college degree or more who had a baby in the prior year were unmarried. In comparison, this share was about four times as high (43%) for new mothers with some college but no college degree. Almost 20% of women near the end of their childbearing years have had children by more than one partner, as have about 3 in 10 (28%) of those with two or more children also see a diversity of family patterns with more fluid gender roles.[10]

Further, men in many countries are increasingly engaged in child-rearing and daily household activities and their former status is challenged. Families can no longer be described as a fixed set of roles. Couple relationships have become less stable and more diverse, and in many countries the proportion of extramarital births has increased significantly. As pointed out by Olah and coworkers,[10] the existing research about family transitions tends to pay limited attention to the role of men, despite the clear gender differences in the mechanisms behind the transitions.[11]

The declining economic position of men in modern relationships, the change in decision-making, as well as the expectations that modern fathers play a more active role in child-rearing, are all challenges and may have an impact on male mental health that is far from sufficiently investigated.

Masculinity, Sexual, and Gender Orientation

The large body of anthropological research related to gender is to great extent equated to women's studies,[12] and a great proportion of men view male identities in comparison to female identities.[13] Masculinity is a construction and encompasses the roles, social norms, and behaviors that men in any society, at any time, are expected to follow.

In the socialization of masculinity, boys in most cultures are told to reject what is considered as stereotypically feminine, and are encouraged to be tough and competitive, and to distance themselves emotionally and physically from other men.[14] Later they are rewarded—in educational institutions as well as the workplace—for fulfilling these expectations, but there are also several negative consequences related to social and health issues. With regard to mental health, a focus on traditional masculinity may be associated with depression, suicide, violence, substance abuse, and stress.[14]

Men in general do not spend a lot of time thinking about what it means to them to be a man. That is because in most societies, being a man is an advantage, one that does not often invite self-reflection. And masculinity is, for many, so much the norm that a separate inventory is not needed. In line with that, we also in biological research see the distribution of various biological parameters based on data from males representing "normalcy." But masculinity also plays an important role in the help-seeking behaviors of men, and efforts should be done to encourage discussions hereof in order to reduce the barriers in male help-seeking behavior in case of mental distress and stress.[15] However, masculinity is not "natural." It is a gender identity that is constructed socially, culturally, historically, and politically, and it reflects how maleness has been interpreted in a given society.

The hegemonic White, heterosexual masculinity is under scrutiny in Western countries and is likely to undergo significant changes. The #MeToo movement is one example of a movement expanding internationally with the purpose to reveal the extent that males—often in superior positions—have abused and sexually harassed women.

Nevertheless, many of the underlying characteristics associated with male supremacy remain quite stable. Hegemonic masculinity consistently represents anti-femininity, success and achievement, independence, and toughness, but the reflection in men's appearance and sexuality is more transitory.[14]

The Precarious Position of Men in Habitat

Work is central to the identity of men. It is their preponderant social role. The capacity to provide for one's self and one's family is at the core of traditional male values. In countries with advanced economies, though, this aspect of male identity is being transformed dramatically. As the structure of the modern economy has shifted away from mass employment in industries based on the extraction of natural resources, the work available to men has shifted too. The change in the market for labor in the formerly industrial countries has dramatically affected men, leading to some of them being casualties of the socioeconomic processes around them. The postindustrial knowledge and service economy offers good opportunities for men with college-level educations, but has been much less generous to men with a high school degree or less. In the United States, for example, these men are making less money than they did in the 1970s. The jobs available to them are also perceived as being less dignified and less "manly." Further, with the waning of the labor movement there is also much less social and political power contained in the jobs these men do. The end results of all these changes are perhaps the only predictable aspects of these developments. Men, especially the White men in question, are not optimistic about the future. For men with high school education or less, the work is more precarious, their participation in the labor market is drastically reduced, and the lives they struggle to live are ending early with the deaths of despair—overdoses, suicides, and deaths related to alcohol use.

Mental Distress: Casualties of Modern Society

Mental illness among men is a public health concern that begs attention.[16] Starting in childhood, a longitudinal US community study of boys[17] documented that childhood risk factors predicted later mental health problems, and in general the more risk factors, the higher likelihood of later distress. In recent years, scholars from domains such as criminology, education, and psychology have agitated for more attention to men's mental health and well-being. And together with epidemiological data showing the high prevalence of mental distress in men, this has led to the development of the specific field of men's mental health.[18]

There is considerable debate about the frequency of common mental health disorders in men and whether men far more frequently than women go undiagnosed. The UK Men's Health Forum[19] has argued that the frequency of clinical diagnoses may be an inadequate measure and that other measures may be more appropriate to provide a picture of men's mental health. Men report significantly lower life satisfaction than women in the UK Government's national well-being survey, and more than 75% of those who commit suicide are men; men are 3 times more likely to report drug abuse than women; men commit 86% of violent crimes and constitute 95% of the prison population, out of which 72% have a mental disorder, and men have clearly less access to social support from friends and relatives. With this in mind, it may be argued that emotional and mental distress in men may not fit within conventional approaches to psychiatric diagnosis, but that a broader social psychiatric perspective is needed.[19]

Mental Illnesses

Depression

In epidemiological surveys, measures of depression and anxiety frequently are based on self-reported severity-based scales, and here gendered differences in the expression of depressive symptoms may influence both the incidence and prevalence reported.[20]

As depression may be expressed differentially in men, particularly in the early stages, it often manifests as irritability, anger, hostility, aggressiveness, risk-taking, and escaping behavior, and other types of acting-out behavior—what has often been named "masked depression"—and can mask more typical "classical" symptoms of depression.[16] It has been suggested[21] that men tend to blunt the reporting of possible depressive symptoms perhaps because such symptoms are inconsistent with dominant notions of masculinity.

In the Swedish Gotland study aimed at reducing suicides by educating general practitioners, a major result was the gender difference in the detection and treatment of depression. One of the reasons was that few suicidal males were known to the medical services, although many of them were known to the police and social welfare services. The reasons why depressed and suicidal men do not show up in the medical services are found to lie in the differences between the male and the female depressive syndrome, leading to difficulties in reaching, diagnosing, and treating these patients, and which resulted in the development of the Gotland Male Depression Scale in order to improve diagnosing depression in males.[22]

Men often avoid addressing their feelings and, frequently, family members, friends, or colleagues are the first to recognize that the person may suffer from a depression—and here it is important that friends and family encourage him to visit a doctor or mental health professional for an evaluation. As regards the treatment, a combination of medication and psychotherapy is effective in most, as well as considering the need for changes in lifestyle.

Suicide

Repeated surveys have demonstrated a higher suicide rate in men compared to women, and this ratio is particularly elevated in some ethnic groups, such as Canadian Inuits; in the United States, African American males show a similar elevated ratio compared to the general population.[18] Among the risk factors, communication is important. In general, males are less likely to open up and share their problems, admitting they are vulnerable, and are less willing to seek help. And if they recognize the mental distress, self-medication in the form of alcohol or drugs may be the remedy of choice. Another risk factor is experiencing job loss, seeing no future opportunities, as is the case in many socially deprived areas. But also divorce, losing contact with children, and subsequent isolation all add to the risk.

Alcohol and Substance Abuse

Epidemiological evidence suggests that nearly 20% of adult males have alcohol abuse or suffer from alcoholism-related complications. On the other hand, only about 5%–6% of adult females are alcoholic or abuse alcohol on a regular basis.[23]

Society has also had the long-held belief that alcoholism and alcohol-related problems are predominantly a male phenomenon, because rates of alcohol dependence are greater in men than in women. However, alcohol dependence does affect an estimated 5% of women in the United States, with serious consequences.[24] In general, women tend to consume less alcohol than men and appear to be less likely to manifest certain risk factors for alcohol use and health problems. Nonetheless, women perceive greater social and health sanctions for drinking, while alcohol and alcoholism may counter desirable feminine traits (e.g., nurturing). Moreover, women are less likely to display characteristics associated with excessive drinking, including aggressiveness, drinking to alleviate distress, behavioral under control, sensation-seeking, and antisociality.[25]

In a population-based study of US male twins, genetic factors played a major role in the development of alcoholism, with similar influence for alcohol abuse and alcohol dependence, and environmental factors shared by family members seemed of little influence on the development of alcoholism in males.[26]

Personality Disorders

Empirical studies on gender differences in personality disorders show divergent results and may depend on the study setting. In a representative Norwegian community sample, males and females were found to have almost the same prevalence of personality disorders,[27] but in analyzing the different categories, men had relatively more antisocial or passive-aggressive disorders, and women had more histrionic, borderline, and dependent disorders. A household survey from the United Kingdom, on the other hand, found a higher prevalence of personality problems in males.[28] Among male prisoners in Sweden, 56% were found to have personality disorders, with a high degree of psychopath personality traits.[29] In a male German prison population, antisocial personality was a predictor of age for first conviction, and this group was found to have had severe childhood traumatic experiences.[30]

Schizophrenia

Many studies indicate that the incidence of schizophrenia is higher in men, and most studies report that the age of onset is earlier in men than in women. As regards the level of cognitive functioning, there is more controversy. On the other hand, men suffering from schizophrenia have a higher level of cannabis consumption and are more likely to have alcohol abuse.

Women also seem to have a better premorbid level of functioning than men.[31] But also later in the course of the illness, women are better adapted, show less disability than men, and have fewer relapses, which may partly be explained by the later onset of illness, but also that female patients tend to show higher compliance.

Trauma, Post-Traumatic Stress Disorder

The lifetime prevalence of post-traumatic stress disorder (PTSD) is about 10%–12% in women and 5%–6% in men. Males experience more traumatic events on average than do females, yet females are more likely to meet diagnostic criteria for PTSD. Men and women experience different types of trauma, both in private life and at work, with women being exposed to more high-impact trauma (e.g., sexual trauma) than men, and at a younger age. War-related mortality and morbidity is very high in men. Examples include 9 million deaths in World War I, 10 million deaths of Soviet soldiers in World War II; 500,000 deaths in the Iran-Iraq war, and 3–5 times higher incidence of PTSD in most of the wars than the number of deaths. It is reported less and diagnosed less in men. Trauma early in life has more impact, especially when it involves type II trauma, interfering with neurobiological development and personality. Traumatic stress affects different areas of the brains of boys and girls at different ages. In the acute phase, women generally score higher than men do on acute subjective responses, e.g., threat perception, per traumatic dissociation and known predictors of PTSD. Women handle stressful situations differently and have evolved differentially to support these different behaviors. For instance, women in stressful situations may use a tend-and-befriend response, rather than the fight-or-flight response that is often assumed. Emotion-focused, defensive and palliative coping are more prevalent in women, while problem-focused coping is higher in men. Women seek more social support, the lack of it being the most consistent predictor of negative outcome of trauma. Women have been shown to benefit more from psychotherapy then men in the reduction of PTSD symptoms.

Sexual Dysfunction and Paraphilias

Sexual dysfunctions are highly prevalent, affecting about 43% of women and 31% of men. Hypoactive sexual desire disorder, erectile dysfunction, and premature ejaculation are common in men. Paraphilia-related experience cannot be regarded as unusual from a normative perspective. Many men experience paraphilias without accompanying problem awareness or distress, even when they are associated with potentially causing harm to others. The percent of men that reported at least one paraphernalia-associated sexual arousal pattern was 62.4%. *Exhibitionism, voyeurism, frotteurism,* and *toucheurism* are some examples of paraphilias. Pedophilia and sexual violence with adult females are the two most harmful offenses against others. In view of the relevance for sex life and relationship satisfaction, the presence of Paraphilia-associated sexual arousal patterns (PASAP) should be assessed in all sexual medical consultations. The etiologic basis for these disorders includes genetic, traumatic, and psychosocial factors. Treatment involves psychological, behavioral, psychopharmacological, and forensic interventions.

Help-Seeking

Men's mental health help-seeking lags far behind women's, with resulting huge personal, relational, physical, mental, and economic costs.[32] WHO reports in their 2018 overview that cultural stigma is one of the greatest barriers for seeking help in the case of mental health problems and that it is particularly pronounced in men.

When it comes to help-seeking in England, only 36% of those accessing psychological therapies are men, and men are also less likely to disclose mental health problems to friends and relatives,[19] and are more likely to use potentially harmful coping methods such as drugs or alcohol in response to stress. Despite huge pain, many men suffer in silence and due to various factors—stigma being prominent, as well as interpreting help-seeking as a sign of weakness—many men decide to avoid mental health services. Furthermore, men are more likely than women to terminate therapy early and generally have negative attitudes toward help-seeking.[33]

In a large US national sample on mental healthcare, an intersectional analysis revealed that men from sexual minorities had a more favorable attitude toward mental health treatment. Considering the income-poverty ratio, it appeared to be unrelated to help-seeking, but when analyzing each racial/ethnic group this became more nuanced, as the ratio was positively associated with help-seeking among White men, unrelated to help-seeking among Mexican American men, and negatively associated with help-seeking among Black men.[34]

Male students represent a group that is less likely to seek mental health treatment than their female counterparts. They have a much higher risk of committing suicide, and reducing help-seeking barriers for this group can have a suicide-preventive function and lead to more positive help-seeking behaviors in adulthood.[35] Based on a focus group model, the research group identified 17 factors influencing help-seeking behaviors. Among them were: "help-seeking is not masculine"; "public-stigma of help-seeking"; "difficulty identifying mental health symptoms"; "unfamiliarity with mental health services"; "symptom severity (i.e., delay until symptoms are unmanageable)"; "preference for proactive therapies"; "availability of services"; and "fear and embarrassment of using mental health services." These are all factors that not only relate to students, but that should be considered for the improvement of mental health services in fulfilling the needs of the male population.

Concluding Highlights

1. The world of today no longer sees humans as divided into two sexes but rather with diversified complexity, as individuals may see themselves no longer identifying with being either male or female. Sexual preferences can change over time, depending on the situation.
2. Males are at greater risk for global burden of disease (GBD), which is responsible for disease and suffering in men, including death.
3. Masculinity, patriarchy, and male power are being examined and challenged mostly due to advancements of society and evolving into healthier, necessary transformations. But at times this contributes to turmoil and conflicts.
4. Changes, advancements, globalization, digitization, and urbanization are changing families, family structures, and family roles, including the role of men in the family. Again, this is not happening without some pain, suffering, and conflict.
5. Culture, nationality, religion, sexual orientation, gender, generational aspects, class, and habitat contribute variations to identity and role differences in men.
6. Mental distress and illness play a significant role in men's distress. Stigma and the various ways it plays a role continue to be major factor in accepting and making use of resources to overcome mental illness. Psychiatrists, and mental health and medical professionals need to play an advocacy role for men and their loved ones to heal, and thus enhance their families and society.

Steps Forward

At times, men are a problem for our societies, and they are a problem for themselves. Indeed, a high proportion of men, not only in Western societies, have acquired psychological coping strategies that are often dysfunctional in the case of mental distress. But men are also an incredible benefit for themselves and other people. It is a mixed bag. Nonetheless, it is clear that if there is to be a resolution of these problems, men themselves must stand up and be a strong source of the solution. There is a need for men to learn more adaptive coping mechanisms and to overcome the barriers in seeking help if we are to overcome the under-utilization of mental health services by men. It is high time to pay more attention—in clinical work, training, and research—to make-tip address men's mental health through: healthcare policy that facilitates access; research on tailoring interventions to men; population-level initiatives to improve the capacity of men to cope with psychological distress; and clinical practice that is sensitive to the expression of mental health problems in men and that responds in a relevant manner.

There are many issues at stake on different levels:

On the *individual level*: men and boys should be encouraged to take better care of their own health, as well as the health of their partners and children.

In *educational facilities*: schools and other educational institutions should have more focus on helping boys to overcome internal barriers in help-seeking and helping them understand that this can be compatible with modern masculinity. Specific approaches to service provision designed to improve men's accessing care.

In relation to *healthcare providers*: the specific needs of men and boys in service delivery should be taken into account, as well as health promotion and clinical practice.

In *research*: efforts should be made to encourage multidisciplinary research into the health of men and boys and to tailor interventions specific to these groups.

On the *policy/governmental level*: global health organizations and national governments.

References

1. Baker P. Men's health: A global problem requiring global solutions. 2016 May–June; www.trendsin menshealth.com.
2. Bilsker D, Fogarty AS, Wakefield MA. Critical issues in men's mental health. *Can J Psychiatry*. 2018 Sep;63(9):590–596.
3. Pateman C. Sexual contract. In: *The Wiley Blackwell Encyclopedia of Gender and Sexuality Studies*. Singapore: John Wiley & Sons; 2016:1–3. doi: 10.1002/9781118663219.wbegss468.
4. Mies M. Sexist and racist implications of the new reproductive technology. *Alternatives*. 1987;XII:323–342.
5. Van Vugt M. Gender differences in cooperation and competition: the male-warrior hypothesis" *Psychol Sci*. 2006;18(1):19–23. doi: 10.1111/j.1467-9280.2007.01842.x. MID 17362372.
6. Edwards T. *Cultures of Masculinity*. London and New York: Routledge, 2006.
7. Kabasakal Ara ZF, Hasan A. Muslim masculinity: what is the prescription of the Qur'an? *J Gender Studies*. 2018;27:788–801.
8. Britton J. Muslim men, racialised masculinities and personal life. *Sociology*. 2019;53:36–51.

9. Ng CJ, Tan HM, Low WY. What do Asian men consider as important masculinity attributes? Findings from the Asian Men's Attitudes to Life Events and Sexuality (MALES) Study. *J Men's Health.* 2008;5:250–255.

10. Oláh LZ, Richter R, Kotowska I. The new roles of men and women and implications for families and societies. *Families and Societies*: Working paper series. 2014;11.

11. Oppenheimer VK. Cohabiting and marriage during young men's career-development process. *Demography.* 2003;40(1):127–149.

12. Gutmann MC. Trafficking in men: the anthropology of masculinity. *Ann Rev Anthropol.* 1997;26:385–409.

13. Gutmann MC. 1996. *The Meanings of Macho: Being a Man in Mexico City.* Berkeley: University of California Press.

14. Mankowski ES, Smith RM. Men's mental health and masculinities In: Friedman HS, ed. *Encyclopedia of Mental Health.* 2nd ed. Elsevier; 2016.

15. Postl C, Jenkins LC. Meditation, yoga and men's health. In: Yafi FA, Yafi NR, eds. *Effects of Lifestyle on Men's Health.* Elsevier; 2019. https://doi.org/10.1016/C2018-0-01154-8.

16. Ogrodniczuk J, Oliffe J, Kuhl D, Gross PA, Mens' mental health. *Can Fam Physician.* 2016 Jun;62(6):463–464.

17. Loeber R, Farrington DP, Stouthamer-Loeber M, Moffitt TE, Caspi A, Lynam D. Male mental health problems, psychopathy, and personality traits: key findings from the first 14 years of the Pittsburgh Youth Study. *Clin Child Fam Psychol Rev.* 2001 Dec;4(4).

18. Affleck W, Carmichael V, Whitley R. Men's mental health: social determinants and implications for services. *Can J Psychiatry.* 2018 Sep;63(9):581–589.

19. UK Men's Health Forum. 2017. https://www.menshealthforum.org.uk/key-data-mental-health. Accessed September 1, 2020.

20. Parker G, Fletcher K, Paterson A. Gender differences in depression severity and symptoms across depressive sub-types. *J Affect Disord.* 2014;167:351–357.

21. Nolen-Hoeksema S, Girgus J. The emergence of gender differences in depression during adolescence. *Psychol Bull.* 1994;115(3):424–443.

22. Rutz R, Wålinder J, Von Knorring L, Rihmer Z, Pihlgren H. Prevention of depression and suicide by education and medication: impact on male suicidality. An update from the Gotland study. *Internat J Psych in Clin Practice.* 1997;1:39–46.

23. Devaud LL, Matthews DB, Morrow AL. Gender impacts behavioral and neurochemical adaptations in ethanol-dependent rats. *Pharmacol Biochem Behav.* 1999;64:841–849.

24. Ceylan-Isik AF, McBride SM, Ren J. sex difference in alcoholism: who is at a greater risk for development of alcoholic complication? *Life Sci.* 2010 Jul 31;87(5–6):133–138.

25. Nolen-Hoeksema S. Gender differences in risk factors and consequences for alcohol use and problems. *Clin Psychol Rev.* 2004;24:981–1010.

26. Prescott CA, Kendler KS. Genetic and environmental contributions to alcohol abuse and dependence in a population-based sample of male twins. *Am J Psychiatry.* 1999;156:34–40.

27. Torgersen S, Kringlen E, Cramer V. The prevalence of personality disorders in a community sample. *Arch Gen Psychiat.* 2001;58:590–596.

28. Coid J, Yang M, Tyrer P, Roberts A. Prevalence and correlates of personality disorder in Great Britain. *Brit J Psychiatr.* 2006;188:423–431.

29. Longato-Stadler E, von Knorring L, Hallman J. Mental and personality disorders as well as personality traits in a Swedish male criminal population. *Nord J Psychiatr.* 2002;56:137–144.

30. Kopp D, Spitzer C, Kuwert P, et al. Psychiatric disorders and childhood trauma in prisoners with antisocial personality disorder. *Fortschr Neurol Psychiatr.* 2009;77:152–159.

31. Ochoa S, Usall J, Cobo J, Labad X, Kulkarni J. Gender differences in schizophrenia and first-episode psychosis: a comprehensive literature review. *Schizophrenia Res Treat.* 2012; Article ID 916198. doi: 10.1155/2012/916198.

32. World Health Organization. *Prevention and Promotion in Mental Health.* Geneva, Switzerland; 2002.

33. Doherty DT, Kartalova-O'Doherty Y. Gender and self-reported mental health problems: predictors of help-seeking from a general practitioner. *Br J Health Psychol.* 2010;15:213–228.

34. Parent MC, Hammer JH, Bradstreet TC, Schwartz EN, Jobe T. Men's mental health help-seeking behaviors: an intersectional analysis. *Am J Mens Health*. 2018 Jan;12(1):64–73.

35. Sagar-Ouriaghli I, Godfrey E, Graham S, June S, Brown L. Improving mental health help-seeking behaviours for male students: a framework for developing a complex intervention. *Int J Environ Res Public Health*. 2020;17:49–65. doi: 10.3390/ijerph17144965. https://www.researchgate.net/publication/342864288s.

Sociocultural Perspectives

Social psychiatry inherently integrates and considers the social and cultural aspects of human behavior. These ranges across cultural values and beliefs, spieirual beliefs, sexual expression, the constructs of families, the phenomenon of human migration across the globe, and the socially related economic factors affecting humans and society. This section reviews these aspects of social psychiatry and hw they impact infdividfual and population mental health.

14

Culture

Normality, Psychopathology, and Treatment

Andres J. Pumariega and Pedro Ruiz

Culture and Human Behavior

Culture is the shared collective knowledge, beliefs, skills, and traditions that allow a group of people and families to adapt successfully to their ecological contexts over multiple generations and often millennia. Culture is central to the understanding and interpretation of human psychological and psychosocial development. Culture influences such concepts and constructs as gender and relational roles, behavioral norms, and normative approaches to child-rearing and discipline. Cultural values determine the cognitive skills (instrumental, analytical, social, etc.) and adaptive psychological skills that are reinforced as children develop (influenced by cultural values). Various protective beliefs, including taboos against certain risky behaviors, are also reinforced by different cultures. Cultural values are transmitted by the family to the child, and later are reinforced by societal institutions such as schools, churches, and other community institutions.

Cultures are not static or reified, and are naturally dynamic, resilient, and constantly evolving, adapting to societal, technological, and environmental changes. A common misconception is that cultures are static and unyielding, but this typically happens when cultures are challenged, such as when they are stressed by external or internal forces, leading to their constituents being overwhelmed by the degree of allostatic load resulting from the degree or pace of changes in their ecological contexts.

The process of learning about and adapting to a new culture is termed *acculturation*.[1] For centuries, traditionalists emphasized *assimilation* as the ideal adaptation, where the native cultural orientation is replaced by that of the host culture. This was the preferred form of adaptation promoted by many nations that received immigrants and refugees. For example, the United States for many decades expected this from multiple waves of European immigrants, with frequent sudden rejections of traditional identifiers (such as names, language, customs, traditions, etc.) in order to assimilate into the host culture. However, potential knowledge and skills are lost in this type of adaptation; as are connections of the individual to their heritage, extended family supports, and many other adaptive resources offered by the culture of origin. Spiegel[2] described psychological problems arising at normal developmental life stages in individuals (including European-origin immigrants) who have assimilated into mainstream American culture, but whose ambivalence becomes manifest in later psychosocial stages of life.

Cultural adaptation is a challenge for immigrants who arrive as adults to the host nation with a fairly established personal, ethnic, and cultural identity, or who are less educated and have greater limitations in learning new concepts and knowledge (including language), especially if their culture of origin greatly differs from the host culture. The traditional ethnic enclave (such as Chinatowns in various cities, South Asian enclaves in London, and Little Habana in Miami) has adaptive value in that it offers an initial base of community support for immigrants and their families, from which they can move into the mainstream society once they obtain new knowledge and skills. Many older immigrants adopt a pattern of cultural *separation* or *enculturation*, where they remain in the ethnic enclave and maintain and prefer the values, beliefs/practices, and language of their native culture and nation while rejecting those of the host culture.[3]

Increasingly, immigrants settle in newer destinations located in relatively homogenous regions, where such same-culture community support is limited, with consequences for higher levels of isolation and stress. Some younger first- and second-generation immigrants may become alienated from both cultures, as a result of living in isolated in homogeneous communities, losing adaptational skills and language from their culture of origin, or both. They may become *marginalized*, and thus lose economic and social opportunities afforded by wider sociocultural contacts and activity.[3]

Culture and Identity Development

Acculturation plays a significant role in the development of immigrant children and children of immigrants. Erik Erikson's[4] work highlighted the significance of culture in psychosocial development. He believed in psychosocial stages of development that spanned the total life cycle and which were both biologically and socioculturally determined. There were common tasks for each stage but variation in how these were expressed and in the timing of their expression or evolution. His major focus was on adolescence; he regarded identity formation as the central psychosocial task of adolescence, and he identified key aspects of optimal identity: (a) experiencing a subjective sense of comfort with the self; (b) having a sense of direction in life as well as continuity of the self from the past, to the present, and to the anticipated future; and (c) expressing an identity that is affirmed by a community of important others.

Erikson was one of the first theorists who saw the importance of adolescence as the key stage for identity consolidation. He conceptualized personal identity as the integration of psychological identity and cultural identity. He was influenced by his observations based on his immigrant experience and psychoanalytic interpretations of the cultural practices, worldviews, and child-rearing of Yurok and Sioux tribes. He was also influenced by Freud, whose only reference to identity was used to denote ethnicity and the impact of the subjugation of Jews in Western culture on his "clear consciousness of inner identity."[4(p20)] Erikson described how a key problem for individuals in identity formation was the degree to which their own cultural identity is nurtured by members of their own culture and how it is validated or mirrored by others in the community, in many ways foreseeing the dilemmas faced by youth from diverse cultural backgrounds living in host cultures. He argued that the central problem for Native Americans (American Indians) was that the powerful psychological salience of their history could not be validated and integrated by non-Indian educators of Native American children. He recognized the importance of racial/ethnic identity, including the value of maturational rituals in traditional cultures, with preparation for social/occupational roles and the development of a stable identity being key adolescent developmental tasks. The processes through which youth learn and internalize these roles and skills are increasingly complex in postmodern societies and cultures and may at times result in an ill-defined adolescent stage and transition process to adulthood. Traditional cultures have clearer proscribed maturational rituals for youth that, even to this day, have been shown to be beneficial to their adaptation and mental health.[5] Phinney[6] proposed a three-stage developmental progression from unexamined ethnic identity, through a period of ethnic exploration, to achieved or committed ethnic identity. This process ultimately results in a deeper understanding and internalization of their ethnicity. This culmination requires coming to terms with two fundamental problems for ethnic minorities: (a) cultural differences between their own group and the dominant group, and (b) the lower or disparaged status of their group in society.

If the dominant culture in a society holds an ethnic group and their characteristics in low esteem, then ethnic group members are potentially faced with a negative social identity and ethnic self-hate. This can be the result of racism and xenophobia, both of which have been recognized as having adverse mental health consequences at both an individual and public health level.[7,8] Individuals may seek to avoid identification with their ethnic group by "passing" as members of the dominant group, but this solution may have negative psychological consequences and is not available to individuals who are racially distinct. Alternative solutions are to develop a sense of ethnic pride, to reinterpret characteristics deemed "inferior" as strengths, and to stress distinctive aspects of one's ethnicity.[9]

Diverse children and youth often face significant pressures to assimilate into mainstream society through media images and implicit threats of social and economic marginalization. A bicultural identity is widely considered the best adaptational outcome, with youth remaining rooted in their culture of origin but having the necessary knowledge and interpersonal skills to successfully navigate mainstream culture. Theorists have postulated that the development of a bicultural identity is the most adaptive resolution for ethnic identity, where the individual is rooted in their own culture but can selectively adopt traits of both traditional and host culture.[9-11] Studies have supported that the development of a strong ethnic identity by minority youth within a host culture[9] and by immigrant groups in various nations[12] that have bicultural elements, including ethnic and national identifications, is associated with positive adaptation. LaFromboise et al.[13] and Rashid[14] proposed that bicultural efficacy (the belief that one can develop and maintain effective interpersonal relationships in two cultures) is directly related to one's ability to develop bicultural competence.[13] Bicultural efficacy is enhanced by parental modeling, particularly how well the parent has *accommodated* to the new culture (adopted certain aspects of the new culture, while still retaining important features of the culture of origin). Those who achieve bicultural efficacy can live effectively and satisfactorily within two groups without compromising their sense of cultural identity and can create and maintain support groups and connections to both minority and majority cultures. It also allows the individual to persist through periods when (s)he may experience rejection from one or both cultures.

However, immigrant and culturally diverse youth (and their families) can also experience other potential outcomes: (1) *marginalization*, with separation from both cultures and some degree of ethnic identity diffusion; (2) *assimilation*, where the culture of origin is rejected and the host culture is largely adopted, with the loss of language and customs of origin; (3) *separation*, where the host culture is rejected and there is a strong adherence to the traditional culture and language, often remaining bound to the "ethnic enclave"; and (4) *negative identification*, a form of marginalization where the youth is openly hostile to both cultures and adopts values and practices antithetical to both (e.g., adoption of gang culture or even extremist ideology or groups). Marginalization and separation can result in lost educational, social, and economic opportunities as the person moves into young adulthood and their generative phase of development. Assimilation may risk their loss of connection with their culture of origin and its sources of identification and support, leading to psychological and mental health difficulties.[2,4]

An even greater challenge is faced by multiracial/multiethnic youth. This is the fastest growing demographic in the United States and many other nations. These youth face stresses around identity formation both within their families and across peer groups, often feeling loyalty conflicts about their different origins. They may often face rejection and even discrimination from their own groups of origin. Multiracial/multiethnic youth need support to determine their own identifications and strengthen their unique racial/ethnic identity.[15]

When Culture Can Be Stressful

Acculturation stress results from adaptation to a host culture, including navigating differences in cultural values and beliefs, internal cultural value conflicts, external pressures to assimilate, as well as facing the host society's adverse reactions. It also results from the loss of protective values and beliefs from the culture of origin that help with psychological and social stresses (e.g., religious prohibition against suicide, norms for public conduct, etc.) while not yet adopting those of the host culture.[10,16] Cultural value differences (or lack thereof) can significantly affect adaptation. For example, Becker and colleagues,[17] in a comparative study of recovery from post-traumatic stress disorder (PTSD) in Bosnian versus Cambodian refugee youth, speculated that fewer cultural differences between the country of origin and the host country accounted for the better adaptation of Bosnian refugees to the United States. Several studies found associations between a stronger ethnic identity with lower acculturative stress, better academic performance, better psychological adaptation, and fewer externalizing and internalizing symptoms, but greater awareness of discrimination. Parental stress and family separations can adversely affect acculturative stress, while positive family relations can ameliorate it.[10,15]

Immigrant and minority children face the challenges of discrimination and bias, which are seen from the earliest stages of development, even among toddlers as they discover "others." In fact, categorization bias (the propensity to categorize "others" of the same species by external characteristics) is seen among many lower species (mammalian and avian), and most acutely in primates.[18] In humans, categorization bias is reified into social constructs, such as racism and xenophobia, within families and in societal institutions. In minority/majority environments, racism and discrimination have been shown to contribute to ethnic self-hate by youth.[19] Additionally, long-standing discrimination/marginalization is often associated with historical trauma related to more overt and systematic oppression of minority populations, which can have multigenerational impact on minority youth.[20] Many social protest movements addressing discrimination and marginalization have sprung up among racial and ethnic minority adolescents and young adults in the United States (such as the Black Lives Matter movement) and in Europe (among marginalized Muslim youth), stemming from the felt impact of discrimination and historical trauma. Such movements are positive in that they provide a sense of agency in the face of social inequities or disparities resulting from historical trauma, discrimination, and marginalization.[21,22]

Adaptation and resilience in the face of acculturation stress is highly dependent on family adaptation. For example, Sullivan et al.[23] found that integrated Latino immigrant adolescents who maintain heritage culture practices and adopt receiving culture practices reported higher parental involvement, positive parenting, and family support, but assimilated adolescents reported the greatest levels of aggressive behavior. Similarly, family adaptation and relationships mediated the impact of Russian immigrant youth's acculturation stress.[24] Youth and families in language-brokering contexts have shown higher levels of family stress, lower parenting effectiveness, poorer academic and emotional adjustment, and substance use in Latino immigrant youth.[25] Greater youth culture and language brokering was linked to less parental acculturation and more family conflict in Vietnamese immigrants.[26] These findings support concerns about the adverse psychological burdens of placing youth in the position of being linguistic interpreters and cultural brokers for their less acculturated immigrant parents. Extended family separations in the process of immigration can also play a role. For example, Mena et al.[27] found that extended parental separations in Latino immigrant youth are linked to problem behaviors, and separations from mothers are particularly linked to depressive symptoms, especially for females.

Acculturative family distancing (AFD) was identified by Hwang[28] to connote a significant acculturation (or cultural adaptation) gap between youth and their more traditional family. It had been described as far back as the 1970s by Szapocznik and colleagues[29] among immigrant Latino youth and their families, and they associated it with higher risk for substance abuse and conduct disturbance. Latter research has confirmed the role of AFD in the mental health of immigrant youth and families. Immigrant families who perceived higher levels of AFD experienced more parenting difficulties,[30] while those perceiving lower levels of AFD reported less family conflict.[31] Asian and Latino immigrant youth who reported higher AFD experienced higher individual and family distress and risk for depression, with the quality of the parenting relationship between fathers and adolescents serving as a mediator.[32,33] Korean Canadian youth identifying with their traditional culture perceived their families as more supportive and less rejecting.[34]

Immigration can often be stressful and even traumatic. These challenges are less frequently experienced by skilled, educated, and non-political immigrants, but they are very frequently faced by poorer immigrants, or those leaving their nations under adverse circumstances, such as refugees. Some of these stressors even start during their lives in their home nations (war, political strife, natural disasters, poverty, and famine) and are often the "push" factors that propel emigration. The migration journey itself can be dangerous (desert and sea crossings; complicated legal processes; surreptitious departures; victimization by smugglers or other travelers; life in refugee camps). Immigrants often suffer separation and immediate (or long-term) loss of extended family (and even nuclear family) or close friends, mitigated by having relatives and friends who have immigrated in advance (or landing in an ethnic enclave) who are available to provide immediate support. When immigrants arrive in the host nation, they then undergo many added stressful experiences: multiple moves in search of economic opportunity or better living environments, new economic pressures (from the prevailing consumer economy), and lengthy and complex legal proceedings (typical even for documented immigrants), all while learning a new language, new customs, and new legal and educational systems. For undocumented families, there is the added risk and stress from traumatic experiences at the hands of immigration authorities, including immigration raids and potential arrest, deportation, and resulting family separation.[10]

A related area that deserves special attention is that of the worst psychosocial outcomes from negative identity formation: gang involvement and radicalization. The former has implications for internal public safety, especially as related to recruitment into human trafficking, the drug trade, and other criminal activities. The latter is even more critical given the threats of recruitment of vulnerable youth into fundamentalism and extremism from outside and within Western nations. Attention to the mental health and welfare of minority youth is critical in preventing such adverse outcomes, in addition to specialized programs designed to identify vulnerable youth and de-programming programs to help re-cruited youth re-enter into mainstream society.[35]

Acculturation and Psychopathology

Risk of mental health problems have been shown to increase in second-generation and generation 1.5 youth (born in the country of origin and raised in the host country/culture) versus first-generation immigrants, with studies demonstrating associations between higher acculturation/assimilation and risk for psychopathology. These studies also clarify the processes through which these generational disparities arise. These findings have included: higher abnormal eating behaviors (among Latina and Asian origin adolescents);[36] higher risk of substance abuse and suicidality (Mexican American youth vs. Mexican youth);[37–39] increasing risk of suicidality and suicide attempts by African American and Latino youth found in the last four biennial CDC Risk Behavior Surveys;[40] higher levels of anxiety in Latino children versus European origin or African American children, with even higher anxiety symptoms in second- versus first-generation Latino youth;[41] acculturation interacting with parent–child conflict to predict suicidality in Asian American youth;[42] and age, acculturation, and cultural adjustment difficulties significantly predicting mental health symptoms in a large study of Japanese, Chinese, and Korean immigrant youth.[43]

More recent studies have further reinforced the relationship between acculturation stress and psychopathology among immigrant youth in the United States. Fenta, Hyman, and Noh[44] found that Ethiopian immigrant youth had rates of depression slightly higher than US Whites (9.8% versus 7.4%), but 3 times higher than their cohorts in Ethiopia (3.2%). Romero et al.[45] found that bicultural stress was higher for Latino and Asian origin youth, and significantly associated with depressive symptoms after accounting for ethnicity, socioeconomic status, gender, and age. In another study of Latina teens, greater differences in traditional gender role beliefs with parents were associated with higher levels of depression.[46] Acculturative stress, self-esteem,[47] and parental acculturation[48] have been correlated to substance abuse risk and antisocial behavior and symptoms of anxiety[49] in Latino youth. Zayas et al.[50] found that parental separation from mothers due to the immigration process and acculturative family distancing increased suicidal risk in Latina youth. Goforth, Oka, and Leong,[51] in a study of Arab American Muslim adolescents, found that acculturation and acculturative stress significantly predicted psychological problems but not overall competence.

Culturally Informed Mental Health Services

The concept of *cultural competence* in mental health services is central in effectively serving diverse populations. Cross, Bazron, Dennis, and Isaacs[52] defined *cultural competence* as the ability to serve people across cultural differences. They identified important provider characteristics in that regard (e.g., awareness and acceptance of differences; awareness of own cultural values; understanding of the dynamics of difference; development of cultural knowledge; ability to adapt practice to the cultural context of the patient). They also identified important service system or organization characteristics in cultural competence (e.g., valuing diversity; cultural self-assessment; management of the dynamics of difference; institutionalization of cultural knowledge; adaptation of policies, values, structure, and services to better address diverse cultural needs). Both types of characteristics are needed in order to deliver culturally competent services effectively.

Expressions of psychological or emotional distress differ across cultures. Idioms of distress are linguistic or somatic patterns of experiencing and expressing illness, affliction, or general stress. Idioms of distress do not generally correspond to diagnostic categories but can at times be alternative means of expression for disorders recognized by psychiatry, such as depression or anxiety disorders. However, they can also be expressions of psychological distress unique to a given culture, even normative expressions of stress. More complex expressions of illness or distress are termed cultural syndromes.[53,54] Idioms of distress and cultural syndromes can often be mistaken for more serious psychopathology. For example, *ataques de nervios* (a reaction combining anxiety, agitation, and dissociation common among Latinos of Caribbean origin) can be confused for a psychotic reaction, while *falling-out* (an expression of emotional stress among Afro-Caribbeans that includes sudden acute paralysis and dissociation) can be confused with catatonia.[55]

The DSM 5 Cultural Formulation[56] guides clinicians to evaluate an individual's cultural conceptualization of illness, which can be based on cultural beliefs or folk beliefs and explanatory model of illness. These include idioms of distress, behavioral/emotional norms, levels of perceived severity, meaning of distressing experiences, and methods of coping and help-seeking (including traditional/alternatives sources), and cultural syndromes.

Level of acculturation is key to understanding patients' conceptualization of illness, since it will determine the relative influence of host cultural values and beliefs versus values from the culture of origin on the expressions, understanding, and help-seeking approaches for psychopathology, as well as the adaptational values or strengths they use or have available. Effective evaluation also requires understanding of their cultural identity formation, impact of acculturative stress (including impact of discrimination/xenophobia, historical trauma and immigration trauma, and family adaptation to cultural transition). The DSM 5 Cultural Formulation and associated interviews/rating scales can assist clinicians to reach a comprehensive formulation that integrates culture, developmental, and other biopsychosocial factors in understanding individual patients and their families.[56]

The Practice Parameter for Culturally Competent Psychiatric Practice from the American Academy of Child and Adolescent Psychiatry[57] provides guidance in the evaluation and treatment of diverse children and adolescents within their cultural context, though it can readily be applied to the care of diverse populations of all ages. The Parameter focuses on these key areas:

- *Linguistic support* is critical for effective service delivery, whether through trained and certified interpreters or (preferably) clinicians who are fluent in the family's native language and familiar with their culture. The use of family members, especially children, as interpreters should be avoided at all costs. There should even be caution about using interpreters from the same community as the family, as doing so may result in a breach of confidentiality.
- *Family involvement* is critical and needs to focus on intergenerational conflicts, bridging the generational acculturation gap, mobilizing family supports, promoting respect for the traditional family structure, promoting cultural flexibility on the part of families, and facilitating the negotiation of confidentiality, so that patients can have some autonomy and privacy but remain engaged with their families. Interventions aimed at enhancing mental health should focus on family and intergenerational relationships, as they are often a predictor of successful outcomes.

- *Psychotherapy* should be practical and problem-solving, addressing immigration traumas, acculturation stress, and ethnic identity conflicts (internal or generational). The use of psychotherapies with evidence for the specific cultural population is preferred, adapted to address culturally specific values/beliefs/expressions, or culturally specific modalities or interventions.

- *Contextual and systemic supports* are important, with clinicians promoting family strengths and community natural supports, avoiding institutionalization and removal from families and communities as much as possible. If available, ethnically specific programs may be particularly effective. Case managers from the ethnic population are needed, who can mobilize such community supports and serve as intermediaries between the family and mainstream community agencies (schools, courts, child welfare, juvenile justice, and mental health) as well as culturally specific community organizations and faith communities.

- *Pharmacotherapy*, if utilized, should reflect ethnically related genetic and dietary factors that impact the metabolism of different medications. Clinicians should de-mystify the use of medications, provide effective education to patients and family members that bridge biomedical information to cultural beliefs that may intersect with the use of medications. At the same time, clinicians should respect the autonomy and decision by patients, parents, and elders around using pharmacotherapy.[58]

There is a growing literature evaluating the efficacy of various forms of evidence-based psychotherapy in the treatment of culturally diverse youth. Psychotherapeutic interventions demonstrating evidence with diverse populations include cognitive-behavioral and interpersonal therapy for treatment of depression in Latinos and African Americans;[59,60] individual and group cognitive-behavioral therapy (CBT) for treatment of anxiety disorders in Latinos and African Americans;[61,62] and trauma-focused cognitive psychotherapy and peer-mediated treatment for traumatic stress for African Americans.[63]

Most of these studies have involved culturally adapted protocols. Culturally adapted treatment modalities have shown some improved effectiveness compared with standard interventions, although the evidence is mixed. Two studies that used a correlational approach indicated that ethnic match between client and therapist was associated with positive outcomes after youth- and family-based treatment.[64,65] A meta-analysis of 76 studies evaluating the benefit of culturally adapted mental health interventions found a moderate benefit for culturally adapted interventions.[66] Another systematic literature review with a smaller meta-analysis, as well as a comparative analysis of effect sizes from culturally modified psychotherapies, found differences in effect sizes to be moderate to nonsignificant.[59]

Several culturally informed evidence-based interventions have been developed to address the special mental health needs of immigrant populations. For example, Brief Strategic Family Therapy[67] is a family-based intervention developed to address acculturative family distancing as a strategy to reduce youth substance abuse and conduct disturbance in Latino youth. It has demonstrated significant improvements in addressing these target symptoms, among not only Latinos but also other racial/ethnic groups, and has been adopted as a NIDA endorsed evidence-based practice. Cognitive Behavioral Therapy for Traumatic

Stress (CBITS)[68] is a school-based, multi-level CBT intervention (group, individual, and psychoeducational) that is delivered by educators and mental health professionals in school settings and addresses acculturation stress and cultural trauma across racial/ethnic populations in inner-city settings. Evaluation has demonstrated significant reductions in PTSD and depressive symptoms.

Culturally based interventions such as storytelling therapies,[69] the use of popular media formats as *telenovelas* (as part of an emergency room intervention with suicidal Latinas),[70] the and adaptation of traditional cultural approaches to services, such as the *promotoras de salud* model of neighborhood healthcare workers[71] and mental health collaboration with cultural healers (*curanderos* and *santeros*),[72] and community programs based on traditional cultural beliefs (Zuni Life Skills Development Program for adolescent substance abuse)[73] have also been used effectively.

There are no randomized controlled trials examining psychopharmacological response in diverse populations, but some studies have offered some indirect evidence. Okuma et al.[74] found that lower therapeutic doses of tricyclic antidepressants and lithium have been noted in Asian populations. Varner et al.[75] found that African American patients needed lower doses of tricyclic antidepressants (TCAs) than White patients to attain a similar response to major depression. They also suggested that African American patients might need lower doses of selective serotonin reuptake inhibitors (SSRIs) to achieve similar levels of response as White patients. The Treatment of Adolescent Depression Study[76] had a 26% minority representation among its participants (principally Latino and African American), and minority status was found not to be a significant moderator of acute treatment outcome using combined cognitive-behavioral psychotherapy and pharmacotherapy. The Multisite Treatment Study of Attention- Deficit/Hyperactivity Disorders found that inner-city African Americans and Latinos required combination stimulant pharmacotherapy and cognitive-behavioral intervention to achieve equal outcomes to White children, who required only stimulant pharmacotherapy.[77] Secondary data analysis from the clinical trials of atemoxetine for treatment of attention deficit hyperactivity disorder (ADHD) indicated that it has equivalent efficacy with Latinos and African Americans as with Caucasians, even though the initial severity of ADHD was more significant in these populations.[78,79]

Conclusions

Culturally diverse populations from non-Western backgrounds will become the majority in the United States by 2050, and a significant percentage of the population of formerly more homogeneous Western European nations. The economic and social future of these nations hinges on the health and welfare of these growing populations. It behooves policymakers to make all possible and expedited efforts to ensure that any disparities in health, mental health, education, and economic potential are addressed for this important segment of youth. The future of the Western world may well depend on it.[80,81]

Additionally, in a world that is rapidly globalizing, we also need to pay attention to the cultural adaptation and mental health of Western-origin populations as they deal with the adverse impact of rapid sociocultural changes,[82] such as economic displacement and increased rates of "deaths of despair" (overdose and suicide deaths) and work to develop new roles as part of multicultural global plurality.

References

1. Berry JW. Acculturation as varieties of adaptation. In: Padilla AM, ed. *Acculturation: Theory, Models, and Some New Findings*. Boulder, CO: Westview; 1980:9–26.
2. Spiegel J. *Transactions: The Interplay Between Individual Family and Society*. New York: Science House; 1971.
3. Berry J. Immigration, acculturation, and adaptation. *Appl Psychology*. 1997;46:5–68.
4. Erikson E. *Identity, Youth, and Crisis*. New York: W. W. Norton; 1968.
5. Markstrom C, Iborra A. Adolescent identity formation and rites of passage: the Navajo Kinaalda´ ceremony for girls. *J Res Adolesc*. 2003;13(4):399–425.
6. Phinney J. Ethnic identity in adolescents and adults: review of research. *Psychol Bull*. 1990;10:499–514.
7. American Psychiatric Association, Committee on Black Psychiatrists. Resolution against racism and racial discrimination and their adverse impacts on mental health. Available at: http://archive.psych.org/edu/other_res/lib_archives/archives/200603.pdf. Accessed May 25, 2016.
8. American Psychiatric Association, Committee on Hispanic Psychiatrists. Position statement on xenophobia, immigration, and mental health. *Am J Psychiatry*. 2010;167:726.
9. Roberts R, Phinney J, Masse L, et al. The structure of ethnic identity of young adolescents from diverse ethnocultural groups. *J Early Adolesc*. 1999;19:301–322.
10. Pumariega AJ, Rothe E. Leaving no children or families behind: the challenges of immigration. *Am J Orthopsychiat*. 2010;80(4):506–516.
11. Alvard M. The adaptive nature of culture. *Evol Anthropol*. 2003;12:136–149.
12. Almqvist K, Broberg A. Mental health and social adjustment in young refugee children 3 1/2 years after their arrival in Sweden. *J Am Acad Child Adolesc Psychiatry*. 1999;38(6):723–730.
13. LaFromboise T, Coleman HLK, Gerton J. Psychological impact of biculturalism: evidence and theory. *Psychol Bull*. 1993;114:395–412.
14. Rashid HM. Promoting biculturalism in young African-American children. *Young Child*. 1984;39:13–23.
15. Kerwin C, Ponterotto JG. Biracial identity development: theory and research. In: Ponterotto JP, Casas JM, Suzuki LA, et al., eds. *Handbook of Multicultural Counseling*. Thousand Oaks, CA: Sage; 1995:199–217.
16. Rothe EM, Tzuang D, Pumariega AJ. Acculturation, development and adaptation. *Child Adolesc Psychiatr Clin N Am*. 2010;19:681–696.
17. Becker DF, Weine SM, Vojvoda D. PTSD symptoms in adolescent survivors of "ethnic cleansing:: results from a one-year follow-up study. *J Am Acad Child Adolesc Psychiatry*. 1999;38:775–781.
18. Sackett G, Holm R, Ruppenthal G. Social isolation rearing: species differences in behavior of macaque monkeys. *Dev Psychol*. 1976;12:283–288.
19. Phinney J. Stages of ethnic identity development in minority group adolescents. *J Early Adolesc*. 1989;9:34–49.
20. Smelser NJ. Psychological trauma and cultural trauma. In: Alexander JC, Eyerman R, Giesen B, Smelser NJ, Stompka P, eds. *Cultural Trauma and Collective Identity*. Berkeley: University of California Press; 2004:31–59.
21. Bandura A. Social cognitive theory: an agentic perspective. *Ann Rev Psychol*. 2001;52:1–26.
22. Earls F. Towards a science of citizenship. *Am J Orthopsychiatry*. 2011;81(4):447–452.
23. Sullivan S, Schwartz S, Prado G, Huang S, Pantin H, Szapocznik J. A bidimensional model of acculturation for examining differences in family functioning and behavior problems in Hispanic immigrant adolescents. *J Early Adolesc*. 2007;27:405–430.

24. Birman D, Taylor-Ritzler T. Acculturation and psychological distress among adolescent immigrants from the former Soviet Union: exploring the mediating effect of family relationships. *Cult Divers Ethnic Minor Psychol*. 2007;13:337–346.

25. Martinez C, McClure H, Eddy J. Language brokering contexts and behavioral and emotional adjustment among Latino parents and adolescents. *J Early Adolesc*. 2009;29:71–98.

26. Trickett E, Jones C. Adolescent culture brokering and family functioning: a study of families from Vietnam. *Cult Divers Ethnic Minor Psychol*. 2007;13:143–150.

27. Mena M, Mitrani V, Muir J, & Santiestaban D. Extended parent-child separations: impact on Hispanic substance abusing adolescents. *J Spec Pediatr Nurs*. 2008;13:50–52.

28. Hwang W. Acculturative family distancing: theory, research, and clinical practice. *Psychotherapy*. 2006;43:397–409.

29. Szapocnik J, Kurtines W, Fernandez T. Bicultural involvement and adjustment in Hispanic-American youth. *Inter J Intercult Relations*. 1980;4:353–365.

30. Buki L, Ma T, Strom R, Strom S. Chinese immigrant mothers of adolescents: Self-perception of acculturation effects on parenting. *Cult Divers Ethnic Minor Psychol*. 2003;9:127–140.

31. Farver J, Narang S, Bhadha B. East meets west: ethnic identity, acculturation, and conflict in Asian Indian families. *J Fam Psychol*. 2002;16:338–350.

32. Hwang W, Wood J. Acculturative family distancing: links with self-reported symptomatology among Asian Americans and Latinos. *Child Psychiatr Human Devel*. 2009;40:123–138.

33. Kim S, Chen Q, Li J, Huang X, Moon U. Parent–child acculturation, parenting, and adolescent depressive symptoms in Chinese immigrant families. *J Fam Psychol*. 2009;23:426–437.

34. Kim U, Choi S. Individualism, collectivism, and child development: a Korean perspective. In: Greenfield PM, Cocking RR, eds. *Cross-Cultural Roots of Minority Child Development*. Hillsdale, NJ: Erlbaum; 1994:227–257.

35. Weine S, Horgan J. Building resilience to violent extremism: one community's perspective. *FBI Law Enforcement Bulletin*. April 8, 2014. https://leb.fbi.gov/2014/april/building-resilience-to-violent-extremism-one-communitys-perspective. Last accessed on May 29, 2016.

36. Pumariega, A. Acculturation and eating attitudes in adolescent girls: a comparative and correlational study. *J Am Acad Child Psychiatry*. 1986;25:276–279.

37. Swanson J, Linskey A, Quintero-Salinas R, Pumariega A, Holzer C. Depressive symptoms, drug use and suicidal ideation among youth in the Rio Grande Valley: a binational school survey. *J Am Acad Child Adolesc Psychiatry*. 1992;31:669–678.

38. Pumariega AJ, Swanson J, Holzer C, Linskey A, Quintero-Salinas R. Cultural context and substance abuse in Hispanic adolescents. *J Child Fam Studies*. 1992;1:75–92.

39. Pumariega AJ, Rothe EM, Swanson J, Holzer CE, Linskey AO, Quintero-Salinas R. Suicidality and acculturation in Hispanic adolescents. In: Sher L, Vilens A, eds. *Immigration and Mental Health: Stress, Psychiatric Disorders, and Suicidal Behavior Among Immigrants and Refugees*. New York: Nova Science; 2010:57–70.

40. Kann L, Kinchen S, Shanklin S, Flint K, et al. Youth risk behavior surveillance: United States, 2013. U.S. Department of Health and Human Services, Centers for Disease Control and Prevention. *Morbid Mortal Weekly Rep*. 2014;63(4):1–168. http://www.cdc.gov/mmwr/pdf/ss/ss6304.pdf. Last accessed on May 29, 2016.

41. Glover S, Pumariega A, Holzer C, Rodriguez M. Anxiety symptomatology in Mexican-American adolescents. *J Child Fam Studies*. 1999;8:47–57.

42. Lau A, Jernewall N, Zane N, Myers H. Correlates of suicidal behaviors among Asian American outpatient youths. *Cult Divers Ethnic Minor Psychol*. 2002;8:199–213.

43. Yeh C. Age, acculturation, cultural adjustment, and mental health symptoms of Chinese, Korean, and Japanese immigrant youths. *Cult Divers Ethnic Minor Psychol*. 2003;9:34–48.

44. Fenta H, Hyman I, Noh S. Determinants of depression among Ethiopian immigrants and refugees in Toronto. *J Nerv Mental Dis*. 2004;192:363–372.

45. Romero A, Carvajal S, Valle F, Orduña M. Adolescent bicultural stress and its impact on mental well-being among Latinos, Asian Americans, and European Americans. *J Community Psychol*. 2007;35:519–534.

46. Cespedes Y, Huey S. Depression in Latino adolescents: a cultural discrepancy perspective. *Cult Divers Ethnic Minor Psychol.* 2008;14:168–172.

47. Zamboanga B, Schwartz S, Jarvis L, Van Tyne K. Acculturation and substance use among Hispanic early adolescents: investigating the mediating roles of acculturative stress and self-esteem. *J Primary Prevent.* 2009;30:315–333.

48. Duarte C, Bird H, Shrout P, et al. Culture and psychiatric symptoms in Puerto Rican children: longitudinal results from one ethnic group in two contexts. *J Child Psychol Psychiatry.* 2008;49:563–572.

49. Suarez-Morales L, Lopez B. The impact of acculturative stress and daily hassles on pre-adolescent psychological adjustment: examining anxiety symptoms *J Primary Prevent,* 2009;30:335–349.

50. Zayas LH, Bright CL, Alvarez-Sanchez T, et al. Acculturation, familism and mother–daughter relations among suicidal and non-suicidal adolescent Latinas. *J Primary Prevent.* 2009;30:351–369.

51. Goforth A, Oka E, Leong F. Acculturation, acculturative stress, religiosity and psychological adjustment among Muslim Arab American adolescents. *J Muslim Mental Health.*2014;8:3–19.

52. Cross T, Bazron B, Dennis K, Isaacs M. *Towards a Culturally Competent System of Care.* Washington, DC: CASSP Technical Assistance Center, Georgetown University, Child Development Center; 1989.

53. Kirmayer L. Cultural variations in the clinical presentation of depression and anxiety: implications for diagnosis and treatment. *J Clin Psychiatry.* 2001;62(suppl 13):22–28.

54. Malgady R, Rogler L, Dharma E. Cultural expression of psychiatric symptoms: idioms of anger amongst Puerto Ricans. *Psychol Assess.* 1996;8:265–268.

55. Guarnaccia PJ, Lewis-Fernandez R, Martinez-Pincay I, et al. Ataque de nervios as a marker of social and psychiatric vulnerability: results from the NLAAS. *Int J Soc Psychiatry.* 2010;56(3):298–309.

56. American Psychiatric Association. *Diagnostic and Statistical Manual of Mental Disorders.* 5th ed. Washington, DC: American Psychiatric Association; 2013.

57. Pumariega AJ, Rothe E, Mian A, et al., and the Committee on Quality Issues. Practice parameter for cultural competence in child and adolescent psychiatric practice. *J Am Acad Child Adolesc Psychiatry.* 2013;52(10):1101–1115.

58. Malik M, Lawson W, Lake J, Joshi S. Culturally adapted pharmacotherapy and the integrated formulation. *Child Adolesc Psychiatr Clin N Am.* 2010;19:791–814.

59. Huey S, Polo A. Evidence-based psychosocial treatments for ethnic minority youth. *J Clin Child Adoles Psychol.* 2008;37,:262–301.

60. Pumariega AJ, Rothe EM, Rogers KM. Treating child and adolescent depression. In: Rey JM, Birmaher J, eds. *Treating Child and Adolescent Depression.* New York: Lippincott, Williams & Wilkins; 2008:321–332.

61. Pina A, Wendy M, Silverman K, Fuentes R, Kurtines W, Weems C. Exposure-based cognitive-behavioral treatment for phobic and anxiety disorders: treatment effects and maintenance for Hispanic/Latino relative to European-American youths. *J Am Acad Child Adolesc Psychiatry.* 2003;42:1179–1187.

62. Ginsburg GS, Drake KL. School-based treatment for anxious African Americans adolescents: a controlled pilot study. *J Am Acad Child Adolesc Psychiatry.* 2002;41:768–775.

63. Cohen JA, Deblinger E, Mannarino AP, Steer RA. A multisite, randomized controlled trial for children with sexual abuse-related PTSD symptoms. *J Am Acad Child Adolesc Psychiatry.* 2004;43:393–402.

64. Halliday-Boykins CA, Schoenwald SK, Letourneau EJ. Caregiver-therapist ethnic similarity predicts youth outcomes from an empirically based treatment. *J Consult Clin Psychol.* 2005;73:808–818.

65. Yeh M, Eastman K, Cheung MK. Children and adolescents in community health centers: does the ethnicity or the language of the therapist matter? *J Community Psychol.* 1994; 22:153–163.

66. Griner D, Smith T. Culturally adapted mental health interventions: a meta-analytic review. *Psychotherapy (Chic).* 2006;43:531–548.

67. Santisteban DA, Coatsworth JD, Perez-Vidal A, et al. Efficacy of brief strategic family therapy in modifying Hispanic adolescent behavior problems and substance use. *J Fam Psychol.* 2003;17:121–133.

68. Kataoka S, Stein B, Jaycox L, et al. A school-based mental health program for traumatized Latino immigrant children. *J Amer Acad Child Adol Psychiat.* 2003;42:311–318.

69. Constantino G, Malgady R, Rogler L. Storytelling through pictures: culturally sensitive psychotherapy for Hispanic children and adolescents. *J Clin Child Psychol.* 1994;23:13–20.

70. Rotheram-Borus M, Piacentini J, Van Rossem R, et al. Treatment adherence among Latina suicide attempters. *Suicide Life Threat Behav.* 1999;29:319–336.

71. Grames H. Depression, anxiety, and ataque de nervios: the primary mental health care model in a Latino population. *J Systemic Therapies.* 2006;25:58–72.

72. Ruiz P, Langrod J. The role of folk healers in community mental health services. *Commun Mental Health J.* 1976;12:392–398.

73. LaFromboise T, Lewis H. The Zuni Life Skills Development Program: a school/community-based suicide prevention intervention. *Suicide Life Threat Behav* 2008;38(3):343–353.

74. Okuma T. Differential sensitivity to the effects of psychotropic drugs: psychotics vs normals; Asian vs Western populations. *Folia Psychiatr Neurol Jpn.* 1981;35:79–87.

75. Varner RV, Ruiz P, Small DR. Black and white patients' response to antidepressant treatment for major depression. *Psychiatr Q.* 1998;69:117–125.

76. Curry J, Rohe P, Simons A, et al. Predictors and modifiers of acute outcome in the Treatment for Adolescents with Depression Study (TADS). *J Am Acad Child Adolesc Psychiatry.* 2006;45:1427–1439.

77. Arnold LE, Elliott M, Sachs L, et al. Effects of ethnicity on treatment attendance, stimulant response-dose, and 14-month outcome in ADHD. *J Consult Clin Psychol.* 2003;71:713–727.

78. Tamayo JM, Pumariega AJ, Rothe E, et al. A comparison of Latino versus Caucasian pediatric outpatients with ADHD in a combined analysis of two acute open-label studies with atomoxetine. *J Child Adol Psychopharm.* 2008;18(1):44–53.

79. Durell T, Pumariega AJ, Rothe E, Tamayo J, Baron D, Williams D. Effects of open-label atomoxetine on African-American and Caucasian pediatric outpatients with attention-deficit/hyperactivity disorder. *Annals Clin Psychiat.* 2009;21(1):26–37.

80. Alegria M, Vallas M, Pumariega A. Racial and ethnic disparities in pediatric mental health. *Child Adolesc Psychiatr Clin.* 2010;19:759–774.

81. Alegria M, Green J, Mc Laughlin K, Loder S. Disparities in child and adolescent mental health and mental health services in the U.S. A William T. Grant Foundation Inequality Paper. March 2015. http://wtgrantfoundation.org/library/uploads/2015/09/Disparities-in-Child-and-Adolescent-Mental-Health.pdf. Accessed on May 29, 2016.

82. Case A, Deaton A. Mortality and morbidity in the 21st century. Brookings Papers on Economic Activity; Spring 2017:397–467. https://www.brookings.edu/wp-content/uploads/2017/08/casetextsp17bpea.pdf.

15

Religion and Social Psychiatry

M. I. López-Ibor and M. Martín Carrasco

Introduction

Religion is part of the life of many individuals worldwide (many more individuals than we sometimes can imagine), and religious and spiritual preoccupations are one of the most relevant values of our own culture.

Social psychiatry pays special attention to the interpersonal and cultural context of mental disorders and mental well-being, and religion and spiritual beliefs are an important component of health. Therefore health professionals in general, but especially psychiatrists, psychologists, and other mental health professionals, need to be trained and to pay attention to religious and spiritual beliefs.

There are 19 major world religions, which are subdivided into a total of 270 large religious groups, and many smaller ones. There are about 2.9 billion Christians (29.9% of the world population); 1.9 billion Muslims (24.4%); 1.5 billion Hindus (14.8%); 0.5 billion practice Chinese folk religion (6%); and 0.36 billion are Buddhist (6%). The rest of religions are practiced by the 10% of the world population. In addition, 1.5 billon people (13%) have no religion (they consider themselves agnostics, freethinkers, humanists, secularists, etc.), and 150 million (2%) are atheists.[1]

Religion plays an important role in every stage of life, such as birth, becoming an adult, marriage, and death. It is also important when confronted with illness and misfortune; many people turn to religion in difficult periods of their life, using a variety of religious styles (for instance, sick persons give more importance to spirituality than the general population, which is well documented in the literature) as coping strategies.

Medicine in general and psychiatry in particular should deal with spiritual and religious questions, as we know that these concerns play an important role in the manifestations, etiopathogeny, course, treatment, prevention, and rehabilitation of many illnesses.

Whether religion has a positive or a negative impact on personal growth and mental health has been a controversial issue. However, there is abundant research evidence that religion, or spirituality (considered as the individual religious experience, as opposed to ritualistic religious practices), is associated with higher levels of subjective well-being and lower levels of anxiety or even depressive symptoms, and may promote both emotional and cognitive growth. This influence is generally positive (71%), although in some cases it is negative (14%).[2,3]

Many severe patients turn to religious beliefs to cope with their disease. In a meta-analysis of 850 studies, those who were religious experienced better health and adapted better to stress.[4] Other studies have shown that religious persons are physically healthier and need to go to healthcare services less frequently.[5]

Studies indicate that religion and spirituality can promote mental health through positive coping strategies, community and support, and positive beliefs. Some studies have found that religious people are less likely to divorce, use less alcohol and drugs, have more access to social support, experience less depression and anxiety, and are less likely to commit suicide.[6]

Koening's[7] first studies point out that religious beliefs and practices improve coping, reduce stress, prevent depression, improve social support, promote healthy behaviors, and prevent alcohol and drug abuse, and these factors will have an impact on physical health. In a recent study, published at the beginning of 2020, religiosity is a factor associated with a healthier lifestyle, including less smoking and alcohol use/abuse, and may have a protective factors on genes associated with cellular aging.[8]

Positive religious coping strategies include searching for spiritual wisdom, and providing spiritual support for others, whereas negative religious coping strategies included feeling dissatisfied, attributing the stressor to the devil, interpersonal conflicts, religious doubts, or perceived failures of faith, guilt associated with failures of virtue, fears. and condemnation.[9] Research also shows that religion and spirituality can be damaging to mental health by means of negative religious coping and misunderstanding, and sometimes can be a source of conflicts and violence, which have had an enormous negative impact on the mental health of thousands of people.[10] We have also to consider that religiousness may be an important factor in clinical decisions; some patients may refuse a treatment for religious convictions.

We also have to take in to account that psychiatrists' and medical and other professionals' personal values, including religious beliefs, have an influence on their relations with patients, and in understanding their own practices. Psychiatrist in general are, among doctors, less religious, but religious physicians and psychiatrists are more likely to discuss religious or spiritual issues with their patients and tend to recommend clergy and pastoral professionals in the care of their patients.[11]

Religion and Psychiatry

Social psychiatry needs to take into consideration religion because mental patients are confronted with spiritual problems; patients suffering from schizophrenia often have delusions related to the sense of life, and those suffering from depression, with the meaning of loss and death.

Relations between psychiatry and religion are influenced by complex belief systems, values, and culture, which are diverse and changing. But this relation has been complicated; it is well-known that philosophers, theologians, anthropologists, psychologists, and psychiatrists have looked for natural and supra-natural explanations for mental disorders. Traditionally, mental diseases are considered as spiritual diseases; in German, mental disorders are called *Geisteskrankheiten*, which means "spiritual illness." In some cultures, mental disorders have been considered as evil spirit possessions, and exorcism or other religious practices have been prescribed as treatment.[12]

Psychiatry has normally ignored the spiritual and religious dimension as a factor that could have an impact in health and illness. Sigmund Freud wrote that religion is a "universal obsessional neurosis of humankind," representing an infantile stage of mental development which prevents human beings from facing the reality of their life.[13]

However, religions have an influence in the treatment and recovery of mental disorders. In a sample of more than 100 patients suffering from schizophrenia, rates of partial or total lack of adherence (determined by analyzing plasma levels of antipsychotics) was 32%, with almost one-third expressing that their religious beliefs were against taking antipsychotics, while in the group with good treatment adherence, only 8% had lack of adherence. And 57% of the patients considered that the representation of their disease was affected by their spiritual beliefs, 31% positively and the remaining 26% negatively.[14]

In spite of this, there is limited bibliography on this subject. A search in PubMed (October 2019) on the subjects of *theology, spirituality, religion* provided 64,406 results, of which only 4,208 correspond to *psychiatry*, 1,280 to *mental disorders*, 687 to *schizophrenia*, and 2,446 to *depression*. On the contrary, there are proportionally higher levels for *cancer* (8,548), *nursing* (7,450), and *palliative* (2,370).

Until recently, religiousness or spirituality was considered something that is too private and personal to be evaluated and, above all, as being difficult and uncomfortable to study in patients. But we have to consider that in most of mental disorders, patients confront the meaning of life and the meaning of illness, and religious, cultural, and social factors undoubtedly have an impact.

Cultural factors may influence the nature of obsessions and compulsions associated with obsessive-compulsive disorder (OCD). In fact, a variety of symptoms related to religious thoughts are more prevalent in clinical populations from countries in which religion is at the central core of the society, particularly in Muslim and Jewish Middle Eastern cultures, as compared with clinical populations from the West. Okasha[12,15] has analyzed in detail the relation between cultural and religious factors in compulsions.

Scrupulosity has been described as a psychological disorder primarily characterized by pathological guilt or obsession associated with moral or religious issues that is often accompanied by compulsive moral or religious observance and is highly distressing and maladaptive. John Moore, Bishop of Ely, wrote in 1691 that scrupulosity is a "Religious Melancholy, that makes people fear that what they do is so abnormal and unfit to be presented unto God."[12(p227)] Abramowitz[16(p826)] considers scrupulosity as a set of "persistent doubts about sin and irresistible urges to perform excessive religious behaviour."

It has been described that between 10.0% and 30% of OCD patients experience religious obsessions,[2,17,18] and that 5.0% of OCD patients experience religious obsessions as their *primary* type of obsession.[19]

Spirituality and religiousness have been shown to be highly prevalent among patients with schizophrenia; however, clinicians are rarely aware of the importance of the religion for patient. Mohr considers that spirituality and religiousness should be integrated into the psychosocial dimension of schizophrenia; in 71% of patients suffering from schizophrenia, religion was a positive way of coping.[20]

Delusional patients generally have some concerns about the meaning of life and of nature, but psychiatrists consider these religious phenomena as symptoms. Data on phenomenology of delusions, hallucinations, or Schneider's first-rank symptoms in schizophrenia demonstrate a remarkable influence of social aspects on the content of psychotic symptoms.

In the depressive states, preoccupations frequently appear regarding the meaning of loss and death, on responsibility and guilt. Jung considered that neurosis "must be understood, ultimately, as the suffering of a soul which has not discovered its meaning."[21]

Religious practice is associated with a lower number of suicide attempts in the general population and in mental patients, regardless of its effects on social supports. That is, it does not have an indirect effect of better social integration.[22]

In a sample of patients with bipolar disorder, 78% stated they had strong religious beliefs and, in fact, 81.5% were practicing their religion. Most of them believed that there was a relation between their beliefs and disease, and one-fifth of them had some type of conflict between their beliefs and the model of the disease and the recommendations of their doctor.[23]

Voluntary starvation has been described since the Hellenistic era, and there are many saints who practiced starvation for spiritual reasons, to have extreme control of their body, including eating abstinence, in order to become close to God.[24] Bell has described how many women whom we would currently diagnose with anorexia nervosa went into convents and were subjected to voluntary fasting to become sanctified. The most significant case is the history of Santa Librada (who also appears with the name of Liberata), who decided to actively fight against her femininity by fasting. She lost a lot of weight, and this weight loss was soon accompanied by the appearance of body hair, including a beard, and she lost her menstruation.[25,12] In current times, there is evidence of religiosity in this disease in studies in which patients with anorexia nervosa significantly respond affirmatively more frequently to the items "I read the Bible several times a week," and "I pray several times a day."[26]

Religiousness is also part of resilience,[27] that is, of the initiation of protective mechanisms against trauma and its consequences. In fact, a traumatic event can give rise to a spiritual crisis and to changes in the scale of values of the person, and may help to recover from post-traumatic stress disorder.

How to Explore Spiritual and Religious Beliefs

It has become clear so far that religious and spiritual issues are relevant for the evaluation and treatment of patients with mental disorders and, therefore, clinicians should be open to consider the effect of religion on the mental health of their patients. Spirituality is highly personal, very central to a person's inner life, and often is inseparable from one's cultural identity. However, it is important that psychiatrists do not exceed professional limits.

The question is, therefore, how can professionals engage in a respectful way in the spiritual life of their patients? Several authors have pointed out the importance of spirituality training in the psychiatric curriculum, with a specific point about spiritual evaluation.

Ideally, the exploration of spiritual problems is integrated into the standard clinical and psychopathological evaluation, and there is no need to rush to religious matters, unless they constitute a central problem. The first step is always to strengthen the doctor-patient relationship. The patient is more likely to discuss spiritual concerns within the context of a positive doctor-patient relationship characterized by empathy, strong communication, and shared decision-making.

Appropriate timing of discussion is crucial. A good starting point can be a routine exploration of support systems (family, friends, hobbies, etc.), in which we can include a question about spiritual resources, which can lead to further discussion. Spirituality issues can also appear naturally when discussing aspects such as death (for example, advance directives, grief, a new diagnosis of serious illness, terminal care planning, suicide, etc.), the purpose of life, or symptoms such as chronic experiences of emptiness or lack of meaning, or the strategies that patients use to appease these experiences, such as addictions or self-aggression.[27] Often, people use a metaphorical or indirect symbolic language when expressing transcendent thoughts, so spiritual evaluation requires careful listening to patients' stories about their life trajectory and key moments of it, particularly related to dual experiences, such as belonging versus exclusion, loneliness versus being together, hope versus hopelessness, or certainty versus uncertainty. If we can perceive these clues and develop them with open or specific questions about the patient's religious beliefs in a gentle way, it can reveal more about spiritual needs than direct interrogation. If the therapist meets resistance by the patient, the topic should be discarded tactfully and maybe addressed at a later time after a stronger therapeutic alliance has developed.

If needed, there are several protocols that can be useful in assessing spiritual aspects, such as the HOPE questionnaire, particularly if the clinician is gaining experience in this type of exploration.

Effects of Spiritual Assessment on Clinical Management

After obtaining the necessary information, it is advisable to take a respectful and neutral position, until a good understanding of the patient's psychopathology and personality structure is achieved.[28] The patient's religious or spiritual beliefs often hold the patient's psyche together. Even strange or clearly pathological religious beliefs must be handled with extreme respect. The psychiatrist should help patients clarify how their religious beliefs and practices influence the course of the disease. If beliefs do not appear obviously pathological and seem to facilitate coping, then the psychiatrist should consider supporting them, without giving explicit spiritual advice. Whatever the attitude toward religiosity, the moral position of the professional must be neutral, without any attempt to influence the beliefs of the patient. However, it has become increasingly clear that such neutrality is more assumed than real, and that many aspects of the therapist's identity are presented to the patient, perhaps in a subtle or surreptitious manner.[29] Obviously, doctors should be aware of how their own attitudes can affect the therapeutic process. A physician needs to understand his or her own spiritual beliefs, values, and biases in order to remain patient-centered and non-judgmental when dealing with the spiritual concerns of patients. This is especially true when the beliefs of the patient differ from those of the physician. In general, shared religious practice is not advisable, even at the patient's request.

It is not necessary that the psychiatrist share the religious beliefs of the patient. Even secular therapists can incorporate the spiritual dimension of the patient into the therapeutic process, provided they are sensitive to religious issues and validate the importance that spirituality has for the patient. Conversely, even if the patient is not religious, the psychiatrist should investigate to gain an understanding of the previous experiences, if any, of the patient with religion. Experiences that may have separated the patient from religion (for example, sexual abuse by clergy, trauma such as sudden death, violence, etc., that altered their religious conviction) could be contributing to current psychiatric problems.

Occasionally, the religious opinions of the patients may conflict with the therapeutic approach, but even in these cases it is important that the doctor try to understand and integrate the patient's particular way of understanding life and consider together with the patient if it makes sense for the patient to turn to members of the religious community or clergy to provide support or specific spiritual advice. If the patient's beliefs are being used defensively to hamper the therapeutic process, they can be questioned tactfully. This is a very sensitive matter and should not be attempted until other strategies have been used, and always within a firm therapeutic alliance.

Conclusions

Religion and spirituality are especially important for many people who turn to religion in difficult periods of their life, using a variety of religious styles as coping strategies. There are two ways in which life flows : one, the everyday form, in which events follow one another in a routinary fashion, without the person stopping to think about them. Another one, in which life itself is perceived and analyzed deeply, through crisis, of which the most revealing symptom is anxiety. Parting from this crisis experience, we start to better understand ourselves and other human beings. The same happens in the way we experience death. There is an external death, which strikes without any preparation. There is another death, a conscious, existential death, which we get to know through events that are experienced intimately.

Spiritual and religious considerations also have important ethical implications for the clinical practice of psychiatry. We have to follow what the World Psychiatric Association[30(pp87–88)] proposes:

> A tactful consideration of patients' religious beliefs and practices as well as their spirituality should routinely be considered and will sometimes be an essential component of psychiatric history taking. . . . Psychiatrists should be expected always to respect and be sensitive to the spiritual/religious beliefs and practices of their patients, and of the families and carers of their patients. . . . Psychiatrists, whatever their personal beliefs, should be willing to work with leaders/members of faith communities, chaplains and pastoral workers, and others in the community, in support of the well-being of their patients, and should encourage their multidisciplinary colleagues to do likewise.

Murthy[12–31] predicts that there will be greater need to base our activities in the religious and spiritual values of different religions.

Religion is one of the ways we give meaning to our lives, and a tool that helps us to understand the world. In psychiatric patients, religiosity may impact psychopathology and the treatment of the patient; therefore it is important for clinicians to pay close attention and to understand the religious beliefs of their patients.

References

1. Regions all over the world. Wikipedia 2019. https://en.wikipedia.org/wiki/List_of_religious_populations
2. Curlin FA, Lawrence RE, Odell S, et al. Religion, spirituality, and medicine: psychiatrists' and other physicians' differing observations, interpretations, and clinical approaches. *Am J Psychiatry*. 2007 Dec;164(12):1825–1831.
3. Oman D, Thoresen CE. Do religion and spirituality influence health? In: Raymond F, Paloutzian CL, eds. *Park Handbook of the Psychology of Religion and Spirituality*. New York and London: Guilford Press; 2005:435–460.
4. Ano GG, Vasconcelles EB. Religious coping and psychological adjustment to stress: a meta-analysis. *J Clin Psychol*. 2005 Apr;61(4):461–480.
5. Weber SR, Pargament KI. The role of religion and spiritual in mental health. *Curr Opin Psychiatr*. 2014;5:358–366.
6. Rasic DT, Belik SL, Elias B, Katz LY, Enns M, Sareen J, Swampy Cree Suicide Prevention Team. Spirituality, religion and suicidal behavior in a nationally representative sample. *J Affect Disord*. 2009 Apr;114(1–3):32–40.

7. Koening HG. Religion and medicine III: developing a theoretical model. *Int J Psychiatry Med.* 2001;31:199–205.

8. Wang L, Koening H, Shoah S, Zhighaong W. Religiosity, depression and telomere length in Chinese older adults. *J Affective Disord.* 2020 Jan;260:624–628,

9. Exeline JJ. The picture is getting clearer, but is the scope too limited: the overlooked questions in psychology of religion. *Psychol Inquiry.* 2002;13:245–249.

10. Winter U, Hauri D, Huber S, Jenewein J, Schnyder U, Kraemer B. The psychological outcome of religious coping with stressful life events in a Swiss sample of church attendees. *Psychother Psychosom.* 2009;78(4):240–244.

11. Korup AK, Sundergraad J, Christensen RD, et al. Religious Values in clinical practice are here to stay. *J Religion Health.* 2020 Feb;59(1):188–194. doi: 10.1007/s10943-018-0715-y

12. Verhagen P, Lopez Ibor JJ, Moussaoui D, Van Pragg HM, Cox J. *Religion and Psychiatry: Beyond Boundaries.* New York: Wiley; 2010.

13. Freud S. Totem and Taboo. In Strachey J, et al. (Trans.), *The Standard Edition of the Complete Psychological Works of Sigmund Freud*, Volume XIII. London: Hogarth Press; 1912–1913.

14. Borras L, Mohr S, Brand PY, Gilieron C, Eytan A, Huguelet P. Religious beliefs in schizophrenia: their relevance for adherence to treatment. *Schizophrenia Bull.* 2007;33:1238–1246.

15. Okasha A, Saad A, Khalil AH, el Dawla AS, Yehia N. Phenomenology of obsessive–compulsive disorder: a transcultural study. *Compr Psychiatry.* 1994 May–Jun;35(3):191–197.

16. Abramowitz JS, Huppert D, Cohen AB, Tolin DF, Cahill SP. Religious obsessions and compulsions in a non–clinical sample: The Penn Inventory of Scrupulosity (PIOS). *Behav Res Ther.* 2002;40:825–838.

17. Eisen JL, Goodman WK, Keller MB, et al. Patterns of remission and relapse in obsessive-compulsive disorder: a 2-year prospective study. *J Clin Psychiatry.* 1999 May;60(5):346–351.

18. Mataix J, Marks IM, Creist JK, Hobeck KX, Baer L. OCD symptom dimensions as predictor of compliance with a response to behaviour therapy: results from a controlled trial. *Psychother Psychosom.* 2002;71:255–262.

19. Tolin DF, Abramowitz JS, Kosok MS, Foa EB. Fixity of belief, perceptual and magical ideation in OCD patients. *J Anxiety Dis.* 2001;15:501–510.

20. Mohr S, Borras L, Betsey C. Delusions with religious content in patients with psychosis: how they interact with spiritual coping. *Psychiatry Res.* 2010;73:158–173.

21. Jung C. Escritos sobre espiritualidad y trascedencia [1913]. In: Jung, *Obras completas*, Dorset B, ed. 2nd ed. Madrid: Trota, 2016:634–636.

22. Mofidi M, Devellis RF, Balzer DG, Devellis BM, Panter AT, Jordan JM. Spirituality and depressive symptoms in a racially diverse US sample of community-dwelling adults. *J Nerv Ment.* 2006;975–977.

23. Vandereyken W, Van Deth R. *From Fasting Saints to Anorexic Girls: The History of Self-Starvation.* New York: New York University Press; 1990.

24. Bell R. *Holy Anorexia.* Chicago: University of Chicago Press; 1985.

25. Graham MA, Spencer W, Andersen AE. Altered religious practices in patients with eating disorders. *Int J Eating Disord.* 1991;10(2):239–243.

26. Meisenhelder J. Terrorism, posttraumatic stress, and religious. *Issues Ment Health Nurs.* 2002 Dec;23(8):771–782. doi: 10.1080/01612840260433659

27. Anandarajah G, Hight E. Spirituality and medical practice: using the, HOPE questions as a practical tool for spiritual assessment. *Am Fam Physician.* 2001;63:81–89.

28. Koenig HG. Religion and mental health: what should psychiatrists do? *Psychiatric Bull.* 2008;32, 201–203.

29. Greenberg D. A religious psychiatrists ethnographic self-report. *Am J Psychother.* 2001;55:564–576.

30. Moreira Almeida A, Sharma A, Cook CH. WPA position statement on spirituality and religion in psychiatry. *World Psychiatry.* 2016;15(1):87–88.

31. Srinivasa Murthy R, Desouza R. Mental Wellbeing, letter to editor. World Psychiatry: Official Journal of the World Psychiatric Association (WPA) 2006;5(3):188.

16

The Impacts of Music, Concerts, and Dance on Mental Health

Jeff Q. Bostic, Kristine Goins, and Basie Bostic

The Impacts of Music, Concerts, and Dance on Mental Health

From an evolutionary perspective, music, concerts, and dance (MCD) serve at least 4 vital social functions: (1) personal and group enjoyment/entertainment; (2) group communication; (3) creative expression, including movement and dance as well as sounds/songs; and (4) group rituals.[1] First, MCD arouse our emotional neural pathways, including our pleasure centers, both when listening alone, and when together, and enhances our liking of others. MCD intensify emotional reactions to events, helping embed and enhance memories (as MCD become associated with one's life events). MCD stimulate multiple brain regions across both hemispheres, far beyond the stimulation associated with words themselves. Second, MCD also allow messages to be transmitted more quickly, accurately, and with specific signals that are more easily remembered and shared with others. Third, MCD help us move in unison, for tasks such as moving items or rowing a ship, yet also inspire us to leap with joy into celebratory dance. Finally, MCD intensify our social rituals, adding meaning to our memory of ritualized content, and accenting the mood of that ritual, be it somber or celebratory. Societies affix MCD to all types of rituals, as MCD are used regularly in sporting events to inspire players, or to signify holiday events. MCD make social groupings not just cohesive but adhesive, bringing individuals together who might have otherwise maintained solitary lives, randomly scattered across the landscape).[2]

Through all these vital social functions, MCD create and sustain strong social bonds, from the early cooing between parent and child, the chanting or dancing of "tribal" members during work, the preparation rituals for hunts and celebrations, and the stretch for new creative expressions pursued by each generation. MCD more than improve intra-tribal communications, moving social interaction into shared meanings and alliances between peoples in ever widening regions).[3]

MCD appear "universal" in the sense that similarities exist across environments: large human predators emit lower, louder sounds *everywhere*, so humans across the globe have largely emulated these sounds in music to evoke power and fear in others. A review of 8,200 field recordings from 137 countries showed that 80% of the music across the globe is familiar to all humans.[4] Cambodians unfamiliar with Western rock music have the same emotional reactions to this music as the Westerners who created it.[5] This "universal" appeal or social magnetism of music is perhaps most visible through concerts. Concerts remain prominent over just listening to music in the comfort of one's home with personally selected speakers, because the social experience is more meaningful and intense to most people, who will spend much more to share a musical experience with strangers than to purchase a song for a fraction of the cost. Dance adds to the social experience of music, and the integration of music with movement has remained embedded in social groups for at least 20,000 years.

MCD connect people, through sharing preferred music, the exhilaration of playing music together, dancing to music, or attending concerts. People of all ages report increased interpersonal trust and bonding while listening to music.[6,7] Biologically, singing raises oxytocin levels immediately following a 30-minute singing experience,[8] and women listening to romantic music are more likely (52% v. 28%) to agree to go out on a date.[9]

Music and Concerts
Impacts of Music on the Developing Brain

Listening to Music

Humans appear wired to *understand* music; humans across diverse cultures naturally make sense of music, following chord changes and remembering melodies.[10] Humans further appear wired to *enjoy* music, naturally releasing dopamine at peak moments in music.[11] The brain begins to enjoy music within the first year of life during passive listening.[12] By age 20–30 years, brain pathways are associated with musical responses,[13] summarized in Table 16.1.

Stimulating music *increases* activity in the nucleus accumbens (NA), ventral tegmental area (VTA), orbitofrontal cortex (OFC), and insula, and *decreases* activity in the amygdala (reducing fear or anticipation of danger). So music stimulates primary pleasure pathways in humans, intensifying positive emotions and reactions to music, and simultaneously decreases the harm/avoidance pathways, resulting in the greater receptivity to dating when music is in the background (as described above).[9]

The type of music one *prefers* is more important than particulargenres. Listening to prior favorite songs triggers pleasure pathways (even decades later) more than preferred genres (e.g., rock, country, classical, rap, opera, etc.), and is associated with greater

TABLE 16.1 Brain Regions Responsive to Music

Brain Regions Responsive to Music

Neural Pathways	Brain Regions
INCREASED REACTIVITY TO POSITIVE ENVIRONMENTAL INPUTS	
Euphoria/pleasant emotion	Nucleus accumbens (NA); ventral tegmental area (VTA); anterior cingulate (AC); insula
Rewards (similar to responses to food/sex/substances)	Dopaminergic stimulation in NA, VTA, and at opioid receptors in periaqueductal gray and pedunculopontine nucleus
Arousal	AC, insula, thalamus
Evaluation of reward/punishment	Orbitofrontal (OFC) regions
DECREASED REACTIVITY TO NEGATIVE ENVIRONMENTAL INPUTS	
Harm/avoidance/risk appraisal	Decreased cholinergic in the amygdala, hippocampus, and ventral medial prefrontal cortex

connectivity between the precuneus and other brain regions.[14] So listening to certain genres is not as harmful as listening to particular genres that one dislikes.

Sad Music

The beneficial purposes and attractions of "sad music" seem counter to positive mental health. However, "sad music" enhances human connection with others by directly releasing endorphins which induce prolactin release, associated with gratification and relaxation.[15] Sad music also indicates that one is not alone, providing comfort that someone else also shares a similar feeling.[16] While melodies intensify both positive and negative emotions, lyrics *detract* from happy/positive emotion-inducing melodies, but *enhance* sad/negative emotion-inducing melodies).[17] Suicidality appears more related to other personality traits or psychiatric symptoms of those who suicide than to their musical preferences.[18]

Playing Music

Playing music is more beneficial than only listening, just as playing sports yields more benefits than watching.[19] Over half of households have someone playing music, and 82% began playing by the age of 14. About 77% of children will play an instrument during childhood, peaking at age 8–10 and then declining to approximately 60% by age 16–17.[20] Music exposure enhances skill development across multiple brain areas, as shown in Table 16.2.

Concerts

Despite the substantial costs associated with concerts, they provide value beyond just hearing music. Those who attend concerts or dance report greater well-being and enjoyment,[30] and concertgoers show lower mortality rates.[31] Concertgoers specifically report high enjoyment in (1) listening to and sharing music with others in a group experience, and *liking, trusting, and cooperating* with others there more; and (2) participating in a unique (potentially historic) musical event with performers and attendees interacting to produce

TABLE 16.2 Impacts of Playing Music on Cognitive and Social-Emotional Skills

Cognitive Skills	Music Impacts
General cognitive abilities	6-year-olds improved after 36 weeks of practicing instrument[21]
Attention	Cortical thickness greater in those practicing instrument, particularly attention, premotor and motor brain regions[22]
Reading ability	3rd graders reading ability improved after 24 weeks of practicing musical instrument;[23] 7–10-year-olds improved reading ability after practicing instrument 28–39 hr/year (compared to those listening in music appreciation class)[19]
Visual spatial abilities	Meta-analysis of children/adolescents showed VS skills improved in those playing instruments[24]
Social-Emotional Skills	
Behavior control	Music instrument training improved self-control and reduced behavioral difficulties[25]
School engagement	Improved among students who play musical instruments[26]
Self-esteem	Improved self-esteem in those who play instruments;[27,28] particularly performing for others over rehearsing[29]

something special in that moment.[32] Body movements become more vigorous and contagious at concerts,[32] and brain waves become particularly "in sync" to music where a dancing type beat occurs (regardless of volume). Attendees with this synchrony reported greater pleasure and greater group connection.[33] Levitin et al.[3] found music exerted a profound effect on social cohesion by (1) synchronizing the internal rhythms of those listening, while (2) promoting feelings of group affiliation through modulation of oxytocin.

Substances and Concert Attendance

Concerts often tacitly support substance use. Substances such as alcohol are now often available, and toleration of alcohol and other substances is common at concerts and music festivals. Figure 16.1 depicts the substances most frequently *reported* used at live music events. A survey of 976 people age 18–82 years (mean = 37yo), and 51% female, revealed that 57% reported substance use at live music events, most commonly alcohol (>90%) or marijuana (~40%), and less than 10% using hallucinogens. Opioids and benzodiazepines are the least reported agents used at live music events.

The availability of alcohol at most concert events favors this substance being reported most frequently used at live music events. Marijuana users report this agent enhances their comfort level with others and improves their enjoyment of music. Much less frequently used are hallucinogens, likely because of their decreased availability, harsher criminal penalties, and social support for use, even though these agents are perceived to enhance or amplify sensory experiences. Conversely, opiates may blunt one's sensory responses, diminishing the intensity of musical events. Benzodiazepines may diminish the intensity of one's senses for enjoyment of music.

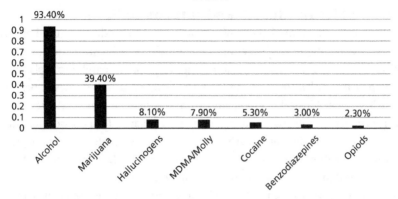

FIGURE 16.1. Substances most frequently reported used at live music events.

By music genre, some types of music are more frequently associated with substance use. Electronic dance music (EDM) is most associated with substance use, as shown in Figure 16.2. The reasons for use of substances at concerts vary widely, both by type of agent and by genre (https://drugabuse.com/featured/substance-use-at-live-music-events/).

EDM is associated with high levels of activity by those attending, such that sustaining energy and hydration likely increase substance use. More passive listening events, emphasizing technical proficiency and large groups playing together, may favor certain concert genres, such as classical, jazz, or pop, to dissuade substance use. Audience demographics also vary by genre, with pop often including minors, while classical music and jazz often for older age groups less likely to use substances.

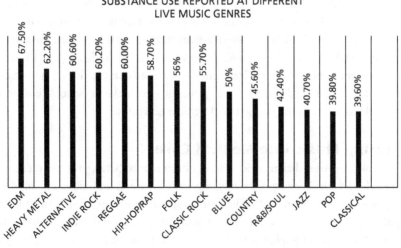

FIGURE 16.2. Music genre and reported substance use at live music events.

Clinical Implications of Music and Concerts

Promoting Mental Health and Improved Function

The evolution of music technology allows music to now be readily produced by anyone to increase positive emotions. No longer *must* one develop specific instrument techniques to play diverse instruments, as commercial software (e.g., Garageband, ProTools, etc.) allows one to *compose using all instruments* and to take existing musical phrases or beats and add to/personalize them. Musical components or phrases may be used to create a "song," but original lyrics may be integrated during every performance to increase spontaneity and greater social participation. Particular musical phrases, beats, etc., can be integrated with lyrics, music, or rhythms *from other cultures*, allowing people from everywhere to access all types of music and to make music more culturally relevant.

Concerts are perhaps the most notable social ritual to allow use of substances to enhance the experience. How such substances should be addressed, and how young members of that society should be taught about concertgoing behaviors, including exposure to intoxicants, warrants attention. Harm reduction efforts at festivals include "kits" to detect substances so attendees can identify specific substances at events. While concerns abound that this promotes substance use, Prohibition in the United States illuminated that (a) people will ingest substances in social gatherings despite social and even legal deterrents, and (b) the dangers of unknown/illicit substances represented a significant public health risk sufficient to repeal Prohibition. *Balance in identifying alternatives to substances to enhance these group experiences with optimizing safety and preparation at such events may improve concert experiences.*

Music is now commonly used among athletes to manage their emotions during games and to *improve their performance*. Athletes show an 18%–20% improvement in running when using music over no music. Adding music playlists to sports activities and exercise regimens at early ages enhances performance and stamina.[34]

The inclusion of music in social rituals, such as school activities, has received increased attention. Evidence is unclear on *using music within the classroom to optimize academic performance*. Music distracts most students from active instruction, and can compete for attention needed for academic tasks; however, for some students (e.g., those in difficult environments where hypervigilance may be favored), music during non-instruction times (e.g., doing individual classroom assignments) may make the school classroom more pleasant and less prone to trigger fight-flight-freeze reactions.

Integrating Music into Medical Care

Music stimulates diverse brain regions across both hemispheres, and has medical implications, such as with those aging, struggling with memory, and experiencing dementia. Music appears to slow memory loss by stimulating different, perhaps better functioning, brain pathways. Creech[35] found that elderly patients, including those with dementia, preferred music (with photographs) over other digital technologies (including videos, movies, etc.). With minimal training, even those with dementia could pick and choose preferred music to play frequently. So at an age when social contributions may give way to narratives of decline, music may strengthen the social fabric of its members. Music improves distress and anxiety for those, including pediatric patients, awaiting[36] or undergoing medical procedures, rivaling medication interventions.[37,38]

Dance

Whether music (sound) or movement (dance) occurred first, MCD have become intertwined in most cultures. Dance involves physical activity, including motor, cognitive, visuospatial, social, and emotional engagement.[39] In addition to artistic and aesthetic components, dance represents a *cultural* innovation with symbolic social meaning for its members. Early body paintings, group dances (members just moving in unison to rhythmical musical sounds), may have initially been applied for practical purposes, such as communication or working together in unison, and only later became symbolic as an art form. Zaidel[40] suggests that group dance arose from neural pathways controlling *entrainment* (the human body synchronizing with external sounds), as well as the hearing and feeling of rhythmical sounds. Natural and spontaneous rhythmical body rocking to inner (in the mind) or outer (external) beats is observed in some animals (e.g., birds, elephants, sea lions, bonobos), babies, children, and adult humans.[41] The transformation of this inherently biological state of *cotiming* (entrainment) into an expressive art form such as group dance appears to be a natural social act.[40] These art expressions would have also advanced and expanded opportunities for symbolically displaying group unity, enhancing cooperation and survival.[40]

Shared synchronized touching, shuffling, and clapping enhance emotional *closeness*.[40] Group dance formations express group identity, social cohesion, and shared values.[42] The synchrony and interdependent group movements of dances (e.g., ballet, line dances), which augment cultural practices and display of one's identity, retain natural appeal across cultures.[40]

Dance and the Developing Brain

Dance appears universal across human cultures,[43] practiced for thousands of years in rituals and for leisure. The impacts of dancing on cognition, brain structure, and function are shown in Table 16.3.[39] Neuroimaging studies show that dancers activate frontal, parietal, and occipitotemporal regions, collectively called the action observation network (AON), involved in *processing others' actions or movements*,[44] particularly when watching visually or physically familiar actions.[45] Dancers also show increased prefrontal activity, with enhanced motor representations of an observed movement.[43] Differences in the AON of dancers is related to the degree of dance training, although short-term dance training improves brain plasticity even in nondancers.

Since the AON is most responsive to familiar actions, chaining *familiar* movements together is easier for dancers to do than creating completely new movements. Similarly, dances comprising familiar movements are also likely more readily understood and appealing to observers.[46] Observers show more brain reactivity to live (vs. recorded) dance

TABLE 16.3 Primary Brain Regions Involved in Dance

Brain Regions	Functions
Action observation network (AON): Sensorimotor brain regions (premotor, parietal, and occipitotemporal)	Engaged when watching others in action, when observing actions that have been physically practiced, visually experienced, or when listening to the sounds associated with specific actions
Inferior parietal lobule	Involved in the perception of emotions in facial stimuli, and interpretation of sensory information
Middle temporal gyrus	Involved in visual perception, and sensory integration
Superior temporal gyrus	The primary auditory center processing sounds
Precentral gyrus	The primary motor center controlling voluntary motor movement on the body's contralateral side
Cerebellum	Coordinates voluntary movements (e.g., posture, balance), to yield smooth and balanced muscular activity
Putamen	Prepares and aids in movement of the limbs
Superior parietal lobule	Involved with spatial orientation
Frontopolar cortex (FPC)	Involved in complex, higher order, organized behaviors
Premotor cortex	Prepares the body's muscles for the exact movements
Supplementary motor area	Controls movements
Internal capsule	Transmits information to and from the cerebral cortex
Corpus callosum	Integrates motor, sensory, and cognitive performances on one side of the brain and sends to the other side
Corticospinal tract	Controls voluntary motor performance and modulates sensory information from the body
Superior longitudinal fasciculus (SLF)	Connects frontal, occipital, parietal, and temporal lobes

performances. Dance video game performance was correlated with gray-matter thickness in the superior temporal gyrus as well as white-matter diffusivity in the corpus callosum, signaling the importance of these regions in dance performance. These studies suggest that long-term dance training is associated with brain plasticity in both gray- and white-matter regions related to motor and auditory functions.[43]

Amateur tango dancers use the *cerebellum* in the entrainment of dance steps to music, while the *putamen* is activated in metric motion, and the *superior parietal lobule* is associated with spatial guidance of leg movements.[47] As tasks became more challenging, activity increases in the superior temporal gyrus and superior parietal lobule. These findings illuminate the network of brain regions involved in dance.[43]

Clinical Implications of Dance

Promoting Mental Health and Improved Function Through Dance

As music facilitates movement,[48] dance facilitates balance, flexibility, endurance, mobility, muscular strength, and coordination.[49] Both mental health disorders and chronic diseases are common (and often comorbid) and disabling.[50] Chronic pathologies are usually associated with reduced social interactions and social inclusion.[51] *Overcoming sedentariness*, such as through familiar movements such as dance, is essential to managing and diminishing chronic pathologies, including mental health disorders, such as depression, schizophrenia, and substance use disorders.[49,52]

Dance is associated with positive behavioral effects in psychiatric conditions across the age span.[53] Young individuals with autism have shown improvements in body awareness, self-other awareness, psychological well-being, and social skills.[43,54] Adults with schizophrenia showed improvements in balance, walking, muscular strength, quality of life, and body mass index after dancing.[49] Patients with fibromyalgia[55] showed a decrease in pain and improvements in walking, mental health and quality of life.[49]

Integrating Dance into Medical Care

Older patients with Parkinson's disease have shown benefits of dance through the accessible, social, and appealing (stimulating alternative, still more functional, brain pathways) aspects of dance, and slowed deterioration of physical abilities such as balance and gait.[49] Those individuals who dance regularly are less likely to develop dementia, and demonstrate better memory performance than people who do not exercise.[56]

Conclusion

Music, concerts, and dance (MCD) are strongly associated with mental health benefits through pleasure pathways, through positive impacts on group cohesion and communication, and development of extensive cognitive, physical, and social abilities. MCD can contribute substantially to positive mental and physical health integration, and provide an embedded daily treatment (preventive as well as healing). Using MCD in common daily activities and rituals increases human interactions, augments social encounters, and amplifies social events, even those shared with strangers. As findings accumulate on the positive contributions of MCD, evolving applications to bridge cultural differences and to expand shared positive emotional experiences with others can improve social events to promote mental health.

References

1. Montagu J. How music and instruments began: a brief overview of the origin and entire development of music, from its earliest stages. *Front Sociol.* 2017;2:8. doi: 10.3389/fsoc.2017.00008.
2. Mithen S. *The Singing Neanderthals.* Cambridge, MA: Harvard University Press; 2005.
3. Chanda M, Levitin D. The neurochemistry of music. *Trends Cogn Sci.* 2013;17(4):179–193.
4. Panteli M, Benetos E, Dixon S. A computational study on outliers in world music. *PLoS ONE.* 2017;12(12):e0189399. https://doi.org/10.1371/journal.pone.0189399.
5. Sievers B, Polansky L, Casey M, Wheatley T. Music and movement share a dynamic structure that supports universal expressions of emotion. *Proc Natl Acad Sci.* 2013;110:70–75.
6. Huron, D. Is music an evolutionary adaptation? *Ann NY Acad Sci.* 2001;930:43–61.

7. Levitin, DJ. *The World in Six Songs: How the Musical Brain Created Human Nature.* New York: Plume/ Penguin; 2009.

8. Grape C, Sandren M, Hansson LO, Dricson M, Theorell T. Does singing promote well-being? An empirical study of professional and amateur singers during a singing lesson. *Integr Physiol Behav Sci.* 2003;38:65–74.

9. Guéguen N, Jacob C, Lamy L. Love is in the air: effects of songs with romantic lyrics on compliance with a courtship request. *Psychol Music.* 2010;38:303–307. https://doi.org/10.1177/0305735609360428.

10. Koelsch S, Gunter TC, Friederici AD, Schröger E. Brain indices of music processing: "nonmusicians" are musical. *J Cognitive Neurosci.* 2000;12:520–541.

11. Salimpoor VN, Benovoy M, Larcher K, Dagher A, Zatorre RJ. Anatomically distinct dopamine release during anticipation and experience of peak emotion to music. *Nature Neurosci.* 2011;14:257–262.

12. Chen, JL, Penhune VB, Zatorre RJ. Listening to musical rhythms recruits motor regions of the brain. *Cerebral Cortex.* 2008;18:2844–2854.

13. Blood AJ, Zatorre RJ (2001). Intensely pleasurable responses to music correlate with activity in brain regions implicated in reward and emotion. *Proc Natl Acad Sci.* 2001;98:11818–11823. doi: 10.1073 pnas.191355898.

14. Wilkins RW, Hodges DA, Laurienti PJ, Steen M, Burdette JH. Network science and the effects of music preference on functional brain connectivity: from Beethoven to Eminem. *Sci Rep.* 2014 Aug 28;4:6130. doi: 10.1038/srep06130. Erratum in: Sci Rep. 2014;4:6667. PMID: 25167363; PMCID: PMC5385828.

15. Huron D. Why is sad music pleasurable? A possible role for prolactin. *Musicae Scientiae.* 2011;15(2):146–158.

16. Good M, Anderson GC, Ahn S, et al. Relaxation and music reduce pain following intestinal surgery. *Res Nurs Health.* 2002;28:240–251.

17. Ali SO, Peynircioglu ZF. Songs and emotions: are lyrics and melodies equal partners? *Psychol Music.* 2006 Oct 1;34(4):511–534. doi: https://doi.org/10.1177/0305735606067168.

18. Litman RE, Farberow NL. Pop-rock music as precipitating cause in youth suicide. *J Forens Sci.* 1994;39:494–499.

19. Kraus N, Slater J, Thompson EC, Hornickel J, Strait DL, Nicol T, White-Schwoch T. Auditory learning through active engagement with sound: biological impact of community music lessons in at-risk children. *Front Neurosci.* 2014 Nov 5;8:351. doi: 10.3389/fnins.2014.00351. PMID: 25414631; PMCID: PMC4220673.

20. ABRSM (Associated Board of Royal Schools of Music). Making music: teaching, learning, and playing in the UK. 2014. https://gb.abrsm.org/en/making-music/4-the-statistics/.

21. Schellenberg, EG (2004). Music lessons enhance IQ. *Psychol Sci.* 2004;15:511–514.

22. Hudziak JJ, Albaugh MD, Ducharme S, et al. Music and cortical thickness development. *JAACAP* 2014;53(11):1153–1161.

23. Moreno S, Marques C, Santos A, Santos M, Castro SL, Besson M. Musical training influences linguistic abilities in 8-year-old children: more evidence for brain plasticity. *Cereb Cortex.* 2009 Mar;19:712–723. doi: 10.1093/cercor/bhn120.

24. Hetland L. Listening to music enhances spatial-temporal reasoning: evidence for the "Mozart effect." *J Aesthet Educ.* 2000;34:105–148.

25. Aleman X, Duryea S, Guerra N et al. The effects of musical training on child development: a random-ized trial of *El Sistema* in Venezuela. *Prev Sci.* 2017;7:865–878. doi: 10.1007/s11121-016-0727-3.

26. Eerola PS, Eerola T. Extended music education enhances the quality of school life. *Music Educ Res.* 2014;16(1):88–104. doi: 10.1080/14613808.2013.829428.

27. Choi A-N, Lee MS, Lee J-S. Group music intervention reduces aggression and improves self-esteem in children with highly aggressive behavior. *Evid Based Complement Alternat Med.* 2010;7(2):213–217. doi: 10.1093/ecam/nem182.

28. Rickard NS, Appleman P, James R, et al. Orchestrating life skills: the effect of increased school-based music classes on children's social competence and self-esteem. *Int J Music Educ.* 2013;31:292–309.

29. Beck RJ, et al. Choral singing, performance perception, and immune system changes in salivary immunoglobulin-a and cortisol. *Music Percept.* 2000;18:87–106.

30. Weinberg MK, Joseph D. If you're happy and you know it: music engagement and subjective wellbeing. *Psychol Music.* 2017;45(2):257–267.

31. Bygren LO, Konlaan BB, Johansson SE. Attendance at cultural events, reading books or periodicals, and making music or singing in a choir as determinants for survival: Swedish interview survey of living conditions. *Br Med J.* 1996;313:1577–1580.

32. Swarbrick D, Bosnyak D, Livingstone SR, et al. How live music moves us: head movement differences in audiences to live versus recorded music. *Front Psychol.* 2019;9:2682. doi: 10.3389/fpsyg.2018.02682.

33. Rajendran VG, Bouwer FL, Henry MJ, Cirelli LK, Grahn J. What makes musical rhythm special: cross-species, developmental, and social perspectives. Presented at the Cognitive Neuroscience Society meeting, March 2018.

34. Karageorghis CI, Priest DL. Music in the exercise domain: a review and synthesis (Part II). *Int Rev Sport Exerc Psychol.* 2012;5:67–84. doi: 10.1080/1750984X.2011.631027.

35. Creech A. Using music technology creatively to enrich later-life: a literature review. *Front. Psychol.* 2019;10:117. doi: 10.3389/fpsyg.2019.00117.

36. DeMarco J, Alexander JL, Nehrenz G, Gallagher L. The benefit of music for the reduction of stress and anxiety in patients undergoing elective cosmetic surgery. *Music Med.* 2012;4:44. doi: 10.1177/1943862111424416.

37. Bringman H, Giesecke K, Thome A, Bringman S. Relaxing music as pre-medication before surgery: a randomized controlled trial. *Acta Anaesthesiol Scand.* 2009;53:759–764.

38. Dileo C, Bradt J. Music therapy: applications to stress management. In: Lehrer P, Woolfolk, R., Sime, W. eds. *Principles and Practice of Stress Management.* New York: Guilford Press; 2007:519–544.

39. Burzynska AZ, Finc K, Taylor BK, Knecht AM, Kramer AF. The dancing brain: structural and functional signatures of expert dance training. *Front Hum Neurosci.* 2017 Nov 27;11:566. doi: 10.3389/fnhum.2017.00566. PMID: 29230170; PMCID: PMC5711858.

40. Zaidel D. Culture and art: importance of art practice, not aesthetics, to early human culture. *Prog Brain Res.* 2018;237:25–40.

41. Ravignani A, Cook PF. The evolutionary biology of dance without frills. *Curr Biol.* 2016;26(19):R878–R879. doi: 10.1016/j.cub.2016.07.076.

42. Christensen U, Schmidt L, Budtz-Jørgensen E, Avlund K. Group cohesion and social support in exercise classes: results from a danish intervention study. *Health Educ Behav.* 2006 Oct;33(5):677–689. doi: 10.1177/1090198105277397. Epub 2006 May 31. PMID: 16740506.

43. Karpati F, Giacosa C, Foser N, et al. Sensorimotor integration is enhanced in dancers and musicians. *Exp Brain Res.* 2016;234:893–903. doi: 10.1007/s00221-015-4524-1.

44. Caspers S, Zilles K, Laird AR, Eickhoff SB. ALE meta-analysis of action observation and imitation in the human brain. *Neuroimage.* 2010;50:1148–1167.

45. Bläsing BE, Coogan J, Biondi J, Schack T. Watching or listening: how visual and verbal information contribute to learning a complex dance phrase. *Front Psychol.* 2018;9:2371. Published 2018 Nov 30. doi:10.3389/fpsyg.2018.02371.

46. Gardner T, Goulden N, Cross ES. Dynamic modulation of the action observation network by movement familiarity. *J Neurosci.* 2015;35:1561–1572. doi: 10.1523/JNEUROSCI.2942-14.2015.

47. Brown S, Martinez MJ, Parsons LM. The neural basis of human dance. *Cereb Cortex.* 2006;16:1157–1167. doi: 10.1093/cercor/bhj057.

48. Dos Santos Delabary M, Komeroski IG, Monteiro EP, et al. Effects of dance practice on functional mobility, motor symptoms and quality of life in people with Parkinson's disease: a systematic review with meta-analysis. *Aging Clin Exp Res.* 2018 Jul;30(7):727–735. doi: 10.1007/s40520-017-0836-2. Epub 2017 Oct 4. PMID: 28980176.

49. Bruyneel AV. Effects of dance activities on patients with chronic pathologies: scoping review. *Heliyon.* 2019 Jul 20;5(7):e02104. doi: 10.1016/j.heliyon.2019.e02104. PMID: 31372555; PMCID: PMC6657024.

50. Centers for Disease Control and Prevention. *Disability and Health Overview.* Atlanta, GA: Centers for DiseaseControl and Prevention, U.S. Department of Health and Human Services. Last updated September 16, 2020. https://www.cdc.gov/ncbddd/disabilityandhealth/disability.html. Accessed on December 17, 2022.

51. Dismuke C, Egede L. The impact of cognitive, social and physical limitations on income in community dwelling adults with chronic medical and mental disorders. *Glob J Health Sci.* 2015;7:183–195.
52. Sporinova B, Manns B, Tonelli M, et al. Association of mental health disorders with health care utilization and costs among adults with chronic disease. *JAMA Netw Open.* 2019 Aug 2;2(8):e199910. doi: 10.1001/jamanetworkopen.2019.9910. PMID: 31441939; PMCID: PMC6714022.
53. Anderson S, Hencke J, McLaughlin M, Ripp M, Tuffs P. Using background music to enhance memory and improve learning. Masters dissertation. Saint Xavier University, 2000. Washington D.C: ERIC Clearinghouse. https://eric.ed.gov/?id=ED437663
54. Koch SC, Mehl L, Sobanski E, Sieber M, Fuchs T. Fixing the mirrors: a feasibility study of the effects of dance movement therapy on young adults with autism spectrum disorder. *Autism.* 2015 Apr;19(3):338–350. doi: 10.1177/1362361314522353. Epub 2014 Feb 24. PMID: 24566716.
55. Baptista AS, Villela AL, Jones A, Natour J. Effectiveness of dance in patients with fibromyalgia: a randomized, single-blind, controlled study. *Clin Exp Rheumatol.* 2012 Nov-Dec;30(6 Suppl 74):18–23. Epub 2012 Dec 14. PMID: 23020850.
56. Klimova B, Valis M, Kuca K. Dancing as an intervention tool for people with dementia: a mini-review dancing and dementia. *Curr Alzheimer Res.* 2017;14(12):1264–1269. doi: 10.2174/1567205014666170713161422. PMID: 28714391.

17

Good Sport

The Importance and Potential of Sports in Mental Health

Jacob Swartz

Introduction

Sports, activities involving physical exertion and skill where an individual or team competes against another or others for entertainment, have emerged prominent across most cultures and civilizations. French cave paintings over 15,000 years ago glorified wrestling, running, and swimming.[1] The Mayans and the Romans positioned their sports arenas in the centers of cities, and the original Greek Olympic Games resulted in suspending war activities so that everyone could enjoy the game.[2] In modern times, sports remain a significant, esteemed cultural and social aspect of life. Numerous television channels are dedicated solely to sports, and nearly every state's highest-paid public employee is a coach.[3] The power of sports may be exemplified by the National Basketball Association's decision to postpone their season for the COVID-19 pandemic, propelling the United States to go into lockdown.[4]

Sports are also an integral part of childhood, particularly in the United States, with an estimated 72% of middle schoolers (6–12 years old) regularly participating.[5] The benefits of exercise are well documented in terms of improving both physical and overall mental health,[6] and sports participation reduces mortality from all causes by 20%–40%.[7] However, while nearly all sports include physical activity, there is a distinction between physical exercise/activity and a sport. Sports have additional meaning, with a set of rules to follow, specific skills required, and a goal to achieve. Sports contribute to the culture, as competing against others, both individually and as part of a team, creates profound and lasting social connections both within and across generations. Moreover, people participate in sports not just as active participants, but also as invested observers—as fans. The current sports industry in the United States alone is valued at approximately $75 billion.[8] Sports are embedded in current social and cultural life, so the impact and implications of sports on mental health from participation and observation, and strategies to better align sports to promote mental health and well-being, will be described in this chapter.

The Evolution and Meaning of Sports in Society

Luck Favors the Prepared Mind (and Body)

Evolutionary psychology and anthropology indicate that traits or behaviors that offer evolutionary benefit, through improved survival and improved procreation opportunities, will selectively rise and thereafter shape the behaviors of a species.[9] Adaptations to a specific, but sometimes changing, environment can eventually lead to advantages that persist as evolutionary changes developing over thousands of years. For example, "the runner's high" refers to a euphoric sense felt after sustained intense aerobic activity. The *proximate*, or seemingly closely connected, "how" explanation for this phenomenon may be that "exercise induced endocannabinoid signaling " leads to euphoria.[9] The *ultimate*, or deeper, more long-term evolutionary favored, "why" explanation may be that this signaling reinforces and sustains aerobic exercise, which increased successful hunting stamina and thus survival at that time.[10] But as conditions (from environmental to social) change, new survival traits may be favored; for instance, the technological advance of projectile weapons altered hunting skills needed beyond the runner's high. Hunting success now relies on technology, calculation skills, as well as aiming and stealth, more than aerobic capacity for sustained chasing of prey, yet the mechanism (runner's high and endocannabinoid signaling) persists.[9] The runner's high now rewards current athletes who derive benefit from this trait in different, less hunting-like situations more commonly practiced in the current environment where aerobic capacity remains favored. Sports have emerged which align with persisting traits that allow individuals to practice still needed physical skills, originally for combat, as well as mental skills such as assessing the capabilities of allies and foes. As both hunting and combat experiences have decreased in recent times, sports have remained, and became themselves the measure by which individuals attain prominence, show strength, and can "safely" demonstrate their prowess to potential allies or foes.[11]

Sports have expanded to many activities far beyond hunting, gathering, and combat, as the primary motivation for sports, for both participants to observers, has become that sports are themselves *enjoyable and entertaining*,[2] and more so to most than survival/hunting skills. The *proximate* ("how") explanation for sports being enjoyable lies in our reward pathways, including opioid, dopamine, and endocannabinoids, yielding the physiological reason why both participating and observing sports yields pleasure.[10] The *ultimate* ("why") explanation for *enjoying sports* appears to be that sporting behaviors reinforced by pleasurable responses also increase our "fitness" to survive in hunting/combat situations, and to appeal more to potential reproductive mates. The *ultimate* ("why") explanation for *observing sports* appears to be influenced by changing social circumstances. As groups became larger, attributes which could be recognized by the group that improved hunting and defending the community also became favored, as these attributes could lead to larger communities, space supporting more offspring, and an increased chance to pass on genes.[2]

Sizing Up the Competition to Improve the Odds

While exercise can be enjoyable, sports have added competition, whether the individual against self ("against the clock") or against others, alone, or in teams. In early hunter-gatherer societies, 30%–40% of males died from tribal warfare.[12] Exercising individually became an inadequate strategy, as it became vital to also discern the abilities of potential rivals or allies.[9] Sports replicated real-life battle situations where winning became increasingly mental, choosing battle circumstances that favored one's strengths while also exploiting the foe's weaknesses. No longer was having more warriors enough; rather, increasing the advantage by extolling one's strengths while exposing the vulnerabilities of a foe better tipped the scales in one's favor. Mental strengths, such as assessing situations accurately, quickly, and identifying and enacting clever, novel, unexpected tactics, became increasingly important (and ultimately led to creating weapons that minimized hand-to-hand skills emphasizing physical strength). Use of both mental and physical strengths occurs in competitive sports, not only for the competitors, but also for the observers, keen to gamble on their own skills in evaluating all the players.

Fandom: Feeling like Part of the Team

The phenomenon of fandom arose from fans collectively feeling a greater ("1 + 1 = 3") vicarious energy when supporting their tribe/team, and which exceeded simple enjoyment or entertainment. Fans frequently exclaim, "we won," or lament that "we lost" (or leave the stadium early when losing), despite not being on the team or having any significant role in a team's success. Joining a team, even if watching the game from hundreds of miles away or having never played that sport before, etc., is experienced vividly and deeply by vested observers. Indeed, the incidence of cardiovascular events such as strokes and heart attacks *decrease* when countries win the (soccer) World Cup and *increase* after a country is eliminated.[13] For (football) fans of teams in the Super Bowl, up to 25% increases or decreases in cerebrovascular and cardiovascular incidents have similarly been observed for cities that win or lose, respectively.[14]

These fandom reactions likely reflect, at a simple (*proximate*) level, the engagement of reward pathways, sympathetic pathways, and stress pathways (cortisol), related to the exaggerated elation, devastation, and medical complications described above. However, more complex neurological mechanisms accentuate engagement and shared experience. Brain regions compared by functional magnetic resonance imaging (fMRI) for hockey players, fans, and novices (with no prior hockey experience playing or observing,[15] revealed that while listening to hockey-related terminology, the novice's expected language areas were activated, but those with hockey knowledge or experience demonstrated increased activity in additional areas of the brain, including the premotor cortex. This suggests an enhanced comprehension and cognitive engagement when fans/athletes watch or discuss sports events.

As to the *ultimate* ("why") explanation, it would have been imperative even up until recent times to quickly identify an encountered group of strangers and categorize them as members of the clan, likely allies, or likely enemies.[9] Psychological mechanisms for quickly discerning "friend versus foe" increased survival and were selected for over time.[16] In the modern world, identifying whether a stranger is a fan of the Yankees or the Red Sox is rarely a life or death matter. Instead, it reflects a tempered version of this previously vital survival skill, and which fulfills a primitive urge toward rivalries, sustaining this social categorization skill.[9] Significant mental health benefits occur for fans, who report feeling more connected, higher self-esteem, and less loneliness.[17] Sports offer a socially acceptable arena for expression of tribal instincts, but now without life or death consequences, while providing intense connections to like-minded others.

Sports and Mental Health

Sports and exercise are beneficial to mental health. Recreational exercise is superior to physical activity (housework, occupational tasks) in decreasing symptoms of depression and anxiety, and improving coping with stress[7] across the life span.[18] Research relying on more objective accelerometers instead of self-reports also shows increased levels of activity correlated with decreased symptoms of depression.[19]

Individual vs. Team Sports

Benefits to sports for youth extend to social domains as well. Organized activities for young adolescents involved in sports, art, or music have been associated with healthier development, better health, and decreased sadness.[20] The activity with the strongest positive correlation was sports, particularly in boys. Involvement in group, but not individual, sports is related to larger hippocampal volume in both boys and girls.[21] This hippocampal volume is further correlated with decreased symptoms of depression in boys, and decreased hippocampal size has been consistently reported in depression.[22] The hippocampus role in mental health appears related to long-term potentiation of memory (particularly relational), and secondly in the hypothalamus-pituitary-adrenal (HPA) axis. Impaired memory formation and the preferential recall of negative memories are common hallmarks of depression.[23] One hypothesis for decreased hippocampal size in depression is that cortisol levels become excessive, and toxic to hippocampal cells which inhibit cortisol.[21] Excessive cortisol is also associated with an altered stress reactivity which potentiates depression from heightened stress reactions. Conversely, exercise promotes brain-derived neurotrophic factor, neuronal resistance to injury, and increased size in the hippocampus, all protective against depression.

The increased hippocampal volume team observed from team sports participation indicates that increased social exposure accentuates mental health benefits.[24] Team participation in adolescents resulted in lower depression and anxiety symptoms compared to the general population, and these symptoms were about 50% lower for team sports than individual sports. Team sports participants are more likely to indicate that their primary motivation in continuing sports is "fun" than individual sport athletes, who were more likely to report they are "goal oriented."

Sportsmanship: The Thrill of Social Victory—and the Agony of Social Defeat

Sports have become a very complex social event, far beyond demonstrations of physical superiority on a given day where victors live for another day while the defeated do not. Promoting good sportsmanship has significant effects on the mental health of participants. The win-at-all-costs mentality is associated with higher levels of depression, anxiety, and eating disorders, especially at higher-level athletics.[25] Learning to win gracefully and learning from defeats are among the most important social components inherent in sports. There is even a special term, *sportsmanship*, denoting the inherent social and ethical rules. Sportsmanship is essentially balancing the will to win with fairness and respect for all participants and the sport itself.[26] Sports are often the first competitive experiences that children and adolescents have with defined winning and losing. Thus, sports can have significant impacts on learning prosocial and antisocial behaviors, both toward competitors and teammates.[27] As direct participants, athletes who are intrinsically motivated are more focused on improvement/mastering a skill and likely to engage in prosocial behaviors toward opponents and teammates.[28] So, coaches and parents can promote good sportsmanship by focusing on each individual's success and by rewarding personal progress. Conversely, antisocial behaviors, such as cheating and intimidation, aggression, or abuse of other participants (poor sportsmanship skills), are associated with preoccupation with winning, motivation for external rewards/prizes, feeling pressured to compete by others (parents, coaches, etc.), and a desire to prove superiority to others.[27] Coaches/parents contribute to an antisocial environment by pressuring players to win rather than focusing on making good plays and demonstrating teamwork, and by modeling antisocial/intimidation tactics. Athletes preoccupied with winning at all costs learn moral disengagement that allows them to justify and cultivate antisocial behaviors which usually expand to other spheres of their daily lives (in dating relationships, cheating at school, exploitation of others, etc.). Interventions to decrease poor sportsmanship include modeling and explicitly discussing moral identity ("more important to win by playing fair than to cheat") and empathy for teammates and opponents related to sports. A school-based program teaching these elements of good sportsmanship was found to decrease acts of violence such as bullying, threatening, and stealing from others.[29] As a parent, this includes modeling good sportsmanship while watching sports as a fan and spectator (encouraging and appreciating both teams' good plays, not chiding their child or intimidating opponents, etc.) of their child's events. Parents and coaches can also praise instances of prosocial behavior and discuss poor sportsmanship, explicitly discussing empathy (e.g., how teammates feel when he/she doesn't pass the ball to them, or how the other team feels when they lose) and morality (is winning by cheating/lying really a victory?). They can also teach children to handle losing by validating disappointment while praising the athlete's effort to compete despite difficult odds, and developing and improving skills for subsequent games.

Sports in Vulnerable Populations

Sports can also benefit psychosocial development for vulnerable populations, such as those with developmental disorders. Young adolescent boys with developmental coordination disorder reported higher loneliness and lower self-esteem, with an inverse relationship between physical coordination ability and loneliness.[30] Participating in team sports such as soccer and basketball appeared to help mediate this inverse relationship. No other activity, including individual sports such as gymnastics, tennis, and cycling, or non-physical group activities such as choir, band, or chess, was found to be significant. For young people, team sports may still be oriented toward participation rather than focusing on winning and competition, as the differing abilities of children with disorders must be considered.

For children and adolescents with more severe disabilities, engagement in appropriate sports programs continues to show psychosocial benefits. However, the difference between individual and team-oriented sports appears less important. A study looking at children and adolescents with intellectual disability (mean IQ = 59) participating in Special Olympics programs found strong correlations with social competence and confidence and the amount of time involved in Special Olympics or similar sports programs.[31] There was no significant difference between the types of events/sports activities.

Good Practices for Good Sports: Clinical Implications

Healthy habits can be instilled beginning in childhood to build more physically active adults. Longitudinal research following children over almost 40 years indicated that the greatest predictors for being physically active later in life were, after socioeconomic status, participating in various sports and engagement in physical education at school.[32] A similar study following 13- to 23-year-olds found that the earlier and longer adolescents engaged in organized sports, the more physically active they remained 10 years later.[33] A number of practices can help promote positive mental, as well as physical, health at all ages, and are summarized in Table 17.1.

Adulthood

A significant goal in for adulthood is to get back into the game. Participation in sports goes from almost 72% in childhood (Project Play, 2019)[5] to less than 20% among adults.[2] Several factors play into this disengagement. Time becomes a limiting factor, as responsibilities like employment and possible family responsibilities take center stage.[2] However,

TABLE 17.1 Recommended Sports Activities Across the Life Span

Young Children (under 6 years old)	
Activities (*be active*)	Early games can include typical physical activities such as hopping, jumping, skipping, running, water play, and cycling (tricycle or bicycle). Problem-solving (mental skills) can be added to activities, such as hop-scotch and simple obstacle courses that require multiple skills.
Sportsmanship (*modeling*)	Children may start exploring fandom and watching sports, particularly if his/her parents do. Parents should model good sportsmanship as spectators by praising prosocial behaviors and participants' efforts, even in defeat.

TABLE 17.1 Continued

Middle Childhood (7–12 years old)	
Activities (*get into the game*)	Most organized sports begin to be available.
	This is the age when physical activity appears optimal at (at least) 30 minutes 5 times per week, which largely continues throughout life.
	Children are encouraged to explore multiple and diverse sports.
	The International Olympic Committee[34] and American Orthopaedic Society for Sports Medicine[35] recommend multiple sports, as this was associated with decreased rates of sports-related injuries, long-term participation, increased motivation to play, and superior psychosocial outcomes.
	There is a lack of evidence that early specialization improves success at the elite level.
	Include at least one team sport (*especially if child is a boy or has coordination disorder*).
	Individual sports such as cycling, swimming, rowing, and sliding type leg movements (e.g., skating, cross-country skiing, elliptical machines, etc.) have been preferred and recommended for children by the American Academy of Pediatrics, as these can be practiced across the life span.
	Caution should be given to the level of violence and risk for traumatic brain injury in selecting sports (particularly for vulnerable children with ADHD, anxiety, PTSD, or depression).
	If there is no inherent interest from the child, consider more readily available aerobic intense sports such as soccer and basketball.
	Particularly for neurologically vulnerable children with mental health concerns such as anxiety and depression.
	If the child is more severely disabled, encourage participation in Special Olympics or related organizations.
Sportsmanship (*concrete*)	This is a critical period in brain and psychosocial development for a concrete understanding of rules and morals.[36]
	Coaches/parents should explicitly teach behaviors (i.e., *congratulating the opponents on a good game in victory or defeat*).
	Parents/coaches should promote prosocial behaviors by praising individual development and effort over outcome, emphasize having fun and respecting others.
	This is often the first time that children compete with discreet winning and losing:
	Promote resilience by validating the sting of losing but praise effort and emphasize developing and improving skills for next game.
	Model prosocial behaviors as spectators/fans.
Adolescence	
Activities (*keep them in the game*)	Organized sports often become more competitive and the focus may shift from participation to performance and winning, and these leagues may become exclusionary to players without a certain level of skill.
	This can be beneficial in teaching adolescents about hard work and effort, improving skills and success.
	It also *increases* the risks of developing a "win at all cost" antisocial mentality and disengagement from sports.[25]
	If he/she is excluded or dislikes competitive leagues, he/she *should be encouraged to continue sports by finding better fits:*
	More inclusive varsity sports such as track and cross country
	Locally organized intramural sports
	Semi-organized/leisure sports (pickup basketball, swimming, running, cycling, hiking, rock climbing, and others).
Sportsmanship (*abstract and agency*)	Parents/coaches can engage in more abstract conceptualizations such as moral identity and empathy.
	Continue to build resiliency by emphasizing improvement and effort, but enjoyment and fun should continue to be highlighted, as well as the adolescents gaining further agency as they age.

the motivation for sports is still apparent, as adults in sports clubs were more likely to regularly engage in leisure-time physical activity than those attempting to stick to exercise plans.[25] Additionally, participating in sports is significantly more emphasized in youth, with afterschool and summer camp sports readily available. In adulthood, it takes more effort to seek out sport opportunities, and they can differ in quality. In high school, college, or for those few able to play professionally, sports are held in significant esteem, which can confer a significant sense of self-worth and pride for athletes. In adulthood, this sense of meaning is often held in careers and/or family. Including other factors, this may lead to disengagement from sports and thinking of youth sports as the glory days. Further contributing to this disengagement, many sports, such as football, lacrosse, track, or rugby, may not be available in similar organized forms for adults.

One safeguard is the encouragement of multiple sports as described above, including some sports that can be practiced across the lifetime. For those who play only one sport that doesn't readily translate to adulthood, there should be examination into what is enjoyable or motivates them in the sport. It could be the rush of competition or physical exertion, a sense of accomplishing a goal, or the comradery with teammates. Identifying motivations can help select other sports to explore. If the rush of physical activity was most motivating, consider strength and/or endurance-based activities, including weight lifting, obstacle courses like "Tough Mudders," skiing, running races, or cycling. If athletes enjoy competition, consider activities like golf (emphasize walking over carting), squash, or tennis. If it was primarily to accomplish a goal, activities like climbing, hiking, and previously mentioned sports like golf, running, or weight lifting may hold interest. If it was the social aspect of being on a team, the athlete may benefit from exploring more structured adult competitive leagues or intramurals. This could include exploring new activities or leagues related to their chosen sport, such as flag football. Similar approaches may help adults who have already disengaged from sports, but barriers should also be explored. For example, if the adult worries about managing time with family life, consider incorporating family and friends in sport activities.

As patients age, physical activity remains important to health. It is recommended that adults over 65 years old do at least 150 minutes of moderate aerobic activity a week. This may include a shift to more physically appropriate sports like golf, walking, soccer, or shuffleboard clubs. If a preferred sport becomes physically problematic, revisiting motivations and matching to new or similar but more physically feasible sport may help keep the person engaged in benefiting physically and mentally from sports.

References

1. Capelo, H. Symbols from the sky. *Seed Magazine*, May 7, 2012. Retrieved from: https://www.seedmagazine.com/content/article/symbols_from_the_sky/.
2. Apostolou M, Lambrianou R. What motivates people to do and watch sports? *Evol Psychol Sci.* 2017;3:20–33.
3. Gibson C. Who's highest paid in your state. *ESPN*, December 31, 2019. Retrieved from: http://www.espn.com/espn/feature/story?id=28261213&_slug_=dabo-swinney-ed-orgeron-highest-paid-state-employees&redirected=true.

4. Thomas L. The day the games stopped. *The New Yorker*, March 12, 2020. https://www.newyorker.com/sports/sporting-scene/the-day-the-games-stopped-coronavirus.
5. Project Play. *State of Play: Trends and Developments in Youth Sports*. The Aspen Institute; 2019.
6. Chekroud SE. Association between physical exercise and mental health in 1.2 million individuals in the USA between 2011 and 2015: a cross-sectional study. *Lancet Psychiatry*. 2018;739–746.
7. Stephens T. Physical activity and mental health in the United States and Canada: evidence from four populations surveys. *Prevent Med*. 1988 Jan;17:35–47.
8. Heitner, D. Sports industry to reach $73.5 billion by 2019. *Forbes*, October 19, 2015. Retrieved from: https://www.forbes.com/sites/darrenheitner/2015/10/19/sports-industry-to-reach-73-5-billion-by-2019/#b5caeb71b4b9.
9. Balish SM, Eys MA, Schulte-Hostedde AI. Evolutionary sport and exercise psychology: integrating proximate and ultimate explanations. *Psychol Sport Exerc*. 2013;413–422.
10. Bramble DM, Lieberman DE. Endurance running and the evolution of Homo. *Nature*. 2004;432:345–352.
11. Lombardo MP. On the evolution of sport. *Evol Psychol*. 2012;10(1):1–28.
12. Keeley LH. *War Before Civilization: The Myth of the Peaceful Savage*. New York: Oxford University Press; 1996.
13. Wilbert-Lampen U, Leistner D, Greven S, Pohl TS. Cardiovascular events during World Cup soccer. *N Engl J Med*. 2008;358:475–483.
14. Schwartz BG, McDonald SA, Kloner RA. Super Bowl outcome's association with cardiovascular death. *Clin Res Cardiol*. 2013;807–811.
15. Beilock SL, Lyons IM, Mattarella-Micke A, Nusbaum HC, Small SL. Sports experience changes the neural processing of action language. *Proc Natl Acad Sci U S A*. 2008;105(36):13269–13273. doi:10.1073/pnas.0803424105.
16. Winegard BM, Deaner RO. The evolutionary significance of Red Sox Nation: sport fandom as a by-product of coalitional psychology. *Evol Psych*. 2010;8(3):432–446.
17. Wann DL. *Sports Fans: The Psychology and Social Impact of Spectators*. New York: Routledge; 2019.
18. Biddle SJ, Asare M. Physical activity and mental health in children and adolescents: a review of reviews. *Br J Sports Med*. 2011;45:886–895.
19. Choi KW, Chen C-Y, Stein MB. Assessment of bidirectional relationships between physical activity and depression among adults. *JAMA Psychiatry*. 2019;76(4):399–408.
20. Badura P, Geckova AM, Sigmundova D, van Dijk JP, Reijneveld SA. When children play, they feel better: organized activity participation and health in adolescents. *BMC Public Health*. 2015;15:1090.
21. Gorham LS, Jernigan T, Hudziak J, Barch DM. Involvement in sports, hippocampal volume, and depressive symptoms in children. *Biol Psychiatry Cogn Neurosci Neuroimaging*. 2019;4(5):484–492.
22. Bremner J, Narayan M, Anderson E, Staib LM. Hippocampal volume reduction in major depression. *Am J Psychiatry*. 2000;157(1):1158.
23. Chaddock L, Erickson K, Prakash R, Kim J, Voss M, Vanpatter M. A neuroimaging investigation of the association between aerobic fitness, hippocampal volume, and memory performance in preadolescent children. *Brain Res*. 2010;1358:172–183.
24. Pluhar E, McCracken C, Griffith KL, Christino MA, Sugimoto D, Meehan WP. Team sport athletes may be less likely to suffer anxiety or depression than individual sport athletes. *J Sports Sci Med*. 2019;18(3):490–496.
25. Malm C, Joakobsson J, Isaksson A. Physical activity and sports—real health benefits: a review with insight into the public health of Sweden. *Sports (Basel)*. 2019 May23;7(5):127.
26. Abad D. Sportsmanship. *Sport Ethics Philos*. 2010;4(1):27–41.
27. Kavussanu M, Stanger N. Moral behavior in sport. *Curr Opin Psychol*. 2017;16:185–192.
28. Boardley I, Kavussanu M. The influence of social variables and moral disengagement on prosocial and antisocial behaviours in field hockey and netball. *J Sports Sci*. 2009;27(8):843–854.
29. Sánchez-Alcaraz Martínez BJ, Gómez-Mármol A, Valenzuela AV, De la Cruz Sánchez E, Díaz Suárez A. The development of a sport-based personal and social responsibility intervention on daily violence in schools. *Am J Sports Sci Med*. 2014;2(6A):13–17.
30. Poulsen AA, Ziviani JM, Cuskelly M, Smith R. Boys with developmental coordination disorder: loneliness and team sports participation. *Am J Occupat Ther*. 2007;61(4):451–462.

31. Dykens E, Cohen DJ. Effects of Special Olympics International on social competence in persons with mental retardation. *J Am Acad Child Adolesc Psychiatry*. 1996;35(2):223–229.
32. Engström L-M. Who is physically active? Cultural capital and sports participation from adolescence to middle age—a 38-year follow-up study. *Phys Educ Sport Pedagogy*. 2008;4(13):319–343.
33. Kjonniksen L, Anderssen N, Wold B. Organized youth sport as a predictor of physical activity in adulthood. *Scand J Med Sci Sports*. 2009;19:646–654.
34. Bergeron MF, Mountjoy M, Armstrong N, et al. International Olympic Committee consensus statement on youth athletic development. *Br J Sports Med*. 2015;49:843–851.
35. DiFiori JP, Benjamin HL, Brenner JS, et al. Overuse injuries and burnout in youth sports: a position statement from the American Medical Society for Sports Medicine. *Br J Sports Med*. 2014;48:287–288.
36. Davies D. *Child Development: A Practitioner's Guide*. New York: Guilford Press; 2010.

18

Psychosexual Disorders

Social Perspective

Shivananda Manohar, Abhinav Tandon,
Suman S. Rao, and T. S. Sathyanarayana Rao

Introduction

The World Health Organization (WHO) defines sexual health as a state of physical, mental, and social well-being in relation to sexuality. It requires a positive and respectful approach to sexuality and sexual relationships, as well as the possibility of having pleasurable and safe sexual experiences, free of coercion, discrimination, and violence. The World Psychiatric Association has defined sexual health as "a dynamic and harmonious state involving erotic and reproductive experiences and fulfillment, within a broader physical, emotional, interpersonal, social, and spiritual sense of well-being, in a culturally informed, freely and responsibly chosen and ethical framework; not merely the absence of sexual disorders."[1] Sexual health has been neglected by both health professionals and patients alike—health professionals being hesitant to conduct proper assessment usually on an uncooperative patient. Social psychiatry deals with interpersonal, social, and cultural context of mental health and its associated problems, and education in this regard can help in the promotion of mental health and the prevention of mental illness. The WHO has defined social determinants of health as "the circumstances in which people are born, grow up, live, work, and age and the system put in place to deal with illness, which is shaped by with various social, economic and political factors and by access to resources like safe environment, education, and health."[1] Social determinants of mental illness include poverty, unemployment, and limited access to healthcare.[2]

As per the *Merriam-Webster* dictionary, the term *psychosexual* is used to describe (i) the mental, behavioral, and emotional aspects of sexual development (the term "psychosexual" was first used in this sense in 1892); (ii) or relating to mental or emotional attitudes concerning sexual activity. It includes the development of personality of an individual under the influence of his/her sexuality. Psychosexual is not synonymous with libido in the broad Freudian sense. Sexuality involves four factors: (i) sexual identity, (ii) gender identity, (iii) sexual orientation, and (iv) sexual behavior.

There is a bidirectional relationship between social determinants and mental health. Sexual health is influenced by a number of social factors, including poverty, healthcare access, social and cultural norms, education, and economic status. Sexual dysfunctions are influenced by the sociocultural milieu of the society. Certain cultural beliefs may lead to anxiety, affecting the sexual performance of the individual. Social expectations from both sexes may be one of the determinants of sexual dysfunctions.[3]

Culture and Sexuality

Culture plays a significant role in determining the attitude toward sexuality and also sexual variations. Cultural determines gender role, which in turn determines the relationship between different sex partners. The definition of what is sexually deviant behavior depends on the cultural norms. Some of the important aspects of culture and sexuality include explanatory models of sexuality, gender role expectations, models of healing, and ways of healing. The prevalence of sexual dysfunction varies in different cultures. Modes of presentation to the professional are also culture specific. Norms of behavior and threshold for abnormality are shaped by culture.

Virginity is prized in some cultures and has no value whatsoever in others. Masturbation is considered unhealthy and unnatural in some cultures, while it is considered a natural release of sexual tension in others. Some cultures consider homosexuality as crime, while others consider it as a natural variation of sexuality. Similarly, acceptance of orogenital sex, adultery, and pornography is different in different cultures.

Based on these factors, Bullough classified cultures into two broad categories; sex negative and sex positive cultures. Sex negative cultures consider sex fundamentally for procreation and reject hedonistic and recreational aspects of sex. Sex positive cultures look at sex beyond procreation.[4]

Psychosocial Factors

Marriage

Sexual expectations flaunted by mass media may lead to conflict with religious prohibitions and restrictive upbringing; this in turn results in guilt or false expectations.

Problems may arise during the honeymoon because of lack of communication, unusual expectations, and exhaustion. Power struggle, hostility, and conflicts lead to a destructive interaction pattern. Struggle for domination leads to sexual sabotage, including arguments before sex, being repulsive, or frustrating the partner's desire. At times, sex can be used as a weapon, where one partner consciously or subconsciously forgoes sexual pleasure rather than give satisfaction to the other. The other partner has to show good behavior for sexual favors. Anger and anxiety are all anti-erotic stimuli and act as blocking mechanisms.

After the birth of a child, the mother will be preoccupied with the child and finds less time for her husband. This may lead to a feeling of rejection in the partner. This sets up a vicious cycle of approach-refusal-dysfunction.

The availability of a sexually willing, societally sanctioned partner is one of the most important factors in determining the sexuality of women. The problem arises as women outlive men. These differences are narrowing as society is moving away from double standards for men. More than three-quarters of couples who complain of sexual dysfunction also have marital disharmony.[5]

Marriage After Living Together

A couple may start taking one another for granted after marriage. When marriage happens after a period of open relationship due to social pressure, they may feel trapped.[5]

Divorce

Divorce rates have increased in both the young and middle-aged in recent years. It typically requires social, emotional, and sexual readjustment. Many people are so adjusted to thinking of their adult life as a couple, they need time to get used to singlehood. It is perplexing and confusing for people to learn the divorced role. Divorce in some people leads to a decline in style of living. Some people believe that divorce leads to new sexual liberty. The education level and the spiritual values a person harbors determine the number of partners as well as the frequency of sexual intercourse post-divorce.[6]

Remarriage

Various factors influence the likelihood of remarriage. The younger the person, the more probability of remarriage; 89% who separate under the age of 25 remarry, but it decreases to 31% after the age of 40. The shorter the duration of the first marriage, the higher the chances of remarriage.[6]

Families

The individual's upbringing and the attitude of his/her parents about sexuality have a significant impact on sexual well-being. The attitude of parents as well as of siblings about nudity, masturbation, and willingness to discuss sex and homosexuality all contribute to the development of sexuality of an individual. The relationship of the parents with the individual as well as the partner also influences sexuality. Distorted intrafamilial relationship, lack of discipline, overcrowding, lack of warmth, unusual helplessness, and withdrawal from society may lead to certain deviant sexual behaviors.[7]

Socioeconomic Status

There is a link between poverty and abuse of sexual rights, which determines the course of life of countless women. Poverty has long-lasting irreparable psychophysiological effects.[8]

Sexuality, Education, and Awareness

Although sex is no longer a taboo, there is much misinformation, which creates many problems. These include unwanted pregnancy, sexual dysfunction, and sexually transmitted diseases. There is need for parents' participation in sex education of their children instead of waiting for teachers or the media to do so. It is necessary for parents to meet teachers as well as counselors in school to discuss about doubts and fears about sexuality. Schools play an important role in sex education, and teachers must be prepared to meet their students' needs and requests for information. Youth centers can be instrumental in sex education if they are able to find information about sexuality and discuss the topic with health professionals. Education improves communication, which in turn has a positive effect on sexual relationships.[9]

Disparity in Desire

Disparity in desire among couples may increase over the years; difficulties arise if one is content to hold hands and the other has strong sexual urges.[7]

Sexual Interest

Individuals who enjoyed sex in younger years continue their sexual interest when they grow older and remain sexually active in later years. Couples tend to become less inhibited and feel free to explore varying types of sexual stimulation as age advances.[7]

Regular Sexual Expression

Regular sexual expression is important, especially for women. Lack of regular sexual expression and privacy correlate with a decreased interest in coitus.[8]

Sexual Response Cycle

In 1966, Master and Johnson described the EPOR (Excitement, Plateau, Orgasmic, and Resolution phases) Model of the sexual response cycle. Kaplan elaborated the DEOR (Desire, Excitement [Arousal], Orgasm, and Resolution phases) Model.[10] Traditionally sexual dysfunction has been referred to a problem during any phase of the sexual response cycle that prevents the individual or couple from experiencing satisfaction from sexual activity[11]

Nosology

What is "normal" or "healthy" sexual behavior, and when does it become a disorder? A patient-centered approach is the most acceptable one; an individual is said to be suffering from a sexual problem when he/she presents with behavioral issues, and/or cognitive or emotional problems associated with sexual functioning.

The DSM-5 (*Diagnostic and Statistical Manual of Mental Disorders*, 5th edition) defines sexual dysfunctions as "a heterogeneous group of disorders that are typically characterized by a clinically significant disturbance in a person's ability to respond sexually or

TABLE 18.1 DSM-5 Classification of Problems Related to Sexual Functioning (Sexual Dysfunctions, Gender Dysphoria, and Paraphilic Disorders)

Sexual Dysfunctions	Gender Dysphoria
➢ Delayed Ejaculation#	➢ Gender Dysphoria (Note: diagnosis is there in DSM-5, but no corresponding numbers are there in DSM-IV or ICD 10)
➢ Erectile Disorder#	
➢ Female Orgasmic Disorder+	
➢ Female Sexual Interest/Arousal Disorder+	➢ Gender Dysphoria in Children+
➢ Genito-Pelvic Pain/Penetration Disorder+	➢ Gender Dysphoria in Adolescents and Adults+
➢ Male Hypoactive Sexual Desire Disorder#	➢ Other Specified Gender Dysphoria+
➢ Premature (Early) Ejaculation#	➢ Unspecified Gender Dysphoria+
➢ Substance/Medication induced Sexual Dysfunction+#	+ Seen in both males and females
➢ Other Specified Sexual Dysfunction+#	
➢ Unspecified Sexual Dysfunction+#	

+Female sexual disorders
#Male sexual disorders

Paraphilic Disorders

➢ Voyeuristic Disorder#	➢ Exhibitionistic Disorder#
➢ Frotteuristic Disorder#	➢ Sexual Masochism Disorder#
➢ Sexual Sadism Disorder#	➢ Pedophilic Disorder #
➢ Fetishistic Disorder**	➢ Transvestic Disorder#
➢ Other Specified Paraphilic Disorder#	➢ Unspecified Paraphilic Disorder#

Seen in both males and females
** Nearly exclusively reported in males.

to sexual pleasure."[12,13] Subtypes include: primary vs. secondary; lifelong vs. acquired; and generalized vs. situational.

Table 18.1 gives an overview of the DSM-5 classification of problems related to sexual functioning. Sexual disorders mentioned in the DSM-5 and the ICD-10 (*International Classification of Diseases*, 10th edition) classifications of mental and behavioral disorders are described in Table 18.2.

A more comprehensive approach in the classification of sexual disorders uses the multiaxial system. Axis I includes sexual dysfunction and comorbidity; Axis II includes disabilities (social functioning); Axis III includes contextual factors (acute or chronic psychosocial problems); and Axis IV is quality of life.[14]

Epidemiology and Etiology

Social and cultural factors strongly influence the presentation of sexual dysfunctions; thus many epidemiological studies may have actually unknowingly underreported sexual dysfunctions. In 1970, Masters and Johnson concluded that sexual problems exist in 50% of all Americans during some point in their lifetime.[15] A Southeast Asian study conducted by Natera, Wig, and Verma in 1977 at Chandigarh, India, found sexual problems to be present in 10% of males attending OPD (outpatient department) of psychiatry and medicine. An epidemiological study of sexual disorders in general medical practice, supported by the Italian Andrological Association (ASS.A.I.) found sexual disorders to be present among 33.0% of

TABLE 18.2 Brief Description and Comparison of Sexual Dysfunctions Mentioned in DSM-5 and ICD-10

DSM-5 (*Diagnostic and Statistical Manual of Mental Disorders*, 5th edition)	ICD-10 (*International Classification of Mental and Behavioral Disorders*, 10th edition)
Delayed Ejaculation: "Marked delay of ejaculation; infrequent or absence of ejaculation:*" Specify: lifelong vs. acquired; generalized vs. situational; mild, moderate, or severe.	
Erectile Disorder "Marked difficulty in obtaining an erection during sexual activity or maintaining an erection during sexual activity or marked decrease in erectile rigidity:*" Specify: lifelong vs acquired; generalized vs situational; mild, moderate, or severe.	**Sexual Dysfunction not caused by organic disorder or disease** **Failure of Genital Response** (includes female sexual arousal disorder; male erectile disorder; psychogenic impotence) Male erectile disorder: "Problem in developing or sustaining erection during sexual activity which is suitable for satisfactory intercourse." In females, vaginal dryness can be psychogenic or as a result of infection or estrogen deficiency.
Female Orgasmic Disorder "Marked delay, infrequent, reduced intensity or absence of orgasm:*" Specify: lifelong vs acquired; generalized vs situational; mild, moderate, or severe.	**F52.3 Orgasmic Dysfunction** (includes inhibited orgasm: male/female and psychogenic anorgasmy) It may be psychological or organic and is more common in women.
Female Sexual Interest/Arousal Disorder "Significantly reduced or absence of sexual interest or arousal which may include any 3 of the following: (1) Absent/reduced interest (2) Absent/reduced erotic thoughts (3) Absent/reduced initiation of sexual activity or no response to partner's attempt to initiate the same (4) Absent/reduced sexual excitement in 75%–100% encounters (5) Absent/reduced response to erotic cues (6) Absent/reduced genital or non-genital sensations during sexual activity in 75%–100% encounters." Symptoms mentioned above are present for a minimum period of 6 months and cause clinically significant distress. Specify: lifelong vs acquired; generalized vs situational; mild, moderate, or severe.	**Lack or Loss of Sexual Desire** (includes hypoactive sexual desire disorder) Initiation of sexual activity is diminished. Loss of sexual desire is the principal problem and is not secondary to other sexual difficulties like erectile dysfunction. **Sexual Aversion and lack of sexual enjoyment** "In Sexual Aversion the idea or thought of sexual interaction is associated with strong negative emotions and the fear associated leads to avoidance of sexual activity." In some cases, sexual responses may occur normally with orgasm but pleasure is lacking, which leads to lack of enjoyment."
Male Hypoactive Sexual Desire Disorder "Persistently deficient or absent sexual thoughts or fantasies and desire for sexual activity. The judgement is made by taking into consideration the age and socio-cultural factors. The symptoms are present for a minimum period of 6 months and cause significant distress."[13] Specify: lifelong vs acquired; generalized vs situational; mild, moderate, or severe.	
Premature (Early) Ejaculation "Persistent or recurrent ejaculation occurring during sexual activity with partner, within 1 minute of vaginal penetration and before the individual wishes:*" This diagnosis may be applied in cases of non-vaginal sexual activities. Specify: lifelong vs acquired; generalized vs situational; mild, moderate, or severe.	**Premature Ejaculation** "The inability to hold ejaculation for sufficient time during sexual activity, for both partners to enjoy sexual interaction; mostly psychogenic." If erection requires prolonged stimulation the time duration between adequate erection and ejaculation is shortened: delayed erection.

TABLE 18.2 Continued

DSM-5 (*Diagnostic and Statistical Manual of Mental Disorders*, 5th edition)	ICD-10 (*International Classification of Mental and Behavioral Disorders*, 10th edition)
Genito-Pelvic Pain/Penetration Disorder "Persistence of any of the following symptoms: (1) Difficulty in vaginal penetration (2) Significant pain during vaginal intercourse/penetration (3) Fear/ anxiety or pain in anticipation during vaginal penetration (4) Significant contraction of pelvic floor muscles during vaginal penetration attempt. The symptoms are present for a minimum period of 6 months and cause significant distress." [13] Genito-pelvic pain disorder can be further classified into (1) Lifelong vs. acquired; (2) Mild, moderate, or severe.	**Nonorganic Vaginismus** "Spasm of the muscles surrounding the vagina, making penile entry impossible or painful." **Nonorganic Dyspareunia** "Pain during sexual intercourse in males or females." **Excessive sexual drive** (includes nymphomania, satyriasis) Seen in males or females during teenage or adulthood. When associated with an affective disorder the primary mood disorder should be quoted.
Other Sexual Dysfunctions mentioned in DSM-5 **Substance/Medication induced Sexual Dysfunction** (specify whether onset is during intoxication, during withdrawal or after medication use) **Other Specified Sexual Dysfunction** **Unspecified Sexual Dysfunction** For making any of the above diagnosis as per DSM-5, a non-sexual mental disorder, substance abuse/ general medical cause leading to sexual dysfunction and severe relationship distress should be ruled out. [13]	**Other sexual dysfunction, not caused by organic disorder or disease** **Unspecified sexual dysfunction, not caused by organic disorder or disease**
	***Dhat* Syndrome**: A culture-bound syndrome of sexual dysfunction which is seen in the Indian subcontinent, as a mixture of neurotic features of anxiety, depression, and hypochondria in young patients; the symptoms are attributed to loss of semen, in nocturnal emission, "bad dreams," semenuria, masturbation, or sexual intercourse.

*On almost all or greater than 75% occasions of sexual activity with a partner (in identified situations or, if generalized, in all situations). The symptoms are present for a minimum period of 6 months and cause significant distress.

people visiting doctors' offices.[16] A Chinese study conducted in Beijing on 6,000 women concluded that female sexual problems are highly prevalent. This was associated with dissatisfaction of the individual with the spouse's sexual ability and poor marital relationship. Not satisfied with one's marriage, rural life, chronic pelvic pain, and postmenopausal status are other factors for FSD (female sexual dysfunction).[7] A few of the epidemiological studies are briefly described in Table 18.3.

In the study done by TSS Rao and colleagues[17] in South India (Suttur Village) among males, erectile dysfunction was the most common disorder, whereas arousal disorder was the most common female dysfunction noted, implicating that biology plays an important role in men, whereas psychology plays an important role in women's sexual functioning.

Bagadia and colleagues in 1959 reported ignorance, superstitions, and guilt feelings about sex as major areas of concern.[19] Bagadia et al. in 1972 reported anxiety over nocturnal emission (65% of the study group [sg]) and passing semen in urine (47%) as main problems in the unmarried group; while impotence (48% of the sg), premature ejaculation (34% of

TABLE 18.3 Epidemiological Studies on Sexual Dysfunction

TSS Rao and colleagues[17] in South India: Suttur Village (above 60 years and sexually active)	• 43.5%: erectile dysfunction • 10.9%: premature ejaculation • 0.77%: male hypoactive sexual desire disorder • 0.3 8%: male anorgasmia.
TSS Rao and colleagues[17] in South India: Suttur Village (above 60 years and sexually active)	• Prevalence: female hypoactive sexual desire disorder: 16% • Female sexual arousal dysfunction: 28%, female anorgasmia: 20% • Dyspareunia: 8% • 43.5% of the male subjects had erectile dysfunction • 10.9% premature ejaculation • 0.77% male hypoactive sexual desire disorder • 0.3 8% male anorgasmia.
Singh and colleagues (2009),[18] (cross-sectional survey; 149 married women; medical outpatient clinic of a tertiary care hospital)	• Female sexual dysfunction (FSD): 73.2% • Difficulties with desire: 77.2% • Arousal problems in 91.3% • Lubrication problem in 96.6% • Orgasmic problems in 86.6% • Dissatisfaction in 81.2% • Pain in 64.4% of the subjects.

the sg), and passing semen in urine (47% of the sg) were common in the married group. Anxiety (57% of the sg), schizophrenia (16% of the sg), and reactive depression (16% of the sg) were common psychiatric diagnosable conditions in that sample.[20] Sexual problems were noted in 10% of males attending psychiatry and medical OPD (study by Nakra, Wig, and Verma in 1977, Chandigarh).[21] Kendurkar et al. in 2008 [22] concluded that premature ejaculation was the most common complaint and the most commonly diagnosed clinical entity, followed by male erectile problems and *dhat* syndrome (retrospective study; 1,242 patients attending a marriage and sex clinic; medical records from 1979 to 2005).

Avasthi and his colleagues in 2008[23] (in a tertiary care hospital, 100 women attending pediatrics outpatient department for the care of children who were not critical were interviewed) concluded that 17% of the subjects encountered difficulties during sexual activity, including painful intercourse (7%), difficulty in reaching orgasm (9%), lack of vaginal lubrication (5%), vaginal tightness (5%), bleeding after intercourse (3%), and vaginal infection (2%).

Etiology of Sexual Disorders

Human sexual response is a complex phenomenon, and therefore sexual dysfunctions are of multifactorial origin and involve biological and psychosocial factors. Masters and Johnson in 1970 described a two-tier model for etiology of sexual dysfunction (Box 18.1). Table 18.4 gives an overview of the etiology of sexual dysfunctions.[24–27] The National Health and Social Life Survey study concluded that there is a strong association between problems of sexual desire, arousal, and pain with decreased physical satisfaction, emotional satisfaction, and overall life satisfaction. Arousal disorders in females were strongly predictive of diminished relationship satisfaction and overall life satisfaction.[28]

BOX 18.1 Masters and Johnson Two-Tier Model for Etiology of Sexual Dysfunction

Immediate Causes
- Performance fear
- Adoption of spectator role
- Observer vs participant

Distal (historical) causes
- Sociocultural
- Biological
- Sexual trauma
- Homosexual orientation

Sexual Learning and Psychological Factors

Childhood is the time when sexual learning begins, through child-parent interaction reinforcing or discouraging gender-associated activities. Genital self-stimulation is considered to be a normal activity of babies between 15 and 19 months of age. Abusive incidents may negatively affect sexual learning during childhood. Sex play during early adolescence may include experiments among the same sex for a short period. Establishing a sexual identity in adolescence is a conflicting process, and controlling sexual impulses produces a physiological sexual tension, which is released by masturbation as a part of normal sexual development. In adolescence the body image is more firmly established and sexual desire begins to develop. Peer acceptance forms an important part, and experimenting with a partner or partners is part of the normal learning process. Traumatic sexual experiences during childhood may contribute to later sexual and relationship preferences, though there is no correlation between particular experiences of early abuse and later problems. In adults a mature sexual relationship includes strong bonding, intimacy, and love for one's partner. Sexual desire constitutes three interactive components, which include sexual drive (biological component), sexual motivation (psychological component), and sexual wish (social component).[29] Psychological factors such as body image disturbances, intimacy, knowledge about the sexual needs of the partner, and self-esteem have an impact on sexual functioning. Drugs leading to sexual dysfunction in males and females are mentioned in Table 18.5.

TABLE 18.4 Etiology of Sexual Disorders

Psychological factors	Depression/anxiety
	Performance pressure/monotonous routine
	Poor self-esteem/rigid attitude/negative thoughts
	Lack of privacy
	Relationship issues
Physical factors	Cardiovascular morbidity, diabetes, vascular insufficiency, penile disease
	Neurological problems, urogenital disorders, endocrinal disorders
	Alcohol/smoking
	Drugs
Sociocultural factors	Conflict with religious, personal, or family values
	Societal taboos

TABLE 18.5 Drugs Leading to Sexual Dysfunction

Males	Females
Antihypertensive medications	**Antihypertensive medications**
Diuretics, beta blockers	Diuretics,
Antiandrogenic	beta blockers, calcium channel blockers
Digoxin, H2 blockers	**Psychotropics**
Others: Alcohol, ketoconazole, phenytoin/other antiepileptics	Antipsychotics, antidepressants, benzodiazepines
Psychotropics	Buspirone, lithium
Antipsychotics	**Other Drugs**
Antidepressants	Digoxin, histamine H2-receptor blockers
Benzodiazepines	Alcohol, ketoconazole
	Phenobarbital/other antiepileptics
	GnRH agonists
	Oral contraceptives

Other Sexual Disorders/Dysfunctions in the Indian Context

The nosological systems don't include all sexual disorders that are influenced by culture and commonly seen in the Indian subcontinent. Indian researchers have consistently found certain sexual clinical conditions such as *dhat syndrome* and *apprehension about potency.* Dhat syndrome finds mention in ICD-10 under other neurotic disorders (F48.8) category, whereas the diagnosis of apprehension about potency doesn't find mention.

Dhat syndrome (first described in 1960)[30] refers to a clinical condition which is culture bound and characterized by guilt about loss of semen, particularly in young men. This is associated with excessive concern over loss of semen causing a debilitating effect on physical and psychological health. There is subjective reporting of loss of semen during micturition or while straining to pass stools, with no evidence regarding the same. Patients present with vague and multiple somatic complaints, pain, generalized fatiguability, poor memory, anxiety, or depressive symptoms.

Diagnostic Evaluation and Treatment Issues

The evaluation and treatment of sexual dysfunction should be patient centered. Assessment should focus on medical, sexual, and psychosocial history. Complete privacy for the couple should be ensured. Establishing a strong rapport is one of the key components in history taking. Making the patient comfortable, with a nonjudgmental attitude, helps to address many sensitive issues.

History Taking of Sexual Problems

A comprehensive sexual history should inquire about the duration of the problem in relation to time, place, and partner; any stress factors; decreased interest in sexual contact or loss of sex drive; interpersonal problems, anxiety, or physical problems.[31] The principles of sexual history taking are given in Table 18.6.[5] Important questions for males/females are mentioned in Table 18.7.[32-35]

TABLE 18.6 History Taking in Sexual Medicine

Sociodemographic data	• Name, age, sex, education, socioeconomic status, occupation, address, current relationship status, sexual orientation
Current sexual functioning	• Whether there is normal functioning or dysfunctions with reference to each phase of sexual response cycle. • Details of typical sexual interaction which includes initiation, duration of foreplay, coital positions preferred, verbal exchanges during the act and afterplay.
(III) Past sexual history Childhood and adolescence Adults	• Assessing the knowledge about sexuality, how it was acquired, any myths or misinformation about sexuality. Attitude of parents about sexuality during childhood. Any instances of viewing sexual act of parents/other persons/animals. • Sexual activities during childhood including self-stimulatory behavior, any sexual play, masturbatory practices, homosexual activity. Perception about self, masculine/feminine. • Any premarital sex, first sexual intercourse with the partner, pregnancy and its effects on sexual relationship in couples.
Psychosocial history	Myths about sexuality, cultural factors influencing sexuality.
Psychiatric and medical history	Any past or present psychological problems. Medical disorders and specific treatment given for the same.
Other important issues	Separation, divorce, widowhood, sexual abuse, abortion and their impact on person's perception about sexuality.

It is important to take into account the fact that women play different roles at different times in their lives, such as professional, daughter, wife, and mother. Time spent in various activities like family time, work time, extended family time (with parents and relations), social time, personal time, and relationship time (time spent together alone, as a couple) during different phases of life can help in the evaluation of sexual problems.[36]

Differentiating features between psychogenic and organic erectile dysfunction are given in Table 18.8.[37]

A thorough physical examination corroborating with history is important.[37,38] Laboratory studies (as and when indicated) should include a urine analysis, blood tests for complete blood count, lipid profile, fasting blood sugar, liver and kidney function tests, thyroid function, and other endocrinal tests. Nocturnal penile tumescence, intracavernous pharmacologic injection using a vasodilating agent, and duplex color ultrasonography are the other tests in some selected cases.[38]

TABLE 18.7 Important Questions to be Asked in Males/Females

Males	Females
• Changes in sexual interest, fantasy • Performance-related problems; difficulty in either achieving or maintaining erection • Difficulty in ejaculation or orgasm	• Desire difficulty • Any arousal difficulty • Pain during coitus

TABLE 18.8 Differentiating Features Between Psychogenic and Organic Erectile Dysfunction

Parameters	Psychogenic	Organic
Onset	Precipitated by psychological stress	Usually insidious onset with progression of disease (e.g. vascular insufficiency); sudden onset in case of trauma
Response to sexual stimuli	Erection usually present; nocturnal or morning erection present usually	Absent; nocturnal or morning erection usually absent or reduced in frequency and intensity
Course of disorder	Episodic or transient loss of erection	Persistent and progressive
Ejaculation	Premature ejaculation or intermittent loss of ejaculation	Retrograde or absent ejaculation

Treatment

Treatment of sexual dysfunction is tailor made for each individual. One of the key factors is that the couple should be involved in all phases of treatment. The PLISSIT model was given Annon in 1974. PLISSIT stands for permission giving, limited information, specific suggestions, intense therapy.[39]

Nonpharmacological Therapies

Relationship issues should be addressed before starting any specific therapy. If the relationship is characterized by hostility, dishonesty, or lack of love, any specific therapy is unlikely to be helpful.

Relationship therapies are indicated when sex is used as a weapon. The basic essence of this therapy is to make the couple realize they need to be on the same side to be happy. Positive aspects of the relationship should be emphasized and the patient should realize that the partner is not a sex maniac.

Sensate focus exercises include structured exercises of 3–5 sessions assigned between the visits. This form of therapy helps couples to understand that sexual activity is not limited to sexual intercourse. It helps couples to enjoy pleasuring and receiving pleasure, without it being regarded as foreplay or a preliminary to intercourse.[40]

Systematic sensitization and desensitization are particularly effective in premature ejaculation. The start-stop technique is another psychological technique to prolong the pleasure of intercourse. In this technique the partner provides manual stimulation to the male and stops after a signal from him when orgasm is imminent.[41]

Pharmacotherapy of Sexual Dysfunction

Erectile Dysfunction

Phosphodiesterase (PDE)-5 inhibitors are found to be effective in the treatment of erectile dysfunction, irrespective of the etiology. There are four PDE-inhibitors available: Sildenafil, vardenafil, tadalafil, and udenafil. They differ in terms of their median half-life. Dose adjustments are required when used in patients beyond the age of 60 years.[42]

Premature Ejaculation

Tricyclic antidepressant clomipramine in doses of 25–50 mg 4–20 hours before intercourse has been found to be effective. Dapoxetine, because of its shorter half-life, can be used as an on-demand treatment for premature ejaculation. There are reports of usefulness of non-specific selective serotonin reuptake inhibitors (SSRIs) like fluoxetine (5–20 mg/day), paroxetine (10–40 mg/day), and sertraline (25–200 mg). Topical lidocaine/prilocaine creams are also effective.[10]

Other Methods

Testosterone is effective when there is hypogonadism to increase desire. In menopausal women, hormone replacement therapy with estrogen may be beneficial. Bromocriptine is useful if there is hyperprolactinemia. Intracavernous injection with vasoactive drugs like phentolamine, phenoxybenzamine, and papaverine have been found to be effective. Prostaglandin E1 has also been reported to be effective. Central alpha 2 adrenergic antagonist yohimbine, serotonin partial agonist trazadone, dopamine receptor stimulant apomorphine, and nitric oxide precursor L-arginine are helpful drugs.[43–48] Flibanserin, which is now available in India, is a United States Food and Drug Administration (UD-FDA) approved drug for hypoactive sexual desire disorder in premenopausal women.[49]

Homosexuality

Homosexuality is now considered as a variation of sexual activity rather than deviation. A component of identity that includes a person's sexual and emotional attraction to another person and the behavior and/or social affiliation that may result from this attraction. Sexual orientation categories include attraction to members of one's own sex (gay men or lesbians), or to members of the other sex (heterosexuals), and attraction to members of both sexes (bisexuals). Few people identify themselves as pansexual (or queer) in terms of their sexual orientation, which means that their sexual orientation lies outside of the gender binary of "male" and "female" only. Current understanding is that sexual orientation is a continuum. There is also research suggesting that sexual orientation is fluid, especially in women.

Some individuals have conflicting biological indicators, and the lived role in society cannot be attributed to the biological characteristics of the individual. The term "gender" refers to the lived role of the individual as a boy (or man) or girl (or woman) in the society. *Gender dysphoria* refers to the cognitive or affective discontent with the assigned gender; it is the distress with the incongruence between one's experienced (or expressed) gender and one's assigned gender. Many individuals are distressed because of non-availability of the physical interventions. The current term is more descriptive than the term *gender identity disorder* of DSM-IV and focuses on dysphoria rather than identity.

Gender dysphoria in children has to be differentiated from that in adults. For 6 months any of the following 6 symptoms should be present for diagnosis in children: (i) desire to be of the other gender; (ii) cross-dressing; (iii/iv) cross-gender fantasy or play; (v) cross-gender playmates; (vi) rejection of toys, games, or activities of his/her assigned gender; (vii) dislike of anatomy; (viii) desire to have other sex characteristics. For diagnosing gender dysphoria in adults/adolescents, any of the following 2 symptoms should be present for 6 months: (i) incongruence between gender identity and primary/secondary sex characteristics; (ii/iii) profound desire to change and desire to have sex characteristics of the other gender; (iv/v) desire to be of other gender and desire to be treated as other gender; and (vi) conviction that one has the feelings of the other gender.

Paraphilia

As per DSM-5, "The term *paraphilia* denotes any intense and persistent sexual interest other than sexual interest in genital stimulation or preparatory fondling with phenotypically normal, physically mature, consenting human partners." At times, particularly in elderly and medically ill, the criteria "intense and persistent" may be difficult to apply; in such cases the term *paraphilia* may apply to any sexual interest greater than or equal to normophilic sexual interests. A *paraphilic disorder* is a paraphilia causing distress to the individual with or without risk of harm to self or others. A paraphilia is a necessary but not sufficient condition for diagnosing a paraphilic disorder, and paraphilia per se may not require clinical intervention. Paraphilic disorders included in DSM-5 are subdivided as mentioned in Table 18.9.

TABLE 18.9 Classification of Paraphilic Disorders in DSM-5

1st Group: *Disorders with anomalous activity preferences*	**(1) Courtship disorders**: distorted components of human courtship behavior **(2) Algolagnic disorders**: these involve pain and suffering	(i) Voyeuristic disorder (sexual gratification from spying on others in private activities); lifetime prevalence: 12% males, 4% females (ii) Exhibitionistic disorder (sexual arousal from exposing one's genitals to an unsuspecting person); prevalence: males: 2%– 4%; females: uncertain (iii) Frotteuristic disorder (touching or rubbing a nonconsenting person); prevalence up to 30% adult males in the general population (iv) Sexual masochism disorder (sexual gratification from self-humiliation); 12-month prevalence: 2.2% (males), 1.3% (females) (v) Sexual sadism disorder (sexual gratification from inflicting humiliation); prevalence: 2%–30%
2nd Group: *Disorders with anomalous target preferences*	(1) Directed at other humans (2) Directed elsewhere	(i) Pedophilic disorder (sexual focus on children aged 13 or younger); prevalence 3%–5% in males (ii) Fetishistic disorder (using non-living objects or having a highly specific focus on non-genital body parts) (ii) Transvestic disorder (getting sexually aroused from cross-dressing); prevalence less than 3% in males.

Treatment with cognitive behavioral therapy (CBT) is sometimes helpful. Behavior therapy (aversion and reconditioning) and psychotropic drugs have shown very poor evidence of being effective in the treatment for paraphilic behaviors. Gonadotropin-releasing hormone treatment works in a way similar to physical castration. However, with a lack of well-designed studies, data and research for treatment of paraphilias are still in the nascent stages.[51]

References

1. World Health Organization. Commission on Social Determinants of Health. *Closing the Gap in a Generation: Health Equity through Action on the Social Determinants of Health.* Geneva: World Health Organization; 2008.
2. United Nations. General Assembly. *Resolution A/RES/70/1—Transforming our World: The 2030 Agenda for Sustainable Development.* New York: United Nations; 2015.
3. Mezzich JE, Hernandez-Serrano R. Comprehensive definition of sexual health. In: Lanham MD, Aronson J, eds. *Psychiatry and Sexual Health: An Integrated Approach.* Lanham, MD: Jason Aronson; 2006:3–13.
4. Finegold JA, Asaria P, Francis DP. Mortality from ischaemic heart disease by country, region, and age: statistics from World Health Organisation and United Nations. *Int J Cardiol.* 2013 Sep 30;168(2):934–945.
5. Kinsey AC, Pomeroy WB, Martin CE, Gebhard PM. *Sexual Behavior in the Human Female.* Philadelphia: Saunders; 1953.
6. Bumpass L, Sweet J, Martin TC. Changing Patterns of Remarriage. *J Marriage Fam.* (August 1990);52(3):747–756.
7. Kinsey AC, Pomeroy WB, Martin CE. *Sexual Behavior in the Human Male.* Philadelphia: Saunders; 1948.
8. Desjarlais R, Eisenberg L, Good B, Kleinman A. *World Mental Health: Problems and Priorities in Low-Income Countries.* Oxford: Oxford University Press; 1995.
9. Haffner DW. Facing facts: sexual health for America's adolescents: the report of the National Commission on Adolescent Sexual Health. *SIECUS Rep.* 1995 Aug–Sep;23(6):2–8.
10. Avasthi A, Rao TSS, Grover S, Biswas P, Kumar S. Clinical practice guidelines for management of sexual dysfuntions. In: Gautham S, Avasthi A, eds. *Clinical Practice Guidelines for Management of Substance Abuse Disorders, Sexual Dysfunctions and Sleep Disorders.* Indian Psychiatric Society; 2006:144–32.
11. Hatzichristou D, Rosen RC, Broderick G, et al. Clinical evaluation and management strategy for sexual dysfunction in men and women. *J Sexual Med.* 2004;1:49–57.
12. Bhugra D, DeSilva P. Sexual dysfunction across cultures. *Int Rev Psychiatry.* 1993;5(2–3):243–252.
13. *Diagnostic and Statistical Manual of Mental Disorders: DSM-5.* 5th ed. Washington, DC: American Psychiatric Publishing; 2013:423–460, 685–706.
14. World Health Organization. The World health report: 2001: Mental health: new understanding, new hope. World Health Organization; 2001. https://apps.who.int/iris/handle/10665/42390
15. Kolodny RC, Masters WH, Johnson VE. *Textbook of Sexual Medicine.* Boston: Little, Brown; 1979.
16. De Rose AF, Gallo F, Bini PM, Gattuccio I, Chiriacò V, Terrone C. Epidemiology of sexual disorders in general medical practice: an Italian survey. *Urologia.* 2019 May;86(2):79–85.
17. Sathyanaryana Rao TS, Shajahan I, Darshan MS, Tandon A. Sexual disorders among elderly: an epidemiological study in South Indian rural population. *Indian J Psychiatry.* Jul-Sep 2015;57(3):236–241.
18. Singh JC, Tharyan P, Kekre NS, Singh G, Gopalakrishnan G. Prevalence and risk factors for female sexual dysfunction in women attending a medical clinic in South India. *J Postgrad Med.* 2009;55:113–120.
19. Bagadia VN, Vardhachari KS, Mehta BC, Vahia NS. Educational group psychotherapy for certain minor sex disorders of males. *Indian J Psychiatry.* 1959;1:237–240.

20. Bagadia VN, Dave KP, Pradhan PV, Shah LP. Study of 258 male patients with sexual problems. *Indian J Psychiatry*. 1972;14:143–151.

21. Nakra BR, Wig NN, Varma VK. A study of male potency disorders. *Indian J Psychiatry*. 1977;19:13–18.

22. Kendurkar A, Kaur B, Agarwal AK, Singh H, Agarwal V. Profile of adult patients attending a marriage and sex clinic in India. *Int J Soc Psychiatry*. 2008;54:486–493.

23. Avasthi A, Kaur R, Prakash O, Banerjee A, Kumar L, Kulhara P. Sexual behavior of married young women: a preliminary study from North India. *Indian J Community Med*. 2008;33:163–167.

24. Butcher J. ABC of sexual health Female sexual problems I: Loss of desire—what about the fun? *BMJ*. 1999a;318:41–43.

25. Fazio L, Brock G. Erectile dysfunction: management update. *CMAJ*. 2004;170:1429–1437.

26. Levine LA. Diagnosis and treatment of erectile dysfunction. *Am J Med*. 2000;109:3S–12S.

27. Swerdloff RS, Kandeel FR.*Textbook of Internal Medicine*. Lippincott; 1992.

28. Laumann EO, Paik A, Rosen RC. Sexual dysfunction in the United States; prevalence and predictors. *JAMA*. 1999;281:537–544.

29. Levine SB. Sexual disorders. In: Tasman A, Kay J, Liberman JA, eds. *Psychiatry*. 2nd ed. New York: John Wiley & Sons; 2003:Vol. 2, Ch. 74:1475.

30. Wig N. Problems of mental health in India. *J Clin Soc Psychol (India)*. 1960;17:48–53.

31. Tomlinson J. ABC of sexual health: taking a sexual history. *BMJ*. 1998 Dec 5;317(7172):1573–1576.

32. Lue TF, Giuliano F, Montorsi F, et al. Summary of the recommendations on sexual dysfunctions in men. *J Sexual Med*. 2004;1:1–23.

33. Basson R, Althof S, Davis S, et al. Summary of the recommendations on sexual dysfunctions in women. *J Sexual Med*. 2004;1:24–34.

34. Gregoire A. ABC of sexual health: assessing and managing male sexual problems. *BMJ*. 1999; 318:315–317.

35. Kandeel FR, Koussa VKT, Swerdloff RS. Male sexual function and its disorders: physiology, pathophysiology, clinical investigation, and treatment. *Endocr Rev*. 2001;22(3):342–388.

36. Butcher J. ABC of sexual health. Female sexual problems II: sexual pain and sexual fears. *BMJ*. 1999b;318:110–112.

37. Ralph D, McNicholas T. U.K. management guidelines for erectile dysfunction. *BMJ*. 2000;321:499–503.

38. Feldman HA, Goldstein I, Hatzichristou DG, Krane RJ, McKinlay JB. Impotence and its medical and psychosocial correlates: results of the Massachusetts Male Aging Study. *J Urol*. 1994;151:54–61.

39. Meuleman EJ, Diemont WL. Investigation of erectile dysfunction: diagnostic testing for vascular factors in erectile dysfunction. *Urol Clin North Am*. 1995;22:803–819.

40. Montague DK, Barada JH, Belker AM, Levine LA, Nadig PW, Roehrborn CG, Sharlip ID, Bennett AH. Clinical guidelines panel on erectile dysfunction: summary report on the treatment of organic erectile dysfunction. *The American Urological Association*. 1996 Dec;156(6):2007–2011. doi: 10.1016/s0022-5347(01)65419-3.

41. Guiliano F, Jardin A, Gingell CJ. Sildenafil (VIAGRA), an oral treatment for erectile dysfunction: a 1-year, open label extension study. *Br J Urol*. 1997;80:93.

42. Hatzimouratidis K (chair), Eardley I, Giuliano F, et al. Guidelines on male sexual dysfunction: erectile dysfunction and premature ejaculation. *Eur Assoc Urol*. 2019:14–56.

43. Costa P. Multidimensional nature of Apomorphine SL therapy. *Int J Impotence Res*. 2003;15(2):S13–S15.

44. Dula E, Keating W, Siami RF, Edmonds A, O'Neil J, Buttler S. Efficacy and safety of fixed-dose and dose optimization regimens of sublingual Apomorphine versus placebo in men with erectile dysfunction. The Apomorphine Study Group. *Urology*. 2000;56:130–135.

45. Van Ahlen H, Piechota HJ, Kias HJ, Brennemann W, Klingmuller D. Opiate antagonists in erectile dysfunction: a possible new treatment option? Results of a pilot study with Naltrexone. *Eur Urol*. 1995;28:246–250.

46. Padma-Nathan H. Efficacy and tolerability of Tadalafil, a novel phosphodiesterase 5 inhibitor in treatment of erectile dysfunction. *Am J Cardiol*. 2003;92:19M–25M.

47. Linet OI, Ogrinc FG. Efficacy and safety of intracavernosal alprostadil in men with erectile dysfunction. The Alprostadil Study Group. *N Engl J Med*. 1996;334:873–877.

48. World Health Organization. *ICD-10 Classification of Mental and Behavioural Disorders: Diagnostic Criteria for Research*. Geneva: World Health Organization; 1993.

49. Sathyanarayana Rao TS, Andrade C. Flibanserin: approval of a controversial drug for a controversial disorder. *Indian J Psychiatry*. 2015;57(3):221–223.

50. American Psychological Association. Guidelines for psychological practice with transgender and gender nonconforming people. *Am Psychol*. 2015;70(9):832–864. doi: org/10.1037/a0039906.

51. Thibaut F, La Barra F de, Gordon H, Cosyns P, Bradford JMW. The World Federation of Societies of Biological Psychiatry (WFSBP) guidelines for the biological treatment of paraphilias. *World J Biol Psychiatry*. 2010;11:604–655.

19

Marginalized People

Marianne Kastrup

Introduction

According to the *Oxford English Dictionary*,[1] marginalization" means "treatment of a person, group or concept as insignificant or peripheral." The word "marginalize" is an example of how the figurative use of a word takes over the literal one. The original meaning, "to write notes in the margin of," has declined in use since 1968, and the sense that is most commonly encountered today is "to relegate to an unimportant or powerless position."[2]

Marginalized persons and groups are found in all corners of the world and have existed long before the concept became part of the vocabulary in the 1960s.

Delineation of Populations

Marginalized groups change in size and composition over time and place. The underlying reasons are many and differ accordingly. Those who are characterized in one country as marginalized may in another live as part of the mainstream, but some are likely to be marginal in any society. The consequences of marginalization may be long-lasting, and irrespective of background have certain communalities. From a social psychiatric point of view there is increasing awareness that marginalization is one of the prominent social determinants of mental health.

Marginalization is complex, including historical, social, cultural, and economic factors with the objective of pushing a specific population toward the edge of society and isolating the marginalized population from services and opportunities.[3]

There is increasing awareness that mental health is determined by factors outside the traditional healthcare setting. When analyzing social determinants, the significance of non-clinical conditions must be taken into consideration to reduce the inequity of marginalized populations.[4] The question remains how this will affect the formation of political actions to reduce health inequalities.[5]

This textbook includes chapters on immigrants, refugees, and displaced persons; poverty, hunger, and homelessness; women; sexuality; and culture, which include discussion of marginalized populations, but the present chapter will focus solely on marginalized aspects. The objective is to analyze marginalized groups in the context of the World Health Organization (WHO) health for all initiative, the UN Sustainable Developmental Goals, and the increasing inequity in health, and to link this to right to health and social psychiatric aspects.

WHO Alma Ata Declaration

When WHO was founded in 1948, a challenging task was for countries to collaborate in the pursuit of health for all. The first Director-General Brock Chisholm was a psychiatrist who stated thatwithout mental health there can be no true physical health[6] A commitment to the principles of equity and social justice was present, as was the aim to extend good healthcare to marginalized populations with the highest attainable standard of health without distinction of race, religion, political belief, economic, or social conditions.[7] At the International Conference on Primary Health Care in 1978, a need was expressed for urgent action by governments, health workers, and the world community to promote health for all. The inequality in the mental health status of people between developed and developing countries, as well as within countries, was politically, socially, and economically unacceptable and of concern to all countries.[8]

Despite being criticized and accused of being too ambitious and without clear targets, the declaration with its urge toward governments and the world community to focus on inequity in fighting for social justice is as valid as ever—also in social psychiatry.[9] This point was supported by the Lancet Series on Global Mental Health from 2007,[10] aiming to change the way policymakers and other stakeholders thought about mental health. However, the goals pointed out in 2007 have in no way been reached,[11] and equity in mental health is far away.

WHO established in 2005 a Commission on Social Determinants of Health[12] to work for action on health equity and social determinants, linking relevant stakeholders. From the work of the Commission,[12] strategic directions are provided to sensitize governments on the relevance of addressing health inequities and Social Determinants of Health; but the question remains to what extent different marginalized groups have benefited hereof.

UN Sustainable Developmental Goals

In 2015 the United Nations adopted 17 Sustainable Development Goals (SDGs)[13] with the aim to build a better world by 2030 and issued a call for action by all countries.[13] The 17 goals focus on improving the situation for different groups of the global population, but several goals are of particular relevance for marginalized groups.

SDG 1 deals with ending poverty. People exposed to extreme poverty are overtly marginalized, and more likely to be victims of violent conflicts. We witness an extremely skewed geographical distribution of poverty, and social protection systems are needed to help provide a safety net for the marginalized poor.

SDG 2 refers to ending hunger. Hunger and undernutrition continue to affect millions, and many marginalized groups run a greater risk of belonging to the group exposed to hunger.

In relation to the marginalized, SDG 3 on ensuring healthy lives and promoting well-being is essential. A large proportion of the global population has inadequate access to essential health services, and urgent action is needed to address the burden of non-communicable diseases, including mental health. Many aspects are important from a social psychiatric point of view. Suicide is a major public mental health problem and the second-highest cause of death among people age 15 to 29 globally, but with a geographically skewed distribution and the large majority found in low- and middle-income countries.[14] Ensuring reproductive and sexual health requires contraceptive methods and access to modern contraception and has significant consequences for the mental health of the women and families involved. Adolescent fertility is one further aspect often related to marginalized groups and with clear social psychiatric implications.

SDG 4 focuses on equitable education and lifelong learning opportunities. We are far from this goal and need to improve learning outcomes, especially for women, girls, and marginalized people in various vulnerable settings.

Gender equality and empowering women and girls is the focus of SDG 5. Indicators of gender equality are progressing, such as decline in female genital mutilation and early marriage, but the overall numbers continue to be high. Moreover, there is insufficient progress on structural issues causing gender inequality, such as legal discrimination, and social norms marginalizing women.

SDG 8 aims to promote sustainable economic growth. However, more progress is needed to increase employment opportunities, particularly for the young, to reduce informal employment and the gender pay gap, and to promote safe working environments—all factors with a particular impact on marginalized vulnerable groups.

SDG 10 deals with reducing inequality, that within and among nations, which continues to be a significant concern despite efforts at narrowing disparities. The Lancet editorial[15] finds that those leading global discussions (e.g., the World Economic Forum) need to engage with the human realities of globalization. Health for all can only be achieved if those at the margins of society are targeted with appropriate interventions and included in all services. Greater emphasis should be placed on reducing inequalities and supporting those marginalized.

SDG 16 promotes inclusive societies with access to justice for all. Advances in ending violence, promoting the rule of law, and strengthening institutions are unevenly distributed and continue to deprive millions of their security and rights.

Rights to Health

The UN Universal Declaration on Human Rights from 1948[16] states the right and freedom of everyone without distinction of any kind, such as race, sex, language, religion, or political opinion. The improvement of one right facilitates the advancement of others. Likewise, the deprivation of one right adversely affects the others.

Seeing health as a human right, we expect states to have a moral obligation to provide mental healthcare that is acceptable and affordable for all, and that mental health programs reach those marginalized as a priority.[17] Puras[18] recently reaffirmed the right of everyone to the enjoyment of the highest attainable standard of physical and mental health, without distinction of any kind; and further that the distinction between health and ill-health is heavily influenced by culture and context, and health determinants such as poverty, inequality, discrimination, and violence result in chronic stressors.

The right to health has two aspects: the right to have control over your health, but also to be entitled to equal opportunities to reach the highest level of health.[17] Marginalized groups are less likely to enjoy good physical and mental health. Communicable diseases are more common among the most disadvantageous populations and are linked with other inequalities, and non-communicable diseases—if related to lifestyle factors and behavior—are exacerbated by factors linked to, for example, migratory background, sexual orientation, or gender.[17]

Healthcare inequities experienced by marginalized groups are complex and are influenced by multiple factors, such as interrelated stigma and racism[19] and the multiplicity of social locations and lived experiences.[20] The focus of primary healthcare and the social determinants should be kept foremost in policy, and communities—also those of the marginalized—should be empowered to be part of that.[21]

Access to Mental Healthcare

The core components of the rights to health as described by the Committee on Economic Cultural and Social Rights include availability, accessibility, acceptability, and quality. Among marginalized groups, access to services is often reduced.[19] Marginalized populations have in general several barriers in accessing appropriate mental healthcare. Services may be insufficient, resulting in treatment gaps or structural reasons; for example, restrictive policies may further add to the marginalization. Services may not be affordable, or geographically out of reach. They may not be acceptable, exhibiting discrimination toward certain populations, but by strengthening the awareness of cultural values, barriers preventing the participation of the marginalized may be reduced.[22]

Most investigations of mental health disparities focus on one dimension.[23] But many are marginalized in multiple ways. If we look at mental health disparities along single axes of social inequality, we may overlook the excess risk faced by populations at the intersection of multiple marginalized social categories, and such populations may fare worse than disparities along single axes indicate. As emphasized by Bowleg,[24] the many social categories characterizing individuals intersect at the micro level of individual experience to reflect the multiple systems of privilege or oppression at the macro, social-structural level. People experience multiple forms of adversities simultaneously, not piece by piece, with possibly synergistic effects,[23] but despite increasing focus, public health studies reflecting intersectionality are rare.[24] Based upon 272 articles on interventions, multicomponent interventions were in general more successful than single interventions. Barriers to overcome include cultural barriers, negative stereotyping by the media, legal status, and judgmental attitude of services.[25]

Who Are Marginalized Groups?

Social inequalities are associated with an increased risk of several mental disorders, and certain subgroups are at higher risk of mental disorders because of greater exposure and vulnerability to unfavorable social, economic, and environmental circumstances.[26]

Looking at marginalized populations, we find groups characterized by race, color, ethnicity, gender, language, religion, political opinion, national or social origin, poverty, physical or mental disability, health status, sexual orientation, or status as prisoners, homeless, and sex workers. The causes of excess morbidity and mortality in these groups resemble largely the causes of health inequalities more generally, but they differ in degree. It is the multiple intersecting causes and the multiple forms of morbidity that characterize social exclusion.[27]

Ethnic and Racial Factors

In many Western countries—in particular the United States—ethnic and racial minorities experience inequity in access to mental healthcare, even among minorities who have lived in the country for generations.[28–31] British institutions have for decades been scrutinized by their racial bias, and there is a silent acknowledgment of problems linked to race in psychiatry.[32]

In fact, being non-white is a significant determinant in the access to mental healthcare and may be closely related to increased use of coercive psychiatric measures, and the inequity cannot be explained by differences in social status.[9] But ethnic minorities may experience the inequity in other ways, for example limited possibility to get a qualified interpreter when required. Having another ethnic or racial background may result in a double marginalization. Moskovitz and coworkers[33] showed that primary care providers had less trust in non-white compared with white socially marginalized drug users, which affected the therapeutic alliance.

One of the most marginalized ethnic groups is the Roma population. Long-term neglect of Roma health needs is reported by the European Roma Rights Centre, and results often in public health threats.[34] This population is frequently deprived the most basic preventive interventions and primary healthcare.

Culture-sensitive primary care may be decisive in providing accessible, high-quality care to vulnerable migrants and should be universal, and recognizing the importance of inter-cultural communication.[35]

Gender

In many cultures, women have marginalized positions under the control of their husbands or fathers, with limited control over their own life. In relation to mental health, there may be barriers in receiving adequate help simply due to their sex, as cultural and traditional factors in many societies prioritize males' health over that of females.[36]

Migrant women often carry a triple burden linked to their sex, class, and ethnic background, and prejudices may be part and parcel of their daily life,[37] as well as exposure to family and domestic violence, which adds to marginalization.[38]

Women are as likely to have been exposed to torture as men,[39] which contrasts with the general perception that men are the primary target, and may reflect that for many atrocities, women's experiences go unnoticed. The European Parliament[40] concludes that "policies aimed at guaranteeing asylum seekers and refugees' rights and wellbeing cannot be gender-neutral, because women have to face gender-specific challenges in the host country." WHO[41] has recommended that primary care providers develop sensitivity to both gender and migrant issues. Refugee women are often forced to provide sexual services to secure survival for themselves and their dependents, and once arrived in new country, their social control by men is often strict since these may feel threatened by the autonomy of Western women.[42]

The former UN Secretary General Kofi Annan[43] once called violence against women the most pervasive, yet least recognized, human rights abuse. And violence prevails; in a population-based study from India, nearly half of women reported physical violence.[44] Also, European women face violence, and according to Amnesty International, domestic violence is a major cause of death and disability for European women age 16–44.[45]

Another large group of females risking marginalization is the increasing number of unskilled women from deprived parts of the world, migrating to richer countries looking for work and often among those forced into trafficking or other abuse.[46] Trafficking is claimed to be the fastest-growing criminal industry in the world,[47] and each year hundreds of thousands of women and girls are sold into sexual slavery and prostitution.[48]

Marginalization may also be related to societal roles, as women's representation in elected bodies varies from less than 1% to 48%, and even though women represent 39% of world employment, they occupy only 27% of managerial positions.[13]

LGBTQ

Media and the public focus increasingly on the inequities that the LGBTQ population experiences. Whether you are homosexual, bisexual, transgender, or other gender-variant, you are likely in many countries to be met with health discrimination, and inequity in access to care, if not direct violation of your human rights, which again may lead to traumatic conditions and the development of psychiatric problems.[9]

The rights of gay and lesbians have in most Western countries been secured, but lack of legal recognition and discrimination are among the major barriers for transgender people to access adequate health services or if their identity document does not coincide with their sex.[49] Approximately 0.3%–0.5% of the global population are estimated to have a gender identity that differs from the sex they were assigned at birth. Member States of WHO have committed themselves by 2030 to provide coverage of health services as part of SDGs, which will be significant for transgender persons, for instance. The transgender population has a higher risk of homelessness, frequently because their families reject them, or due to general marginalization.[50]

When it comes to determinants of mental health among bisexuals, determinants of emotional well-being could be seen either as part of social structure, interpersonal level, or individually,[51] and health disparities are found among gay and bisexual persons already in adolescence.[52]

Homeless, Poor, and Imprisoned Groups

Aldridge and coworkers[53] carried out a meta-analysis with a focus on the homeless, sex workers, prisoners, and persons with substance abuse who experience extreme health inequities, and found that the extent of the health inequity greatly exceeded what was found in populations with low socioeconomic status.

Marginalized people often live in deprived neighborhoods characterized by indicators such as unemployment, low income, and low education.[54] The health of individuals varies according to neighborhood characteristics, and several studies report that socioeconomically poor areas have higher morbidity than other areas, but also that lack of trust and coping abilities may result in that the marginalized populations lack the courage and desire to participate in the available health program.[54]

It is well-known that prisoners have a high rate of mental illness. Change in prisoners' mental health status may require changes in organizational structure to improve access to adequate care.[55] However, the prison setting often provides a possibility to address health inequities, but once out of prison any benefit may be lost again[56] and marginalization reappears.

Those who experience homelessness and mental illness occupy a position near the bottom of the social gradient in health, with experiences that could be described as a complex interplay of individual and structural factors that perpetuate cycles of inequity.[57] Much of the research on homelessness has its primary focus on the individual, thereby increasing our understanding of risk factors for homelessness but failing to grasp the complex social structures that contribute to income disparity, and ultimately homelessness.[57]

Indigenous Populations

Indigenous populations represent groups that in many settings experience inequity in access to mental healthcare. Mental healthcare providers must understand the structural and historical forces that influence racial disparities in healthcare and personal attitudes when treating indigenous populations.[19] Despite the Canadian public healthcare system, aboriginals are faced with inequalities in access to healthcare and service utilization, and similar findings are reported among Maori in New Zealand and Aboriginals in Australia.[19] Marrone[58] found that inequalities in access and utilization of healthcare may contribute to the fact that despite public health interventions, disparities still exist in indigenous populations in different continents. To have an exclusive focus on health disparities between indigenous and non-indigenous people is not adequate, as ethnic group per se does not operate as a single determinant of health, and it overlooks the huge diversity in the experiences of indigenous groups.[20]

Children and Adolescents

Violence against children persists, and sexual violence is perhaps the most disturbing of children's rights violations. Birth registration plays a primary role in ensuring individual rights and access to justice and social services. Many regions have reached near universal birth registration, but in Sub-Saharan Africa less than half of children under 5 have their births registered.[13]

Child labor also violates children's rights and represents a health hazard. Such children belong to marginalized populations, but changes in this complex worldwide problem require infrastructural changes in the incentives to child labor as well as enlightened public health policies.[59]

In marginalized adolescents, the social determinants of health affecting them comprise factors including education, gender, identity, homelessness, poverty, family structure, culture, religion, and racism, but there is little solid evidence as to how to best address these factors. They have less access to health promotion and health services, and if available, these tend to overlook the crucial social and cultural factors that affect their health.[60] Yet, there has been insufficient focus on how to measure, evaluate, or prove the impact of social determinants on the health of marginalized adolescents.[60]

Perspectives

Many approaches may be taken to fight marginalization in mental health. It is time to call for an ethical, scientific, and humanistic standpoint and to request that responsible authorities show concrete acts of solidarity.

The Lancet Commission on Global Mental Health[61] emphasizes the need to improve the mental health of entire populations, including the marginalized groups, and emphasizes that all persons have a right to mental health and that good mental health can lead to a fairer world.[11] Similarly, the *Lancet* editorial, "A shared future for all,"[15] stresses that it is high time for decision-makers to recognize that health and well-being for all can only be achieved if those currently at the margins of society are targeted with appropriate interventions and are included in all available services.

Public consultation with marginalized persons, the teaching of ethics in departments of public health, and the use of health equity impact assessments might help protect against policies that disadvantage marginalized populations.[62]

Achieving health goals in a setting of inequality and marginalization requires going beyond the simple expansion of mental health services and working with developing trusting relationships. Involving marginalized members of the community in decision-making processes contributes to empowerment. Still, findings show that tackling these issues may prove complicated and will require going beyond the health system, as lack of trust and discrimination permeate public policies that deal with indigenous and rural populations.[3]

To overcome the inequity in care for marginalized groups, Browne and coworkers[63] emphasized the complexity in equity-oriented primary healthcare services. Emphasis should be given to medical education, as knowledge about social determinants of health are not necessarily seen by future doctors as conditions to be changed;[64] major structural and cultural transformations within medical education need to occur to make educational institutions truly socially responsible.

What can governments and civic society do to reduce inequities for marginalized groups? Stakeholders' actions may take three forms: guaranteeing human rights and essential services; facilitating policy frameworks that provide the basis for equitable health improvement; and gathering data related to health equity.[65]

In order to reduce health disparities among the marginalized, cultural competence of healthcare providers and diversity within the workforce should be prioritized to better serve those with diverse cultural, social backgrounds.[4]

When it comes to overcoming health disparities, there is still a long way to go.[66] Scientists and policymakers should be guided by human rights values and ethical principles. And yet we see little progress in eliminating health disparities by socioeconomic status, and it is high time to work for that to ensure a more just society.

Ryn and Fu[67] stress that due to institutional racism there is a reluctance to investigate racial and ethnic health disparities, and they question whether health providers contribute to these inequities by, for example, expressing lower expectations for disadvantageous groups and offering them less sophisticated treatment options.

We in the mental health profession need to become more critical and see medicine in a social, cultural, and historical context. Time has come to recognize societal problems, to search for appropriate solutions, and to show political will to implement them if we want to change the mental health inequity of marginalized groups. This is one of the major future tasks of social psychiatry.

References

1. *Oxford English Dictionary*. https://global.oup.com/academic/product/the-oxford-english-dictionary-9780198611868?cc=dk&lang=en&.
2. *Websters Dictionary*. https://www.paperwhitecollections.com/websters-dictionary/
3. Ruano AL, Sánchez S, Jerez FJ, Flores W. Making the post-MDG global health goals relevant for highly inequitable societies: findings from a consultation with marginalized populations in Guatemala *Int J Equity Health*. 2014;13:57. Published online 2014 Oct 10. doi: 10.1186/1475-9276-13-57.
4. Chazeman S, Jackson J, Gracia, N. Addressing health and health-care disparities: the role of a diverse workforce and the social determinants of health. *Public Health Rep*. 2014 Jan;.129(Supplementum 2): .

5. Carlsson J, Kastrup M. Separate services or integrated services. In: Bhugra D, ed. Oxford *Textbook of Migrant Psychiatry*. Oxford: Oxford University Press; 2021, pp 581-587.

6. Kolappa K, Henderson DC, Kishore SP. No physical health without mental health: lessons unlearned? *Bull WHO*. 2013;91:3–3A. doi: 10.2471/BLT.12.115063.

7. WHO. https://www.who.int/governance/eb/who_constitution_en.pdf.

8. WHO Alma Ata Declaration International Conference on Primary Health Care, Alma Ata, USSR, 6–12 September 1978. http://www.who.int/publications/almaata_declaration_en.pdf.

9. Kastrup M. Inequity in mental health: an issue of increasing public health concern. *World Ass Soc. Psychiatr*. 2019;1:36–8.

10. Lancet series of Global Mental Health. https://www.thelancet.com/series/global-mental-health.

11. Frankish H, Horton R. Mental health for all: a global goal. *Lancet*. 2018;392:1493–1494.

12. WHO. *Social Determinants of Health*. Geneva: WHO; 2008. https://apps.who.int/iris/bitstream/handle/10665/206363/B3357.pdf.

13. United Nations. Sustainable Developmental Goals. https://sustainabledevelopment.un.org/partnerships/unsummit2015.

14. WHO. https://www.who.int/westernpacific/news/detail/04-09-2014-who-calls-for-coordinated-action-to-reduce-suicides-worldwide.

15. Editorial. A shared future for all. *Lancet*. 2018;391:179. Available from: https://linkinghub.elsevier.com/retrieve/pii/S0140673618300862.

16. United Nations. https://www.un.org/en/universal-declaration-human-rights/.

17. WHO. December 2017. https://www.who.int/news-room/fact-sheets/detail/human-rights-and-health29.

18. Puras D. Special Rapporteur on the right of everyone to the enjoyment of the highest attainable standard of physical and mental health. 74th session of the UN General Assembly, October 29, 2019.

19. Goodman A, Fleming K, Markwick N, Morrison T, Lagimodiere L, Kerr T. "They treated me like crap and I know it was because I was Native": the healthcare experiences of Aboriginal peoples living in Vancouver's inner city. *Soc Sci Med*. 2017;178:87–94.

20. Hankivsky O, Christoffersen A. Intersectionality and the determinants of health: a Canadian perspective. *Critical Publ Hlth*. 2008;18(3):271–283.

21. Rasanathan K, Montesinos EV, Matheson D, Etienne C, Evans T. Primary health care and the social determinants of health: essential and complementary approaches for reducing inequities in health. *J Epidem Comm Hlth*. 2011;65:656–60.

22. Montesanti SR, Abelson J, Lavis JN, Dunn JR. Enabling the participation of marginalized populations: case studies from a health service organization in Ontario, Canada. *Health Promot Int*. 2017 Aug 1;32(4):636–649. doi: 10.1093/heapro/dav118.

23. Jackson JW, Williams DR, Van der Weele TJ. Disparities at the intersection of marginalized groups. *Soc Psychiatr Psychiatr Epidemiol*. 2016;51(10):1349–1359.

24. Bowleg L. The problem with the phrase *women and minorities*: intersectionality—an important theoretical framework for public health. *Amer J Publ Hlth*. 2012;102(7):1267–1273.

25. Luchenski S, Maguire N, Aldridge RW, et al. What works in inclusion health: overview of effective interventions for marginalized and excluded populations. *Lancet*. 2018;391:266–268.

26. Allen JMM. *Social Determinants of Mental Health*. World Health Organization. Fundação Calouste Gulbenkian;Lisbon 2014 2014.

27. Marmot M. Inclusion health: addressing the causes of the causes. *Lancet*. 2018;391(10117):186–188.

28. Alegría M, Canino G, Ríos R, et al. Mental health care for Latinos: inequalities in use of specialty mental health services among Latinos, African Americans, and non-Latino Whites. *Psychiatr Serv*. 2002;53(12):1547–1555.

29. Joint Commissioning Panel for Mental Health. *Guidance for Commissioners of Mental Health Services for People from Black and Minority Ethnic Communities* [Internet]. 2014. Available from: http://www.jcpmh.info/wp-content/uploads/jcpmh-bme-guide.pdf.

30. Bhui K, Bhugra D, McKenzie K. Specialist Services for Minority Ethnic Groups? Maudsley Discussion Paper no. 8. 2000.

31. Bhui K, Sashidharan SP. Should there be separate psychiatric services for ethnic minority groups? *Br J Psychiatry*. 2003 Jan 1;182(1):10–12. Available from: http://bjp.rcpsych.org/cgi/doi/10.1192/bjp.182.1.10.

32. Sashidharan SP. Institutional racism in British psychiatry. *Psychiatr Bull*. 2001;25:244–247.

33. Moskowitz D, Thom D, Guzman D, Penko J, Miaskowski C, Kushel M. Is primary care providers' trust in socially marginalized patients affected by race? *J Gen Int Medicine*. 2011;26:846–851.

34. Loewenberg S. The health of Europe's most marginalized populations. *Lancet World Rept*. 2006 Dec 16;368(9553):2115-2115.

35. O'Donnell CA, Burns N, Mair FS, et al., RESTORE Team. Reducing the health care burden for marginalized migrants: the potential role for primary care in Europe. *Health Policy*. 2016 May;120(5):495–508.

36. Niaz U. Impact of violence, disasters, migration and work. In: Chandra P, et al., eds. *Women's Mental Health*. Chichester: John Wiley; 2009:359–368.

37. Ekblad S, Jaranson J. Psychosocial rehabilitation. In: Wilson J, Drozdek B, eds. *Broken Spirits: The Treatment of Traumatized Asylum Seekers, Refugees, War and Torture Victims*. New York, Brenner-Routledge Press; 2004:609–636.

38. Rees S, Pease, B. Refugee Settlement, Safety and Wellbeing: Exploring Domestic and Family Violence in Refugee Communities, 2007. Paper Four of the Violence Against Women Community Attitudes Project. VicHealth, Immigrant Women's Domestic Violence Service.

39. Jaranson JM, Butcher J, Halcon L. et al. Somali and Oromo refugees, correlates of torture and trauma history. *Amer J Publ Health*. 2004;94:591–598.

40. European Parliament. Female refugees and asylum seekers: the issue of integration. Directorate-General for Internal Policies. Policy Department. Citizens' rights and constitutional affairs, 2016.

41. World Health Organization. Stepping up action on refugee and migrant health: towards a WHO European framework for collaborative action. Outcome document of the High-level Meeting on Refugee and Migrant Health November 23–24, 2015, Rome. Copenhagen: Regional Office for Europe. 2016. http://www.euro.who.int/__data/assets/pdf_file/0008/298196/Stepping-up-action-on-refugee-migrant-health.pdf.

42. Kastrup M, Arcel L. Gender specific treatment of refugees with PTSD. In: Wilson J, Drozdek B, eds. *Broken Spirits: The Treatment of Traumatized Asylum Seekers, Refugees, War and Torture Victims*. New York, Brenner-Routledge Press; 2004:547–571.

43. Annan, K. Review of the Implementation of the Beijing Platform for Action and Women 2000: Gender, Equality, Development and Peace for the 21st Century, 2004. E/CN.6/2002, p. 22.https://press.un.org/en/1999/19990308.sgsm6919.html

44. Jejeebhoy S. Wife battering in rural India: husband's right? Evidence from survey data. *Economic Political Weekly*. 1999;33:855–862.

45. Amnesty International. http://web.amnestyorg.

46. Kastrup M. Abuse and trafficking among female migrants and refugees. In: Garcia-Moreno C, Riecher A, eds. *Violence Against Women and Mental Health*. Basel: Karger Verlag; 2013:118–128.

47. Haken J. Transnational crime in the developing world. *Global Financial Integrity*. Retrieved June 25, 2011.https://www.gfintegrity.org/wp-content/uploads/2014/05/gfi_transnational_crime_high-res.pdf

48. Krug EG, Dahlberg LL, Mercy JA, Zwi AB, Lozano R, eds. *World Report on Violence and Health*. Geneva: WHO; 2002.

49. Balakrishnan VS. Growing recognition of transgender health. *Bull WHO*. 2016;94:790–791.

50. Spicer SS. Healthcare needs of the transgender homeless population. *J Gay Lesbian Mental Health*. 2010;14:320–339.

51. Ross LE, Dobinson C, Eady A. Perceived determinants of mental health for bisexual people: a qualitative examination. *Amer J Publ Health*. 2010;100:496–502.

52. Bruce D, Harper GW. Operating without a safety net: gay male adolescents and emerging adults' experiences of marginalization and migration, and implications for theory of syndemic production of health disparities. *Health Educ Behav*. 2011;38:367–738.

53. Aldridge RW, Story A, Hwang SW, et al. Morbidity and mortality in homeless individuals, prisoners, sex workers, and individuals with substance use disorders in high-income countries: a systematic review and meta-analysis. *Lancet*. 2018;391(10117):241–250.

54. Rasmussen M, Poulsen EK, Rytter AS, Kristiansen TM, Bak CK. Experiences with recruitment of marginalized groups in a Danish health promotion program: a document evaluation study. *PLoS ONE*. 2016 Jun 23;11(6):e0158079. doi: 10.1371/journal.pone.0158079. eCollection 2016.

55. Newman L, Baum F, Javanparast S, O'Rourke K, Carlon L. Addressing social determinants of health inequities through settings: a rapid review. *Health Promot Int*. 2015;30(Suppl 2, 1):126–143. https://doi.org/10.1093/heapro/dav054.

56. Kinner S, Streitberg L, Butler T, Levy M. Prisoner and ex-prisoner health. *Austral J Family Physician*. 2012;41:535–537.

57. Patterson M, Markey M, Somers J. Multiple paths to just ends: using narrative interviews and timelines to explore health equity and homelessness. *Int J Qual Methods*. 2012;11:132–151.

58. Marrone S. Understanding barriers to health care: a review of disparities in health care services among indigenous populations. *Int J. Circumpolar Health*. 2007;3:188–198.

59. Woolf A. Health hazards for children at work. *J Toxicol: Clin Toxicol*. 2002;40:477–482.

60. Mohajer N, Earnest J. Widening the aim of health promotion to include the most disadvantaged: vulnerable adolescents and the social determinants of health. *Health Educ Res*. 2010;25:387–394.

61. Lancet Commission on Global Mental Health. 2018. https://www.thelancet.com/commissions/global-mental-health.

62. Silva DS, Smith MJ, Upshur RE. Disadvantaging the disadvantaged: when public health policies and practices negatively affect marginalized populations. *Can J Public Health*. 2013;104(5):e410–e412.

63. Browne AJ, Varcoe CM, Wong ST, et al. Closing the health equity gap: evidence-based strategies for primary health care organizations. *Int J Equity Health*. 2012;11:59. doi: 10.1186/1475-9276-11-59.

64. Sharma M, Pinto AD, Kumagai AK. Teaching the social determinants of health: a path to equity or a road to nowhere? *Acad Med*. 2018;93:25–30.

65. Blas E, Gilson L, Kelly MP, et al. Addressing social determinants of health inequities: what can the state and civil society do? *Lancet*. 2008;372(9650):1684–1689.

66. Braveman PA, Kumanyika S, Fielding J, et al. Health disparities and health equity: the issue is justice. *Am J Public Health*. 2011;101(S1):149–155.

67. van Ryn M, Fu SS. Paved with good intentions: do public health and human service providers contribute to racial/ethnic disparities in health? *Am J Public Health*. 2003 Sep 24;93(2):248–255.

20

Family Matters

The Family as a Resource for the Mental, Social, and Relational Well-Being of Migrants, Asylum Seekers, and Other Displaced Populations

Vincenzo Di Nicola and Suzan Song

Introduction: The Figure of the Migrant

A specter haunts the world and it is the specter of migration.
—Michael Hardt and Antonio Negri[1(p13)]

We are all becoming migrants. . . . This general increase in human mobility and expulsion is now widely recognized as a defining feature of the twenty-first century.
—Interview with Thomas Nail[2]

The reasons why people migrate away from their home country to a new one are extremely varied. Some voluntarily seek new economic opportunities and social mobility; others are forced out of their homes from persecution due to race, religious beliefs, sexual orientation, and social or political membership (see Grinberg and Grinberg[3] for a classic psychoanalytic study of this subject). Some directly experience the collective violence of war, armed conflict, gang violence, or organized crime, and others indirectly experience the potential of these types of violence, or the harm to loved ones. Understanding the types of displacement that people undergo is important, as they may have different levels of moral stigma attached.[4] Immigrants who voluntarily leave their homes for better opportunities elsewhere may be marginalized and discriminated against by citizens in the host country who are competing for similar resources (for example, housing and jobs). Survivors of torture, who are forced to flee their countries due to persecution, are seeking safe haven. The host community may look more favorably on those who are arriving to a host country due to unjust human rights violations and abuses than those arriving for work. Refugees and asylum seekers as well are migrating out of safety concerns due to persecution in their home country and real fears of threatened death should they stay. The difference between the refugee and asylum seeker are that refugees are given legal status while in their home country and are told where they can migrate to, whereas asylum seekers come to a new country seeking safety and legal status while in the host country. Some forcibly displaced people travel alone, unaccompanied and separated from parents or caretakers, and others travel with a family member or intact family units. Some have the economic and social means to travel via train or plane, whereas others have treacherous journeys via foot or buses. Hence, we use the term "migrants" for the reader's ease, while aware that the term is extremely general and does not adequately portray individual variance.

The term "migrant" is consciously nonspecific, invoking multiple types of human movement. The *Oxford English Dictionary* defines migrant as "one who moves, either temporarily or permanently, from one place, area, or country of residence to another." Therefore, the term incorporates well-resourced voluntary immigrants relocating for employment, as well as asylum seekers forced to flee their country due to persecution and violence, and other displaced populations. The different definitions of the term have significant consequences for the number and which types of migrants are counted as entering a country, which affects the analysis and understandings of the impact of migration. In the past, the term "migrant" had a neutral connotation, but recently has become controversial, with some believing that the term "migrant" is used pejoratively to conjure images of entering a country to create threat, as people moving abroad to pursue career or financial interests are rarely called "migrants," but rather "expats" or "immigrants." Labeling an immigrant who voluntarily chooses to migrate for personal convenience the same as one who flees persecution may devalue the life-threatening experiences of the latter. We will use the term "migrants" for the reader's ease, while aware that the term is general and covers many different types of movement, from voluntary migration to asylum seekers and other displaced populations.

A signal aspect of the 21st century is that we are now a world of migrants. Migration can no longer be considered an exception, and philosopher of motion Thomas Nail[2,5] calls migration the norm in human history such that the "figure of the migrant" is the new *nomos* or paradigm for our times. In this light, our goal here is to provide humanitarian workers on the frontline with basic skills for assessing migrant and refugee families.

This requires two epistemological shifts:

- From the *individual* to the *family*[6,7]
- From seeing children and families as *stable and stationary* to understanding human existence as *migratory and in flux*.[5,8]

The exposure to and experience of trauma are consequently more hazardous and more complex.[9] On the other hand, families are the crucible for socialization and belonging, providing crucial resources for the care and support of their members.

Negative and Positive Conceptions of Cultural Encounters

In the nature of the migratory or refugee experience, families come into contact with a series of new cultural encounters.[10,11] These can be experienced in many ways, but the literature in the human and social sciences is filled with overwhelmingly negative conceptions of cultural encounters. So let's deal with this right away. The most common popular term for cultural encounters is "culture shock," and displaced persons are said to react to new cultural encounters with shock, even trauma, and to respond with anxiety and mourning at the loss of their previous cultural contexts. From shock to trauma to anxiety to mourning—the overall theme of negative conceptions of cultural encounters is one of dislocation and loss (see Table 20.1). Public perceptions of the migrant as vagabond,[2,5] ascendant today, also add to their burdens.

Now, while displaced families need to be prepared as much as possible for all eventualities, we may orient them toward more positive conceptions of their cultural encounters. Instead of shock, the displaced person may respond with surprise and see new cultural experiences as opportunities to learn, replacing anxiety with delight and mourning the old with celebration of new possibilities. From surprise to the delight of new learning experiences, displaced people can learn to celebrate their new cultural encounters with the overall theme of discovery and growth (see Table 20.1).

Family Functioning

> Family therapy provides one of the most fruitful areas of cooperation between psychology, psychiatry and medical anthropology.
> —Cecil Helman[12(p291)]

First, it is important to understand the difference between individual and family functioning, using relational psychology. The family genogram is presented as an information-gathering tool.[13] A brief overview of this approach based in systems theory, family therapy, and other relational therapies is offered, noting that these approaches were founded on more or less stable social and cultural contexts. The first challenge for clinicians with displaced

TABLE 20.1 Negative and Positive Conceptions of Cultural Encounters

Negative Conceptions	Positive Conceptions
Shock	Surprise
Trauma	Learning
Anxiety	Delight
Mourning	Celebration
Overall theme: Dislocation and loss	*Overall theme: Discovery and growth*

Adapted from Di Nicola.[6,19]

families is to add a sociocultural dimension to sensitize them to working with families across cultures,[6,14–16] appreciating changing definitions of families and understanding families in light of globalization and global mental health.[17–19] A cultural genogram helps the worker understand the family's culture of origin. The second challenge is to appreciate how family functioning is affected by disasters and conflicts leading to displacement, including migration and refugee status. These dislocations not only disrupt family functioning in the culture of origin (enculturation), but demand adaptation to other cultures (acculturation). This is often not a unitary process but a sequential one, requiring multiple adaptations, leading to the creation of a new, synthetic refugee culture.

Relational Psychology

The first distinction to be made is between *individual* and *family functioning*. We can go so far as to say that traditional Western psychology is based on the individual and has three I-centered ethnocentric assumptions:[19(p52)]

- The *individual* as the subject of psychology;
- *Introspection* as the vehicle of psychological development and the privileged method of inquiry in psychological therapy;
- *Insight* as the Holy Grail of psychological therapy.

These have heuristic value in Western psychotherapy but are not easily portable across cultures, as the issues of attachment and belonging require us to include relationships in our conception of human being. A Zulu saying captures the heart of what family therapy, relational psychology, and social psychiatry all affirm: *Umuntu ngumuntu ngabantu*—"A person is a person through other persons."[20,21]

 Relational psychology allows us to think about individuals and their relationships in families and how they relate to their culture. With this schema, we can expand the notion of the individual's adaptation (called "defense mechanisms" in psychotherapy) to other levels—familial and cultural adaptation (see Table 20.2). Family level adaptations or "defenses" include *family myths, rules, and rituals*. These are the ways in which families organize life to give structure and meaning to daily challenges.[6,22] Examples of family myths are that Italians are warm and family-centered, or that Americans are independent and tough-minded. A family rule may state that when the going gets tough, the tough get going. A family ritual is a way of organizing myths and rules around sanctioned events such as mealtimes, going to church, or leisure time and holidays.

TABLE 20.2 Levels of Adaptive Functioning

Level	Adaptive Functioning
Individual	Adaptive (defense) mechanisms
Family	Family myths, rules, and rituals
Culture	Cultural costume and camouflage

Adapted from Di Nicola.[6,19]

Cultural Costume and Camouflage

> Families of all cultures have a tendency to select or emphasize from their
> culture's repertoire of customs and ceremonies those modes of behavior that
> fit their own style.
> —Edwin Friedman[23(p522)]

Just as each individual is socialized by her family with recognizable rules and rituals for daily life, there is a larger cultural level of adaptation.[6] Each culture furnishes its members with *cultural costume* (how we present ourselves to the world), including *camouflage* (like individual defenses).[6,23] You can spot cultural camouflage because it sounds like an ethnic stereotype, but with a twist, since it used by people to describe themselves: *It's not my fault, I'm Irish; we were raised on the other side of the tracks; that's how we talk in New York/East LA/Mississippi/Montreal.* It camouflages underlying personal or family issues by projecting them onto social or cultural stereotypes that do not explain or enlighten the problem.

Family Studies and Family Therapy

Family studies includes family psychology (and related areas such as family history and family sociology), family medicine and family psychiatry, as well as family therapy. The study of families and family therapy arose in the United States in the mid-20th century and has spread around most of the world.[24,25]

As a field, family therapy offers a comprehensive understanding of three basic things:

1. *Normal family functioning* (the role and functions of family members);
2. *How family problems arise* (including individual mental disorders as well as relational disorders); and
3. *A theory of change* (along with techniques for inducing change in therapy).

The *task* of family therapy is to *give structure and meaning* to a family's predicament. Whether a family evaluation proceeds to a form of therapy or not, all caregivers need to think about how to interact with families to make sense of their experiences of adversity across cultures.

Every contact with displaced people is a kind of intervention, and it is difficult to separate assessment and evaluation from therapy. That is why it is important to understand the basics of family interventions. Across all the theoretical and specialized techniques, a family-based approach offers three basic interventions:[6]

1. *Enhance uncertainty* (asking whether their usual beliefs, thoughts, or practices are working as well as they hoped).
2. *Introduce novelty* (offering a new perspective about their situation).
3. *Encourage diversity* (trying new ways of thinking about or working on their problems).

And this starts with the first clinical encounter with a displaced person.

The Family Genogram

The *family genogram* is a practical, easy-to-understand information-gathering tool[13] for family assessment. Rather than examining functions or tasks of the family,[26,27] it draws a schematic map of the family by looking at three or more generations of family members and the quality of their relationships, including warm and abiding ties, tense and conflictual relationships, and "emotional cutoffs" that result from life's adversities such as separation and loss. The family genogram creates a map of the "relational DNA" of the family system. It has several uses: it is a way to get to know people in a nonjudgmental and unobtrusive way that demonstrates curiosity and empathy. It structures the first meeting and the initial assessment interview. It may be kept as a record of the interview and for future reference at later sessions. It can be revisited and revised as the family feels safer and more trusting of the interviewers, revealing themselves more intimately over time. As the family members experience a degree of differentiation, they may offer different affective and relational maps of the same basic relationships.

An excellent training exercise is to invite trainees to present their own family genograms in a gentle, encouraging small-group context, guided by a teacher or supervisor. It can also be used to guide trainees at all levels when they encounter challenging situations that may parallel their own family stories or conflicts, or when they encounter very new, alienating family configurations and relationships.

"Meeting Strangers"

Two challenges commonly arise in doing family assessments.

The first is working with children and families across cultures[28-33] or "meeting strangers."[6] Sometimes, the experience of the interviewer being "a stranger in the family"[6] echoes the experience of the family as "strangers in a strange land" in their new circumstances, and, all-too-often, the estranging experiences of a family member with alienating or "strange" personal experiences, ranging from adaptational difficulties to serious mental illness. To guide these estranging experiences toward more positive ones, a second cultural map based on the family genogram can be drawn with them. Examining the family's "culture of origin" provides the *cultural genogram* in parallel with the family genogram to give a richer understanding of their cultural experiences. This tool can be used both for assessing families and as a training tool for caregivers to know themselves. Again, it may be useful to do or review the trainees' and interviewers' cultural genogram when conflicts and discomfort arise.

For more detailed cultural assessments, there is the well-developed "Cultural Formulation Interview" (CFI)[34,35] and the well-established toolkit of "Cultural Competence"[36,37] that set out a skills-based approach to cultural interviewing and understanding.

Enculturation vs. Acculturation

The second challenge in assessing the health of a displaced family is how disasters and conflicts impinge on the family functioning of displaced persons.[38,39] This is true both in the culture of origin through the *enculturation* of families into their native contexts. Their social standing may interfere with becoming fully enculturated with a secure sense of belonging, or this may become challenged due to social and cultural changes in their home countries due to a civil war or being part of a marginalized or targeted group. When families then migrate by choice or through constraints, their *acculturation* to new social and cultural circumstances is difficult enough on its own, but may be amplified by challenges in their culture of origin.[10,11]

Clinical Challenges

Some of the clinical challenges for the clinician include family fragmentation and new family configurations, exposure to traumatic incidents, and differential effects of fragmentation and trauma across the domains of age (with unique challenges for refugee youth, elderly and special needs), gender (with special sensitivity to how LGBTQ+ issues morph across culture), culture (including language, religion, and social class), and other aspects of identity and belonging. Critical issues include the need to balance dealing with loss while promoting healthy adaptations to new realities, using the resources of the family, including all of its members and the community of care in its new contexts.

Disasters, conflicts, and other adverse events should not be conceived of as discrete events but as processes. These adverse events push people onto different and unexpected trajectories. It is also important to understand their ongoing nature as a sequential process. Trauma is thus best understood as "sequential trauma," meaning that the experience and impact of traumas are multiple and create a cascade of consequences.[40]

Especially among family members, the issue of directly experienced trauma versus indirectly observed or vicarious trauma is very significant. A child may be just as traumatized by witnessing an attack on a family member as a direct attack on herself. In fact, watching a loved caregiver being attacked is a multiple threat because not only is the child's protector and loved one attacked, but their own integrity is at stake. Such a vicarious attack undermines their most basic sense of security and leaves them fearful for their lives.

Family Fragmentation

Further nuances of this idea are in the differential effects of family fragmentation[10,11] and trauma across the domains of age, gender, culture, and other aspects of identity and belonging. Each of these factors will change the experience of dislocation and loss and how potential traumas are lived and processed throughout their lives. In the cross-cultural encounter, healthcare workers must be sensitive to new and different family forms, including those that arise out of displacement and trauma. Trauma survivors often gravitate to each other for mutual support and understanding based on shared experiences, and the foundation of their relationships may be quite different from what even they would have expected under more ordinary or normal life circumstances. Furthermore, the exposure to traumatic incidents may be unacknowledged and unspoken.

In dealing with all of this, we must always be sensitive to the family's lived experience while guiding them to more positive constructions and possibilities. Critical issues include: dealing with loss, promoting healthy adaptations to new realities, and identifying the family's own resources without imposing such expectations as a burden.

Vignette: "At the Memory Clinic"

Samya, a 14-year-old adolescent refugee from a Near Eastern conflict zone, was referred for a child psychiatric evaluation for possible post-traumatic stress disorder (PTSD), which the Canadian psychologist involved in her refugee process had diagnosed. Seeing her more than 2 years later, no signs of PTSD were evident at all in this rather bubbly, even cheeky teen. Accordingly, I asked her why she was there and what she wanted. "I want to forget," she answered readily. The war in her home country? The separation from her family, her culture, her language? No, she insisted, she wanted to forget how her aunt in Canada with whom she had been placed had mistreated her. I explained that this was a kind of "memory clinic" where we helped people remember things and learn to live with them. "I want the other kind of clinic," she demanded, "the forgetting clinic." So, I recommended that she watch a film called The Eternal Sunshine of the Spotless Mind, *which is about the kind of forgetting clinic she was looking for. When she returned, she mentioned in the most casual way that she had seen the film: "These people go to a clinic to forget painful things," Samya recalled, "It begins with two people who meet and fall in love, when in fact, they have already fallen in love. Since they went to the forgetting clinic, they don't remember that they love each other." And what did the film mean to her? She blushed, recalling the conflicts she had with her group home over dating inappropriate boys. "That if you really love somebody, even if you erase the memory and even if you're not allowed"—she shot a meaningful look toward her youthcare worker—"you will still love them!" And now she asked me what it meant. This was a therapeutic opening, so I quoted a famous paper by John Bowlby,[42] the founder of attachment theory. "What this film is about, Samya," I told her, "is something you already know from your own life—it's about remembering what you are not supposed to remember and saying what you are not supposed to say"* (adapted from Di Nicola).[41]

What this vignette highlights is the need to understand this adolescent in terms of both her family and culture of origin. She lived a fragmented family and cultural reality. The "family" assessment was done through her experience of it. Yet, that is the critical component. The task that all cross-cultural work emphasizes, whether by anthropologists, cultural psychiatrists, or cross-cultural workers, is *cultural translation*, that is, an accurate understanding of where they come from.[6] Conducting such work requires refined interviewing skills,[34,35] competent language translators,[43] cultural mediators or brokers,[44] and the worker's own comfort with meeting people across cultures.[6,7] Now, the other part of the task is *therapeutic translation*, translating how their original enculturation and their current acculturation into a new culture shape their experience in order to negotiate therapeutic goals.[6] While the great majority of the literature in cross-cultural psychology and therapy and cultural psychiatry addresses cultural translation, much fewer studies and approaches address therapeutic translation.

TABLE 20.3 Tools for Family Interviewing and Interventions

Tool	Task
Spirals	**Meeting strangers**
Masks	**Cultural costume and camouflage**
Roles	Cultural insiders (*emic*) and cultural insiders (*etic*)
Codes	**Cultural and therapeutic translation**
Cultural Strategies	**Adaptation and acculturation**
Bridges	The family life cycle across cultures
Stories	The evolving narratives of family life
Suturing	Cultural family therapy as story repair

Adapted from Di Nicola.[6,19]

Tools for Listening to the Family's "Trauma Story"

Everything caregivers do should be focused on helping them listen to the family's "trauma story."[45] Psychiatric trauma specialist Richard Mollica affirms that "trauma is a story that must be told." Let's add the emphasis that trauma is a story that must be told *to another person, face to face.*

Here are tools that everyone can learn with a minimum of training and time because they are based on how we live, rather than what we know. (The "tasks" in bold in Table 20.3 are discussed in this chapter.)

The Relational Dialogue

In the *face-to-face encounter* (cf. philosopher Emmanuel Levinas[46]), where we aim to create the conditions for youth and families to tell their stories, which are often trauma stories, we use these ways of being with other families in order to witness their suffering.

Finally, we come to the real goal of family work. If we can create an atmosphere of safety, trust, and confidence, where family members may reveal their pain and suffering, along with their anxieties and doubts, fears, and shame, through experiences of humiliation and exclusion, negligence and mistreatment—in short, all their adversities and traumas—we can be witnesses to their testimony, which is the beginning of healing.

Witnessing requires these elements—*a face-to-face encounter*[46] that creates a safe environment to hear the *trauma story*,[45] and acknowledging that their trauma story has been heard and validated by active listening in a *relational dialogue.*[7]

Primo Levi, who survived the Auschwitz death camp, repeatedly asserted that the value of his own survival was to serve as a witness to those who did not. This need to witness the suffering of others is reported in many narratives in the trauma literature.

If healing, forgiveness, and the rebuilding and repairing of lives are possible, it all starts with active listening in a relational dialogue to witness the pain of others and to acknowledge their stories.

It's as simple and as hard as that. Not everyone can do this work, but if you are chosen to do it, these tools may make it more bearable for you as a caregiver.

Do not forget to create a healing environment and to do regular and frequent self-care.

For caregivers to be able to do their work, they must create a healing environment for the families they evaluate and treat. Regular and frequent self-care is also necessary for caregivers dealing with displaced families. A colleague who was supervising the first elections in Iraq after the war told me he would spend a week in Baghdad and a week in Jordan as a reprieve, and only gradually extended his time in Baghdad as conditions improved and his own capacity for dealing with the situation increased.

Conclusion

> I think of humanity as a family that has hardly met.
> —Theodore Zeldin[47(p465)]

In their declaration of the Global Mental Health movement, Prince and associates[48,49] declared that there is "no health without mental health." Agreed, but mental health is first social and relational.[19] We must place all human functioning in the meaningful contexts of *family, cultural, and psychosocial worlds*, which are social and require relational bonds and resources.

In working with displaced families, we are simultaneously getting to know them and their worlds and introducing ourselves as unknown, often foreign caregivers.[6,50] As we learn about their painful predicaments and traumas to offer them new solutions, we do our best to understand how their cultures shape them and introduce them to ours or other cultures to help them to adapt to their new worlds.[51–53]

The family, so difficult to define with its protean manifestations, remains a cornerstone not only for society, but for the clinician dealing with families under conditions of adversity. The best tool we can offer under these conditions is to remember that "meeting strangers"[6] is always a very human encounter and, as Theodore Zeldin concludes in his masterful overview of human history, these strangers that we are about to meet are just family members we have hardly met.[47] And they need the same attention, care, and understanding that all families need.

References

1. Hardt M, Negri A. *Empire*. Cambridge, MA: Harvard University Press; 2000.
2. Rosales J. On destroying what destroys you: an interview with Thomas Nail. 2015. http://criticalle galthinking.com/2015/06/30/on-destroying-what-destroys-you-an-interview-with-thomas-nail/. Accessed November 10, 2018.
3. Grinberg L, Grinberg R. *Psychoanalytic Perspectives on Migration and Exile*. Foreword by O Kernberg. New Haven, CT: Yale University Press; 2004.
4. Song SJ, Ventevogel P, eds. *Child, Adolescent and Family Refugee Mental Health: A Global Perspective*. New York, NY: Springer Nature; 2020.
5. Nail T. *The Figure of the Migrant*. Stanford, CA: Stanford University Press; 2015.
6. Di Nicola V. *A Stranger in the Family: Culture, Families, and Therapy*. New York, NY and London, UK: W.W. Norton & Co.; 1997.
7. Di Nicola V. *Letters to a Young Therapist: Relational Practices for the Coming Community*. New York, NY and Dresden: Atropos Press; 2011.

8. Di Nicola V. The Global South: An emergent epistemology for social psychiatry. *World Soc Psychiatry.* 2020;2:20–26.

9. De Haene L, Rousseau C, Kevers R, Deruddere N, Rober P. Stories of trauma in family therapy with refugees: supporting safe relational spaces of narration and silence. *Clin Child Psychol Psychiatry.* 2018;23:258–278.

10. Sluzki CE. Migration and family conflict. *Family Process.* 1979;18:379–390.

11. Sluzki CE. Disruption and reconstruction of networks following migration/relocation. *Family Systems Med.* 1992;10:359–363.

12. Helman C. *Culture, Health and Illness.* 3rd ed. Oxford, UK: Oxford University Press; 1994.

13. McGoldrick M, Gerson R, Petri S. *Genograms: Assessment and Intervention.* 3rd ed. New York, NY and London, UK: W.W. Norton & Co.; 2008.

14. Di Nicola VF. Family therapy and transcultural psychiatry: an emerging synthesis. Part I: The conceptual basis. *Transcult Psychiatr Res Rev.* 1985;22(2):81–113.

15. Di Nicola VF. Family therapy and transcultural psychiatry: an emerging synthesis. Part II: Portability and cultural change. *Transcult Psychiatr Res Rev.* 1985;22(3):151–179.

16. Di Nicola V. Children and families in cultural transition. In: Okpaku SO, ed. *Clinical Methods in Transcultural Psychiatry.* Washington, DC: American Psychiatric Press; 1998:365–390.

17. Cohen A, Patel V, Minas H. A very brief history of Global Mental Health. In: Patel V, Minas H, Cohen A, Prince MJ, eds. *Global Mental Health: Principles and Practice.* Oxford, UK: Oxford University Press; 2013:3–26.

18. Patel V, Prince M. Global mental health: a new mental health field comes of age. *JAMA.* 2010 May 19;303(19):1976–1977.

19. Di Nicola V. Family, psychosocial, and cultural determinants of health. In: Sorel E, ed. *21st Century Global Mental Health.* Boston, MA: Jones & Bartlett 2012:119–150.

20. Birhane A. Descartes was wrong: "A person is a person through other persons." *Aeon Magazine*, April 7, 2017. Available from: https://aeon.co/ideas/descartes-was-wrong-a-person-is-a-personthrough-other-persons. Last accessed September 1, 2021.

21. Di Nicola V. "A person is a person through other persons": A social psychiatry manifesto for the 21st century. *World Soc Psychiatry.* 2019;1(1):8–21.

22. Andolfi M, Angelo C, De Nichilo M. *The Myth of Atlas: Families and the Therapeutic Story* (Di Nicola V, ed. & trans.). New York, NY: Brunner/Mazel; 1989.

23. Friedman EH. The myth of the shiksa. In: McGoldrick M, Pearce JK, Giordano J, eds. *Ethnicity and Family Therapy.* New York, NY: Guilford Press; 1982:499–526.

24. Minuchin S. *Families and Family Therapy.* Cambridge, MA: Harvard University Press; 2009.

25. Selvini M, ed. *The Work of Mara Selvini Palazzoli.* New York, NY: Jason Aronson; 1988.

26. Bray JH. Family assessment: Current issues in evaluating families. *Fam Relat.* 1995;44(4):469–477.

27. Staccini L, Tomba E, Grandi S, Keitner G. The evaluation of family functioning by the family assessment device: a systematic review of studies in adult clinical populations. *Fam Process.* 2015;54(1):94–115.

28. Canino IA, Spurlock J, eds. *Culturally Diverse Children and Adolescents: Assessment, Diagnosis, and Treatment.* 2nd ed. New York, NY: Guilford Press; 2000.

29. Johnson-Powell G, Yamamoto J, eds. *Transcultural Child Development: Psychological Assessment and Treatment.* Hoboken, NJ: John Wiley & Sons; 1997.

30. Kaslow, NJ, Celano M, Dreelin ED. A cultural perspective on family theory and therapy. *Psychiatr Clin N Am.* 1995;18(3):621–633.

31. Super CM. Cognitive development: looking across at growing up. *New Direct Child Devel.* 1980;8:59–69.

32. Valsiner J, ed. *Child Development in Cultural Context.* Toronto, ON: Hogrefe & Huber; 1989.

33. Vargas LA, Koss-Chioino JD, eds. *Working with Culture: Psychotherapeutic Interventions with Ethnic Minority Children and Adolescents.* San Francisco, CA: Jossey-Bass 1992.

34. American Psychiatric Association. Cultural formulation. In: *Diagnostic and Statistical Manual of Mental Disorders.* 5th ed. Washington, DC: American Psychiatric Association; 2013:749–759.

35. DeSilva R, Aggarwal NK, Lewis-Fernández R. The DSM-5 Cultural Formulation Interview and the evolution of cultural assessment in psychiatry. *Psychiatric Times*, 2015;2(6):1–3.

36. Beach MC, Price EG, Gary TL, et al. Cultural competence: a systematic review of health care provider educational interventions. *Med Care.* 2005;43:356–373.

37. Brach C, Fraser I. Can cultural competency reduce racial and ethnic health disparities? A review and conceptual model. *Med Care Res Rev.* 2000;57(suppl 1):181–217.

38. Karageorge A, Rhodes P, Gray R, Papadopoulos R. Relationship and family therapy for newly-resettled refugees: a qualitative inquiry of an innovative, needs-adapted approach in Sydney, Australia. *Eur Psychiatry.* 2017;41:S622–S623.

39. Matlin SA, Depoux A, Schütte S, Flahault A, Saso L. Migrants' and refugees' health: Towards an agenda of solutions. *Public Health Rev.* 2018;39:27.

40. Keilson, Hans. *Sequential Traumatisation in Children: A Clinical and Statistical Follow-up Study on the Fate of the Jewish War Orphans in The Netherlands.* Trans. Bearne Y, Coleman H, Winter D. Jerusalem: The Magnes Press, Hebrew University; 1992.

41. Di Nicola V. Letter to young psychiatrists. "At the memory clinic"—remembering what you are not supposed to remember. *Washington Psychiatrist Magazine.* 2017 Spring, 14–15.

42. Bowlby J. On knowing what you are not supposed to know and feeling what you are not supposed to feel. In: *A Secure Base: Parent-Child Attachment and Healthy Human Development.* New York, NY: Basic Books; 1988:99–118.

43. Leanza Y, Miklavcic A, Boivin I, Rosenberg E. Working with interpreters. In: Kirmayer LJ, Guzder J, Rousseau C, eds. *Cultural Consultation: Encountering the Other in Mental Health Care.* New York: Springer Science & Business Media; 2013:89–114.

44. Miklavcic A, Leblanc MN. Culture brokers, clinically applied ethnography, and cultural mediation. In: Kirmayer LJ, Guzder J, Rousseau C, eds. *Cultural Consultation: Encountering the Other in Mental Health Care.* New York, NY: Springer Science & Business Media; 2013:115–137.

45. Mollica RF. *Healing Invisible Wounds: Paths to Hope and Recovery in a Violent World.* Nashville, TN: Vanderbilt University Press; 2009.

46. Levinas, E. *Ethics and Infinity: Conversations with Philippe Nemo.* Trans. Richard A. Cohen. Pittsburgh, PA: Duquesne University Press; 1985.

47. Zeldin T. *An Intimate History of Humanity.* New York, NY: Random House; 2012.

48. Prince M, Patel V, Saxena S, et al. No health without mental health. *Lancet.* 2007;370:859–877.

49. Patel V, Minas H, Alex C, Prince MJ (eds.). *Global Mental Health: Principles and Practice.* Oxford, UK: Oxford University Press; 2013.

50. Di Nicola V. De l'enfant sauvage à l'enfant fou: A prospectus for transcultural child psychiatry. In: Nathalie G, Liliane S, Pierre M, eds. *Transcultural Issues in Child Psychiatry.* Montreal, QC: Éditions Douglas; 1992:7–53.

51. Di Nicola V. Ethnocultural aspects of PTSD and related stress disorders among children and adolescents. In: Marsella AJ, Friedman M, Gerrity E, Scurfield R, eds. *Ethnocultural Aspects of Posttraumatic Stress Disorder: Issues, Research, and Clinical Applications.* Washington, DC: American Psychological Association; 1996:389–414.

52. Di Nicola V, Leslie M, Haynes C, Nesbeth K. Clinical considerations for immigrant, refugee, and asylee youth populations. *Child Adolesc Psychiatr Clin N Am.* 2022;31:679–692.

53. Guzder J. Family systems in cultural consultation. In: Kirmayer LJ, Guzder J, Rousseau C, eds. *Cultural Consultation: Encountering the Other in Mental Health Care.* New York, NY: Springer Science & Business Media; 2013:139–161.

21

Poverty, Hunger, Homelessness

Social Psychiatry

Andres J. Pumariega and Rama Rao Gogineni

Introduction

Everyone has the right to a standard of living adequate for the health and well-being of himself and of his family, including food, clothing, housing and medical care and necessary social services, and the right to security in the event of unemployment, sickness, disability, widowhood, old age or other lack of livelihood in circumstances beyond his control.
    —Article 25; The Universal Declaration of Human Rights adopted by the United Nations General Assembly on December 10, 1948

The world's population is approximately 7 billion. About 925 million people go to bed hungry every night, and approximately a billion are homeless. Poverty globally, regionally, and for all ages, genders, ethnicities, and nationalities has been a major social, physical, and mental health issue for decades, if not centuries. The following is a summary of the myriad effects of poverty, homelessness, and hunger on children and youth, mothers, women, and men all over the world. This chapter reviews some of the literature associated with the psychosocial impact of poverty, hunger, and homelessness, and their effects on psychology and mental health, and recommendations to advocates and care providers.

Poverty

Poverty is roughly defined as not being able to afford the basic necessities of life that would provide a minimum standard of living. The World Bank reports that 736 million people worldwide live on less than $1.90 a day. While poverty rates have declined in all regions of the world, progress has been uneven. More than half of the extreme poor live in Sub-Saharan Africa. The majority of the global poor live in rural areas and are poorly educated, employed in the agricultural sector, and under 18 years of age. Access to good schools, healthcare, electricity, safe water, and other critical services remains elusive for many people, often determined by socioeconomic status, gender, ethnicity, and geography. Currently, 1,000 children under the age of 5 die every day from illnesses like diarrhea, dysentery, and cholera, caused by contaminated water and inadequate sanitation associated with poverty.[1]

Poverty is endemic, even in the richest nation on Earth. United States Census Bureau data[2] show that the poverty rate rose to 15.9% (46.2 million) in 2010. The percentage of people in deep poverty was 13.5% of all Blacks and 10.9% of all Hispanics, compared to 5.8% of Asians and 4.3% of Whites. Deepening poverty is inextricably linked with rising levels of homelessness and food insecurity/hunger for many Americans, and children are particularly affected by these conditions. U.S. Census data reveal the total number of children under age 18 living in poverty increased to 22% in 2010 and was the highest at that time since 1993. The sudden and severe economic impact of the COVID pandemic has resulted in a rapid increase in poverty in the United States and worldwide.[3] Racial and ethnic disparities in poverty rates persist, and are especially highest among children. The poverty rate for Black children was 38.2%; 32.3% for Hispanic children; 17% for non-Hispanic White children; and 13% for Asian children. In the United Kingdom, 14 million people (one-fifth of the population) live in poverty, 4 million are more than 50% below the poverty line, and 1.5 million are classed as destitute, unable to afford even basic life essentials.[4] Poorer children and teens are also at greater risk for several negative outcomes, such as poor academic achievement, school dropout, abuse and neglect, behavioral and socioemotional problems, physical health problems, and developmental delays. Additionally, the multiple stressors associated with poverty (divorce, domestic violence, lack of parental monitoring, parental mental illness) result in significantly increased risk for developing psychiatric and functional problems.[5]

Poverty remains one of the most pressing problems facing the world; the mechanisms through which poverty arises and perpetuates itself are not well understood. But poverty may have particular psychological consequences that can lead to economic behaviors that make it difficult to escape poverty. The evidence indicates that poverty causes stress and negative affective states, which in turn may lead to short-sighted and risk-averse decision-making, possibly by limiting attention and favoring habitual behaviors at the expense of goal-directed ones. Together, these relationships may constitute a feedback loop that contributes to the perpetuation of poverty. In 2020, it was estimated that 88 million to 115 million additional people would be pushed into absolute poverty worldwide by the COVID pandemic, bringing the total to between 703 million and 729 million living on less than $1.90 a day. The absolute poverty rate will be 9.1%–9.4%, taking us back three years to 2017 levels.[6] This is affecting developing nations disproportionately, where some recent gains had been made in reducing poverty. For example, the World Bank[6] indicated that South Asia was set to plunge in 2020 into its worst-ever recession as the devastating impacts of

COVID-19 on South Asian economies lingered on, taking a disproportionate toll on informal workers and pushing millions of South Asians into extreme poverty.

Poverty and mental illness are linked together in a complex manner. Poorer persons have been shown to be at higher risk of developing mental illnesses, possibly both as a result of the physical and psychosocial impact of lower socioeconomic status leading to greater disease burden and the lack of access to health resources to manage precursors of illness. Conversely, people with poor mental health are more susceptible to the main factors that can lead to poverty and homelessness: loss of productivity, disaffiliation, and personal vulnerability for social stigmatization with negative stereotyping that exacerbate deprivation.[5,7-9]

Neuropsychiatric Sequelae of Poverty

Poverty in children is damaging to their mental, physical, emotional, and spiritual development. For example, Kishiyama et al.[10] reported that prefrontal-dependent electrophysiological measures of attention were reduced in lower socioeconomic status (SES) children compared to high SES children in a pattern similar to that observed in patients with lateral prefrontal cortex (PFC) damage, including self-regulation and behavioral difficulties and reasoning. Poverty has been found to be associated with smaller white and cortical gray matter and hippocampal and amygdala volumes. The effects of poverty on hippocampal volume were mediated by caregiving support/hostility on the left and right, as well as stressful life events on the left. Findings that these effects on the hippocampus are mediated by caregiving and stressful life events suggest that attempts to enhance early caregiving should be a focused public health target for prevention and early intervention.[11]

Hair et al.[12] conducted a longitudinal cohort study analyzing 823 magnetic resonance imaging scans of 389 typically developing children and adolescents age 4 to 22 years from the National Institutes of Health Magnetic Resonance Imaging Study of Normal Brain Development, with complete sociodemographic and neuroimaging data. One-quarter of sample households reported the total family income below 200% of the federal poverty level. Poverty was associated with structural differences in several areas of the brain associated with school readiness skills, with the largest influence observed among children from the poorest households. As much as 20% of the gap in test scores could be explained by maturational lags in the frontal and temporal lobes. Some of these effects are also related to disparities in information and language exposure. Children in poor families hear about 30 million fewer words by the time they are 4 than children from middle-class families.[13]

Regardless of the contributing factors, these impacts can be long-lasting. A longitudinal study, published by Evans,[14] found that childhood poverty predicted multimethod indices of adult psychological well-being at age 24 when controlling for outcomes at age 9, manifesting greater allostatic load, an index of chronic physiological stress, higher levels of externalizing symptoms (e.g., aggression) but not internalizing symptoms (e.g., depression), and more helplessness behaviors. In addition, childhood poverty predicts deficits in adult short-term spatial memory. In a longitudinal study of nearly 4,000 families in Canada, Hastings et al.[15] found that growing up in a poor urban neighborhood was associated with a doubling in the risk of developing a psychosis-spectrum disorder by middle adulthood.

Children raised in low SES families also tend to go on to have relatively high rates of chronic physical illness in adulthood.

Hunger

The United Nations Food and Agriculture Organization estimated that about 815 million people of the 7.6 billion people in the world, or 10.7%, were suffering from chronic undernourishment in 2016. Almost all the hungry people live in lower-middle-income countries, with only 1 million undernourished people living in developed countries. Africa has the highest prevalence of undernourishment, but as the most populous region in the world, Asia has the highest number of undernourished people.[16]

One in three children in low- and middle-income countries suffers from chronic undernutrition. Surveys showed that approximately 45% of all child deaths worldwide are from causes related to undernutrition. At least 17 million children suffer from severe acute malnutrition around the world. Severe acute malnutrition is the direct cause of death for 2 million children every year. and every day.[1]

Physiological and Neuropsychiatric Impact of Hunger/ Malnutrition

The beginning of the understanding of the neurocognitive impact of hunger and malnutrition began in November 1944, when 36 young men took up residence in the corridors and rooms of the University of Minnesota football stadium as volunteers for a nearly yearlong experiment on the psychological and physiological effects of starvation. The Minnesota Starvation Experiment was a project of the newly established Laboratory of Physiological Hygiene at the University of Minnesota. At the time, World War II was raging around the world, and so, too, were hunger and starvation, with the prospect of finding even more severely starved victims in liberated concentration and prisoner of war camps. The research protocol called for the men to lose 25% of their normal body weight. They spent the first 3 months of the study eating a normal diet of 3,200 calories a day, followed by 6 months of semi-starvation at 1,570 calories a day, then a restricted rehabilitation period of 3 months eating 2,000 to 3,200 calories a day, and finally an 8-week unrestricted rehabilitation period during which there were no limits on caloric intake. They were required to work 15 hours per week in the lab, walk 22 miles per week, and participate in a variety of educational activities for 25 hours a week. Throughout the experiment, the researchers measured the physiological and psychological changes brought on by near starvation. During the semi-starvation phase the changes were dramatic, with significant decreases in strength and stamina, body temperature, heart rate, and sex drive. The psychological effects were significant as well, with food obsessions, fatigue, irritability, depression, and apathy. The men also reported decreases in mental ability, although mental testing of the men did not support this belief. The Minnesota Starvation Experiment, which ended in October 1945, painted a vivid picture of the physical and psychological decline caused by starvation and offered guidelines on rehabilitation.[17]

Children are the most visible victims of undernutrition. It is estimated that undernutrition—including stunting, wasting, deficiencies of vitamin A and zinc, and fetal growth restriction—are a cause of 3.1 million child deaths annually, or 45% of all child deaths in 2011.[1] Undernutrition magnifies the effect of every disease, including measles and malaria. Maternal undernutrition during pregnancy increases the risk of negative birth outcomes, including premature birth, low birth weight, smaller head size, and lower brain weight. Babies born prematurely are vulnerable to health problems and are at increased risk for developing learning problems when they reach school age. The first 3 years of a child's life are a period of rapid brain development. Too little energy, protein, and nutrients during this sensitive period can lead to lasting deficits in cognitive, social, and emotional development. Protein-energy malnutrition, iron deficiency anemia, iodine, zinc, and other vitamin deficiencies in early childhood can cause brain impairment. Failure to thrive, the failure to grow and reach major developmental milestones as the result of undernutrition, affects 5%–10% of American children under the age of 3. Hunger reduces a child's motor skills, activity level, and motivation to explore the environment. Movement and exploration are important to cognitive development, and more active children elicit more stimulation and attention from their caregivers, which promotes social and emotional development.[18]

Numerous studies have demonstrated the negative effects of poverty on children's health outcomes. Findings from studies conducted on a broader range of family incomes showed that not only poverty but also factors associated with it (race, gender, education, and employment status) are related to hunger, which in turn is associated with negative health outcomes. For example, a community sample of 328 low-income children age 6–12 who were classified as "hungry," "at-risk for hunger," or "not hungry" found that hungry children were significantly more likely to receive special education services, to have repeated a grade in school, and to have received mental health counseling than at-risk-for-hunger or not-hungry children. In this same study, hungry children exhibited 7 to 12 times as many symptoms of conduct disorder (such as fighting, blaming others for problems, having trouble with a teacher, not listening to rules, stealing) than their at-risk or not-hungry peers. Among low-income children, those classified as "hungry" show increased anxious, irritable, aggressive, and oppositional behavior in comparison to peers.[19] Weinreb et al.,[20] in a study of 180 preschool and 228 school-age poor children, found that, for school-age children, severe hunger was a significant predictor of chronic illness after controlling for housing status, mother's distress, low birth weight, and child live events. For preschoolers, moderate hunger was a significant predictor of health conditions while controlling for potential explanatory factors. For both preschoolers and school-age children, severe child hunger was associated with higher levels of internalizing behavior problems. After controlling for housing status, mother's distress, and stressful life events, severe child hunger was also associated with higher reported anxiety/depression among school-age children.

Families often work to keep their food insecurity hidden, and some parents may feel shame or embarrassment that they are not able to feed their children adequately. Children may also feel stigmatized, isolated, ashamed, or embarrassed by their lack of food.[5] Most research has shown strong associations between depression and food insecurity. Though most studies are cross-sectional, longitudinal analyses suggested bidirectional relationships (with food insecurity increasing the risk of depressive symptoms or diagnosis, and depression in turn predicting food insecurity). Several studies have focused on vulnerable subgroups, such as pregnant women and mothers, women at risk of homelessness, refugees, and those who had been exposed to violence or substance abuse. Overall, studies support a link between food insecurity and mental health (and other factors, such as housing circumstances and exposure to violence) among women in high-income countries and underscore the need for comprehensive policies and programs that recognize complex links among public health challenges.[5]

Homelessness

It is estimated that no less than 150 million people, or about 2% of the world's population, are homeless. However, about 1.6 billion, more than 20% of the world's population, may lack adequate housing.[21] Homelessness affects individuals of all ages, genders, and ethnicities. We often consider homelessness to be a result of poverty, lack of housing or government support, and economic challenges such as raising a child alone; however, homelessness can also be caused by physical, sexual, and emotional trauma, such as domestic violence, or trauma resulting from disasters. Trauma is considered by many to be the root cause of homelessness, and that most cases of homelessness result from a series of losses and resulting learned helplessness. Homelessness itself can lead to further trauma. The loss of a home is often accompanied by loss of community, possessions, and security. Those with severe and persistent mental illness or those who have experienced multiple traumas can experience an internal, ongoing terror, loneliness, fear, and dread. Even the lives of their family are affected negatively.

Homelessness is the direst state of deprivation. Homelessness exists when people do not have access to safe, stable, and appropriate places to live. A homeless person is deprived of security, safety, dignity, and liberty. Periods of homelessness often have serious and lasting effects on personal development, health, and well-being. The U.S. government defines a chronically homeless individual as an unaccompanied person who has been homeless for a consecutive year (or 4 or more periods of homelessness within the last 3 years) with a disability preventing them from working,[22] but chronic homelessness can exist in the absence of disabilities in parts of the world affected by war, disasters, or famine. Homelessness is one of the most extreme manifestations of poverty. There is both national and international evidence that highlights the link between poverty and homelessness. Homelessness is ubiquitous; only a very few countries are not facing this issue at the moment. Countries with better safety nets and social policies such as Finland and Sweden have zero homelessness.[21]

In the United States, an estimated 567,715 people experienced homelessness on a given night in January 2019, according to the National Alliance to End Homelessness.[23] An estimated 2.3 million to 3.5 million Americans experience homelessness at least once a year. Homelessness affects people of all ages, geographic areas, occupations, and ethnicities, but occurs disproportionately among people of color. In 2009–2010 school year, 939,903 homeless children and youth were enrolled in public schools, a 38% increase from the 2006–2007 school year. More than 1.6 million children (1 in 45 children) in the United States are home-less and approximately 650,000 are below age 6. Approximately 47% of children in homeless families are Black, although Black children make up just 15% of the U.S. child population. Hispanic children make up 13%, whereas Native American children make up 2% of the homeless children population.[24,25]

Homelessness often has serious and lasting effects on personal development, health, and well-being. It can cost society approximately $50,000 per year for a single chronically homeless individual who is cycling in and out of treatment facilities, jails, hospitals, and other institutional care facilities. Homeless children confront abject poverty and experi-ence a constellation of risks that have a devastating impact on their well-being. The research reviewed here links homelessness among children to hunger and poor nutrition, health problems and lack of health and mental health care, developmental delays, psychological problems, and academic underachievement. Homelessness has particularly adverse effects on children and youth, including its association with poor physical and mental health and missed educational opportunities. Schooling for homeless children is often interrupted and delayed, with homeless children twice as likely to have a learning disability, repeat a grade or to be suspended from school. Homelessness and hunger are closely intertwined. Homeless children are twice as likely to experience hunger as their non-homeless peers. Hunger has its own additive negative effects on the physical, social, emotional, and cogni-tive development of children.[26]

Economic changes resulting in lack of affordable housing are also a risk factor for homelessness. This can be a result of economic conditions impoverishing large sectors of the population, or scarcity of housing driving housing prices beyond the means of many poorer individuals, as is seen in the gentrification of urban centers. The COVID pandemic has led to massive unemployment as a result of quarantines and lockdowns to mitigate the virus, with many individuals and families living paycheck to paycheck, unable to make their rent and risking eviction. Though there was some financial assistance in the United States early in the pandemic, as well as a moratorium on the eviction of renters, this aid was in the process of running out by the end of 2020, with upward of 18 million people at risk of being evicted.[27]

Psychosocial and Psychiatric Consequences of Homelessness

Most mental health literature on homelessness has focused on characteristics that may be risk factors for homelessness. But homelessness itself is a risk factor for emotional dis-orders, psychological trauma, social disaffiliation, and learned helplessness. Psychological trauma is likely among homeless individuals and families for three reasons: (a) The sudden or gradual loss of one's home can be a stressor of sufficient severity to produce symptoms of psychological trauma. (b) The conditions of shelter life may produce trauma symptoms. (c) Many homeless people—particularly women—become homeless after experiencing physical and sexual abuse and consequent psychological trauma.[28] A study by Toro et al.[29] showed that never-homeless poor individuals were significantly more likely to be receiving public benefits, were less likely to have a diagnosed mental disorder or problems with substance abuse, and showed lower levels of self-rated psychological distress. A number of other studies from the United States provide similar evidence, suggesting that those who are homeless (in the sense that they are roofless or sleep in shelter facilities) tend to be a particularly vulnerable subgroup of individuals within the poor.

Homeless mothers were found to have higher levels of unmet need for mental health services; 72% of sheltered homeless mothers reported high current psychological distress or symptoms of major mental illness or substance abuse. The relationship between maternal and child problems underscores the need for homeless family interventions that promote access to psychiatric care for both generations. Homeless single mothers often have histories of violent victimization, with over one-third having post-traumatic stress disorder (PTSD) and over half experiencing major depression while homeless. An estimated 41% develop dependency on alcohol and drugs and are often in poor physical health. Maternal depression and parental substance abuse have a series of negative outcomes for children.[30]

A quarter of homeless children have also witnessed violence, and 22% have been separated from their families. Exposure to violence can cause a number of psychosocial difficulties for children, both emotionally (depression, anxiety, withdrawal) and behaviorally (aggression, acting out). Half of school-age homeless children experience problems with depression and anxiety, and 1 in 5 homeless preschoolers have emotional problems that require professional care. Homelessness is linked to poor physical health for children, including low birth weight, malnutrition, ear infections, exposure to environmental toxins, and chronic illness (e.g., asthma). Homeless children also are less likely to have adequate access to medical and dental care.[26,30]

In the United States, unaccompanied youth (sometimes referred to as runaway youth or street youth) number between 575,000 to 1.6 million annually, and typically range from age 16 to 22, while worldwide they likely number in the tens of millions.[31] The major causes of homelessness for unaccompanied youth are poverty/lack of affordable housing, family conflict, mental illness, and substance abuse. Family conflict is the primary cause of homelessness in developed nations, with 46% having experienced abuse and an estimated 20%–40% identifying as lesbian, gay, bisexual, or transgendered (LGBT). In the developing world, extreme poverty is the strongest predictor of homelessness for street youth as well as for families.[31] Homeless families are often forced to choose between housing and other necessities for their survival. Female-headed households are also particularly vulnerable. Teen parents are also particularly at risk of homelessness. Substance abusing or physically violent parents and stepparents are the major drivers of homelessness in runaway youth, particularly for those who identify as LGBT.[28]

Unaccompanied homeless youth are often more likely to grapple with mental health (depression, anxiety, and PTSD) and substance abuse problems. Many runaway youths, most of them pushed out and rejected by their families because of their differences (sexual orientation, gender identity, or mental health problems), engage in sexually risky behaviors (sometimes for their own survival), which places them at risk of HIV, other sexually transmitted diseases (STDs), and unintended pregnancies. Also, emerging research has shown that LGBT homeless youth are 7 times more likely to be victims of violent crime.[32] Studies on homeless youth in the United States have shown high rates of risk-taking behaviors (smoking, alcohol, marijuana abuse, physical fights, truancy, high sexual behaviors, low use of birth control measures, running away, sexual abuse); they face additional barriers to access of healthcare, and suffer from a high burden of poor health.

Similar patterns are also seen in other nations. Homeless youth in Australia are found to have extremely high rates of psychological distress and psychiatric disorders. Homeless youth have scored significantly higher on standardized measures of psychological distress than all domiciled control groups. Youth homelessness studies have also reported very high rates of suicidal behavior. Rates of various psychiatric disorders are usually at least twice as high among homeless youth than among youth from community surveys. As homeless youth are at risk of developing psychiatric disorders and possibly self-injurious behavior the longer they are homeless, early intervention in relevant health facilities is required.[33]

Homelessness and Serious Persistent Mental Illness

According to the Substance Abuse and Mental Health Services Administration, 25%–33% of the homeless population in the United States suffers from some form of severe mental illness. In comparison, only 6% of Americans are severely mentally ill.[34] Serious mental illnesses disrupt people's ability to carry out essential aspects of daily life, such as self-care and household management. Mental illnesses may also prevent people from forming and maintaining stable relationships, or may cause people to misinterpret others' guidance and to react irrationally. This often results in pushing away caregivers, family, and friends who may be the force keeping that person from becoming homeless. As a result of these factors and the stresses of living with a mental disorder, people with mental illnesses are much more likely to become homeless than the general population. Patients with schizophrenia or bipolar disorder are particularly vulnerable. In addition, half of the mentally ill homeless population in the United States also suffers from substance abuse and dependence. Minorities, especially African Americans, are overrepresented in this group. Some mentally ill people self-medicate using street drugs, which can lead not only to addictions, but also to disease transmission from injection drug use.[34]

Schizophrenia is much more prevalent among homeless persons than in the population at large. The rate of schizophrenia in homeless persons reported in 33 published reports, representing 8 different countries, ranged from 2% to 45%. Rates were higher in younger persons, women, and the chronically homeless. Slightly less than half of the homeless persons with schizophrenia were not currently receiving treatment.[35]

The combination of mental illness, substance abuse, and poor physical health makes it very difficult for people to obtain employment and residential stability. In major cities from New York to San Diego, homeless people with severe mental illness are now an accepted part of the urban landscape and make up a significant percentage of the homeless who ride subways all night, sleep on sidewalks, and hang out in public facilities such as libraries and bus stations. In the United States, homelessness emerged as a national issue in the mid-20th century as one of the unintended consequences of closing state mental hospitals without providing replacement treatment for people with the most serious mental illness. Six studies reported that lifetime rate of victimization in the population ranged from 74% to 87%. The same survey examined 15 studies and found that mentally ill homeless individuals had a lifetime risk for arrest ranging between 63% and 90%. Homelessness and incarceration increase the risk of each other. A 2008 study reported recent homelessness to be 8 to 11 times more common in jail inmates; the increased risk was attributed in part to mental illness.[34]

Systemic Causes of Poverty, Hunger, and Homelessness

The systemic causes of poverty and homelessness are diverse, complex, interwoven, and related to many institutional structures within our world and societies. Social and economic policies, wars, immigration, the impact of technology, and many other socioeconomic and political forces contribute to poverty, hunger, and homelessness. Low- and middle-income nations have larger challenges dealing with this triple threat as a result of limited resources, and often population growth that is unsustainable. Corruption and governmental/political mismanagement in such nations can complicate efforts to deal with these challenges due to the diversion of resources or concentration of wealth within elites.

Developed and developing nations have made major strides in reducing the percentages of poverty, hunger, and homelessness, as witnessed in Europe in the 17th through 20th centuries, in the United States in the 19th and 20th centuries, and especially many emerging nations in Pacific and Central Asia in the 20th and 21st centuries. According to 2015 estimates, 10 % of the world's population lived on less than US$1.90 a day (world level of absolute poverty), compared to 11% in 2013, but that is down from nearly 36% in 1990. Nearly 1.1 billion fewer people were living in absolute poverty, down from 1.85 billion in 1990. Two regions, East Asia and the Pacific (47 million extreme poor) and Europe and Central Asia (7 million) have reduced extreme poverty to below 3%, achieving the 2030 United Nations development target.[6] In China, the most populous and formerly one of the poorest nations on Earth, policies that promoted more liberal economic development have resulted in almost 1 billion people being lifted out of absolute poverty over the last 50 years. The Chinese government just announced the elimination of absolute poverty in China, including rural remote regions.[36] However, more than half of the extreme poor live in Sub-Saharan Africa. The number of extreme poor in the region increased by 9 million, with 413 million people living on less than US$1.90 a day in 2015, more than all the other regions combined. If the trend continues, by 2030, nearly 9 out of 10 extreme poor will be in Sub-Saharan Africa.[6] A combination of economic and business development, governmental social safety net programs, international aid programs, and nonprofit nongovernmental assistance organizations have been successful in these poverty-reduction efforts.

An overwhelming majority of people with mental and psychosocial disabilities are living in poverty, poor physical health, and are subject to human rights violations. People with mental and psychosocial disabilities are a vulnerable group as a result of the way they are treated by society. They are subjected to stigma and discrimination on a daily basis, and they experience extremely high rates of physical and sexual victimization. Frequently, people with mental disabilities encounter restrictions in the exercise of their political and civil rights, and in their ability to participate in public affairs. They also are restricted in their ability to access essential health and social care, including emergency relief services. Most people with mental disabilities face disproportionate barriers in attending school and finding employment. As a result of all these factors, people with mental disability are much more likely to experience disability and to die prematurely, compared with the general population.[8]

Vulnerable groups often targeted by development groups also have high rates of mental disabilities. For instance, up to two-thirds of people with HIV/AIDS have depression, while rates of mental disability among the homeless can be greater than 50%, but their mental health needs are commonly not addressed. People with mental disabilities are not only missed by development programs, but can be actively excluded from these programs. This is in spite of the fact that an explicit goal of development is to reach the most vulnerable.[8]

However, it is important to note that there has been a growing trend toward income inequality and concentration of wealth in fewer hands in the United States and other developed and developing nations, which has slowed and even regressed the progress that had been made in addressing these challenges. Cultural values and beliefs around individualism, glorification of wealth, and mistrust in government as a social agency have contributed to these trends. The COVID-19 pandemic has aggravated this more recent trend, with those well off being able to often work from home, while pooper front-line workers risk either infection and illness (or death) or unemployment.[6]

There are also added challenges that the world is facing that are unique and global in nature. The growing threat of climate change and its impact on economic activity, agriculture, and even housing along coasts and flood-prone regions are presenting new threats to the well-being of humans and threatening to lead to the serious impoverishment of large areas of the globe.[37] Additionally, a growing lack of international cooperation in an increasingly polarized world threatens to undermine international efforts in growing economic activity and trade, addressing climate change, and lending assistance to nations and regions in need.

Conclusions

Technological advances in agriculture and in global productivity have particularly contributed to feeding and housing larger numbers of humans worldwide than was ever thought possible. Cooperation in the late 20th century among governments through international agencies such as the United Nations/UNICEF, the World Health Organization, and the World Bank, in collaboration with nongovernmental organizations, has contributed to large-scale efforts to ameliorate hunger and poverty in many low- and middle-income countries and nations affected by adverse conditions such as war and famine. Though there continues to be a strong tradition of charitable nongovernmental organizations (lay and religious) that seek to address these challenges within and across national boundaries, government action in concert with the business sector in addressing economic development so far has been the most effective vector of change to ameliorate these conditions.[6] Nonprofit organizations that serve the needs of the world's poor currently use social marketing strategies and techniques to create greater awareness of poverty conditions and increase giving by more affluent citizens and organizations. Advocacy groups, such as the Red Cross, Save the Children, and Catholic Charities, tend to focus their attention on the "innocent victims" within poor communities, especially children.[3]

National efforts are also critical in achieving the amelioration and eradication of poverty, hunger, and homelessness. For example, in the United States, food insecurity and hunger can be prevented through effective programs such as Supplemental Nutrition Aid for Persons (SNAP), Women Infant and Children (WIC) benefits, the National School Lunch Program, and the Summer Food Service Program, all of which focus on children and families and have been especially critical during the COVID-19 pandemic.[38] In developing nations, the United Nations is addressing youth poverty and hunger through programs that support rural and urban youth in entering farming and promote collaboration between rural and urban youth.[39]

Multiple studies have demonstrated success in reducing the homeless population, as well as the harmful financial and societal effects of homelessness, by providing these individuals with a combination of housing (without preconditions) and supportive care. Programs that provide long-term (a year or longer) stable housing for people with mental illnesses can help to improve mental health outcomes, including reducing the number of visits to inpatient psychiatric hospitals. Multiple studies have demonstrated success in reducing the burden of mental illness with innovative treatment models and care delivery to the poor and homeless. There is widespread agreement that services to the homeless severely mentally ill population must be comprehensive and coordinated and provide for clients' mental health, housing, and support needs. Anecdotal evidence suggests that an individual's compassionate attitude toward this intractable problem can go a long way in rebuilding lives.[34]

The world should renew its commitment to achieving to the UN's Sustainable Development Goals which include, at number one, "no poverty", with "zero hunger" at number two by 2030. Many nations have already reached those goals or have made major strides, even in the face of global challenges. International collaboration, as well as national commitment and dedication, will be needed to reach them. Ultimately, political will is what is needed to meet these commitments; poverty can be reduced drastically if governments— through taxes, etc.—work to reduce inequity, support public free schooling, and in many areas of the world support strong family planning so millions of children are not born to teenage mothers or families who cannot afford to feed them.

In conclusion, an entire generation of children faces truly unacceptable risks that jeopardize their future potential. In the long run, the monetary costs of neglecting children's needs are likely to substantially exceed the costs of combating poverty and homelessness. The human costs will be much more tragic. Our nations must develop an appropriate and effective response.

References

1. United Nations Children's Fund (UNICEF), World Health Organization (WHO), and the World Bank. *Levels and Trends in Child Malnutrition: Key Findings of the 2019 Edition of the Joint Child Malnutrition Estimates.* Geneva: World Health Organization; 2019. License: CC BY-NC-SA 3.0 IGO.
2. Bishaw A. *Poverty: 2010 and 2011.* American Community Survey Briefs. September 2012. https://www2.census.gov/library/publications/2012/acs/acsbr11-01.pdf. Last accessed January 3, 2021.
3. UNICEF. *Impact of COVID-19 on children living in poverty.* December, 2021. https://data.unicef.org/resources/impact-of-covid-19-on-children-living-in-poverty/. Last accessed November 13, 2022.
4. Full Fact. *Poverty in the UK: A Guide to the Facts and Figures.* September 27, 2019. htpps://fullfact.org/economy/poverty-uk-guide-facts-and-figures/. Last accessed January 3, 2021.
5. American Psychological Association. *Effects of Poverty, Hunger, and Homelessness on Children and Youth.* 2016. Retrieved from http://www.apa.org/pi/families/poverty.aspx; Accessed November 29, 2020.
6. World Bank, International Bank for Reconstruction and Development. *Reversals of Fortune: Poverty and Shared Prosperity.* Geneva: World Bank; 2020.
7. Organisation for Economic Co-operation and Development (OECD), World Health Organization (WHO). *Poverty and Health.* DAC Guidelines and Reference Series. World Health Association, Parism, France, 2003. IBSN 92 4 156236 6. Accessed through https://www.google.com/books/edition/_/ykriGmCkWOkC?hl=en&gbpv=1&pg=PP1, Last accessed November 13, 2022.
8. World Health Organization (WHO). *Breaking the Vicious Cycle Between Mental Ill-Health and Poverty.* Geneva: World Health Organization; 2007. Mental Health Core Information Sheet, Sheet 1. http://www.who.int/mental_health/policy/development/en/intex.html. Last accessed January 3, 2021.
9. Kuruvilla A, Jacob KS. Poverty, social stress & mental health. *Indian J Med Res.* 2007 Oct;126(4):273–278.
10. Kishiyama M, Boyce T, Jimenez A, Perry L, Knight R. Socioeconomic disparities affect prefrontal function in children. *J Cogn Neurosci.* 2009;21(6):1106–1115.
11. Luby L, Belden A, Botteron K, et al. The effects of poverty on childhood brain development: the mediating effect of caregiving and stressful life events, *JAMA Pediatr.* 2013; 167(12):1135–1142.
12. Hair N, Hanson J, Wolfe B, Pollak, S. Association of child poverty, brain development, and academic achievement. *JAMA Pediatr.* 2015;169(9):822–829.
13. Fernald A, Marchman V, Weisleder A. SES differences in language processing skill and vocabulary are evident at 18 months. *Dev Sci.* 2013;16(2):234–248.
14. Evans G. Childhood poverty and adult psychological well-being. *PNAS.* 2016;113(52):14949–14952.
15. Hastings P, Serbin L, Bukowski W, et al. Predicting psychosis-spectrum diagnoses in adulthood from social behaviors and neighborhood contexts in childhood. *Dev Psychopath.* 2020;32(2):465–479.
16. United Nations Food and Agriculture Organization (FAO), International Fund for Agricultural Development (IFAD), UNICEF, World Food Program, and World Health Organization (WHO). *The State of Food Security and Nutrition in the World 2017: Building Resilience for Peace and Food Security.* Rome: FAO; 2017. www.fao.org/3/a-I7695e.pdf. Last accessed January 3, 2021.
17. Keys A, Brozek J, Henschel A, Taylor H. *The Biology of Human Starvation.* Vol. I and II. Minneapolis, MN: University of Minnesota Press and Oxford Press; 1950.
18. Nyaradi A, Li J, Hickling S, Foster J, Oddy W. The role of nutrition in children's neurocognitive development, from pregnancy through childhood. *Front Human Neurosci.* 2013;7(97):1–16.
19. Kleinman R, Murphy M, Little M, et al. Hunger in children in the United States: potential behavioral and emotional correlates. *Pediatrics.* 1998;101(1):e3.
20. Weinreb L, Wehler C, Perloff J, et al. Hunger: its impact on children's health and mental health. *Pediatrics.* 2002;110(4):e41.
21. U.N. Department of Economic and Social Affairs. Expert Group Meeting, Affordable Housing and Social Protection Systems for All to Address Homelessness. Nairobi, Kenya, May 22–24, 2019. https://www.un.org/development/desa/dspd/2019-meetings/homelessness.html. Last accessed November 13, 2022.

22. United States Interagency Council on Homelessness. *Opening Doors: Federal Strategic Plan to Prevent and End Homelessness, as Amended in 2015.* 2015. https://www.usich.gov/resources/uploads/asset_library/USICH_OpeningDoors_Amendment2015_FINAL.pdf. Last accessed February 6, 2021.

23. National Alliance to End Homelessness. *State of Homelessness: 2020 Edition.* https://endhomelessness.org/homelessness-in-america/homelessness-statistics/state-of-homelessness-2020/. Last accessed January 3, 2021.

24. U.S. Conference of Mayors. *Status Report on Hunger and Homelessness: A Status Report on Hunger and Homelessness in America's Cities: A 25-City Survey.* December 2008. www.ncdsv.org/images/USCM_Hunger-homelessness-Survey-in-America's-Cities_12%202008.pdf. Last accessed January 3, 2021.

25. Child Trends. *Children and Youth Experiencing Homelessness.* 2019. Retrieved from https://www.childtrends.org/indicators/homeless-children-and-youth. Last accessed January 3, 2021.

26. Rafferty Y, Shinn M. The impact of homelessness on children. *Am Psychologist.* 1991; 46(11):1170–1179.

27. Farmer B. A wave of evictions is on the horizon: what impact could they have on kid's education? *CBS 60 Minutes Overtime.* November 22, 2020. https://www.cbsnews.com/news/eviction-moratorium-covid-19-schools-60-minutes-2020-11-22/. Accessed November 29, 2020.

28. Goodman L, Saxe L, Harvey M. Homelessness as psychological trauma, broadening perspectives. *Am Psychologist.* 1991;46(11):1219–1225.

29. Toro PA, Bellavia CW, Daeschler CV, et al. Distinguishing homelessness from poverty: a comparative study. *J Consult Clin Psychol.* 1995;63(2):280–289.

30. Zima B, Wells K, Benjamin B, Duan, N. Mental health problems among homeless mothers: relationship to service use and child mental health problems. *Arch Gen Psychiat.* 1996;53(4):332–338.

31. Embleton L, Lee H, Gunn J, Ayuku D, Braitstein P. Causes of child and youth homelessness in developed and developing countries: a systematic review and meta-analysis *JAMA Pediatr.* 2016;170(5):435–444.

32. Moore J. *Unaccompanied and Homeless Youth Review of Literature (1995–2005).* National Center for Homeless Education, 2005. https:// files.eric.ed.gov/fulltext/ED489998.pdf. Last accessed January 3, 2021.

33. Kamieniecki G. Prevalence of psychological distress and psychiatric disorders among homeless youth in Australia: a comparative review. *Aust N Z J Psychiatry.* 2001 Jun;35(3):352–358.

34. Substance Abuse and Mental Health Services Administration (SAMHSA). *Behavioral Health Services for People Who Are Homeless. Treatment Improvement Protocol (TIP) Series 55.* HHS Publication No. (SMA) 13-4734. Rockville, MD: Substance Abuse and Mental Health Services Administration; 2013. Last accessed January 3, 2021.

35. Folsom D, Jeste D. Schizophrenia in homeless persons: a systematic review of the literature. *Acta Psychiatr Scand.* 2002 Jun;105(6):404–413.

36. China Global Television Network (CGTN). Zero poverty: China eliminates absolute poverty one month before self-imposed deadline. 2020. https://news.cgtn.com/news/2020-11-23/China-eliminates-absolute-poverty-one-month-before-schedule-VEp8VAJJS0/index.html. Last accessed November 13, 2022.

37. Organisation for Economic Co-operation and Development (OECD). *Poverty and Climate Change: Reducing the Vulnerability of the Poor through Adaptation.* Geneva: OECD; 2003.

38. Dunn C, Kenney E, Fleischhacker S, Bleich S. Feeding low-income children during the Covid-19 pandemic. *N Engl J Med.* 2020;382(18):e40(1)–e40(3).

39. United Nations Department of Economic and Social Affairs: Youth. Hunger and poverty WPAY (World Programme of Action for Youth). 2020. https://www.un.org/development/desa/youth/hunger-and-poverty-wpay.html. Last accessed February 6, 2021.

Clinical Perspectives

On clinical perspectives focuses onsocial aspects of Nero biology, neuroscience, Brain and Biology and clinical syndromes of Neurodevelopmental Disorders, Depressive and Anxiety Disorders, Trauma and Trauma Disorders, Psychotic Disorders Substance Use Disorders, Neurocognitive Disorders and disorders. Also presents on social psychiatric aspects of Medical Illness, Child Maltreatment and incarceration.

22

Social Psychiatry

Brain and Biology

Basant Pradhan

An important part of social intelligence is the ability to predict someone else's response and use that prediction to successfully navigate the social exchange.
—Humphrey, Bateson, and Hinde, 1976:303–317[1]

Like the Mind and the Brain, Social Psychiatry and the Social Brain Are Linked Inseparably

It will not be an exaggeration to say that humans are party animals: social interactions are an essential aspect of being human. In fact, humans spend on average 80% of their waking time in the company of others, and 80%–90% of our conversations are spent talking about ourselves and gossiping about other people.[2] Compared to the brains of other animals, human brains have something different that allows us to be so social. Comparative studies reveal that the brain size of the great ape species (such as bonobos/pygmy chimpanzees), our closest in the evolutionary ladder, is only 25%–35% of that of the modern human, although the body sizes are comparable. Part of this can be explained by selection pressures exerted by evolution in this regard. The particular evolutionary selection pressures that the human species faced while adapting to myriad social interactions, ranging from cooperation, deception, and the countless ways of obtaining food and ensuring offspring, etc., explain partly this extraordinary size and complexity of the human brain compared to closely related species.[3,4,5] The parts of the brain especially responsible for these social interactions are called the *social brain*. The various social processes, social cognition, social behavior, and the myriad social functions are governed by the social brain.

Social Brain

The *social brain* refers to those brain structures that subserve the various social processes and social phenomena such as social cognition, social behavior, and social functioning. The National Institute of Mental Health (NIMH) group defined social cognition as *the mental operations that underlie social interactions, including perceiving, interpreting, and generating responses to the intentions, dispositions, and behaviors of others.*[6(pp1211–1220)]

Interestingly, and as elaborated later, these phenomena are governed by the social brain often in relatively domain-specific ways. For example, regions in the temporal lobe such as the fusiform facial area (FFA) are implicated in processing faces, whereas the temporoparietal junction and medial prefrontal cortex (mPFC) are implicated in representing other people's beliefs, and so forth.[7,8,9] In her seminal review, Brothers[10] proposed that there was a circumscribed set of brain regions that were dedicated to social cognition, which she called the *social brain*. She proposed the amygdala, orbital frontal cortex, and temporal cortex as its major components. Later work by others has expanded this list of social brain regions and has included the mPFC and the adjacent paracingulate cortex[11] and the *mirror neuron system*. The latter is an intricate neuronal network involved in *mentalization* (otherwise known as the *theory of mind*, ToM): our unique ability to infer the mental state of others from their observed behavior.[12] These areas have also been consistently implicated in studies involving *empathy*, our unique ability to understand and internally share the experiences/feeling states of another person. Mentalization and empathy are quintessential for our social functioning and are considered to be higher order abilities unique to human beings, although some other primates show precursors to this ability.[13] Thus, *the social brain forms the organ of our social interactions, the organ that makes meaning of our social environment, the organ that interprets the social signals and responds to them*. It is the social brain that allows us to interact with other people. Broadly encompassed in *social cognitive neuroscience* (SCN), a fascinating and emerging field, the social brain attempts to understand and explain how the brain function supports the cognitive processes underlying social behavior. Social brain is *the biological substrate of our social behavior*, and one of its main functions is to enable us to make predictions during social interactions. No wonder that, as a field of study, it has strong relevance and connections to *social psychiatry*.

Social Psychiatry in the Context of Social Cognitive Neuroscience (SCN)

Social psychiatry was the dominant form of psychiatry in the 20th century, and with new insights coming from quite diverse disciplines, it is now being integrated into an ever-growing discipline, social cognitive neuroscience (SCN). SCN, which contains within it the concept of social brain and social psychiatry, has resulted due to the recent marriage between social psychology, neurobiology, and cognitive neuroscience and also the comparative studies mentioned before. It differs from cognitive neuroscience in that, unlike the former, its emphasis is on social situations, social contexts, and social processes, all of which determine how we act or think.[14] SCN refers to domains such as social cognition, social perception, and social information processing. As an integrative discipline, *social psychiatry* focuses on the interpersonal and cultural context of mental disorders and mental well-being. This important branch of psychiatry has been particularly associated with the development of therapeutic communities. In its therapeutic, preventive, as well as advocacy domains, social psychiatry attempts to study, teach, and promote consciousness of how social factors contribute to the maintenance of psychological well-being, and establishes the understanding that social factors are often core to many behavioral health issues. Social psychiatry involves a disparate set of theories and approaches, fuses core psychiatry with important public health perspectives, and thus bridges across many disciplines such as social anthropology, social psychology, cultural psychiatry, sociology, socioeconomic factors, seminal life events, and the community aspects of mental health and illnesses. Social psychiatry can be contrasted with biological psychiatry, with the latter focused on genetics, neurochemistry, neurocircuitry etc., and psychotropic medications. SCN, including the social brain and the related biology, can be conceptualized as the biological aspects of social psychiatry.[15] As a growing field, social cognitive neuroscience concerns itself with understanding the neural representation of self and others, and also social signals and social knowledge, including social rules and procedures. The social brain implements social cognition, which in turn causes social behavior, which in turn constitutes social functioning when integrated over time and context. Social cognition refers to the various psychological processes (both conscious and non-conscious) that underlie the social behavior. Social cognition includes any cognitive processing, perception, reasoning, memory, attention, motivation, and decision-making that underlie social behavior. Social behavior, the anchor for all these different levels of explanations, comprises the readily observable interactions between an individual and other people. Social functioning is broader than social behavior and refers to the long-term, contextualized ability of an individual to interact with others (e.g., a person's behavior within a community over the past months). The relationships between these different levels (social functioning, social behavior, social cognition, social brain) are systemic rather than unidirectional. With the accumulating evidence on the social brain, one can no longer think of the brain in isolation; rather, it is conceptualized in terms of interacting domains and networks. Rooted in the broader concept of SCN, social psychiatry is closely linked with the various social phenomena and related processes, which in turn are influenced by the social brain and group mind. The myriads of social processes and social phenomena serve as the operational domains for both the social brain and social psychiatry.

Biology of the Social Brain: The Neuronal Hubs, Neuronal Networks and Neurochemicals

One's notion of self and others are very important dimensions that contribute to the creation and maintenance of one's social world. The notion of self, in turn, is governed by one's *self-perception*, *self-feelings*, and *self-memories*. In general, the brain areas that are more involved in *self-perception* are the prefrontal cortex (PFC: both the dorso-lateral as well as medial and ventromedial parts), the posterior cingulate cortex (PCC), and also the medial as well as lateral parts of the parietal cortex. The *self-feelings* are orchestrated by the orbitofrontal cortex (OFC), the anterior cingulate cortex (ACC), insula (right), the auto-nomic nervous system, the hypothalamo-pituitary adrenal (HPA) axis, and the endocrine systems, whereas in the creation of *self-memories*, the medial temporal lobe plays a crucial role. To understand the biology of our sociality, it is important to know more about the major neuronal hubs, the neuronal networks, and the neurochemicals that orchestrate the various aspects of the social brain.

The Neuronal Hubs

It is important to note that there is no well-delineated brain area specifically devoted to the social brain. The major neuronal hubs implicated in our social and cognitive-emotive func-tioning are the following:[16,17]

   (i)   the medial prefrontal cortex (MPFC);
   (ii) the anterior cingulate cortex (ACC);
   (iii) the lateral prefrontal cortex (LPFC);
   (iv) the insular cortex (mostly the right insula); and
   (v)   the amygdala.

The LPFC is the *assessment center* of the brain because it decreases the brain's tendency to take things personally and overrides the automatic behaviors/habits/biases/prejudice, etc. Thus, the LPFC allows us to look at things from a more rational and balanced perspec-tive. The MPFC is rightly called the *Me center*, or the *self-referencing center* of the brain. It is the storehouse of autobiographical memories and is deeply involved in building one's sense of self and also plays an important role in self-reflection and empathy, some of the core attributes essential for one's sociality. The MPFC engages us in social interactions and helps in inferring other people's state of mind (*theory of mind* or *mentalizing ability*). The MPFC has two parts: the ventromedial part (VMPFC) and the dorsomedial part (DMPFC). The former is involved in processing information related to us and others that we view as *similar* to us, whereas the latter is involved in processing information related to people we perceive as being *dissimilar* from us. From a social brain and social functioning perspec-tive, the former can be conceptualized as the "unhelpful part" of the MPFC because it is often activated when we take things too personally, and thus can contribute to creation of strong reactions, emotional alienation, prejudice, and so forth, in us. On the other hand, the DMPFC, which is involved in feeling empathy, especially for people whom we perceive as not being like us, and which also helps in maintaining social connections, can be con-sidered the "helpful part'"of the MPFC. In our day-to-day social life, the LPFC (*the assess-ment center*) acts like a *brake* for the unhelpful parts of the MPFC (i.e., *the Me center*).

The insula is the part of the brain that is involved in experiencing "gut-level" feelings by monitoring one's bodily sensations and also helping guide how strongly we will respond to what we sense in our bodies (i.e., are these sensations dangerous or benign?). Insula, especially the right one, is also heavily involved in experiencing empathy. Amygdala is the alarm system (otherwise called the *fear center*) of the brain. It works closely with cingulate cortex and the autonomic system to coordinate the emotional orchestra in the brain. It is responsible for many of our initial emotional responses and reactions, including the "fright-fight-or-flight" response, seen more in anxiety disorder including post-traumatic stress disorder (PTSD), social anxiety disorder, etc.

The four major/core functional neural networks implicated in our social and cognitive-emotive functioning are as follows:[18–20]

(i) the default mode network (DMN) that focuses on our internal world (self and others);
(ii) the salience network (SN) that integrates the internal and external stimuli, and from a constant stream of incoming sensory inputs, dynamically selects only specific stimuli for additional processing;
(iii) the central executive network (CEN), which is primarily an externally focused network and manages our action perceptions and action-execution; and
(iv) the reward circuit network, which works closely with the CEN and plays a crucial role in maintaining the motivation, appetitive, and sexual functions, as well as social functioning.

The CEN brain areas are primarily centered dorsally (above), i.e., in the DLPFC, whereas the *risk–reward evaluation circuits* are located ventrally (below), i.e., in OFC and the ACC. Additionally, the *risk–reward evaluation circuits* include hubs within the amygdala (fear detector) and nucleus accumbens (reward center). The ACC is strategically connected, sandwiched between the DLPFC (associated with attention and executive functions) and the OFC (the area that elicits risk evaluation and impulse control). Because of its role in reward and motivation, ACC–nucleus accumbens circuitry plays a significant role in the social reward system, in addition to addiction-related rewards. These reward circuits work closely with the prefrontal CEN and the autonomic nervous system, thus allowing the thinking, feeling, and somatic functions, as well as planning dimensions of the risk–reward situation, to operate flexibly and appropriately as per the needs of the situations demanded by one's environments, both internal and external. The salience network (SN) brain areas are the anterior insula (AI), dorsal ACC (dACC), and three key subcortical structures: the amygdala, the ventral tegmental area (VTA, which is involved in the reward pathway), and the substantia nigra (the major source of mid-brain dopamine involved in cognitive/executive and reward functions). The major functional areas in the DMN are the posterior cingulate cortex (PCC), the posterior parietal cortex (PPC), the precuneus which is an important part of the PPC and is involved in memory recollection and retrieval, the mPFC, and the angular gyrus.[21]

Typically, in healthy individuals, the SN and CEN increase in activation during cognitive tasks requiring attention to external stimuli,[22] whereas DMN activity is suppressed.[18,23] The SN is thought to be responsible for detecting and filtering information necessary to maintain goal-directed behavior by shifting attention between external and internal processes.[20,24] Mechanistically, SN serves as an on-off switch between the CEN and DMN.[20,24] These patterns are observable during cognitive tasks as well as the resting state.[25] Although interactions among all these core neurocognitive networks are relevant for efficient cognition, *functional coupling between the SN and the DMN in particular is critically important* for performing tasks requiring cognitive control, or switching attention between externally and internally salient stimuli,[19,25,26] and is necessary for successful cognition across domains.[27]

As mentioned before, the DMN is more involved with our internal world and is generally active when the individual is not focused on the outside world. It is involved in generation and sustenance of internal trains of thoughts (internally driven cognitions) unrelated to the external reality. Day-dreaming is an example of the work of the DMN, and in this state, the brain is at wakeful rest. Smallwood et al.[28] propose that these internally driven cognitions are produced as a result of cooperation between the default mode network and a frontoparietal control network (the top-down control system). The engagement of the internally guided trains of thoughts depends mainly upon the internal-perception-guided cognitions (imagery) and less upon the external physical referents for these cognitions. Because access to the top-down attentional control system (from cerebral cortex downward) is generally a prerequisite for our conscious experiences, during periods of internally guided thoughts, the frontoparietal top-down attentional control system and the default mode system often operate simultaneously. The default mode network provides the autobiographical information of the individual that acts like a scaffold for the frontoparietal network to further sustain the internal trains of thought and buffer them from the disturbances of the external world. In the process, the attention generated by the frontoparietal network suppresses the irrelevant external (perceptual) information. Though the DMN was originally noticed to be deactivated in certain goal-oriented tasks, it can be active in other goal-oriented tasks, such as social working memory or autobiographical tasks (elaborated below).[29]

The Salience Network Deserves Special Mention

The SN functions as a key brain network for integrating cognition, action, and feelings by helping with the switching between the lateral frontoparietal central-executive network and the medial frontoparietal default-mode network to keep attention focused on task-relevant goals. The SN, with its saliency detection mechanisms, contributes to a variety of complex brain functions, including communication, social behavior, and self-awareness through the integration of sensory, emotional, and cognitive information.[19,30] The close connection between the SN and attention is clearly evident in classic definition of *attention* more than a century ago by James:[31(pp403-404)] attention is "the taking possession by the mind, in clear and vivid form, of one out of what seem several simultaneously possible objects or trains of thought." Being situated at the interface of the cognitive, homeostatic, motivational, and affective systems of the human brain, and by identifying the most biologically and cognitively relevant endogenous and external stimuli in order to adaptively guide behavior, it critically contributes to a highly coordinated integration of sensory, emotional, and cognitive information in the brain.[19,20,25] In SN, the functional coupling of the AI (the dynamic hub of SN) with the dACC facilitates rapid access to the motor system.

Functional neuroimaging research points to the role of the insula and cingulate gyrus in the development of the (*visceral*) representations of our experiences. The insula plays a crucial role in processing the information that integrates interoception (the ability to perceive and respond to stimuli from one's own body/organs, such as feeling one's stomach rumbling, timing one's own heartbeat) with emotional salience. This integration generates a subjective representation of the body and bodily self-awareness, like one's sense of body ownership.[32] In addition to the insula and the cingulate gyrus, the OFC and the amygdala assist in determining the salience of objects within our awareness by rating their emotional significance. The amygdala projects to the same sites in the OFC that receive direct sensory input, thus allowing the OFC to extract the emotional significance of sensory events.[33] Both the amygdala and the OFC ignore the neutral sensory inputs, those which bear no implications of risk or reward, and function to cease response to any input lacking motivational value.[33] Thus, motivation plays a critical role in building our social experiences: adequate motivation in the suitable context can reinforce our social experiences via activity of the facilitative pathways, which not only can reinforce social learning, but also can assist in maintaining our social representations within the brain, allowing one to *own* these experiences, thus contributing to our *social self*. A unifying framework presenting large-scale network connectivity of the brain allows a systematic examination of brain functions as well as dysfunctions, including those of the social brain.[34] These large-scale networks are disrupted across many neuropsychiatric disorders, including the disorders involving the social brain, such as the autism spectrum disorders.[24]

Neurochemicals Involved in Sociality

Within the context of motivation, incentive salience, and the facilitated neural transmission of information, including social information, Berridge and Robinson[35] propose an *incentive salience hypothesis* and elaborate on the role of dopamine, *the pleasure chemical*, in the reward and salience system.[35-38] In addition, primate sociality involves the neuroendocrine system (mostly endorphin system and probably oxytocin as well), which provides a psychopharmacological platform off which the social-cognitive and social-behavioral components are then built. Of note, endorphins play a central role in creating and servicing the social relationships.[39] The endorphin activation is triggered by social grooming: the more frequently this is activated, the stronger and more enduring the relationship becomes. In contrast, the oxytocin system, although helping with socialization (especially on affiliation), appears to be insensitive to relationship quality or quantity. Also, the oxytocin response habituates very quickly and in social interactions it does not allow individuals to influence the responses of the other individuals with whom they interact.

The Social Brain and Social Psychiatry in the Context of the Higher Order Human Functions Such as Mentalization and Empathy

As mentioned before, two crucial functions of the social brain are *mentalization* (also known as *theory of mind*[13]) and empathy.[40] Mentalization is our ability to infer the thoughts or mental states of others based on their observable behavior, whereas empathy is the shared emotional experience when one tries to put oneself in another's shoes. These two unique and higher order abilities are quintessential for our social functioning. Mentalization involves the whole cognitive-affective construct, including empathy, anticipation, prediction, some executive functions, etc., whereas empathy pertains to only the (shared) affective portion of this whole construct. Empathy can be conceptualized as affective mentalization. Empathy is a *spontaneous emotive* simulation experience, whereas mentalization (otherwise called the *theory of mind*) is a *deliberate cognitive* ability. Empathy involves brain regions such as the premotor cortex and the insula (especially the right insula), whereas mentalization also involves regions such as the mPFC and the temporoparietal junction as well.[41]

To be able to infer the thoughts or mental states of others (i.e., to mentalize), one must translate what is observable (i.e., the behavior of the other person) into an inference about what is unobservable (i.e., the other person's psychological state). The mentalization system has three components which are consistently activated during both implicit and explicit mentalizing tasks, and these components form an important part of the social brain.[42] These three components are:

(i) the medial prefrontal cortex (MPFC): this brain area distinguishes the mental state representations from the physical state representations,

(ii) the posterior superior temporal sulcus (STS): this area lies between the superior and middle temporal gyrus. The STS is probably the basis of our social perceptions and also detection of the social agency (i.e., it helps to distinguish between the human voice vs. environmental sounds, stories vs. nonsensical speech, moving faces vs. moving objects, etc.). Thus, the perception of *biological motion* (as opposed to *inanimate motion*) and the attribution of intention and other mental states share a common neural basis via the neural activities in the STS.

(iii) the temporal poles: these might be involved in accessing the social knowledge in the form of the *social scripts* stored in the various areas of the brain.

The three areas mentioned above are also the locations rich in *mirror neurons*, the mind-reading neurons which serve as the biological basis of empathy.[12] Mirror neurons are also abundant in the *inferior parietal lobule*—a structure that underwent an accelerated expansion in the great apes and, later, in humans. As the brain evolved further, this lobule split into two gyri—the anterior one is the supra-marginal gyrus, which allows us to "reflect" on our own anticipated actions, whereas the posterior one is the angular gyrus that allows us to "reflect" on our body (function of the right angular gyrus) and perhaps on other more social and linguistic aspects of ourselves (function of the left angular gyrus). In the context of face and emotion recognition, the important role of the fusiform gyrus needs special mention. Otherwise called the lateral occipitotemporal (LOT) gyrus, this fusiform face area (FFA) is located in the inferior aspects of both occipital and temporal lobes. Impairment of the *right* FFA causes prosopagnosia, or facial blindness (inability to recognize faces). This important area has been implicated in autism spectrum disorders, a known pathological condition involving impaired sociality.

Of note, the face- and object-processing areas in the brain are necessary for developing social cognition, and these two aspects can develop independently of one another (i.e., the ability to process objects is not a prerequisite to process faces, and vice versa).

Developmentally, the mentalizing system of the brain is probably in operation implicitly from around 18 months of age, whereas between the ages of 4 and 6 years, the explicit mentalizing becomes possible,[43] thus allowing the *implicit and explicit* attribution of intentions and mental states of others, respectively. As an important part of the social brain, the *mentalization* network mentioned above governs the various aspects of our social functioning and related processes. These core functions become altered in pathological conditions such as autism spectrum disorders and severe psychopathological states such as antisocial- and schizoid personality disorders.

The Social Brain and Social Psychiatry in the Context of Understanding the Self and Others

From the viewpoint of an information-processing model, the neurobiological processes that contribute to social cognition and social information processing are often grouped into two broad categories: those related to *automatic processing*, driven more by the stimuli; and those related to *controlled processing*, driven more by the person's goals and intentions. Thus, the automatic processing is a *bottom-up* process, whereas the controlled processing is a *top-down* process. The neural science of understanding the self, otherwise called *self-referential processing*, is a crucial functional domain of the social brain. The three main sub-domains inside the self-referential processing are: *self-perception, self-feelings, and self-memories*.[15] Self-perception is a unique social cognitive process because *self is simultaneously the perceiver and the perceived*. Also, our sense of self relies partly on seeing the differences between our self-knowledge, other's feedback about us, and the knowledge we have about other people's characteristics, thoughts, and desires. These notions about *perception of self* (self-image), *perception of others* (worldview), and *our perception about how others are perceiving us* constitute the three major constituents of our personality. All of these elements are governed by the social brain.

The Dynamic Relationship Between the DMN and the SN in the Context of Social Memories and the Social Self

In the DMN, the PCC and precuneus combines the sensory-driven bottom-up (not controlled) attention with information from the memory and perception. The dorsal (upper) part of the PCC involves involuntary awareness and arousal, whereas its ventral part becomes activated in all tasks related to thinking about self (self-referential thinking), thinking related to others, remembering the past, and thinking about future (part of autobiographical memory), etc. The mPFC is involved in decisions about self-processing, such as personal information, autobiographical memories, future goals and events, and decision-making regarding those people who are personally very close, such as family. In the work of the DMN, the angular gyrus connects perception, attention, spatial cognition, and action, and helps with parts of recall of episodic memories, whereas the precuneus is involved in visual, sensorimotor, and attentional information.[21] During activation of the DMN, the attentional networks of the brain are temporarily uncoupled from the external sensory/

perceptual inputs (perceptual decoupling). It is important to note that such decoupling oc-curs temporarily. However, the internally and externally driven streams may compete, and attention can be rapidly recoupled to perceptual events *if the SN becomes activated due to salient external events.*

The DMN is known to be involved in many seemingly different functions, such as information regarding the self (*autobiographical information, self-referential thinking,* and reflecting about one's own emotional state), *Theory of mind* (inferring other's mental states by thinking about them and observing their behavior), *moral reasoning* (determining just and unjust results of an action), *social evaluations* (good–bad judgments about social con-cepts), etc. Many of these functions are closely related to our social cognition and social functioning. Thus, it will not be an exaggeration say that the DMN is a very important net-work that critically *contributes to the neurological basis for the self,* including the *social self/ social identity.*

Is Social Information Processing Different from Non-Social Information Processing?

Although many of the same brain structures involved in the general perception, cogni-tion, and behavior are also involved in processing social perception and social cognition as well, it is increasingly being recognized that social information processing is different from non-social information processing in many respects. This has provided support for some schemes that claim that *social cognition and social information processing are modular.*[41] What then is it that distinguishes human social cognition from that of other species? Three prominent differences are:

(i) the ability to shift one's conscious experience to places and times outside the here-and-now, and into the viewpoint of another mind (i.e., mentalization);[44,45]

(ii) the association of our evaluation of others with strong *moral emotions* that motivate particular aspects of social behavior, such as altruistic punishment;[46] and

(iii) the capacity to use these abilities flexibly as a function of the context, across consider-able time intervals, and with the help of a prodigious episodic memory that helps us to keep track of a large number of other individuals and their past behavior.[47] When the demands on social cognition become severe, these three abilities taken together may define much of the nature of human conscious experience and indeed provide an argument for its emergence.

Towards a Universal Self: Social Psychiatry and the Social Brain in the Context of Globalization

Globalization refers to the process of the integration and intensification of economic, polit-ical, social, and cultural relations across international boundaries.[48] It is principally aimed at the universal homogenization of ideas, cultures, values, and even lifestyles.[49] Globalization opens people's lives to other cultures, their creativity and the flow of ideas and values. In the past, globalization has often been seen as a more or less economic process. However, today it is increasingly perceived as a more comprehensive phenomenon that includes three major categories: economic, political, and social. These three are interdependent: the economic and political forces are usually the driving factors of globalization, whereas the social changes generally occur as effects of the former two. Social globalization pertains to human interaction within cultural communities, encompassing topics such as family, religion, work, and education. Social globalization is evident in the similarities of social trends between cultures and it is marked by the increase in association among people from separate parts of the world. Globalization can be viewed as sociocultural, sociopolitical, or socioeconomic interdependence and in that very sense is influenced by the social brain and the group mind. This interdependence is again associated with world peace and intercultural growth and assimilation and social harmony. As the world around us is becoming progressively interconnected and complex, human health is being increasingly perceived as the integrated outcome of its ecological, sociocultural, economic, and institutional determinants. Thus, globalization is incrementally affecting the institutional, economic, sociocultural, and ecological determinants of population health.[50] In addition, sociocultural globalization, involving powerful global communication methods such as social media and internet, global mobility, cross-cultural interaction, etc., deeply influences the prevailing cultural norms and values. The informal social networks are gaining tremendous importance and as a result, distance is no longer a barrier for social interactions. Like-minded people now are not only able to interact at distance through, for example, the internet, but also are able to make important life decisions in order to actualize many goals of their lives. These crucial aspects underscore the impact (actual as well as potential) of the social brain and social psychiatry on the current globalized world culture and vice versa.

Therapeutic Manipulations of the Social Brain: Some Implications

The interdependence of mental health and social life, and hence that of social psychiatry and the social brain, cannot be emphasized enough. Stable and supportive social life is crucial for healthy human development and well-being, whereas altered social functioning over time results in changes in the brain and cognition, and vice versa. Concepts of social psychiatry and the social brain provide the "language" for discussing illness with the patient. The various sociocultural contexts of human life serve as the language and media for the expression of psychiatric symptoms and related dysfunctions. These contexts do possess interactional meanings that have relational and functional repercussions that can be tapped into therapeutically so that treatment outcomes can be enhanced, both psychotherapeutically and psychopharmacologically as well. A social brain and social psychiatry focus allows clinicians to formulate the pertinent interactional/relational narratives as the etiological and interventional hypotheses which are quite rich, meaningful, holistic, and resonating, compared to just focusing on some mere "chemical imbalances" which, more often than not, is a rather vague and unduly reductionistic approach in treating mental illnesses. The quality of the doctor-patient relationship can enhance or undermine even the most effective "biological" treatments in psychiatry.[51] The sociocultural narratives and images of the illnesses and the related lived experiences provide the springboard to establish a shared understanding of the problem and the proposed therapeutics between the doctor and the patient, to trust in and commit to a treatment plan, and more importantly, facilitates the formation of a trusting therapeutic alliance and therapeutic success, which is independent of the specifics of a particular intervention. The social brain has been extensively studied in autism spectrum disorders in which social skills deficits have been identified as the core deficits.[52] Psychotherapy affects the social brain via verbal and nonverbal engagements and also alters the input from the individual or family or other social networks. The social role can lead to molecular changes and vice versa, which provides the rationale for pharmacological and psychotherapeutic treatment.

The Role of Yoga, Meditation, and Brain Stimulation in Enhancing Social Functioning

Yoga and meditation practices are ancient, relatively inexpensive, and quite rich experiences with tremendous empowerments to its practitioners. These are grounded on some of the very fundamental principles and philosophies of the human body and mind. These multidimensional interventions have effects not only on illnesses, but also upon our very existence, our perceptions, attitude, and worldviews as humans. The powerful effects of these interventions, including some of their far-reaching health benefits, are beginning to be understood in terms of their effects on *neuroplasticity*, which is now known to occur in a wide variety of neural circuits with many different simultaneous mechanisms, involving the immensely active *neurodynamic model of the human brain*, and has been a major focus of recent research. In the past two decades or so, major scientific advances have shown positive effects of yoga and meditation on physical and emotional health, including not only functional changes in brain hemodynamics or metabolism, but also permanent changes in brain structures as well. Other rather unexpected results of these practices include alterations in cellular DNA, including increase in the telomerase enzyme activity, changes in immune factors, etc.[53] Yogic and meditative traditions, many honed over millennia, can serve as a very good platform for generating new hypotheses regarding the mind-body interactions, and may also provide important ways of inducing healthier mental states that can serve as a springboard for applying psychotherapeutic methods in targeted ways.[54]

From a social psychiatry standpoint, an important aspect in this regard is the development of evidence-based interventions using the focused brain stimulation methods (e.g., repetitive transcranial magnetic stimulation, rTMS) and yoga-mindfulness methods for the maladies of the mind and brain, including the social brain. Among all the Eastern spiritual practices (e.g., yoga, meditation, qi gong, tai chi, mindfulness, etc.), there need to be culturally accepted and scientifically validated therapy models which are optimally customized and targeted for their use in disorder-specific ways. Standardized yoga and mindfulness interventions can be used alone or in combination with other interventions (both medications and psychotherapies). In our ongoing work, we find these interventions efficacious and high-yield, when used in a standardized and customized manner.[54-56] In this regard, Pradhan et al. have developed an evidence-based and biomarker-informed (serum D-serine and EEG-based markers) standardized yoga and mindfulness-based cognitive therapy approach called TIMBER (Trauma Interventions using Mindfulness-Based Extinction and Reconsolidation of trauma memories) which has shown efficacy in chronic PTSD, treatment-resistant depression, traumatic psychosis, and opioid use disorders as well.[57] Another important aspect in this regard is the development of targeted brain stimulation methods (e.g., rTMS) to therapeutically manipulate the social brain network for disorders of the social brain, e.g., autism spectrum disorders.[58] Transcranial magnetic stimulation (TMS) is beginning to be used by a number of centers worldwide and may represent a novel technique with both diagnostic and therapeutic potential.[59]

Conclusions and Future Directions

Despite some of the amazing advancements in our knowledge of social psychiatry and the social brain, many crucial and unanswered questions still remain. For example, despite all the advances in neuroimaging and cognitive neuroscience, we still know very little about the precise causes of the individual differences in social abilities and their genetic basis. Can medications such as oxytocin be used to improve social abilities in autism?[60] Can they be used to enhance social ability even in otherwise healthy people? Can studies of this type have application in the resolution of social conflicts? And so on. One of the most challenging frontiers for the biological sciences now is to understand if the human brain "produces" the mind: if yes, how exactly? The brain has evolved to enable us to interact and communicate with each other: finding the precise and accurate basis of this ability will be the key for more translational applications of those insights.

Although many neural structures and networks participate in social behavior, future research into the social dysfunctions of psychiatric disorders can be more meaningful by shifting the focus on the core set of brain structures that constitute the "social brain" and their connectivity, which may provide a good base to explore answers to many unanswered questions on social brain.[42] Careful design and contrast of tasks to isolate social processing, and establishing links across the levels of the social brain, cognition, behavior, and functioning will help to keep social neuroscience domain-specific to some extent and hopefully in the future, will result in interventions for the various psychiatric maladies of the social brain that we touched upon elsewhere.[53]

A widely recognized disparity in modern neuropsychiatry is the wealth of novel information regarding the pathophysiology of psychiatric disorders derived from basic neuroscience research, on the one hand, and the lack of successful translations into effective treatments, on the other hand. This disappointing situation is partly rooted in the biological complexity of the brain and mind and of the psychiatric conditions, but arguably also in some conceptual limitations. We urgently need to know more about these aspects. New translational research strategies are needed to delineate the neural outcomes of the complex underlying gene-environment interactions. The in-depth understanding of these mechanisms holds the key for development of novel strategies for pharmacology, psychotherapy, and social policy that target and converge on the identified neural circuits. Hopefully, this rapidly expanding field, that has so far provided rich and exciting data, will be able to provide pragmatic and meaningful answers in the distant future, if not sooner.

References

1. Humphrey NK, Bateson PPG, Hinde RA. The social function of intellect: growing points in ethology. Cambridge: Cambridge University Press; 1976:303–317.
2. Emler N. Gossip, reputation and adaptation. In: Goodman RF, Ben-Ze'ev A, eds. *Good Gossip*. Lawrence: University of Kansas Press; 1994:117–138.
3. Allman, JM. *Evolving Brains*. New York: Scientific American Library; 1999.
4. Barrett L, Henzi P. The social nature of primate cognition. Proc Biol Sci. 2005;272:1865–17=875.
5. Dunbar RI. The social brain hypothesis. *Evol Anthropol*. 1998;6:178–190.
6. Green MF, Penn DL, Bentall R, et al. Social cognition in schizophrenia: an NIMH workshop on definitions, assessment, and research opportunities. *Schizophr Bull*. 2008;34:1211–1220.
7. Kanwisher N, Yovel G. The fusiform face area: a cortical region specialized for the perception of faces. *Philos Trans R Soc Lond B: Biol Sci*. 2006;361:2109–2128.
8. Van Overwalle F. Social cognition and the brain: a meta-analysis. *Hum Brain Mapp*. 2009;30:829–858.
9. Kennedy DP, Adolphs R. The social brain in psychiatric and neurological disorders. *Trends Cogn Sci*. 2012 Nov;16(11):559–572. doi: 10.1016/j.tics.2012.09.006. Epub 2012 Oct 6. PMID: 23047070; PMCID: PMC3606817.
10. Brothers L. The social brain: a project for integrating primate behavior and neurophysiology in a new domain. *Concepts Neurosci*. 1990;1:27–61.
11. Amodio DM, Frith CD. Meeting of minds: the medial frontal cortex and social cognition. *Nat. Rev. Neurosci*. 2006;7:268–277.
12. Rizzolatti G, Craighero L. The mirror-neuron system. *Annu Rev Neurosci*. 2004;27:169–192. doi: 10.1146/ annurev. neuro.27.070203.144230)\.
13. Premack D, Woodruff G. Does the chimpanzee have a theory of mind? *Behav Brain Res*. 1978;1(4):515–526. https://doi.org/10.1017/S0140525X00076512
14. Ochsner, KN. Social cognitive neuroscience: historical development, core principles, and future promise. In: Kruglanski A, Higgins E, eds. *Social Psychology: A Handbook of Basic Principles*. New York: Guilford; 2007:39–66.
15. Gazzaniga MS, Ivry RB, Mangun GR. *Cognitive Neuroscience: The Biology of the Mind*. New York: W. W. Norton; 2014.
16. Newberg AB, Iversen J. The neural basis of the complex mental tasks of meditation: neurotransmitter and neurochemical considerations. *Med Hypotheses*. 2003;61:282–291.
17. Newberg AB. *Principles of Neurotheology*. Farnham, Surrey, UK: Ashgate; 2010.
18. Greicius MD, Krasnow B, Reiss AL, Menon V. Functional connectivity in the resting brain: a network analysis of the default mode hypothesis. *Proc Natl Acad Sci U S A*. 2003;100:253–258. https://doi.org/10.1073/pnas.0135058100
19. Menon V, Uddin LQ. Saliency, switching, attention and control: a network model of insula function. *Brain Struct Funct*. 2010;214(5–6):655–667. doi: 10.1007/s00429-010-0262-0.
20. Seeley WW. The salience network: a neural system for perceiving and responding to homeostatic demands. *J Neurosci*. 2019 Dec 11;39(50):9878–9882.
21. Andrews-Hanna JR, Smallwood J, Spreng RN. The default network and self-generated thought: component processes, dynamic control, and clinical relevance. *Ann NY Acad Sci*. 2014;1316 (1):29–52.
22. Dosenbach NU, Visscher KM, Palmer ED, Miezin FM, Wenger KK, Kang HC, . . . Petersen SE. A core system for the implementation of task sets. *Neuron*. 2006;50(5):799–812. S0896-6273(06)00349-7.
23. Raichle ME, MacLeod AM, Snyder AZ, Powers WJ, Gusnard DA, Shulman GL. A default mode of brain function. *Proc Natl Acad Sci U S A*. 2001;98(2):676–682.

24. Menon V. Large-scale brain networks and psychopathology: a unifying triple network model. *Trends Cogn Sci.* 2011;15(10):483–506. S1364-6613(11)00171-9.

25. Sridharan D, Levitin DJ, Menon V. A critical role for the right fronto-insular cortex in switching between central-executive and default-mode networks. *Proc Natl Acad Sci U S A.* 2008;105(34):12569–12574.

26. Fransson P, Marrelec G. The precuneus/posterior cingulate cortex plays a pivotal role in the default mode network: evidence from a partial correlation network analysis. *Neuroimage.* 2008;42(3):1178–1184.

27. Putcha D, Ross RS, Cronin-Golomb A, Janes AC, Stern CE. Salience and default mode network coupling predicts cognition in aging and Parkinson's disease. *J Int Neuropsychol Soc.* 2016;22(2):205–215. doi: 10.1017/S1355617715000892.

28. Smallwood J, Brown K, Baird B, Schooler JW. Cooperation between the default mode network and the frontal–parietal network in the production of an internal train of thought. *Brain Res.* 2011;1428:60–70.

29. Spreng RN. The fallacy of a "task-negative" network. *Front Psychol.* 2012;3:145. doi: 10.3389/fpsyg.2012.00145.

30. Gogolla N, Takesian AE, Feng G, Fagiolini M, Hensch TK. Sensory integration in mouse insular cortex reflects. *GABA Circuit Maturation.* 2014 Aug 20;83(4):894–905. doi:10.1016/j.neuron.2014.06.033. Epub 2014 Jul 31. PMID: 25088363.

31. James W. *The Principles of Psychology*, vol 1. New York: Henry Holt; 1890.

32. Karnath HO, Baier B, Nagele T. Awareness of the functioning of one's own limbs mediated by the insular cortex? *J. Neurosci.* 2005;25:7134–7138.

33. Barbas H, Saha S, Rempel-Clower N, et al. Serial pathways from primate prefrontal cortex to autonomic areas may influence emotional expression. *BMC Neurosci.* 2003;4:25. https://doi.org/10.1186/1471-2202-4-25

34. Bressler SL, Menon V. Large-scale brain networks in cognition: emerging methods and principles. *Trends Cogn Sci.* 2010;14(6):277–290. doi: 10.1016/j.tics.2010.04.004.

35. Berridge KC, Robinson TE. What is the role of dopamine in reward: hedonic impact, reward learning, or incentive salience? *Brain Res Rev.* 1998;28:309–369.

36. Schultz W, Dayan P, Montague PR. A neural substrate of prediction and reward. *Science.* 1997;275:1593–1599.

37. Berridge KC, Robinson TE. Parsing reward. *Trends Neurosci.* 2003;26(9):507–513.

38. McClure SM, Daw ND, Montague PR. A computational substrate for incentive salience. *Trends Neurosci.* 2003 Aug;26(8):423–428. doi: 10.1016/s0166-2236(03)00177-2.

39. Dunbar R. The social brain hypothesis and human evolution. Oxford Research Encyclopedia of Psychology. 2016. https://doi.org/10.1093/acrefore/9780190236557.013.44

40. Decety J, Jackson PL. The functional architecture of human empathy. *Behav Cogn Neurosci Rev.* 2004 Jun;3(2):71–100.

41. Adolphs R. The social brain: neural basis of social knowledge. *Annu Rev Psychol.* 2009;60:693–716.

42. Meyer-Lindenberg A, Tost H. Neural mechanisms of social risk for psychiatric disorders. *Nat Neurosci.* 2012;15:663–668.

43. Frith CD, Frith U. Interacting minds: biological basis. *Science.* 1999;286:1692–1695.

44. Buckner RL, Carroll DC. Self-projection and the brain. *Trends Cogn Sci.* 2007;11(2):49–57.

45. Suddendorf T, Corballis M. Mental time travel and the evolution of the human mind. *Genet Soc Gen Psychol Monogr.* 1997;123:133–167.

46. Fehr E, Gaechter S. Altruistic punishment in humans. *Nature.* 2002;415:137–140.

47. Stevens JA, Cushman F, Hauser M. Evolving the psychological mechanisms for cooperation. *Annu Rev Ecol Evol Syst.* 2005;36:499–518.

48. Akindele ST. Colonialization and economic dependence: the case of Nigeria. In: Bamisaye OA, Egbuwalo MO, eds. *Readings on the Political Economy of Nigeria Since Independence.* Lagos: Ventures; 1990:1–15.

49. Ohiorhenuan, JFE. The South in an era of globalization. *Cooperation South.* 1998;2:6–15.

50. Huynen MMTE, Martens P, Hilderink H. *The Health Impacts of Globalisation: A Conceptual Framework.* Bilthoven, Netherlands: Environmental Assessment Agency; 2005.

51. Smith TC, Thompson TL. The inherent, powerful therapeutic value of a good physician-patient relationship. *Psychosomatics.* 1993;34:166–170.

52. Baron-Cohen S, Leslie AM, Frith U. Does the autistic child have a "theory of mind"? *Cognition.* 1985;21:37–46.
53. Pradhan B, Gogineni RR, Sharma S. Mind, mindfulness, and the social brain: psychobiological understandings and implications. *Indian J Soc Psychiatry.* 2018;34(4):313.
54. Pradhan BK. *Yoga and Mindfulness Based Cognitive Therapy: A Clinical Guide.* Gesterbrasse, Switzerland: Springer; 2014.
55. Kabat-Zinn J, Massion AO, Kristeller J, et al. Effectiveness of a meditation-based stress reduction program in the treatment of anxiety disorders. *Am J Psychiatry.* 1992;149:936–943.
56. Pradhan BK, Pinninti N, Rathod S, eds. *Brief Interventions for Psychosis: A Clinical Compendium.* Gesterbrasse, Switzerland: Springer International; 2016.
57. Pradhan BK, Pinninti NR, Rathod SR. *TIMBER Psychotherapy: For PTSD, Depression and Traumatic Psychosis.* Gesterbrasse, Switzerland: Springer International; 2019.
58. Pascual-Leone A, Freitas C, Oberman L, et al. Characterizing brain cortical plasticity and network dynamics across the age-span in health and disease with TMS-EEG and TMS-fMRI. *Brain Topography.* 2011;24(3–4):302–315.
59. Oberman LM, Rotenberg A, Pascual-Leone A. Use of transcranial magnetic stimulation in autism spectrum disorders. *J Autism Dev Disord.* 2015 Feb;45(2):524–536. doi: 10.1007/s10803-013-1960-2.
60. Ebstein RP, Israel S, Lerer E, Uzefovsky F, Shalev I, Gritsenko I, Yirmiya N. Arginine vasopressin and oxytocin modulate human social behavior. *Ann N Y Acad Sci.* 2009;1167:87–102.

23

Social Psychiatry

Neurodevelopmental Disorders

Rama Rao Gogineni, Prasad Joshi, and
Anthony Rostain

Introduction

The early developmental period spanning birth and childhood and extending to adolescence is characterized by progressive attainment and refinement of social skills, ensuring a successful integration in society; first through successful assimilation in the family unit, followed by a successful passage through the school system, finally leading to occupation and independent living. This developmental trajectory is fueled by complex multisystem changes in a number of neurobiological/functional domains, including speech, vision, and hearing, attention, learning abilities, cognition, and social communication skills. Any derangement in development of any one domain is expected to not only lead to a specific functional deficit (e.g., speech) but also affect the overall developmental trajectory, including family interaction and social integration. Medical, neurological, and neurodevelopmental disorders (NDDs) with origins in childhood often contribute to disturbances in such developmental necessities.

After the historical information, the chapter describes clinical, neurobiological, social aspects, and social treatments of specific NDDs and concludes with key points for social psychiatry.

Historical Background and a Brief Outline

NDDs typically manifest in early childhood before entering first grade. The disorders contribute to deficits in interpersonal, social, academic, and occupational settings. A vast array of NDDs has been described in pediatrics and child neurology. The historical divide between childhood NDDs and disabilities and adult mental illness is increasingly recognized as artificial. The symptoms of various NDDs were described long before the diagnostic concepts were delineated from each other in the mid-20th century. Developmental disorders were included for the first time in DSM-III in the category that comprised autistic disorder. "Neurodevelopmental disorders" (NDDs) were introduced in DSM-5, replacing "disorders usually first diagnosed in infancy, childhood, or adolescence." In ICD-11, published by the World Health Organization (WHO), NDDs gained even more prominence as "mental, behavioral or neurodevelopmental disorders."

In DSM-5, NDDs are defined as a group of conditions with onset in the developmental period, inducing deficits that produce impairments of functioning. NDDs comprise intellectual disability (ID), communication disorders, autism spectrum disorder (ASD), attention-deficit/hyperactivity disorder (ADHD), neurodevelopmental motor disorders, including tic disorders; and specific learning disorders. The classification of NDDs in ICD-11 does not diverge significantly from that in DSM-5. These diagnostic categories show considerable comorbidity and phenotypic overlap. All disorders affect personal, educational, social, and occupational functioning to degrees ranging from small to large. ID and ASD affect multiple neurological systems simultaneously and cause global changes to personal, social, and occupational functioning. ADHD, which involves deregulation of attention and executive functioning, also may lead to significant derangement of functioning, while specific communication, motor, or learning disability may cause a more circumscribed change. In addition to neurobiological, genetic, and developmental factors, deprivation from social and emotional care causes severe delays in brain and cognitive development. Studies with children growing up in Romanian orphanages, under conditions of poverty and hunger, revealed profound effects of social deprivation on the developing brain.[1]

The multitude of neurodevelopmental disorders span a wide range of associated symptoms and severity, resulting in different degrees of mental, emotional, physical, and economic consequences for individuals, and in turn families, social groups, and society. These disorders have an enormous impact on families and society. According to the 1996 book *Learning Disabilities: Lifelong Issues*, children with these disorders have higher rates of mental illness and suicide, and are more likely to engage in substance abuse and to commit crimes as adults.[2]

Specific Disorders

Autism Spectrum Disorder (ASD)

ASD, first described by Leo Kanner in 1943 as autism, is marked by deficits in social communication and social interactions and restricted, repetitive pattern of behaviors (including motor behaviors such as stereotypical behaviors, tics, etc.) and interests. ASD may or may not be accompanied by intellectual disability. Deficit in social communication is marked by deficits in social-emotional reciprocity and failure of shared conversations, emotions, and interests. In addition, individuals with ASD have highly restrictive interests (e.g., trains), which may further prevent development of relationships around shared interests. An individual with ASD has difficulty initiating and maintaining social contact and also displays poor verbal and nonverbal communication. Combined, these deficits significantly affect the ability to form and maintain social relationships across multiple domains, including school, occupation, and community. The diagnosis of ASD is typically made during childhood before age 3. DSM-5 criteria require that a child has persistent impairment in social communications and interactions across multiple contexts, as well as restricted or repetitive patterns of behavior, interests, or activities; that symptoms should present in early childhood and cause significant functional impairments; and that the impairments are not better explained by intellectual disability. The current version of the DSM introduced in 2013, DSM-5, lists "autism spectrum disorder." This version does not distinguish subtypes such as "autistic disorder" or "Asperger's syndrome." The social deficits are more prominent during earlier years, but will continue throughout the course, and can remain in adults as deficits in adaptive or social skills or as eccentricity. Early deficits begin before age of 1 year as nonverbal deficits and include lack of social gestures such as pointing, showing, and giving. Around 15 months of age, deficits are noted in joint attention as well, such as focusing on a person's mouth rather than eyes. Even in higher functioning autism, significant social skills deficits are noted. In this population, several cognitive components, including the theory of mind, pragmatic competence, and cognitive processing speed, all can be impaired. On occasion, language may be superficially normal appearing with adequate vocabulary and grammar skills, though on closer examination, poor ability to draw inference from dialogue and poor comprehension of narrative becomes obvious. Interestingly, an individual with ASD may show lack of a sense of humor in situations involving self, while able to see humor in situations involving others; this can contribute further to social difficulties in this population.[3]

Neurobiology and Etiology

Human social behavior is based on the ability to appropriately communicate with others and involves sensing, processing, and interpreting social cues, as well as responding with appropriate behaviors. These functions have been mapped to brain areas comprising the "social brain," in particular, the medial prefrontal cortex, amygdala, anterior insula, anterior cingulate cortex, inferior frontal gyrus. and superior temporal sulcus. Autism is described as a polygenetic developmental neurobiological disorder with multiorgan system involvement, though it predominantly involves central nervous system dysfunction. The evidence supports autism as a disorder of the association cortex, both its neurons and their projections. In particular, it is a disorder of connectivity, which appears, from current evidence, to primarily involve intra-hemispheric connectivity; intra-cortical connectivity is also likely to be disturbed. In ASD, abnormal sensory integration across these cortical and sub-cortical brain regions results in derailment in processing of social information. Autism is a polygenetic developmental neurobiological disorder with multi-organ system involvement, though it predominantly involves central nervous system dysfunction. Autism is a disorder of the association cortex, both its neurons and their projections. The focus of connectivity studies thus far has been on white matter, but alterations in functional magnetic resonance imaging activation suggest that intracervical connectivity is also likely to be disturbed. Furthermore, the disorder has a broad impact on cognitive and neurologic functioning. Deficits in high-functioning individuals occur in processing that places high demands on integration of information and coordination of multiple neural systems. Intact or enhanced abilities share a dependence on low information-processing demands and local neural connections. This multidomain model with shared characteristics predicts an underlying pathophysiologic mechanism that impacts the brain broadly, according to a common neurobiologic principle. The multiorgan system involvement and diversity of central nervous system findings suggest an epigenetic mechanism.[4]

Diagnosis of ASD is significantly associated with a higher probability of previous occurrence of adverse childhood events (ACEs), with the number of children with ASD who were exposed to 4 or more ACEs reportedly twice as high as the non-ASD population. A combination of ASD phenotype and occurrence of higher ACEs predisposes this population to higher likelihood of development of psychiatric disorders, including anxiety, depression, and worsening of self-injurious behaviors.[5]

Features of ASD Specially Pertaining to Social Deficits

Individuals with a diagnosis of ASD face several social challenges, both as a result of the autism phenotype and as a result of a misfit between individual and societal expectations of "normal" social behavior. A large number of studies have examined social outcomes in autism. These studies have focused on evaluations of social functioning, including independence, social relationships, employment status, and living arrangements. Overall, outcomes, as measured on a 5-point scale, have ranged from poor to very poor. Studies indicate that individuals with ASD display a high degree of dependence, either on family or on support services. Even in individuals with higher functional status, rates of dependence range from 16% to 36%. The presence of an intellectual disability (ID) is associated with much lower rates of independent living, with a large number of studies reporting that less than 5% of individuals with both ASD and ID live independently. Studies of social inclusion have examined housing arrangements and rates of employment as indirect measures. Higher IQ and milder ASD symptoms are associated with higher rates of independent living. In terms of employment, individuals with ASD have low rates of employment overall. Higher IQ and lower ASD severity also correlate with higher rates of paid employment, with 20%–55% of such individuals in paid work. However, overall only about 1 in 5 individuals with ASD diagnosis engages in full-time paid work, and only about 1 in 10 live independently. Social interactions remain impaired in both children and adults with ASD, and factors such as deficits in reciprocal social interaction skills and extent of response to joint attention are associated with level of attainment in social functioning. In more severely affected individuals, daytime activities are primarily scheduled with the help of family or community resources. Daytime activities involve day programs or sheltered workshops. Dependent living arrangements, as well as resources needed to provide structured daytime activities, put considerable stress on family and community resources. ASD individuals often exhibit severe communication deficits, including expressive speech. Problems with pronoun use are frequent. Loud voice volume (prosody) and idiosyncratic language are common. They often have difficulty understanding pragmatic language like humor, sarcasm, irony, etc.[6]

Psychosocial Treatments of ASD

Treatment approaches to ASD include behavioral, educational, and pharmacological interventions. In ASD, social deficits are core feature of psychopathology and are therapeutically targeted with both specific and nonspecific interventions. The mainstay of social intervention is social skills training though experimental pharmacological interventions including oxytocin, propranolol, and vasopressin agonists, and antagonists are under active investigation. Bumetanide and microbiota transfer therapy are also being investigated; other behavioral and pharmacological interventions that decrease maladaptive behaviors and improve communication skills also have an indirect positive effect on improving social engagement. Social skills training includes 3 essential components: (1) behavioral adaptations, including skills needed to develop joint attention, greeting others, and initiating social contact; (2) fostering the development of affective understanding, which includes teaching strategies to recognize emotions in others using images of facial expressions; (3) development of social cognitive skills, including perspective taking and developing the theory of mind. Methods used include use of social stories and asking participants to predict storylines from children's books or movies. Applied behavior analysis (ABA), a treatment based on theories of learning and operant conditioning, has shown remarkable outcomes, including gaining significant IQ points, language development, daily living skills acquisition, and social functioning. Pivotal Response Treatment (PRT) is another useful model that includes a more naturalistic behavioral method that targets specific skills as well as motivations. PRT has shown more widespread/generalizable gains in areas not specifically targeted by the therapy, such as joint attention. It is also less time-intensive than ABA therapies. A supplemental social curriculum to treatment, which included aspects of ABA and PRT, resulted in improved joint attention, shared positive affect, and socially engaged imitation. Other psychosocial interventions include parent-mediated early interventions (teaching parents interventions that they can then apply in the home) and social skills interventions. Social skills interventions include peer-related mediation, social narratives, and video modeling. Goals of social skills training may include emotional regulation, basic conversation skills, nonverbal communication skills, perspective taking, initiating, responding, and maintaining social interactions; these have shown to be promising treatments, especially with targeted skills. Particularly in higher functioning ASD individuals, this has shown to be an effective treatment for comorbid anxiety.[7,8]

Intellectual Deficiency Syndrome (ID)

ID, previously called *mental retardation*, has an onset during the developmental period and includes deficits both in intellectual and adaptive functioning. Deficits in intellectual functioning, such as reasoning, problem-solving, abstract thinking, learning, and judgment are seen. Deficit in adaptive functioning causes inability to reach personal and social-cultural developmental milestones and necessitates the need for support in multiple domains, including activities of daily living (ADLs), communication, and social participation, and help across multiple environments, including home, school, occupation, and community. Social functioning in individuals with ID is correlated with the severity level. In mild ID, the individual is immature and concrete in social interactions, communication, and language, and this is accompanied by difficulty in accurately perceiving social cues from peers. Also accompanied are gullibility, undue risk-taking behaviors, and emotional dysregulation. Combined, these deficits lead to impaired social interactions, which lead to distress and later avoidance of similar situations. However, in mild ID, the individual maintains the capability to form meaningful relationships and with therapeutic interventions can develop a repertoire of social skills, leading to successful integration in society. In moderate ID, significant differences in social and communicative differences from peers exist, and this is reflected in social interactions at school, at work, and in the community. Interactions with typically developing peers may be limited. However, individuals with moderate ID maintain the ability to form relationships with family and friends and are even capable of forming romantic relationships in adult life. However, these individuals need significant help with making personal decisions, and this may affect their ability to navigate complex interpersonal issues. These individuals also need significant communication and social support in both school and at work. In severe ID, language and cognitive abilities are limited, and this significantly affects the ability to form relationships, and social interactions are limited to close family and caregivers.

Clinical Features

ID refers to a disorder that starts during the developmental period. It consists of certain intellectual deficits and challenges handling aspects of daily life like school, work, home, social life, and health, among other things. ID is an explanatory phrase for substandard intelligence that occurs below age 18. While DSM-IV emphasized IQ scores, this is not so with DSM-5. Instead, no particular score is indicated to establish diagnosis, and the assessment is done based on the individual's complete clinical presentation. In some cases, patients with ID also have a bigger medical condition, such as Down's syndrome, fragile X syndrome, or Klienfelter's syndrome, which also require more extensive treatment. Across the world, the prevalence of developmental disabilities has been increasing, but the United States has seen the prevalence of ID decline to 1.5% because of advancements in public health and healthcare facilities.[9]

Individuals with ID have a higher risk of psychiatric disorders than individuals with intelligence in the normal range: prevalence is as high as 40.9% compared to normal range, Based on clinical diagnosis IT IS 15.7%. The most common comorbid psychiatric disorders are problem behavior (18.7%), affective disorder (5.7%), autism spectrum disorder (4.4%), psychotic disorder (3.8%), and anxiety disorder (3.1%).

Neurobiology

Marylyn Bullof Johns Hopkins University who studies Rett syndrome, autism, Down syndrome, and other genetic causes of mental retardation, says: "The idea that ultimately mental retardation is a problem with synaptic connections in the brain is a fair statement to make—albeit admittedly vague. The synapse is where neurons talk to one another, so whenever that process is disrupted, there are going to be consequences. Ultimately, it is going to be an effect that happens at the synapse." Huda Zoghbi,[10] a neuroscientist at Baylor College, reports Rett syndrome and ASD seem to involve reduced branching of dendrites.[10]

Synaptic abnormalities are well recognized in fragile X syndrome and Down syndrome, two of the better-characterized causes of mental retardation from a neurobiological standpoint. Synaptogenesis in various mental retardation syndromes can be traced to the dysfunction of a single gene. Stevenson, who focuses on syndromes arising from defects in specific genes on the X chromosome (X-linked mental retardation), points to three X-linked genes. These defective genes encode for specific brain chemicals or hormones that are essential to some aspect of brain function; for example, a missing molecular transporter prevents creatine, an enzyme that supports energy metabolism in mitochondria, from reaching the brain, or a transporter for a vital thyroid hormone is missing.[11]

Fragile X syndrome occurs in about 1 in 2000 males and roughly half that number of females. The *FMR1* gene carries the code for making a protein called FMRP, and the absence of this protein causes the familiar fragile X symptoms.

William T. Greenough, PhD, a neurobiologist at the University of Illinois at Urbana-Champaign, thinks that a particular kind of protein synthesis at the dendritic spines requires FMRP. "This protein synthesis is not seen in the Fragile X knockout mouse," he says. (The fragile X knockout mouse is bred specifically to lack the *FMR1* gene.) Because new protein synthesis is known to be a requirement for learning and memory, experts believe FMRP is a key player in this process.[12]

Bear now believes that without FMRP, synaptic connections are weakened, a process called long-term depression (LTD). The cause appears to be excessive signaling by a subclass of receptors for the neurotransmitter glutamate. Glutamate, the main excitatory neurotransmitter in the brain, is known to play important roles in learning and memory, and problems with its regulation have been implicated as a potential mechanism in several forms of mental retardation. Bear and his team continued on to investigate how the consequences of the lack of FMRP might be linked to fragile X symptoms. More and more evidence accumulated that seemed to explain everything from cognitive impairment to seizures to sensory hyperarousal and anxiety to loose bowel movements—all symptoms of fragile X syndrome. Bear's theory about the role of the glutamate receptors has since been a focus of research in laboratories worldwide and has become well accepted as a key piece of the molecular puzzle underlying fragile X syndrome, even as scientists continue to work out the details. Sention, Inc., a small biotech firm cofounded by Bear, has recently licensed a family of glutamate receptor antagonists from Merck and is developing the compounds for clinical testing in people with fragile X syndrome.[13]

Social Aspects

Social aspects of ID include systems of healthcare, family dynamics, life events, culture, social anthropology, social psychology, socioeconomic factors, work and occupation, legal issues, and human rights issues. Some of the problems that individuals with ID experience occur when they age out, and are no longer considered minors. Patients with ID face great stigma within the community at large, and children may face bullying both at school and at home. Adults with ID are vulnerable to stressful social interactions Psychological stress occurs as a result of a person-environment interaction in which individuals appraise a situation as threatening their well-being or self-esteem and as exceeding their resources to deal with the situation. Adults with mild ID state that this category of stressful events occurs more frequently and is more stressful when experienced than are other types of negative events.

Documented etiological factors of people with ID in India include genetic disorders, malnutrition, infectious diseases, early or late-age pregnancy, and poor medical care before, during, and after birth as the major contributing factors for ID. Similarly, the major social, environmental, and biological determinates of ID are poverty, poor nutrition, lack of awareness regarding preventive measures, illiteracy, poor healthcare facilities, and lack of access to healthcare services. Overall, these factors negatively affect pre-, peri-, and postnatal care of an individual with ID. To develop a culturally sensitive and need-based public health program, we must first better understand how these key social, environmental, and biological factors influence ID in India. This most probably apples to most developing countries. Down syndrome (trisomy 21) and fragile X syndrome are the 2 most common genetic disorders. Fetal alcohol syndrome is another major contributor.[14]

Treatment

ID is most successfully managed in a holistic, and therefore multidisciplinary, manner. Unfortunately, ID has generally been absent from the political, social, and economic agenda of Latin American and several other countries. Most of the children and adults with ID want to socialize, have friends, and be part of their community. For this to be achieved, they recognize the need to seek some form of support. With appropriate and targeted support, adults with ID can move from social exclusion toward supported inclusion and can experience richer lives. Both being and feeling socially included can have a vital and positive impact on the lives of people with ID. For young adults, the supported social group countered loneliness, expanded the circle of people they could call friends, extended their social life beyond the family, and gave them a sense of greater well-being. The social group reversed what appeared to be a largely sedentary and isolated life, leading to greater social participation and physical activity. Research has shown that family caregivers support over 80% of people with an ID, and that family care remains the predominant type of care until middle age.[15]

Social, Learning, and Communication Disorders

Social (pragmatic) communication disorder is diagnosed based on difficulties with both verbal and nonverbal social communication skills, which include: responding to others; using gestures (like waving or pointing); taking turns when talking or playing; talking about emotions and feelings; staying on topic; adjusting speech to fit different people or situations (e.g., talking differently to a young child versus an adult or lowering one's voice in a library); asking relevant questions or responding with related ideas during conversation; using words for a variety of purposes, such as greeting people, making comments, asking questions, making promises; and making and keeping friends. Primary difficulties are in social interaction, social cognition, and pragmatics. The syndrome can cause persistent difficulties in the social use of verbal and nonverbal communication, as manifested by deficits in using communication for social purposes, impairment in the ability to change communication to match context or the needs of the listener, difficulties following rules for conversation and storytelling, such as taking turns in conversation, rephrasing when misunderstood, and knowing how to use verbal and nonverbal signals to regulate interaction. The etiology of developmental dyslexia is not established. Often there is a positive family history, predominant in males, suggesting an autosomal dominant mode of inheritance. It is widely believed that immature development of the parietal lobe with microscopic developmental anomalies may play a role.

Speech-language pathologists also work with individuals who have problems with the nonverbal aspects of communication and social interaction. Incorporating families to encourage and assist children in social communication skills—which include take turns, read and discuss, talk about the feelings, what's next?, clue into pop culture, plan structured play dates, and use visual supports—can be very helpful.

Specific learning disorders describe deficits in specific domains related to learning abilities (as opposed to global deficits seen in ID). An estimated 5%–15% of school-age children struggle with a learning disability. An estimated 80% of those with learning disorders have reading disorder in particular (commonly referred to as dyslexia). One-third of people with learning disabilities are estimated to also have attention-deficit hyperactivity disorder (ADHD). Other specific skills that may be impacted include the ability to put thoughts into written words, spelling, reading comprehension, math calculation, and math problem-solving. Difficulties with these skills may cause problems in learning subjects such as history, math, science, and social studies, and may impact everyday activities.

Learning disorders and communication disorders, if not recognized and managed, can cause problems throughout a person's life beyond having lower academic and social achievement. These problems include increased risk of greater psychological distress, poorer overall mental health, unemployment/underemployment, and dropping out of school. Neurobiological language learning disorders are due to dysfunctions of corticostriatal systems, more likely to be associated with corticostriatal loops involving the dorsal striatum. Individuals with learning and communication disorders face unique challenges that may persist throughout their lives. Depending on the type and severity of their disability, interventions and technology may be used to help the individual learn strategies that will foster future success. Teachers, parents, and schools can work together to create a tailored plan for intervention and accommodation to aid an individual in successfully becoming an independent learner and performer. Social support may also improve learning and communication difficulties. Working with stigma, accepting these as medical conditions, enhancing self-esteem, and dealing with family issues can be very helpful.[16]

Attention Deficit Hyperactive Disorder (ADHD)

ADHD was first mentioned in 1902. British pediatrician Sir George Still described an abnormal defect of moral control in children. He found that some affected children could not control their behavior the way a typical child would, but they were still intelligent. In 1936

Dr. Charles Bradley stumbled across some unexpected side effects of Benzedrine that enhanced young patients' behavior and performance in school.

Clinical Features

ADHD is a disorder characterized by a persistent pattern of inattention and/or hyperactivity/impulsivity that occurs in academic, occupational, or social settings. Problems with attention include making careless mistakes, failing to complete tasks, problems staying organized and keeping track of things, becoming easily distracted, etc. Problems with hyperactivity can include excessive fidgetiness and squirminess, running or climbing when it is not appropriate, excessive talking, and being constantly on the go. Impulsivity can show up as impatience, difficulty awaiting one's turn, blurting out answers, and frequent interrupting. Although many individuals with ADHD display both inattentive and hyperactive/impulsive symptoms, some individuals show symptoms from one group but not the other. The prevalence of ADHD in the general unscreened school-age population was estimated at 4% to 12%.[17]

Age Specificity and Psychosocial Consequences

ADHD in a preschool child is associated with difficulties, such as delayed development and poor social skills. ADHD during childhood can greatly affect psychosocial and family life. Children experience academic failure, rejection by peers, and suffer from low self-esteem. They often manifest comorbid problems, such as specific learning difficulties and difficulties at home or on outings with caregivers, for example, when shopping, out in the park, or visiting other family members. Parents may find that family members refuse to care for the child, and that other children do not invite them to parties or out to play. Family relationships may be severely strained, and in some cases break down, bringing additional social and financial difficulties. This may cause children to feel sad or even show oppositional or aggressive behavior. The presence of a child with ADHD can result in increased disturbances to family and marital functioning, disrupted parent-child relationships, reduced parenting efficacy, and increased levels of parent stress, depression, and alcohol consumption, particularly when ADHD is comorbid with conduct problems. ADHD can disrupt siblings in three primary ways: victimization, caretaking, and sorrow and loss. Siblings reported feeling victimized by aggressive acts from their ADHD brothers through overt acts of physical violence, verbal aggression, and manipulation and control. In addition, siblings reported that parents expected them to care for and protect their ADHD brothers because of the social and emotional immaturity associated with ADHD. Furthermore, as a result of the ADHD symptoms and consequent disruption, many siblings described feeling anxious, worried, and sad.

ADHD in adolescents and young adults can cause low self-esteem, poor social skills, antisocial behaviors, school problems, motivational difficulties, and learning problems. Teenagers reported having more parent-teen conflict in part due to academic failure, dropping out of school or college, teenage pregnancy, and criminal behaviors. Driving poses an additional risk. Individuals with ADHD are easily distracted from concentrating on driving when going slowly, but driving fast may also be dangerous. It has been shown that, compared with age-matched controls, drivers with ADHD are at increased risk of traffic violations, especially speeding, and are considered to be at fault in more traffic accidents.

As many as 60% of individuals with ADHD symptoms in childhood continue to have difficulties in adult life. Adults with ADHD are more likely to be dismissed from employment and have often tried a number of jobs before being able to find one at which they can succeed. They may need to choose specific types of work and are frequently self-employed. In the workplace, adults with ADHD experience more interpersonal difficulties with employers and colleagues. Further problems are caused by lateness, absenteeism, excessive errors, and an inability to accomplish expected workloads. At home, relationship difficulties and breakups are more common. The risk of drug and substance abuse is significantly increased in adults with persisting ADHD.[18]

Neurobiology and Etiology

There is evidence of a genetic basis for ADHD, but it is likely to involve many genes of small individual effect. Differences in the dimensions of the frontal lobes, caudate nucleus, and cerebellar vermis have been demonstrated, with particular focus on the neurotransmitter dopamine and its actions at the cellular and systems level. Neuropsychological testing has revealed differences in two main domains: executive function and motivation. There is also little evidence to suggest that parenting practices and family stress are important causal factors in the development of ADHD. These factors may influence the severity of a child's symptoms, however. This is important because it highlights the tremendously important role that parents can play in helping to promote the successful development of their child. The following factors also may influence the severity of a child's symptoms: systems of healthcare, family dynamics, life events, culture, social anthropology, social psychology, socioeconomic factors, work and occupation, legal issues, and human rights issues.[19]

Comorbidity

Comorbid disorders may impact individuals with ADHD throughout their lives. It is estimated that at least 65% of children with ADHD have one or more comorbid conditions. The reported incidence of some of the most frequent comorbidities include neurodevelopmental problems, such as dyslexia and developmental coordination disorder, and tic disorders. The core symptoms of ADHD, like impulsivity and inattention, might lead children to behave in ways that can put their health at risk or cause them to forget healthy and protective behaviors, which, if not addressed, can lead to injury, disease, or even an earlier-than-expected death. Having a healthy lifestyle can help children with ADHD deal with stress and difficulties in their daily lives. Physical activity, nutrition, and sleep can help children with ADHD manage their symptoms.[20]

Treatment with Emphasis on Psychosocial Interventions

Treatments range from behavioral, family, social, and other psychosocial interventions to prescription medication. In many cases, medication alone is an effective treatment for ADHD. Several therapy options can help children with ADHD. Psychotherapy can be useful to open up about their feelings, better handle relationships, explore their behavior patterns, and learn how to make good choices in the future. Behavior therapy helps to monitor their behaviors and then change those behaviors appropriately, and to develop strategies for how the child behaves in response to certain situations. Social skills training helps teach the child new and more appropriate behaviors. Support groups are great for helping parents of children with ADHD connect with others who may share similar experiences and concerns. Parenting skills training gives parents tools and techniques for understanding and managing their child's behaviors.

A family-orientated, multidimensional treatment approach for children with ADHD and their families is found to be helpful. The genetic aspects of ADHD mean that adults with ADHD are more likely to have children with ADHD. This in turn causes further problems, especially as the success of parenting programs for parents of children with ADHD is highly influenced by the presence of parental ADHD. Thus, ADHD in parents and children can lead to a cycle of difficulties in ADHD multiplex families (families with child and parents struggling with ADHD). Maternal mental health in general plays a significant role, especially the level of aggression and hostility. Treatment must not only address child symptoms, but also parental psychopathology. Focus should be set on comorbid conditions in particular.

Multimodal treatment of ADHD includes a combination of several of the following procedures: token economy, extinction, response cost and time out, self-instructions, reinforced self-evaluation, training in social abilities, assessment for parents and teachers, and training in study skills or instructional management procedures. Family-based, school-based, academic-based, social skills training, and medication interventions are part of the treatment. Culture, race, ethnicity, gender, and sexual orientation should be included in designing treatments. Community health workers will be working with parents in parent training and with the child in social skills training.

A neurodevelopmental perspectives advocate will be working with secondary preventive interventions for attention deficit/hyperactivity disorder (ADHD). By targeting preschool children, a developmental stage during which ADHD symptoms first become evident in most children with the disorder, many of the adverse long-term consequences that typify the trajectory of ADHD may be avoided. A dynamic/interactive model of the biological and environmental factors that contribute to the emergence and persistence of ADHD throughout the life span is proposed. Based on this model, it is argued that environmental influences and physical exercise can be used to enhance neural growth and development, which in turn should have an enduring and long-term impact on the trajectory of ADHD. Central to this notion are 2 hypotheses: (1) environmental influences can facilitate structural and functional brain development, and (2) changes in brain structure and function are directly related to ADHD severity over the course of development and the degree to which the disorder persists or remits with time. Also a case is made for initiating interventions during the preschool years, when the brain is likely to be more "plastic" and perhaps susceptible to lasting modifications, and before complicating factors, such as comorbid psychiatric disorders, academic failure, and poor social and family relationships emerge, making successful treatment more difficult. Communitybased interventions for Children with ADHD and ASD, including community-based cognitive-behavioral, Executive Functioning (EF) treatment are found to be helpful.[21,22]

Neurodevelopmental Motor Disorders

Introduction and Overview

Tics are sudden twitches, movements, or sounds that people do repeatedly. People who have tics cannot stop their body from doing these things. Tourette syndrome (TS) is a common, chronic neuropsychiatric disorder characterized by the presence of fluctuating motor and phonic tics. The typical age of onset is ~5–7 years, and the majority of children improve by their late teens or early adulthood. DSM-5 categorizes tic disorder as Tourette's disorder (also called Tourette syndrome [TS]), persistent (also called chronic) motor or vocal tic disorder, and provisional tic disorder. Affected individuals are at increased risk for the development of various comorbid conditions, such as obsessive-compulsive disorder, ADHD, school problems, depression, and anxiety. There is no cure for tics, and symptomatic therapy includes behavioral and pharmacological approaches. Evidence supports TS being an inherited disorder; however, the precise genetic abnormality remains unknown. Pathologic involvement of portico-striatal-thalami-cortical (CSTC) pathways is supported by neurophysiological, brain imaging, and postmortem studies, but results are often confounded by small numbers, age differences, severity of symptoms, comorbidity, use of pharmacotherapy, and other factors. The primary site of abnormality remains controversial. Although numerous neurotransmitters participate in the transmission of messages through CSTC circuits, a dopaminergic dysfunction is considered a leading candidate. Several animal models have been used to study behaviors similar to tics as well as to pursue potential pathophysiological deficits. TS is a complex disorder with features overlapping a variety of scientific fields. Despite description of this syndrome in the late 19th century, there remain numerous unanswered neurobiological questions.[23,24]

Psychosocial Aspects

The social impact of TS is varied. Many with TS cope and adapt well, with some using creativity or humor to their advantage, or by focusing on something that they are good at or enjoy doing such as leisure activities, sports, or academic or artistic pursuits. Physical and behavioral manifestations can also contribute to stigma, which subsequently leads to poorer health outcomes, discrimination, and a reduced willingness to seek help. The available evidence suggests that young patients with TS can experience reduced social acceptance from peers and difficulties establishing relationships. Some studies show problems in the domains of self-concept and self-esteem, feelings of isolation, loneliness, and experiences of bullying. For those with severe forms of the disorder and with severe comorbidities, TS may interfere with the individual's everyday life and activities of school, home, or work, such as being educated to their full potential, obtaining a job/career, gaining independence, and having meaningful relationships with family and friends. Severe fidgetiness due to comorbid ADHD, coprolalia, and disruptive behaviors may well attract negative consequences, such as disciplinary action in children or stigma and social embarrassment in adults. In this regard, supportive environments, anticipatory guidance, as well as appropriate emotional, behavioral, and learning supports are indicated to overcome the challenges confronting those with TS. Education of health and other professionals, as well as implementation of community awareness programs, is essential. Pharmacological interventions and improving a sense of personal mastery through skill building in comprehensive behavioral intervention for tics (CBIT) can helpful.[25]

Key Points

1. NDDs produce deficits that ultimately result in deficits in interpersonal, social, academic, and occupational settings. These disorders have an enormous impact on families and society.
2. Most NDDs are polygenetic and cause central nervous system dysfunction.
3. The incidence of comorbidity is very high in all these disorders.
4. NDDs often cause much psychological, educational, occupational, and relational dysfunction that further complicate the clinical picture.
5. Psychosocial, family, educational, and pharmacological interventions are essential for enhancement of functionality in the individuals as well as families.

References

1. Morris-Rosendahl DJ, Crocq MA. Neurodevelopmental disorders—the history and future of a diagnostic concept. *Dialogues Clin Neurosci*. 2020 Mar;22(1):65–72.
2. Shirley C. Cramer, William Ellis. Learning disabilities lifelong issues. P. RH. Brookes Publishing Company 1996. https://books.google.com › ... › Learning Disabilities
3. Rosen NE, Lord C, Volkmar FR. The diagnosis of Autism: from Kanner to DSM-III to DSM-5 and Beyond. *J Autism Dev Disord*. 2021;51(12):4253–4270.
4. Barak B, Feng G. Neurobiology of social behavior abnormalities in autism and Williams syndrome. *Nat Neurosci*. 2016 Apr 26;19(6):647–655.
5. Craig, Newschaffer, Berkowitz, Lee. Examining the association of autism and adverse childhood experiences in the National Survey of Children's Health: The important role of income and co-occurring mental health conditions. *J Autism Dev Disord*. 2017 Jul;47(7):2275–2281.
6. Henninger NA, Taylor JL. Outcomes in adults with autism spectrum disorders: a historical perspective. *Autism*. 2013 Jan;17(1):103–116.
7. Subramanyam AA, Mukherjee A, Dave M, Chavda K. Clinical practice guidelines for autism spectrum disorders. *Indian J Psychiatry*. 2019 Jan;61(Suppl 2):254–269.
8. Volkmar F, Siegel M, Woodbury-Smith M, McCracken J, State M, et al. Practice Parameter for the Assessment and Treatment of Children and Adolescents With Autism Spectrum Disorder. *J Am Acad Child Adolesc Psychiatry*. 2014;53(2):237–257.
9. Patel DR, Carbal MD, Ho A, Merrick J. A clinical primer on intellectual disability. *Transl Pediatr*. 2020 Feb;9(Suppl 1):S23–S35.
10. Zoghbi H. Rett syndrome: a prototypical neurodevelopmental disorder. *J Child Neurol*. 1988;3:576–578. https://journals.sagepub.com
11. Hanson D, Hagerman R. Intractable serotonin dysregulation in Fragile X Syndrome: implications for treatment. *Rare Dis Res*. 2014 Nov;3(4):110–117.

12. Brenda Patoine. Mental retardation: struggle, stigma. *Science.* https://dana.org › article › mental-retardation-struggle-s. April 1, 2005.

13. Bear MF, Huber KM, Warren ST. The mGluR theory of fragile X mental retardation. *Trends Neurosci.* 2004;27:370–377.

14. Ram Lakhan. Profile of social, environmental and biological correlates in intellectual disability in a resource-poor setting in India. *Indian J Psychol Med.* 2015 Jul-Sep;37(3):311–316.

15. Katz G, Lazcano-Ponce E. Intellectual disability: definition, etiological factors, classification, diagnosis, treatment and prognosis. Salud Pública de México. 2008;50(suplemento 2).

16. Johnson CR, Slomka G. Learning, motor, and communication disorders. In: Hersen M, Ammerman RT, eds. *Advanced abnormal child psychology.* Lawrence Erlbaum Associates Publishers; 2000:371–385.

17. The History of ADHD: A Timeline – Healthline https://www.healthline.com › health › adhd › history

18. Haprin V. The effect of ADHD on the life of an individual, their family, and community from preschool to adult life. *Arch Dis Child.* 2005;90(Suppl I):i2–i7. doi: 10.1136/adc.2004.059006

19. Tripp G, Wickens JR. Neurobiology of ADHD. *Neuropharmacolog.* 2009 Dec;57(7-8):579–589.

20. Gnanavel S, Sharma P, Kaushal P, Hussain S. Attention deficit hyperactivity disorder and comorbidity: a review of literature. *World J Clin Cases.* 2019 Sep 6;7(17):2420–2426. Published online 2019 Sep 6. doi: 10.12998/wjcc.v7.i17.2420.

21. Children and Adults with Attention-Deficit/Hyperactivity Disorder (CHADD) Psychosocial Treatments – CHADD https://chadd.org › For Parents 1-5-23

22. Centers of Disease Control and Prevention (CDC). Treatment of ADHD. https://www.cdc.gov › ncbddd › adhd › treatment

23. Shivam Om Mittal MD. Tics and Tourette's syndrome. *Drugs Context.* 2020;9:2019-12-2. Published online 2020 Mar 30. doi: 10.7573/dic.2019-12-2

24. Jones KS, Saylam E, Ramphul K. Tourette syndrome and other tic disorders. Tourette Syndrome And Other Tic Disorders – StatPearls – NCBI https://www.ncbi.nlm.nih.gov › books › NBK499958

25. Eapen V, Cavanna AE, Robertson MM. Comorbidities, social impact, and quality of life in Tourette syndrome. *Front Psychiatry.* 2016;7:97. Published online 2016 Jun 6. doi: 10.3389/fpsyt.2016.00097

24

Social Psychiatry

Depressive and Anxiety Disorders

Sami Pirkola, Sari Fröjd, and Kirsti Nurmela

Introduction

In the history of social psychiatry, so called severe mental illnesses have been an important focus of interest for good reasons. The impact of psychotic disorders, for example, on the adaptation of individuals to society and the major role of societal and socioeconomic factors in the development of long-term psychiatric problems have emphasized the need to study and develop the interaction of society and severe psychiatric disorders.

The role and importance of the more common, but initially less severe depressive and anxiety disorders have not been very clear in the agenda of global social psychiatry. Particularly in the developing countries, the urgency of taking care of the most severe mental illnesses has understandably overcome in priority these less devastating but still very burdensome psychiatric disorders.

Recently, these so-called common mental disorders have gained attention, particularly due to their effect on the everyday and social life, general functioning, and occupational capacity of many people. They have historically been less stigmatizing than the more severe mental disorders, but there seems to be a contemporary conflict between their cognitive impact and the demands of society, and the labor market in particular, which expects more social and cognitive skills. Their impact on the quality of life and functioning of people in the developing countries is largely unknown, partly due to lack of research on mental disorders altogether.

Common Mental Disorders

The reason for forming the concept of common mental disorders for depressive and anxiety disorders involves their relative frequency in populations and consequent "commonness." Their symptoms as such are more than common, since they belong to our everyday experiences or reactions to the challenges we meet. These include anxiety and a lowered mood for many reasons. When proceeding into disorders, they become persistent, distressing, and harmful. This category of disorders typically includes depressive and anxiety disorders, but occasionally and depending on the context, substance use disorders are classified as belonging to the common mental disorders, as well. In our context, we focus here on the depressive and anxiety disorders, due to their convergence and characteristic comorbidity. The symptoms of depressive and anxiety disorders overlap, and these disorders typically affect the same persons, either simultaneously or temporally separately.

Diagnostic Categorizing

The history of descriptive diagnostics of psychiatric disorders altogether extends to the first DSM (*Diagnostic and Statistical Manual*) classification by American Psychiatric Association in 1980. Critical debate occasionally wails around the usefulness of this kind of a categorical diagnosing system, although for the purposes of research and prognostic evaluation of the patients, the need for it is obvious. The classification into diagnostic categories is based on described symptoms, estimated to exist, by a diagnosing clinician. The most widely used diagnostic classification system in the world is the *International Classification of Diseases*, currently in its 10th version. It is maintained by the World Health Organization (WHO), and in it mental and behavioral disorders form a main category titled with F. The codes for mental and behavioral disorders thus range from F00 (organic brain disorders) to F99 (a mental disorder not otherwise specified).

Depressive disorders have sometimes been argued to be a way to give a diagnosis to normal distress or suffering, such as bereavement. In the new DSM-5, and also in the forthcoming ICD-11, there are separate diagnoses for prolonged or complicated bereavement (DSM-5 diagnosis, persistent complex bereavement disorder, PCBD, and ICD-11 prolonged grief disorder, PGD). It should be emphasized that especially moderate and severe depression are disturbing and disabling states, and labeling them merely justified of natural reactions may cause reasonable confusion and shame to individuals.

The current descriptive diagnostic classifications do not include biological markers for psychiatric disorders, or on the other hand, measures for social or other functioning other than that these are most often expected to be disturbed. All medical disorders, psychiatric disorders in particular, affect patients' psychological—including cognition and affects—and social functioning, in addition to the suffering they involve.

Depressive Disorders

A depressive mood is one of the core components in the list of typical symptoms, which form the concept of a depressive disorder, when appearing simultaneously in a dominant and disturbing manner. The validity and reliability of the concept are based on epidemiological and clinical research. In its mild form, a depressive disorder may not be recognized by other people, but a moderate disorder disturbs functioning, and in a severe depression the subject is unable to perform well occupationally or otherwise.

In the current *International Classification of Diseases*, the ICD-10, depressive disorders include single or recurrent major depressive disorders, persistent (dysthymic) depressive disorder, and unspecified depressive disorders. In addition, the concept of mood disorders includes the diagnosis of bipolar disorder with both depressive and manic episodes, but it is usually not included in this class of common mental disorders.

There are no known directly etiological or causal risk factors for depressive disorders. However, genetic factors contribute to the pathophysiology, as well as many environmental, short- or long- term precipitants. Socioeconomical disadvantage, distress, traumas, and adversities associate with the likelihood of developing a depressive disorder. The development of depressive disorders is often seen as a process, in which the genetic liability, interacting with environmental factors during lifetime, as well as more recent adversities, leads to a full-blown syndrome. A particular form of adversities is interpersonal loss, like partnership breakups or bereavement, which emphasizes the importance of social life, bonds, and commitments.

Clinical Picture and Diagnostic Criteria for a Major Depressive Episode

A clinical description by WHO states:

> In typical mild, moderate, or severe depressive episodes, the patient suffers from lowering of mood, reduction of energy, and decrease in activity. Capacity for enjoyment, interest, and concentration is reduced, and marked tiredness after even minimum effort is common. Sleep is usually disturbed, and appetite diminished. Self-esteem and self-confidence are almost always reduced and, even in the mild form, some ideas of guilt or worthlessness are often present. The lowered mood varies little from day to day, is unresponsive to circumstances and may be accompanied by so-called "somatic symptoms," such as loss of interest and pleasurable feelings, waking in the morning several hours before the usual time, depression worst in the morning, marked psychomotor retardation, agitation, loss of appetite, weight loss, and loss of libido. Depending upon the number and severity of the symptoms, a depressive episode may be specified as mild, moderate or severe.[1]

A typical but not exclusive feature of a depressive disorder is significantly lowered mood. The disorder may involve a feeling of intense sadness or depressiveness, loss of pleasures, or a constant and deep tiredness. Following the WHO ICD-10 classification that is used worldwide, the most common clinical manifestation is a depressive episode with at least 2 of the 3 key symptoms of depressive mood, loss of pleasure, and fatigue, complemented by a variety of additional symptoms ranging from changes in sleep and appetite to suicidal thoughts. Concentration, appetite, sleep, and self-confidence are typically disturbed in various ways. The severity of depression is assessed by the number of symptoms, so that a mild depression presents with 4–5 symptoms, moderate with 6–7, and severe with 8–10. The disorder may also include psychotic symptoms, like unrealistic negative beliefs or even auditory hallucinations (Box 24.1).

A parallel classification system for mental disorders is the diagnostic and statistical system for mental disorders (DSM-5) maintained by the American Psychiatric Association. The ICD and DSM systems are thought to differ from each other only slightly, and their basic concepts for depressive and anxiety disorders are fairly similar.

The typical symptom profile for adolescent major depression differs from that of the adult symptom profile. The core symptom of adolescent depression appears to be loss of energy, followed in prevalence by insomnia. Contrary to earlier findings, new evidence shows irritable mood being rare in adolescent depression. In this regard, the possibility of an underlying bipolar disorder should also be taken into consideration when evaluating adolescent mood symptoms.

The severity and clinical manifestation of depressive disorders vary greatly. In dysthymia, often mild symptoms of depression may cause subjective misery, but the ability to function may be rather well-preserved, although typically the course of the disorder is chronic. Conversely, in severe depression, a person may be totally unable to function, but the state can remit into normal mood and functioning. Occasionally depression may involve symptoms of irritation and anxious activity, which may cause diagnostic confusion. Similarly, sleep or appetite may both be either decreased or increased.

BOX 24.1 ICD-10 Diagnostic Criteria for a Major Depressive Episode

Key Symptoms

Persistent sadness or low mood

Loss of interests or pleasure

Fatigue or low energy

Associated Symptoms

Disturbed sleep

Poor concentration or indecisiveness

Low self-confidence

Poor or increased appetite

Suicidal thoughts or acts

Agitation or slowing of movements

Guilt or self-blame

Anxiety Disorders Diagnoses and Clinical Picture

Another diagnostic category of the common mental disorders is anxiety disorders. The ICD-10 anxiety disorders include as separate entities: agoraphobia, social phobia, specific-, and other or unspecified phobias, panic disorder, and generalized anxiety disorder (F40–F41). In addition, the forthcoming ICD-11 will also classify separation anxiety disorder and selective mutism. Stress-related disorders, like post-traumatic stress disorder (F43.1), are included in the same ICD-10 main division (F40–F48) with anxiety disorders as well as obsessive-compulsive disorder (F42). The ICD-10 also includes a category of a mixed depressive and anxiety disorder (F41.2). The diagnosis refers to a state where both depressive symptoms and anxiety dominate simultaneously, but the symptoms are milder and do not fulfill the diagnostic criteria for either depressive or other anxiety disorders.

There is a clear genetic liability for anxiety disorders; and a tense or anxiety-related family upbringing increases the risk for these disorders, too. In many cases, these genetic and environmental factors interact in a synergistic manner. In addition, distressful or traumatic experiences can reportedly contribute to the emerging of anxiety disorders. The ICD also classifies a separate category of reactive- or stress-related disorders.

The clinical picture of anxiety disorders constitutes a disturbing and often intensive sense of anxiety or fears, and its consequences on an individual's behavior. The sense of anxiety, tension, or worry may appear as attacks, or a prevailing state. Attacks can be triggered by either social situations or feared objects or situations (social phobia or specific phobias), or they can appear without preceding triggers (panic disorder).

A typical and clinically important consequential symptom is the development of avoidance of the experienced cause of the anxiety, e.g., social situations or places that cause phobic fears. Anxiety disorders typically emerge in adolescent years and may disturb the individual's social life or occupational career. Anxiety in social situations or fear of panic attacks can significantly affect choices made at a relatively young age, and have thus serious long-term, or even lifelong consequences. General anxiety disorder (GAD) involves intensive, overwhelming, and disturbing worrying over stressors, like personal health or economy. Anxiety disorders may cause remarkable subjective suffering, while not being particularly recognizable by peers and other people, but avoidance of social situations may cause social degradation.

Risk Factors for the Common Mental Disorders

Causal risk factors for mental disorders in general hardly exist. These disorders are typically multifactorial and complex, involving a genetic predisposition, a variety of external long- and short-term precipitating factors, and their interactive combinations. However, epidemiological research has been continuing to find relative risk factors that are estimated to increase the probability of the disorders. Several national and multinational epidemiological surveys have been conducted in order to estimate the prevalence and burden of mental disorders, and their so-called epidemiological risk factors.

Depressive disorders in general are more common among socioeconomically disadvantaged people, and females are almost at 2-fold risk. Being employed and married decreases the risk, whereas lower education associates with increased prevalence. These associations are most likely reciprocal, meaning that environmental or external distress contributes to the development of depressive symptoms, and on the other hand, severe depression can cause role impairment and drift toward socioeconomical adversity. On the other hand, these risk factors are not exclusive, and depressive and anxiety disorders are prevalent comprehensively all over the adult population, regardless of socioeconomic or other status.

Anxiety disorders, particularly panic disorders and phobias, generally start at a younger age than depressive disorders, typically at young adulthood. Their course is somewhat fluctuating, by remitting often easily, but relapsing over time, partially precipitated by external stress and adversities.

Reported childhood adversities also associate with depressive and anxiety disorders in cross-sectional studies. Although recall bias and "effort after meaning" are likely to increase retrospective reporting of adversities, many adversities and traumas most likely add to the risk of developing a depressive or anxiety disorder later on.

Epidemiology of the Common Mental Disorders

Depressive and anxiety represent the most prevalent categories of mental disorders. An estimate by the WHO World Mental Health Study (WMSH) of the global prevalence of a major depressive disorder involves a point prevalence of 4.7% (3.7%–5.5%) with observable, but statistically nonsignificant regional differences.[2]

In a systematic review and meta-analysis, Steel and colleagues estimated that 1 in 5 of the global population suffered from a common mental disorder during the last 12 months, when substance use disorders were included.[3] In a World Mental Health Survey report covering 65 countries, depressive episodes were relatively the most frequent in low-income countries and the least frequent in middle-income countries. Among high-income countries, the incidence of depressive episodes was associated with economical inequity as measured by the Gini index.[4]

The global prevalence of anxiety disorders was estimated in a review including 87 epidemiological studies across 44 countries, between 1980 and 2009. After adjustments for confounding factors, the global point prevalence of anxiety disorders was 7.3% (4.8%–10.9%), ranging from 5.3% (3.5%–8.1%) in African cultures to 10.4% (7.0%–15.5%) in Euro/Anglo cultures.[5]

WHO estimates that some global variation exists in the prevalence of depressive and anxiety disorders:

Prevalence of common mental disorders (% of population by WHO Region)

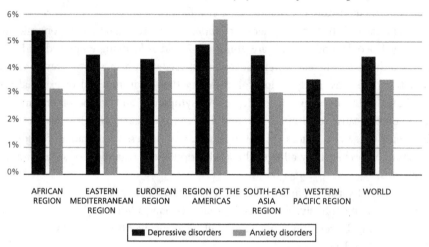

Source: Global burden of Disease Study 2015 (*http://ghdx.healthdata.org/gbd.result.tool*)
Regional data shown are age-standardized estimates.

Course and Outcome

In general, the prevalence rates peak in older adulthood, meaning that females age 55–70 years have the highest prevalence of above 7.5%. Depression is usually 2-fold more common among females than males in most populations.[6] In adult populations, the median age of onset for mood disorders is 32 years, and gender differences in prevalence of depressed mood seem to develop before that age. The first episode of major depression may occur in childhood, and pediatric depression is suggested to have high risk of recurrence.[7,8] Comorbid psychopathology is also highly common in clinical juvenile populations. The prevalence of mood disorders increases in adolescence, with lifetime prevalence of US adolescents being 14%.[7,9] The detrimental effects on neuropsychological functioning of depressive symptoms may be stronger in early adolescence.

As common mental disorders, depressive and anxiety disorders are easily recurring, or in part of the cases, chronic in nature. Anxiety disorders begin at a relatively younger age—the median of age of onset being 13 years—but during adolescent development, may remit fully and permanently. However, a fluctuating course is also common. Initiation of depressive disorders occurs typically in the thirties or forties, but variation is wide, as is the severity. Recurring major depression that starts at a younger age is thought to be either relatively more severe, or appears to switch into a bipolar affective disorder in follow-up.

Both of these disorders have a high risk of comorbidity, meaning that either simultaneous or sequential other mental disorders emerge. Depressive and anxiety disorders appear often together, leading to diagnostic and therapeutic challenges. Actually, ICD-10 also describes a mixed depressive and anxiety state. Comorbid substance use disorders are also quite common, up to 30%–40% in both disorders in follow-up, and even half have a personality disorder.[6]

Depressive disorders, in particular, are associated with an elevated suicide risk, especially when comorbid with other disorders. Depression is often considered as the most common so-called gateway disorder in suicidal processes, meaning that it exists in a variety of suicidal paths in some form, and often as a final contributor. Approximately 800,000 people die due to a suicide in the world every year, and suicide is the second leading cause of death among youngsters from 15 to 29 years.[10] In 2015, 78% of suicides occurred in low- and middle-income countries (LAMIC). Compared to the risk to meet another kind of violent death, the risk for suicidal death is nearly 2-fold higher than homicidal death, over 8-fold higher than death in war, and over 40-fold higher than terroristic death.[6]

Treatment and Rehabilitation of the Common Mental Disorders

The treatment of depressive and anxiety disorders is usually divided into biological and psychosocial components. Biological treatments include pharmacological and neuromodulation therapies. The first medication specified for depressive disorders, tricyclic antidepressants, was launched in 1950s. The tricyclic antidepressants have an impact on several neurotransmitters, typically the monoamines. The next huge advancement in the pharmacotherapy among depressive disorders was in 1990s, when the use of selective serotonin reuptake inhibitors (SSRIs) was established. In psychotic or severe depression, without any noteworthy effect of antidepressive medication, the augmentation strategies are recommended. Since the 1990s, SSRIs have been a drug of choice also in the treatment of many anxiety disorders. A consequent reduction of the use of previously used benzodiazepines has been presumed but not constantly seen.

The first neuromodulation treatment for depression was electro-convulsive therapy (ECT). The first ECT session was put into practice in 1930s. There was a quiet phase in the medical use of ECT, but since the 1990s the utilization of ECT has arisen, especially in the care of the most serious or complex cases of depression. Repetitive transcranial magnetic stimulation (rTMS) was introduced in 1985. In rTMS an alternating magnetic field stimulates neurons. Transcranial direct current stimulation (tDCS) is a more recent treatment among neuromodulation treatments. The therapeutic mechanism of tDCS relies on the technique where electrodes induce direct weak current regional changes in cortical excitability. In addition, there are also other electromagnetic methods used, e.g., invasive deep brain stimulation.

Psychotherapies are demonstrated to be an effective treatment for depressive and anxiety disorders. Psychotherapy alone may be effective enough for mild to moderate major depression. In more severe or recurrent depression, a combination of antidepressive medication and psychotherapy is indicated fairly invariably as a more efficient treatment than one of them alone. The clinical evidence is supporting for the use of cognitive-behavioral therapy (CBT), interpersonal, psychodynamic, or problem-solving therapy, or behavioral activation (BA) in the acute phase. For recurrent or complicated depression, there is evidence for the efficacy of CBT, psychodynamic, and interpersonal psychotherapy. In addition, short- or medium-term Cognitive Behavioral Analysis System of Psychotherapy (CBASP) seems to be effective for acute and rehabilitative treatment in long-term depression. Growing evidence points at the unspecific factors being effective in psychotherapies, and the role of the technique relative to that. One could argue that qualified, often eclectic and individualized psychosocial treatment may be the treatment of choice, particularly in case of a lack of formal psychotherapists.

The central symptoms of major depressive disorder (MDD), the lack of energy and interest, are usually bounded up with many behavioral and cognitive changes like lack of initiative, inefficiency, difficulties in concentration, and social withdrawal. Furthermore, when the latency in in help-seeking is from time to time rather long, those dysfunctional modes of experience or action may be at risk for become chronic. For recovery, the positive behavioral changes are crucial in depressive disorders at issue. In many cases, biological or psychological therapies alone or combined are not enough, but rehabilitative interventions are also needed. Social or vocational rehabilitation usually comprises different group activities, individual coaching and support, peer support. and modifications at the workplace. The goal for rehabilitation is to gradually enhance the functional and/or work ability of the patient.

For anxiety disorders like panic disorder, social and other phobias, cognitive behavioral psychotherapeutic techniques are useful. Cognitive reprocessing, hyposensibilization or exposure training, and psychoeducation are possible psychotherapeutic strategies. As pharmacotherapy, SSRIs and other antidepressive agents can be effective for anxiety disorders.

Managing treatment in different societies varies according to resources and cultural and political factors. In societies with low resources, treatment is usually managed in primary care settings. Treatment options like different psychotherapeutic techniques may not be available, but primary community services can provide general support and psychopharmacological treatments. In more resourced settings, so-called secondary level specialized psychiatric services may exist, or even tertiary, which means highly educated and centralized units, like evaluation teams for double diagnosis patients.

Depression and Anxiety in Western Societies

The idea of an increase in the prevalence of the common mental disorders has not been supported by epidemiological research. They do not seem to represent, as implicitly thought, consequences of modernization or distress caused by social or cognitive challenges of contemporary life. However, in Western societies, presented by 27 European countries, despite a relative stability of depressive and anxiety disorders, their effect on occupational disability seems to have been on the rise. The impression of increasing prevalence of mental disorders may be connected to growing care-seeking, especially among young people. However, WHO forecasts that depressive and anxiety disorders will become more frequent in the future because the populations in lower-income countries are growing fast, and at the same time, life expectancy grows. As a result, more people than before reach the age when depression and anxiety disorders break out. Furthermore, their relative importance within all medical conditions is likely to rise during an increasing control of global health threats by infectious diseases, like diarrhea. Globally, a better recognition of the common mental disorders, both in general and in possibly developing mental health services, may reveal a true burden caused by them.

In Western countries, reasons for the discrepancy between the stability of the common mental disorders and the increase in sick leaves and pensioning remain somewhat unclear.

It is likely that when in general mental disorders have become more acceptable or less stigmatizing, people have been more willing to admit that their functioning has been disturbed due to mental health problems. On the other hand, it is possible that the attitudes of the labor market in the case of mental problems have moved toward more demanding and less tolerant.

Particularly in aging Western societies, the occupational disability caused by depressive and anxiety disorders has become an economic and a public health issue. Early intervention strategies, as well as interventions associated with working life, have emerged. Social insurance institutions and private companies have become increasingly interested in workplace support, occupational healthcare, and vocational rehabilitation, which all aim at maintaining the occupational functioning and productiveness of the people.

Global Issues

Most of the research on mental disorders has been conducted in the estern countries. The Mapping Project conducted in the middle of 20th century by Global Forum for Health Research and the WHO revealed that even among the LMICs, the richest three, namely China, India, and Brazil, account for 40% of the mental health publications indexed.[11]. Depressive symptomatology may vary between ethnic groups, and estimating the prevalence with questionnaires may be affected by cultural biases. Thus, it may be argued that depression has been investigated through a Western gaze, emphasizing the symptoms of an individual.

Alonso and a large group of researchers reported in 2018 on a huge project with translation, backtranslation, and harmonization protocol, using culturally competent bilingual clinicians assessing the prevalence of anxiety disorders worldwide with WHO Composite International Diagnostic Interview (CIDI) Version 3.0.[12] They found that 1 in 10 adults had suffered from one or more anxiety disorder during the past year. The prevalence varied between countries, but it was not systematically lower in low-income countries. Despite the symptoms warranting a diagnosis, less than half of the individuals reported a need for treatment. The lack of perceived need for treatment was one of the main reasons for the treatment gap. A similar finding has been made among Finnish adolescents: only a third of depressed individuals reported a need for help, even though help would be easily accessible through school health services.

In 2007 the *Lancet* published a series of papers calling the global community into action to innovate services for people with mental disorders, especially in low- and middle-income countries. A new movement, Global Mental Health, was introduced by the international psychiatric community. The approach stressed the need for evidence-based interventions, sharing knowledge and experiences, and promoting human rights worldwide.[13,14]

In 2016 the WHO developed the second version of the Mental Health Gap Action Programme Intervention Guide (mhGAP-IG) comprising clinical guidelines for providing evidence-based practices by non-specialized healthcare providers, such as family physicians or nurses after a training period.[1]

Here is an example of the Assessment and management guide on how to treat depression:

Assessment and Management Guide

1. Does the person have moderate-severe depression?

» **For at least 2 weeks, has the person had at least 2 of the following core depression symptoms:**
- Depressed mood (most of the day, almost every day), (for children and adolescents: either *irritability or depressed mood*)
- Loss of interest or pleasure in activities that are normally pleasurable
- Decreased energy or easily fatigued

» **During the last 2 weeks has the person had at least 3 other features of depression:**
- Reduced concentration and attention
- Reduced self-esteem and self-confidence
- Ideas of guilt and unworthiness
- Bleak and pessimistic view of the future
- Ideas or acts of self-harm or suicide
- Disturbed sleep
- Diminished appetite

» **Does the person have difficulties carrying out usual work, school, domestic, or social activities?**

Check for recent bereavement or other major loss in prior 2 months.

YES

If **YES** to all 3 questions then: **moderate-severe depression is likely**

» Psychoeducation. » **DEP 2.1**
» Address current psychosocial stressors. » **DEP 2.2**
» Reactivate social networks. » **DEP 2.3**
» Consider antidepressants. ⊕ » **DEP 3**
» If available, consider interpersonal therapy, behavioural activation or cognitive behavioural therapy. » **INT**
» If available, consider adjunct treatments: structured physical activity programme » **DEP 2.4**, relaxation training or problem-solving treatment. » **INT**
» **DO NOT** manage the complaint with injections or other ineffective treatments (e.g. vitamins).⊘
» Offer regular follow-up. » **DEP 2.5**

NO

If **NO** to some or all of the three questions and if no other priority conditions have been identified on the mhGAP-IG Master Chart

» Exit this module, and assess for Other Significant Emotional or Medically Unexplained somatic Complaints » **OTH**

In case of recent bereavement or other recent major loss

*Follow the above advise but **DO NOT** consider antidepressants or psychotherapy as first line treatment.* ⊕ *Discuss and support culturally appropriate mourning/adjustment.*

The Global Mental Health concept, like any other concept, has received some criticism. It has been argued to be yet another form of colonialism or medical imperialism trying to bring Western concepts and interventions into the developing world and ignoring the culturally determined nature of mental illness and traditional healing techniques.[14] On the other hand, in countries struggling to get more resources to establishing a system of modern psychiatric practice, psychiatrists criticize the idea of treating severe mental illness in the communities only. The history of treating mental illness in the community may have included serious violations of human rights.

The rising understanding that mental illness is causing a large proportion of disability and economic burden in the world is not only a good argument for asking for more resources to mental health promotion and treatment of illnesses. It may also be a way to transform complex political issues of poverty and inequality into the medical dilemma of an individual. If people in low socioeconomic status bear the highest proportion of mental suffering, they should perhaps be helped both medically and socially. It is not enough to consider the social determinants of health without attending to greater political and economic processes that lead to inequalities.[15]

New means of treating psychological suffering without labeling have been introduced in developing countries and imported to developed countries as well. An example is the "Friendship Bench" model in Harare, Zimbabwe. This intervention is an application of problem-solving therapy adapted for use by lay health workers. Tools and language with cultural validity were used to reduce symptom severity of depression and anxiety in community settings.[16] The "Granny on the Bench" approach has been introduced in disadvantaged areas of New York, Malawi, Tanzania, and Kenya, and is being scaled up elsewhere, too.

While depression is seen as being associated with economic disadvantage in both regional and global perspective, another point of view is its role in contemporary occupational life. As said, in many Western economies, the proportion of depressive disorders in occupational disability seems to be on the rise. On the other hand, we can expect a substantial amount of reactive and stress-related depressive and anxiety disorders in disturbed and crisis areas, and in refugee and other migrating populations, in addition to other psychiatric disorders.

The Burden of Depression

Depressive disorders are the largest reasons for non-fatal health loss globally, counted as years lived with disability (YLD). Depression accounts 7.5% of all YLD. In addition to decreased capacity to function, depression causes emotional, social. and economic burden to the patients, their families, and their social networks. Unipolar depression is a remarkable factor behind the decreased ability to work.

The costs of MDD increased from US$173 billion to US$211 billion in the United States from 2005 to 2010. Of the total costs, 38% were related directly to MDD and comorbidities, 5% were suicide-related, and 50% were work-related costs. In Europe, costs of anxiety disorders grew from US$41 billion to US$66 billion from 2004 to 2010 and mood disorders from US$106 billion to US$113 billion, respectively. Indirect costs composed over 60% of the total costs in mood disorders and nearly 40% in anxiety disorders in Europe in 2010. The costs and burden of common mental disorders in the LAMIC is still largely un- or underestimated.[6,17]

Conclusion

Depressive and anxiety disorders, conceptualized as the common mental disorders, are a major cause of suffering and disability worldwide, although their impact has often been overlooked by the more severe chronical mental illnesses. In Western countries they have gained increasing attention due to their impact on occupational capacity, and on the other hand, the well-being and development of younger people. In the developing and low- and middle-income countries, the existence of these disorder may be obscured by a range of other problems and scarcity of services available for recognition and actions.

References

1. World Health Organization. *mhGAP Intervention Guide for Mental, Neurological and Substance Use Disorders in Nonspecialized Health Settings, Version 2.0.* Geneva: World Health Organization; 2016.
2. Ferrari AJ, Charlson FJ, Norman RE, et al. Burden of depressive disorders by country, sex, age, and year: findings from the global burden of disease study 2010. PLoS Med. 2013 Nov;10(11):e1001547.
3. Steel Z, Marnane C, Iranpour C, Chey T, Jackson JW, Patel V, Silove D. The global prevalence of common mental disorders: a systematic review and meta-analysis 1980–2013. *Int J Epidemiol.* 2014 Apr;43(2):476–493. Published online 2014 Mar 19. doi:10.1093/ije/dyu038. PMCID: PMC3997379. PMID: 24648481.
4. Cifuentes M, Sembajwe G, Tak S, Gore R, Kriebel D, Punnett L. The association of major depressive episodes with income inequality and the human development index. Soc Sci Med. 2008 Aug;67(4):529–539.
5. Baxter AJ, Scott KM, Vos T, Whiteford HA. Global prevalence of anxiety disorders: a systematic review and meta-regression. *Psychol Med.* 2013 May;43(5):897–910.
6. World Health Organization. *Depression and Other Common Mental Disorders: Global Health Estimates.* Geneva: WHO; 2017. https://apps.who.int›WHO-MSD-MER-2017.2-eng.pdf.
7. Kovacs M, Obrosky S, George C. The course of major depressive disorder from childhood to young adulthood: recovery and recurrence in a longitudinal observational study. *J Affect Disord.* 2016;203:374–381. https://doi.org/10.1016/j.jad.2016.05.042.
8. Wilson A, Hicks BM, Foster KT, McGue M. Age of onset and course of major depressive disorder: associations with psychosocial functioning outcomes in adulthood. *Psychol Med.* 2015; 45(3): 505–514.
9. Merikangas K, He J-P, Burstein M, et al. Lifetime prevalence of mental disorders in U.S. Adolescents: results from the National Comorbidity Survey Replication–Adolescent Supplement (NCS-A). *J Am Acad Child Adolesc Psychiatry.* 2010;49(10):980–989.
10. Turecki G, Brent DA. Suicide and suicidal behaviour. *Lancet.* 2016 Mar 19;387(10024):1227–1239.
11. Mental health systems in selected low- and middle-income countries: a WHO-AIMS crossnational analysis. World Health Organization; January 2009. https://www.who.int/mental_health/publications/research_capacity_mh_low_middle_income_countries/en/.
12. Alonso J, Liu Z, Evans-Lacko S, et al. Treatment gap for anxiety disorders is global: Results of the World Mental Health Surveys in 21 countries. *Depress Anxiety.* 2018 Mar;35(3):195–208.
13. Patel V, Saxena S, Lund C, et al. The Lancet Commission on global mental health and sustainable development. *Lancet.* 2018;392:1553–1598.

14. Cooper S. Global mental health and its critics: moving beyond the impasse. *Crit Public Health*. 2016;26(4):355–358.

15. Gajaria A, Izenberg JM, Nguyen V, et al. Moving the global mental health debate forward: how a structural competency framework can apply to global mental health training. *Acad Psychiatry*. 2019;43:617–620. https://doi.org/10.1007/s40596-019-01073-3.

16. Chibanda D, Weiss HA, Verhey R, et al. Effect of a primary care–based psychological intervention on symptoms of common mental disorders in Zimbabwe: a randomized clinical trial. JAMA. *2016*;316(24):2618–2626. doi: 10.1001/jama.2016.19102.

17. Greenberg PE, Fournier AA, Sisitsky T, Pike CT, Kessler RC. The economic burden of adults with major depressive disorder in the United States (2005 and 2010). *J Clin Psychiatry*. 2015 Feb;76(2):155–162.

25

A Social Psychological Perspective on Trauma and Trauma Disorders

Maryssa Lyons, Daniel Buhalo, and April Fallon

Worldwide, more than 70% of adults will experience at least one stressful event in their lives.[1] Many of these are sudden and unexpected, as on September 11, 2001, when planes crashed into the World Trade Center in New York. However, the places a person frequents or where they reside can increase such a possibility. For example, living in Khorramshahr, Iran, when Iraq invaded the Iranian city (1980–1982) would likely have increased the changes of encountering such an unexpected and negative event. Much attention has been given in the media to the effects and aftermath of natural catastrophes, such as the 2004 Indian Ocean earthquake-tsunami, and to human-induced ones, such as the Sri Lankan civil war, as well as the interpersonal ones such as rape.

An enduring psychological trauma does not automatically result from experiencing such an event. Many exposed to these events respond with an initial acute stress reaction or increased anxiety which remits spontaneously over the course of a few months. A small group of those will present with a more decreased functionality. The proportion of those who have a more enduring and chronic impairment depends upon a number of factors, including how *trauma* is defined, the type of event, social identity and supports, and other individual factors. Why many may endure a number of these events and continue to function, or even experience a post-traumatic growth, and why some become chronically disabled when the experience is only indirectly relayed remains a mystery to many researchers and clinicians.

In this chapter we first explore the nature of the changing definition of trauma, with a brief historical review of the clinical phenomena associated with trauma. We will illuminate how over time sociological and cultural forces have framed our understanding of what and how a negative event impacts the trauma experience, contributing to impairment and functionality. We include the contributions of the psychiatric community in delineating the diagnosis of post-traumatic stress disorder (PTSD). We also review the contributions of psychoanalytic theory to our understanding of trauma. We next consider a sociocultural perspective to frame trauma. We delineate the sociological elements of social identity and social supports that affect the traumatic response. Lastly we discuss treatment, primarily emphasizing the social elements that may aid in the attenuation of the disorders and impairment.

Defining Trauma

In everyday parlance there are two different definitions of trauma. A medical definition of trauma refers to "a body wound or shock produced by sudden physical injury, as from violence or accident" (https://www.dictionary.com/browse/trauma?s=t). In this context, a discrete event results in an observable injury or trauma to the body. From a psychological perspective, a somewhat different definition of trauma emerges; it is "an experience that produces psychological injury or pain (https://www.dictionary.com/browse/trauma?s=t.). While psychiatry has tried to limit and further refine "psychological injury" by the use of *Diagnostic and Statistical Manual* (DSM) and *International Classification of Diseases* (ICD) definitions and diagnoses, both "experience" and "pain" permit a very wide intersubjective berth. This understanding of the term promotes the notion that the individual's interactions with the world (and external events) are passed through an internal and subjective lens and are judged to be dangerous and harmful such that the individual suffers. Thus we see two definitions and two dimensions emerge: the physical-psychological and the direct and inevitable injury versus the experiential lens which interprets a danger.

Both of the medical and psychological definitions describe the negative *impact* on the individual. Yet, in some circles, trauma has come to denote the event that occurs, not its impact. As Summerfield suggests, "In Western societies, the conflation of distress with 'trauma' increasingly has a naturalistic feel."[2(p96)] For example, on the US Department of Veterans affairs website (https://www.ptsd.va.gov/understand/common/common_adults.asp), the first paragraph suggests this confusion in their definition of trauma, "A trauma is a shocking and dangerous event that you see or that happens to you. During this type of event, you think that your life or others' lives are in danger." Such a shift, perhaps subtle, infers that the event equals either physical or psychological injury or both. In these conceptualizations, which are to some extent socially constructed, there is the implication the event is equivalent to the "injury."

Thus, there are two elements to our use of trauma that lead to the confusion. First is the dimension of physicality—whether etiology of trauma is a somatic injury or intraopsychic (not of the soma). Second is whether the event is sine qua non to the impact. Is a traumatic experience the result of an event alone, or of the subjective experience or interpretation? A brief review of the history of trauma will further elaborate the changing sociological conceptions of our notions of trauma and will illuminate the elements of conflation in our understanding.

Brief Medical History of Our Understanding of Trauma

In the mid- to late 1800s, doctors were observing that railway and industrial accidents without physical injury sometimes resulted in otherwise healthy individuals exhibiting behaviors such as intense memories of the event, headaches, and seizures. This came to be labeled as "railway spine" and "traumatic neurosis," which was attributed to an increasingly mechanized society and reckless industrialists.[3a] Deemed to be damaging to the brain or nervous system, the risks of "modern life" were seen as infiltrating the mind. In approximately the same era, Charcot documented similar neurological symptoms that had no physical origins. After studying many cases, he linked male "traumatic hysteria" to traumatic shock rather than sexuality or emotional distress.[4] He was able temporarily to create these symptoms with hypnosis, but the same technique did not permanently reduce symptoms already present. Janet[5] and Freud[6] suggested that these symptoms were psychological in nature—individuals could not tolerate the meaning of the event or their emotional reactions to it and entered an altered state of consciousness (dissociation), which they termed "hysteria."[b] Much of our understanding of trauma originates in the psychoanalytic literature, which we will return to it later in the chapter.

World War I ushered in more widespread trauma response; "shell shock"[c] was viewed as a result of battlefield experiences. Episodes of blindness, deafness, and muteness were initially given an organic explanation, as it was thought to be the result of those having been close to explosions. It was later determined that symptoms occurred for many even though they had not directly experienced the events. In Europe there was widespread belief that well-prepared units with high morale would be immune from it, while those suffering from these symptoms were perhaps either afraid, unprepared, or malingering.[3] British psychiatrist Yealland treated these soldiers with threats and electrical shock, while Rivers used more humane methods that permitted return to the battlefield without the traumatic neuroses (https://newperspectivesinc.com/the-history-of-psychological-trauma/).

Freud originally argued that actual sexual experiences during early life caused the trauma. In his later work, he transitioned to believe that actual experience was important and that soldiers were not prepared for the psychological burdens of war. He distinguished between traumatic neuroses resulting from real experiences and anxiety neuroses caused by

---

a. In DSM I, this concept was introduced as "shell shock" which referred to veterans who were suffering from psychological symptoms cause by their direct experience with life and death experiences during World War I (American Psychiatric Association. *Diagnostic and statistical manual of mental disorders*. Washington, DC; 1952).

b. Freud initially felt that his patients, mostly female, experienced sexual trauma, but later came to believe that these experiences were not based in reality, but were the result of conflict between fantasy and the unacceptable nature of the internal desire.

c. Always an after-the-fact experience, Nachträglichkeit (see Prager).

sexual and aggressive fantasies.[7] As the war ended, doctors continued to ponder the boundaries between cowardice, honor, and psychic injury.[8,9]

During World War II, there was some attempt to prepare young men for the experience of war with pamphlets that suggested. "heroes—apparently tough men . . . even the strongest . . . had his breaking point."[3(p 39)] Kardiner,[10] an American psychiatrist, viewed the symptom reaction as an adaptation when the psychological resources needed to process the event were greater than what the individual was able to muster at that time. He and Spiegel viewed soldiers with these symptoms to be suffering from their loss of attachment to their units and treated them close to their units with recreation and hypnosis. Although symptoms were ameliorated, it was felt that this state would not be permanent due to the "lasting effects of trauma on the mind" (https://newperspectivesinc.com/the-history-of-psychological-trauma/).

Interest in traumatic response waned until the Vietnam War. Lifton testified before Congress unlike the previous wars, it was "dreadful, filthy, unnecessary."[14(p10911)] Domestic protests of the war contributed significantly to the veterans' alienation upon returning home. Vietnam vets returned with understandable guilt as ". . . .all civilized men who have ever been sent to make murder in the name of virtue. . . ."[12(p27)] PTSD was first introduced in the DSM-III,[13] creating the basis of our current understanding of the disorder. Personality and risk factors were less important than the severity of the experience, as a defining feature of the disorder placed the etiology as outside the victim. The DSM-III elaborates that the event needs to be "outside the range of usual human experience."[13(p236)] It has been said that the introduction of ". . . the PTSD diagnosis was recognition and metaphorical restitution for the suffering soldiers endured for the nation in Vietnam."[14(p 114)] This diagnosis allowed for restitution in the form of ongoing service-connected disability monies. The "service-connected" compensation awarded implies that the dangers of war are irreparable and led to permanent psychological dysfunction. In this decision and definition of trauma, the etiology is outside the victim, and predisposition prior to the event is not considered. In the minds of some, "PTSD significantly organizes the current rhetoric of victimhood,"[3(p 40)] and has become a symbol of suffering. We see here the infusion of social realities and injustices into the definitions of an individual psychological disorder. Much of our understanding had previously been influenced by psychoanalytic thinking which began in the previous century but continues to evolve to this day. We pause to review those contributions in the next section.

Psychoanalytic Contributions to Trauma Disorders

Much of our more detailed understanding of the origins and effects of trauma begin with Freud's clinical observations. His initial formulation conceptualized the traumatic reaction as the result of being unable to process actual events that occurred. At a later point, the experience included not only actual events, but fantasies related predominantly to conflicts around sexuality. When the emotion accompanying the frightening event is able to be experienced, it becomes an ordinary recollection. When frightening events cannot be processed (the affect and event too much for the person to bear and the mind is flooded with overwhelming emotion), the event becomes stored in a second consciousness, which is split off or dissociated from conscious awareness.[15] In *Beyond the Pleasure Principle*, Freud suggests that a frightening event, if not processed, could lead individuals to repeat in recurrent intrusive conscious memories some of the most threatening parts of the experience. Edith Jacobson[16] emphasized that a traumatic event (which could also include fantasy and conflict) overwhelms the self (ego) as a previously healthy self-representation, challenged by the inability to control the event, conflicts with a new self that is worthless, humiliated, and dependent. Phyllus Greenacre[17] adds that potentially traumatic experiences occur for all children and adolescents. It is the intensity, timing and kind that impact psychological growth and development. She is one of the first to suggest that later traumatic experiences are impacted by earlier trauma experiences and the individual's previously developed ego resources. The pathogentic pathway from event to symptom development occurs when the individual cannot differentiate psychologically whether there is an impending threat versus an actual life-threatening dangerous situation.[18] Impending threats do not just signal the possibility of helplessness, but become actual threats in the individual's mind.

Later psychoanalytic writers, Scharff and Scharff[19] emphasize the importance of the intrapsychic experience and the role of dependency and helplessness in the trauma experience. Kalsched[20] added that it is the inner world that periodically or unremittingly persecutes the victim with images and sensations. It is not the actual event or experience, but the meaning (determined by previous developmental challenges and accomplishments). In Kohutian language, it is how the event changes the individual's perception of the self in relation to self-objects.[21] "The trauma therefore takes on an unconscious meaning which challenges and undermines the person's sense of self, and a symbolically represented in the symptoms of trauma."[22(p 40)] Individuals must integrate the traumatic event into their comprehension of life's meaning, self-construct, and view of the world.[23] The memory of the trauma is not integrated and accepted as a part of one's personal past; time has not healed these psychic wounds.[24] It is dissociated, existing independent of the conscious ego. Traumatic memory is dominated by imagery and bodily sensation.

Immediately after a dangerous event, almost all people have intrusive thoughts about what happened.[25] The intrusions help them learn from the event and plan for a future with a different outcome. When the individual engages with the memory of the dangerous event, anxiety is generated. Under healthy circumstances, a series of engagements and withdrawals with the memory occur. Individuals either gradually accept what happened, integrate it into their self and world, and perhaps readjust expectations, or the affect and sensation are partitioned off.[26] The traumatic event, which may have begun as a social and interpersonal process, comes to have secondary biological consequences that are difficult to reverse. These biological maladaptations frame the symptoms of arousal, attention, stimulus discrimination, and other psychological defenses. A new event can stimulate the memory of something long forgotten. One not previously distressed by memories develops intrusive thoughts about the earlier experience.[24]

Vulnerability plays a role in the long-term adjustment to new traumas. The security of the early attachment bond protects against the development of trauma-induced psychopathology.[27,28] Winnicott[29] described this in the context of a "good enough mother." The lack of good enough mothering or other supportive environment impacts an individual's capacity to trust and view others supportively. During development, when the danger of an "event" overwhelms the internal capacity of the child to feel invulnerable, the mother physically and psychologically holds the child. Over the course of a healthy development, the child develops greater internal resources and a greater acceptance of the realities of body integrity and psychological wholeness.[30] Gradually, slight disappointments in the sensitivities of the mother to perfectly mirror the child's needs allow for a process of transmuting internalization, which provide the child with opportunities to develop a greater psychological fortitude.[21]

Thus the adolescent and later adult face life events imbued at one extreme with a cohesive self and positive internalized representation of others who will be there to support, or at the other end riddled with representations of self and other as negative, unavailable, and unpredictable. Psychological trauma ensues when there is a loss of faith in order, predictability, and continuity in life. Trauma is accompanied by humiliation, helplessness, and an attack on being able to rely on oneself.[24] Avoidance, numbing, and dissociation are employed defensively. For some, there is a compulsive re-exposing to similar situations. Freud[31] thought that this repetition was to achieve mastery, but this is an unlikely event (repetition compulsion).

As Praeger cogently states, "All phenomenon external to the person are filtered from the inside out . . . both primitive and mature co-existing in the individual: primary process, unconscious thought and affect, timeless and fantastic, with other more conscious rationally based secondary process thinking logical and reasonable."[30(p 436)] The subjective meaning of the event in terms of the potency of the threat, the accompanying loss of life, possessions, integrity, or beliefs and accompanying helplessness impact the trauma experience.[24] When a wounding event occurs, beliefs in personal invulnerability, self-efficacy, and belief in a meaningful and predictability world are challenged, and individuals lose agency over their environment and experience the world as unsafe.[22] Thus we conclude from a psychoanalytic perspective that the internal psychological organization filters the external reality, and when this results in maladaptation in terms of current functioning, treatment must involve attention to the internal world, rather than simply the external environment or the resulting external symptomatology.

Contemporary Understandings of Trauma in the Psychiatry Community

The psychiatry community has focused efforts on developing reliable diagnosis of trauma disorders with their continued development of detailed manuals put together by researchers and scholars in the field. DSM iterations and ICD compendium have supported our continued research and fine-tuning of our understanding. We also must mention that biological research has also proliferated in the past few decades and we would be remiss not to briefly summarize some of that work.

DSM-IV

In 1993, the DSM-IV organized PSTD symptoms, time requirements, and severity for making the diagnosis. Most of the controversy around the disorder, however, is around the etiology of the event. The person has been exposed to a traumatic event in which the person experienced, witnessed, or was confronted with an event or events that involved actual or threatened death or serious injury, or a threat to the physical integrity of self or others, and the person's response involved intense fear, helplessness, or horror. The traumatic event is persistently re-experienced by: recurrent and intrusive distressing recollections of the event, including images, thoughts, or perceptions; and/or recurrent distressing dreams of the event; and/or acting or feeling as if the traumatic event were recurring (including a sense of reliving the experience, illusions, hallucinations, and dissociative flashback episodes) .[32(p424)] The definition is broadened to include not only a direct experience, but also the direct witnessing of a dangerous event or "learning" about such an event. Thus we are left with an array of symptoms that must be present (many overlapping with other anxiety disorders) in the context of a subjective reaction of fear, helplessness, and horror to a dangerous event directly or indirectly experienced.

DSM-5 and ICD-11

At present, the two prominent sets of criteria for the diagnosis of PTSD are found in the *International Classification of Diseases*, 11th edition (ICD-11), and the *Diagnostic and Statistical Manual of Mental Disorders*, 5th edition (DSM-5). While these two entities include largely similar descriptions of PTSD and its signature symptoms, they do have notable differences.

ICD-11 is brief and broad in its description of the precipitating traumatic event for PTSD diagnosis, specifying only that the exposure must have been "extremely threatening or horrific."[33] It lists a set of associated symptoms that are largely focused on an aberrant fear response. ICD-11 defines 3 major groups of symptoms: re-experiencing the event, avoidance of thoughts or triggers, and an increased sense of current threat, and requires at least one symptom from each of the 3 primary groups to be concurrent for a period of at least 2 weeks.[33] Of note, ICD-11 includes a separate diagnosis for what is termed *complex PTSD*. For this diagnosis, the above criteria of PTSD are met, with the added presence of decreased ability to manage one's affect, decreased self-worth, and decreased interpersonal relational functioning.[33] Complex PTSD is conceptualized as a separate disorder that is more severe than PTSD alone.

In contrast, DSM-5 is more specific in its requirements for exposure to a traumatic event, but broader in its list of possible symptoms than ICD-11. DSM-5 specifies that the event must have exposed the individual to "actual or threatened death, serious injury, or sexual violence."[34(p271)] It does allow for certain types of indirect exposure to the event, for example in the case of learning that such an event has occurred to a close family member or friend, but in general the DSM-5 is more stringent in its exposure criteria. It also specifically excludes "exposure through electronic media, TV, movies, or pictures,"[(p271)] with one exception in the case of repetitive exposure to these images through one's job.[34] In addition to the 3 symptom clusters identified in ICD-11, DSM-5 includes mood symptoms as a fourth category. It offers a total of 20 possible symptoms with at least 1 or 2 required from each of the 4 categories for a duration of at least 1 month.[34] DSM-5 does not include the diagnosis of complex PTSD as a separate disorder. Rather, DSM-5 includes some of these complex symptoms in its description of the mood symptoms of PTSD.[34]

Although the DSM explicitly excludes most forms of indirect or media exposure to events in its consideration of PTSD, there is mounting evidence that individuals can experience significant trauma symptoms after secondhand exposure to an event. While witnessing an act of violence as it is reported on television or reading about a terrorist attack in print media would not be experiences which put the individual in any immediate danger, repetition of such experiences does have the potential to impact one's perception of relative safety and threat in a similar way to experiencing traumatic events firsthand. Since trauma is itself a construction of the mind which occurs in response to an event or perception, it stands to reason that a pattern of trauma symptoms develops in certain patients with or without direct exposure to a traumatic event.[35]

Biological Bases of PTSD

Risk factors for PTSD and behavioral changes resulting from traumatic experiences do have a biological basis, with differences seen in hormonal signaling and neurocircuitry. The hypothalamic-pituitary-adrenal axis (HPA axis) is responsible for the stress response, its main hormonal mediator being cortisol. Following cortisol's release from the adrenal cortex, it then acts via binding to produce change in response to stress as well as negative feedback.[36] Studies of this system's relationship to PTSD has shown low basal levels of cortisol and exaggerated negative feedback sensitivity. Additionally, studies of glucocorticoid levels and startle responses in at-risk individuals and those with recently developed PTSD showed that both groups had reduced glucocorticoid signaling, while only those with PTSD had the increased startle response.[37] The evidence seen concerning the HPA axis, combined with elevated catecholamine levels in individuals with PTSD, supports the theory that reduced glucocorticoids at the time of experiencing trauma allow for unopposed catecholamine surge, through stimulation of the sympathetic nervous system, resulting in enhanced consolidation of the trauma memory.[37] The main sympathetic action at play can be understood through the framework of the Polyvagal Theory, where the sympathetic nervous system responds to threats, real or perceived, with "fight, flight, and freeze," driven by the main sympathetic system, and "collapse" or "play dead," mediated by the dorsal vagal branch of the parasympathetic nervous system. These last two, "freeze" and "collapse," relate more to dissociative experience.[38]

Besides the HPA axis and sympathetic nervous system, major neurocircuitry at play includes those involved in fear and memory. Smaller hippocampal volume, the brain region responsible for memory consolidation, has been shown to be a risk factor for developing PTSD, as well for persistence of symptoms.[37,39] The regions involved in fear circuitry, such as the amygdala, the medial prefrontal cortex, the insula, and the cingulate gyrus, have also been shown to show differential activation in those with PTSD. The amygdala has shown overall increased activation and the medial prefrontal cortex has shown decreased activation in those with PTSD compared to healthy controls, meaning that the prefrontal cortex inhibition of fear circuitry is diminished and the circuit is activated, and this activity is increased in PTSD.[37,38] The genetic, neuroendocrine, and neurocircuitry factors involved in PTSD, as well as their modulators, are areas of active current research, not only to better understand the disease, but also to create robust novel therapeutic interventions.[37]

Dissociation and Other Disorders

While much of the discussion of trauma in psychiatry focuses on PTSD as an entity, traumatic events are risk factors for a multitude of other psychiatric disorders and psychological disturbances. In DSM-5 alone, trauma is noted to increase the risk of developing anxiety disorders, specific phobias, hoarding disorder, somatic symptom disorder, dissociative identity disorder, and depersonalization and derealization disorders, among other diagnoses.[34] Additionally, the experience of a traumatic event may result in the experience of psychological symptoms which may not fully meet criteria for any one psychiatric disorder, but still cause distress. Much like the events which engendered them, these symptoms can be wide-ranging and include anxiety, depression, difficulty in interpersonal relationships or functioning, and perhaps most classically, dissociation.[34]

Dissociation has long been observed and studied as a reaction to trauma, one which serves as a coping mechanism for proceeding with day-to-day life after a dangerous event has occurred. There is strong ongoing debate regarding the definition of dissociation, with some scholars arguing that it is a wide-ranging spectrum of experiences which includes memory disturbances, alterations in consciousness, splits in identity, and perceptual changes such as depersonalization and derealization; others argue that dissociation is a more discrete phenomenon separate from some or all of these related phenomena.[40] Traditionally, however, dissociation in the study of trauma refers specifically to a process in which painful, traumatic components of memories are split off and compartmentalized. The aspects of a memory which are too traumatizing to remain in one's consciousness are thus dissociated from the more tolerable components of a memory and are retained in such a way that the individual can no longer access them.[41]

Importantly, dissociation differs from simple amnesia in that the memories are not lost or forgotten, but rather are stored in such a way that they are out of one's reach. Dissociation can also be distinguished from depersonalization and derealization, which are perceptual, sensory changes rather than memory changes.[40] While depersonalization, derealization, and other related experiences may be distressing to the patient, dissociation often goes unnoticed. It serves as a maladaptive defense mechanism meant to protect the patient from the psychological pain of integrating the experienced event with the other components of the self.[42] Dissociation stands in contrast to the recurrent and intrusive memories of PTSD, although both can be conceptualized as failures to adequately integrate the traumatic memory into one's self-concept. The work of uncovering dissociated memories and reintegrating them with a patient's conscious reality is often an essential component of a treatment plan for the patient affected by trauma symptoms. Without adequate treatment, the painful and distressing memory may remain hidden as dissociative symptoms persist, or may return to the surface in distressing and intrusive flashbacks.[42]

Of note, the presence of dissociative symptoms during and after a dangerous event increases the risk of PTSD in these patients, suggesting that these two mechanisms of responding to trauma are intertwined.[34] Additionally, dissociation is recognized as an important component of complex PTSD in ICD-11,[33] and the diagnostic specifier "with dissociative symptoms" is listed in the discussion of PTSD in DSM-5.[34] Where dissociation was once historically considered to be the primary and defining characteristic of trauma disorders, it is now understood to be an important subgroup of a range of possible symptoms and responses which fall under the umbrella of PTSD and other trauma disorders.[43]

Defining, Delineating, and Understanding Trauma from a Sociological Perspective

Thus far we have focused on the psychological and biological foundations of trauma, PTSD, and dissociation. We have also highlighted how psychiatry has viewed the events, experience, and outcome of trauma through the ages and in modern day. But what is trauma? What events cause it?

Definition

As a foundation on which to explore trauma, we begin with Prager's definition of psychological trauma as "an internal psychic response generated after the dangerous event confronted is remembered (whether minutes later, or months, or years2) and that proves emotionally overwhelming."[30] This definition alerts one to consider whether all dangerous events produce trauma. If not, what is the level of physical or psychological danger necessary to produce trauma? Second, his definition encourages the question: what are the mechanisms by which the individual experiences the event as traumatic? His definition allows for the possibility that neurobiological factors, social constructions, historical and cultural determinants, and individual developmental experiences result in a composite of strengths and vulnerabilities. These in turn may fortify and protect the individual, or result in the overwhelmed state. Third, he has indicated the importance of time, and we believe this element implies that the event may not be directly witnessed. Lastly, his definition allows for the possibility that not all dangerous or physical events result in a traumatic response, and conversely that some events never directly experienced produce traumatic symptomatology. In order to explore these elements further, we want to explore the nature of these negative events and how might they differentially impact individuals.

Experiencing Dangerous Events

Event "involves a process, a change in the properties of something."[44(p 839)] Events are not necessarily stressful or abnormal, but are given meaning by the cultural and social interaction and construction of the event. From Durkheim's perspective, dangerous or traumatic events can be viewed as "social facts" which are internal to the individual and expressed through individual thoughts, feelings, and acts, but are framed and defined by a fusion of individual consciousness (collective consciousness), a sui generis reality.[45]

There are four types of events that potentially may trigger a trauma response. The first type is a discrete environmental event that may destroy or injure individuals, their belongings, and their view of their social order. The event may affect a single individual, such as a house fire or an auto accident. Or it may ravage communities such as a volcano, a flood, a hurricane, a forest fire, a tsunami, outbreak of viruses, or a bombing. How these events are conceptualized within the community, identification with that community, and social support from both inside and outside the group affect individual perceptions and responses to the events. With adequate resources and the opportunity to return or build anew a productive community, most people regain their psychological integrity.

The prevalence of PTSD and related trauma symptoms after this first type of event has varied estimates, but is generally thought to be less than 20% of those exposed at 1–2 years after exposure.[34] Studies of PTSD after natural disasters have largely been consistent with this estimate, with a notable study which followed survivors of earthquakes in Turkey in 1999 demonstrating a prevalence of 11.7%, and studies of other natural disasters reporting prevalence as low as 3.7%.[d] Other types of discrete environmental events also have PTSD prevalence generally lower than 20%, for example 6%–12% following industrial accidents and 13%–21% following motor vehicle accidents.[34]

The second type of event is interpersonal in nature. These events vary along the dimension of chronicity. At one end are single events such as rape, robbery, or assault. At the other end are ongoing and chronic events. Examples are systemic racism, sexism, and other cultural and religious ongoing discriminations that range from subtle and unconscious micro aggressions to ongoing threats and dangers to life merely because someone is identified with a particular group. Somewhere in the middle are events that occurred for a discrete time period, but that have more or less ended. Examples of these are wars, the South African Apartheid, child abuse, and domestic violence. Within this latter subgrouping, individuals directly experienced the events or witnessed the events, or the events have been graphically relayed to the individual.

This second, interpersonal category of events is the primary driver of PTSD symptomatology, with the highest rates of development of the disorder following exposure, at 33%–50% on average. Interestingly, interpersonal events which occur at the individual level such as rape, military combat, and assault share these higher prevalence rates with the other, more systemic and society-wide events in this category, such as genocide and political internments.[34] These higher-risk events all share an additional component above and beyond the first, environmental category; not only are these events dangerous, they are also examples of suffering wrought deliberately by another human being or group of human beings. Their interpersonal nature is what sets them apart, and in turn leads to

---

d. Of note, the prevalence of symptomatology seems to correlate with how severely the disaster affected the group, and how close the group was in proximity to the epicenter of the disaster. For severely affected groups, prevalence has been estimated to be as high as 60% in individual studies, but for the vast majority of natural disasters the rule of 20% or less seems to hold true.

higher prevalence of symptoms in a faster timeline; these events are also the highest risk for acute stress disorder, which is a DSM diagnosis categorized by PTSD-like symptoms within the first month of exposure to such an event.[34]

The third category of potential events involves historical happenings. These have never been directly experienced by an individual belonging to the identified victims, but memories of the events have been maintained by subsequent generations. These have been referred to in the literature as historical or intergenerational trauma. Historical trauma is based in legacy. It is not only the event itself but the way the narrative around it evolves, and the meaning takes on a life of its own. It becomes intertwined with identity. Facets of the present serve as reminders of the original trauma, strengthening and perpetuating it. These reminders can be something as mundane as a cartoon illustration or an adage, such as cartoonish depictions of Native people for sports logos. These brief and unremarkable statements and actions communicate, either intentionally or not, bigoted attitudes toward marginalized people. It is in this way that identity remains a salient point for many of the historical traumas we discuss today.[47] This third category has not been studied much in terms of being a direct driver of PTSD symptom development, largely because this type of indirect exposure is insufficient for the diagnosis by DSM criteria. Nevertheless, these historical events are essential to a nuanced and complete understanding of trauma, particularly in marginalized communities. For example, historical trauma theory has been used to highlight the long history of suffering endured by Native American people and to place the current experiences of this group within a broader context.[e]

The fourth type is intergenerational trauma, in which trauma is experienced in multiple instances across multiple generations through reverberations of the sequalae of an original event and then the consequences which continue through the generations. In the instance of Native populations in North America, this can be seen through generation after generation of people experiencing higher rates of violence, sexual abuse, oppression, accidental death, and suicide. This can be related to the aftereffects of colonialism and economic and social dependence, as well as through the perpetuation of complex trauma formed from experiences in childhood, including abuse, neglect, disruptions in attachment, deculturation, and other adverse childhood events. The effects of this trauma are seen in disorganized attachment styles, problems with attention and concentration, and difficulty regulating affect and self-soothing. However, the definitions of historical and intergenerational trauma do overlap and are at times used as synonyms.[49]

As we have now articulated the potential events that may trigger a traumatic reaction, in the following section we will consider the sociological influences of trauma.

The Social Construction of Trauma

Symptoms of dissociation and PTSD appear shortly after potentially traumatic events. However, exposure to physical harm or extreme, suddenly changing environments do not

e. Some studies have estimated a lower prevalence of PTSD among this group compared to the general population, while others have suggested prevalence may be higher; either way, history provides a framework for continuing to make sense of these findings.[48]

necessarily produce a traumatizing experience. The individual's determination of the experience as traumatic is the perception of an event that is then filtered by individual's psychological capacities and then given meaning by the individual. That meaning is also framed by the social and cultural processes by which the dangerous or violent event is given meaning.

There is an unpredictable and chaotic nature to dangerous happenings. Associated with this is existential anxiety of death and personal meaninglessness.[50] Societies from the beginning of time have attempted to construct methods of predicting danger and establishing rituals to mitigate its risk. Engraining meanings of understanding and controlling the environment frees up community energies so that the society is freer to discover and create. Social constructions of benevolent or angry powerful beings as the cause of dangerous events have helped people make these events more tolerable by providing activities to reduce the violence and a socially validated meaning to mediate the impact of it. The violence of a natural disaster can be mediated by the meaning of the event as "God intended it to be as a part of a grand design even if we cannot understand the meaning right now." A study of Bhutanese torture survivors found that few developed PTSD symptoms when imprisoned in Nepal. The study concluded that these Hindus were less likely to develop the symptoms because they believed that their suffering came from bad karma.[3] To the extent that God has less influence and agency in contemporary society, other social constructions are required to reduce vulnerability to overwhelming anxiety and vigilance for impending and unpredictable violence, particularly when it is a relatively peaceful society. Yalom[49] used the metaphor of "staring at the sun." It can only be tolerated in small doses. Even otherwise rational and scientifically inclined individuals who intellectually recognize the unpredictability of violence need to find a reprieve from this unadulterated truth. Thus there is a need to find existential illusions that allow humans to symbolically preserve the self.[51]

Many subgroups witnessing violence develop a group mindset that aids in mediating the boundlessness of violence. For example, there are certain rules of war. Soldiers are entitled to kill other soldiers, but not citizens such as women and children. When one learns of the number of soldiers killed, one is relatively immune from experiencing the effects of violence. However, the killing of women and children invokes an outrage and increased anxiety. Likewise, the shooting of a soldier is not viewed in the same way as a maiming of that soldier's body.

Another mindset to mediate the effects of violence is attributions toward the victim. The most extreme is by dehumanizing the victims. For example, those in Vietnam War often referred to the victims of napalm bombings as "crispy critters," which referred to the way napalm sticks to the skin and chars it. The phrase removes the humanity and pain of another human being. Another common strategy is to blame the victim for the violence. For example, until two decades ago, rape victims were often seen as too beautiful or too sexually provocative as a justified reason for their attacks.

Contemporary political and cultural leaders attempt to replace religion with political ideologies (nationalism, communism, imperialism). Believing in one of these ideologies and identifying with other members who support the ideology allow for the development of an *esprit de corps*. It becomes a social identity.[f] Maintaining a strong commitment to that

f. *Social identity* refers to an individual's perception that they belong to a social group, who through comparison to others see themselves as similar on important dimensions such as values, affective reactions, physical characteristics, and attitudes.[52,53]

ideology seems to protect against the violence experienced, as was the case in the Lebanese civil war where strong commitment to their ethnic group reduced symptoms of PTSD. Similarly, for Palestinians a strong commitment to their group and its future reduced the psychological distress experienced in the face of violence.

Social identities can be antecedents and/or mediators of traumatic experiences. Group membership can place a person at risk for trauma, or it can provide resources to attenuate the traumatic experience.[54] The construction of a group identity for those inside and outside the group accentuates the similarities of members and can minimize differences.[55] From within the group, the characteristics of an individual related to group identity are seen as positive, and those in other groups not possessing the same characteristics are seen as negative. For the individual who identifies with the group, this identity positively affects self-esteem regardless of the social standing of the group within the larger social structure.[53] The more strongly someone identifies with a group, the less likely they are to experience distress and PTSD, when victimization is due to social identity. This has been shown to be true when individuals are tortured for political affiliations.[56] When individuals choose a group membership, their feelings of trust, support, and connection provide psychological resources to protect against the effects of perceived traumatizing events. Having multiple group memberships allows for the possibility of individuals drawing more on more groups for psychological resources.

Social Identity as a Risk for Trauma

While social identity may serve as a buffer to the effects of ongoing discrimination, it can also put an individual at risk for discrimination and resulting trauma experiences which span generations. As mentioned, American Natives are a prime example. Historically, they experienced mass death resulting from illnesses originally brought from Europe, endured forced relocation for the manifest destiny of European colonists, and had children removed from the homes of their parents in order to attend boarding schools.[47] In some iterations, students were from different tribes or even neighboring states. They often were beaten and/or berated for not conforming to European social norms for all manner of things—including speaking their native language or practicing any traditional customs. They were made to cut their hair and change their names for the purpose of "integration" with the dominant culture.[57] These practices deculturated generations of Native Americans, causing them to lose skills and practices around parenting, which led to poor bonding and attachments in the subsequent generations, which continues today. O'Neill[48] summarizes that in the first generation, of those who experienced boarding schools, many experienced symptoms of complex PTSD, including dissociation, intense anger, numbing of emotions, and avoidance. The second generation took on caretaking roles with a high degree of dedication but also exhibiting high levels of distress and many of the same PTSD symptoms their parents had. They also showed low self-esteem, difficulty with affective regulation, and susceptibility to PTSD and depression. The third generation shows mixed evidence, with some studies showing continued attachment and communication difficulties and vulnerability to PTSD, anxiety, and depression; and some showing extinction of the effects of first generations trauma in the third generation. In this generation it was shown that an early attachment to caregiver was the most important mitigating factor in trauma presentation, thus highlighting the importance of attachment trauma in the perpetuation of intergenerational effects of trauma.

A similar and more recent event can be seen in the genocide of the Tutsi people in Rwanda. A dark time in the history of a country that has seen recurrent violence along ethnic lines, the 1994 genocide left approximately 1 million, mostly Tutsi, of the country's 7 million people, dead. One million people were brought before the justice system as alleged perpetrators or conspirators, over 300,000 of whom were sentenced to imprisonment. It is in this way that all families in Rwanda can be seen as affected by this violence. The effects on survivors and those who came after them have been a direct look into how families are affected by large scale violence and how, when it is on the basis of identity—in this case along ethnic lines—the effects are seen for generations.[58]

These effects can be seen in the economic disadvantages and difficulties, feelings of hurt and regret, family conflict, and social exclusion seen in the families of both the victims and perpetrators. These have direct effects on parenting, with parents being unable to provide the education and healthcare they would like for their children due to poverty, and are further exacerbated by illness (both mental and physical) resulting directly from the genocide. These effects are propagated to children through the difficult and worrisome childhood associated with poverty and lack of medical care and education, and even to the point of secondary trauma from their parents' recollection of events. Children were, however, also seen to have been able to form relationships with other children whose relatives have even harmed their own family; this points to resilience at play and further deepens the complexity unfolding as these traumatic events are taken in and reinterpreted in subsequent generations. So while the genocide was on the basis of identity, the trauma extended across the ethnic line.[58]

Some lines of research do elaborate on the ideas of the cycles of violence in Rwanda, such as that by Roth.[59] This research showed that children of mothers who experienced the Rwandan genocide and showed maternal PTSD did not experience increased rates of depression, anxiety, and antisocial behavior—Rather it was the child's own experience with violence and instability, including domestic violence that influenced the child's mental health. This elaborates on the theme of the importance of family support and the cultural and childhood environment for children's mental health.[59]

Taken together, the above examples of the difficult history of Native Americans in the United States and the genocide of the Tutsi people in Rwanda show the importance of having the needs of children met, both physically and emotionally, for trauma not to be handed down through the generations. High among these is the need of secure attachment to an adult caretaker. The reoccurrence of the importance of attachment, connection, and community throughout analyses of these events highlights the importance of supportive environments in the face of traumatic events, which we will touch more on later.

Social Identity as Protective

On the other side of the coin, the relationship between trauma and identity is not unidirectional. Not only does identity modulate the effects of trauma, but collective trauma can also cause identities to be created and maintained. This can be especially true of historical trauma, where the narrative of the trauma can evolve with the potential to become the focus of the group identity. For the victims of collective trauma, strengthening group identity is adaptive, allowing the individual to be part of something that transcends and outlasts their individual life. It allows them to find purpose, worth, self-efficacy, and values. Perpetrators of mass violence undergo a different process for similar reasons. In order to maintain a stable worldview and sense of self, it is necessary that they either distance themselves from the identity now associated with violence and form new identities, or engage in apologetics for their actions to maintain both their identity and their self-image.[60]

Across multiple contexts, however, it has been shown that strong group identification has multiple positive effects for individuals. One particularly pertinent aspect is the beneficial effect on self-esteem. This effect is an outgrowth of positive social interactions, both online and in person, and identity pride. Additionally, improved self-esteem and social supports have been shown to increase resilience, which acts to protect against psychological distress. Furthermore, community connectedness has been shown to be associated with fewer depressive symptoms.[61] Specifically, in the face of collective trauma, a group identity can serve to give the individual member a "bird's-eye view" of the situation, allowing them to place value on the future of the group instead of the current suffering of themselves. This perceptual shift allows for management of the terror that is innate to a traumatizing experience.[60] Individuals can be more resilient to trauma when their social identities are maintained or shifted in response to trauma, and those group ideals are strongly held.[54] Identity allows access to other resources such as a sense of belonging, trust, and solidarity, which also have roles in resilience and resistance to the effects of trauma on mental health.[53] These findings suggest how association with group identity can be protective against the effects of trauma and the development of long-term psychological sequela.

Multiple Social Identities

All of us have multiple social identities, ranging from race to gender to sexual orientation to ability, that interrelate to form our reality and influence the ways in which we navigate the world. They are not additive or multiplicative, but instead inexorably intertwined.[g] Sidika et al.[63] explored "double discrimination" as an ethnic and sexual minority in Canada. It highlighted how LGBTQ people of color (POC) experienced racial micro aggressions within the LGBTQ community and homophobic/transphobic micro aggressions in their racial/ethnic community. This can lead to homonormativity within the queer community as being largely white, resulting in ethnic minorities to suppress their ethnic identity to receive benefits from LGBTQ spaces and support. This is further strengthened in the sexual racism seen in dating contexts. The mere realization of holding multiple identities may cause a wide variety of negative emotions—from shock to inner turmoil. More points of contention are seen when considering the "coming out narrative"; in the dominant Western narrative, LGBTQ people are pressed to "come out" and "live as their authentic selves," which may not be possible or necessary in other cultural contexts. LGBTQ people of color risk losing

g. This describes intersectionality theory.[62]

connections around their racial/ethnic identity by severing familial or communal ties by coming out.[63,64] The taboos around speaking of sex, even heterosexual sex, in cultures such as some in South Asia, further contribute to the inherent difficulty. At times, however, it has been seen that some LGBTQ individuals who have not explicitly come out interpret the silence around their identity as passive acceptance of their sexual or gender minority status.[63] The summation of this "double discrimination" can be seen in feelings of loneliness, displacement, and invisibility in South Asian LGBTQ people, and bisexual people of color had more anxiety than those who did not experience racial or ethnic discrimination. The end result is the potential for a greater amount of minority stress and the associated psychological and health implications in people with multiple marginalized identities.[63]

Much like with those with a single marginalized identity, those with multiple marginalized identities benefit from social support. This support can be from within or outside of identity communities. This is exemplified by the positive effect on mental health seen in LGBTQ children of color when they have a supportive parental figure. The form that support can take can be in person, such as in a support group or meeting those with similar multiple identities at a larger event, or online, through chatrooms and forums.[63] For some with particular marginalized identities, one identity can partly ameliorate the negative experience of the other. This can be seen in some Southeast Asian communities, where gay men might point to historical examples of sexual and romantic minority groups being seen as acceptable in society, as well as having the ability to point to the origination of some negative views on homosexuality being in Christianity and Islam, not the religions of their ancestors. This does not apply to all in an ethnic minority equally, though, as within the same group men can have a difficult time reconciling their sexual identity with the heterosexual norms and expectations to perform masculinity as valued in their ethnic community. In these two simultaneously observed phenomena, the difficulty inherent to intersectionality is fully seen.[63]

A more specific example of the intersection of a marginalized gender or sexual identity with the added variable of displacement is seen in LGBTQ refugees from predominantly Muslim communities to Europe. As conflict in the Middle East has evolved and the numbers of those seeking refuge have increased, anti-Islam and anti-refugee sentiments have increased in Europe, and Islamophobia has been increasingly prevalent even in areas with small numbers of Muslim people.[65] This further compounds the stress innate to seeking refuge in a foreign country—lacking local contacts and social connections, and needing to navigate the legal process, learn a new language, find housing, and employment.[66] For LGBTQ refugees, however, they face additional stressors. To start, many are fleeing countries of origin where their LGBTQ identity put them at increased risk of violence, and many risked being killed.[67] This high level of discrimination carried over to the refugee camps, where they were often harassed and threatened.[67] It was often inescapable due to the need to access services such as classes in English as a second language and centers to facilitate the legal aspects of immigrating as a refugee. Furthermore, some refugees report an immense pressure to conform to the stereotypes of what a queer person "looks like" or "acts like" in order for immigration officials to consider their reason of refuge to escape LGBTQ discrimination as valid. Europe is not a monolith of LGBTQ acceptance either. Even once in Europe, many refugees report European teachers or acquaintances not intervening when other refugees or Europeans harass them for their queer identity. Some even report discrimination from those Europeans who were supposed to be providing them aid.[66]

These multiple fronts of discrimination can result in LGBTQ refugees feeling hopeless and alone. They may feel unaccepted or outright ostracized in the refugee community, and may face problems in the LGBTQ community due to Islamophobia, or their personal lack of identification with LGBTQ as an identity. Some have felt pressured into sex work or using sex as a means to secure necessities such as housing or mailing address. Thus, the LGBTQ refugee community is particularly vulnerable as a result of their intersecting marginalized identities.[66]

Social Support as Protective

Unlike social identity, which seems to both attenuate and exacerbate the trauma experience, social support [h] almost always serves to protect the individual against development of post-traumatic symptoms and disorders following trauma. Social support is a broad term that first gained widespread use in sociology literature in the 1970s and 1980s, and has been used to generally describe those aspects of individuals' relationships with others, and with communities as a whole, which contribute to the individual's well-being.[68] It has been posited as a protective factor against the development or worsening of many conditions, ranging from symptoms of mental illness including depression and anxiety, to more general morbidity and mortality in the medical setting.[69] In this section we provide examples of social support systems and the ways in which they exert their protective effects in the setting of trauma, including the diathesis-stress model and theories of social support's influence on cognitive processing of trauma. We also discuss the ways in which it has been demonstrated to be a protective factor against the development of trauma symptoms.

Social support can take many distinct forms, from engagement in formal group therapy sessions with others who have experienced similar events, to the institution of monetary or resource-based aid in hard-hit communities, to simply relying on the presence of loved ones for comfort and emotional support in the aftermath of trauma.[i] While the different forms that social support can take are wide and varied, they share a common thread in that they involve giving the individual impacted by trauma an outlet in which they can express their experiences and receive assurance that they are valid and supported in return. The recognition and implementation of such social supports can be used as an important therapeutic tool to both aid in management of post-traumatic symptoms and, with early intervention, alter and improve the course of their development after a traumatic experience.

One important way to conceptualize the impact of social support on well-being in the context of trauma comes from what is termed the diathesis-stress model, a framework

---

h. The term "social support" is used here to refer to a resource, relationship, or outlet provided to an individual by members of their community in the aftermath of a traumatic event.

i. Social support is often offered along identity lines, within your familial, religious, location, and/or gender group. One positive aspect of identity is social support.

which posits that stressors and triggering events in the environment interact with the biological and psychological characteristics of individuals to engender an individualized response.[70] Traumatic events constitute significant stressors which are often responded to in maladaptive or debilitating ways at the individual level. However, the presence of social support can serve as a "buffer" in the face of traumatic stressors, providing the individual with a source of comfort and resources which can soften the impact of a terrible event.[70]

There is increasing evidence that even secondhand exposure to dangerous events can be traumatic stressors under the diathesis-stress model. For example, the repetition of relatively uncommon but disastrous events in news media can lead viewers to come to believe that such disasters are far more likely to occur to them than they are in actuality. This misperception can in turn lead to changes in behavior and increased anxious distress.[35] Recent studies have demonstrated that particular trauma symptoms, including hypervigilance, racing thoughts, and negativistic thinking, can develop in the setting of repeated secondhand exposure to discussions of trauma.[35] Early studies of this concept have demonstrated that the more frequently and intensely one engages with media cycles of violent or traumatic content, the more likely it is for one to develop symptoms of anxiety. This anxiety may focus on possible future danger, fear for loved ones' safety, or may result in changes in behavior meant to prepare for a future encounter with the traumatic situation.[35]

Younger age has long been examined as a risk factor for negative psychological outcomes after media exposure to violence. The effects on children of secondhand exposure to various American disasters, including the *Challenger* space shuttle explosion and the September 11 attack at the World Trade Center, have been documented in the literature as including a range of post-traumatic stress symptoms and reactions.[71] Further research in children has demonstrated the importance of the emotional resonance of the observed event in determining the potential for symptom development; for example, in children who were exposed to television, radio, and print media coverage of a bombing, the strongest association with trauma symptoms was in those children who reported an intense emotional reaction on initial exposure to the media.[71] This interplay of a stimulus with an emotional response is consistent with the conceptualization of trauma itself, as not just an event that is experienced or witnessed, but as a perception that is emotionally charged and highly individualized. Importantly, social support can play a buffering role even in cases of secondhand exposure to trauma, helping the individual to mitigate their emotional response to the exposure in a healthier way.

One's individual stress response is highly influenced by one's social networks, social capital, and past social experiences, which can be extended as far back as to an individual's first family and parental relationships.[72] Just as group identity can provide guidance for meaning-making after a traumatic event, so too does one's individual support network play an essential role in making sense of trauma. The individual who has a strong foundation of relationships with others to fall back on in times of distress is better equipped to cope with trauma in a way that will protect against PTSD development, as has been demonstrated by studies which correlate higher levels of perceived help and positive interactions with others following an event, with better outcomes.[72] It is notable that the types of trauma which carry a higher risk for PTSD development, namely intimate and interpersonal trauma, are also those which many individuals find harder to talk about and are less likely to find supports around.[72] A natural disaster, for example, is the sort of trauma that is shared among a group and that garners a more universal level of empathy and support. Meanwhile, the individual affected by an interpersonal trauma such as assault may be less likely to find strong supports from the wider community, whether because of issues around shame, judgment, or lack of specific resources; these types of traumas in turn produce higher rates of trauma symptoms and PTSD.[72]

Beyond impacting the cognitive processing of an event after it has already occurred, there is evidence that the presence of preexisting social support can influence the way trauma is perceived by the individual in the moment. Functional magnetic resonance imaging (fMRI) studies have demonstrated that individuals' fear responses to threatening or traumatic experiences are dampened by the physical touch and presence of loved ones, and further studies have linked the effects of social relationships on fear response to the activity of oxytocin and other neurochemicals in the amygdala circuitry.[72] The presence of intimate and supportive relationships can thus be considered a protective factor against PTSD from the very beginning of the process, in that it influences brain activity and cognition surrounding the experience of trauma itself (Charuvastra & Cloitre, 2008).[72]

Of course, not every trauma victim is equipped with a strong and supportive network of family members, friends, and community resources. The establishment of therapeutic support groups and assurances to survivors that they are not alone, therefore, becomes an essential component of preventive management for PTSD and related symptoms. When providers quickly and effectively match up trauma survivors with appropriate, high-quality support services, the protective effects of such intervention against symptomatology have been noted as far as 2 years after the event and beyond.[73] In the case of natural disaster, for example, timely implementation of supports and services that are perceived by survivors as relevant and accessible has been associated with decreased symptom development. This result is consistent across demographic categories such as gender and economic status.[73] Of note, it is the perceived quality of assistance and support, rather than simply the quantity of referrals or groups provided, that demonstrates such an effect.[73]

There are established disparities in access to support which vary across place and time, but it is intuitive that minority groups or groups lacking political or social power tend to have fewer supportive resources available to them. As was noted following a devastating Mexican flood in 1999, those already facing economic or other hardship prior to a natural disaster face a longer and more arduous road to recovery, with lower quality supports and less accessible resources compared to more privileged groups.[74]

In addition to social support itself, it appears that the individual or psychological factors which determine one's perception of available support also contribute to post-traumatic outcomes. Different individuals in the same community often have vastly different perceptions of how effectively that community can serve them and their needs. The objective readiness of a community to cope with a traumatic event is certainly a factor in how well individuals are protected against the development of trauma symptoms, but those individuals who view their communities as less supportive to begin with may be at higher risk. Interestingly, a survey of individuals impacted by Hurricane Sandy demonstrated that those individuals who had a higher regard and perception of the ability of hospitals and medical providers to cope with a large-scale disaster also tended to rate a higher level of subjective mental health.[75] Beyond just receiving high-quality social support, individual characteristics such as level of trust, biases, and more also serve as protective or exacerbating factors when it comes to development of PTSD.

Even early social support research emphasized the individual's perception of the available resources as being as important as the actual resources themselves. The relationships, resources, and outlets which a community provides in the form of social support are valuable, but the concept of perceived social support also takes into consideration the extent to which the individual finds the support to be useful, relevant, and accessible.[69] Quality of support resources has been demonstrated to take priority over quantity, and an individual will be protected more by supports that are viewed as relevant to the situation.[73] It is this subjective experience that is the impetus for later trauma symptom development, and in turn, the subjective experience of being helped or being accompanied through a difficult time can be protective. Some recent research has extended the concept of perceived social support to include a perceived sense of belongingness, and has identified this experience of belonging to a group in the setting of trauma as an important contributor to continued mental well-being.[76]

An important developing area in social support research involves the massive surge in social media and other internet use as a source of community and support. Online spaces have provided both support and distress for those who interact with it. It can be a valuable social support that boosts resilience, especially in marginalized groups. For example, research surveys have found that while LGBTQ youth often face bullying and harassment in their communities, many participants identify social media platforms such as Facebook and YouTube as spaces in which they can more freely express their ideas and feel supported by peers.[77] Similarly, research on the social media habits of young mothers in Russia has demonstrated that social media sites such as Facebook and Instagram provide communities in which parents can seek out parenting advice as well as validation from others, in a way that boosts confidence in parenting abilities and self-esteem.[78] Social media generally serves as a community which boosts resilience and adaptability for users, much in the way that other forms of social support serve as protective factors.

Of course, the ubiquity of social media platforms in many communities has also been highlighted as a social stressor in some cases. Cyber-bullying in particular is a deleterious and destabilizing experience, turning what could be a source of social support into a system that decreases resilience over time. Analysis of social media use among adolescents in 42 countries indicated that risk factors for cyber-bullying and victimization include increased frequency of internet use and interactions with strangers, and that adolescent girls are at a slightly increased risk compared to boys in the majority of countries.[79] Additionally, a study of social media users in Pakistan demonstrated that increased frequency of social media use actually decreased overall self-esteem in survey participants, with many participants identifying frequent "upward comparisons" between themselves and other users, in which they rate themselves negatively as compared to their peers.[80]

Socially Based Treatments of Trauma-Induced Experiences

There are several evidence-based treatment options for PTSD which are popular, well-established, and provided to patients on an individual basis, including trauma-focused psychotherapy, prolonged exposure therapy, cognitive behavioral therapy for PTSD, narrative exposure therapy, Eye Movement Desensitization and Reprocessing (EMDR), and pharmacotherapy.[38,81–83] While these treatments have demonstrated efficacy in treating individual patients and their symptoms, the field of social psychiatry offers multiple effective interventions which focus on patients' groups and communities, and which providers may otherwise overlook.

Social support can serve as a therapeutic intervention even after symptoms have begun to develop. Social support increases resiliency, motivation, and coping in the face of trauma.[70] In terms of therapeutic efficacy, social support recommendations and referrals are most effective when they are tailored to the individual patient's needs. Ensuring a high standard of quality in each recommendation requires an intimate understanding of the resources available in one's own community. Providers must also be aware of potential pitfalls in recommending and ensuring access to social support, particularly as such support relates to patients' demographic characteristics of gender, race, class, and more. Another important role for the provider, then, is advocating for equitable access to the highest quality social supports across demographic and social lines.[73]

The primary way for providers to implement social support as a therapeutic intervention is through therapeutic support groups. Support groups are forums, either in-person or online, in which patients can interact with and learn from peers who have similar conditions or diagnoses. Peer support groups specific to trauma and PTSD are available for patients to discuss their struggles with the experience in a setting in which the impact of stigma is not as acutely felt. Interactions with peers in a group can provide individuals with education and models for behavior that empower each member of the group to respond and cope in more effective ways. In a supportive group, one feels a sense of community with others who see one's struggles and freely offer help without judgment or shame. This experience of helpfulness is protective in that it alters one's thinking around trauma to make it less isolating and less threatening.

Peer support groups have been studied internationally as an intervention which reduces the functional impact of symptoms and increases resilience. One example of the therapeutic impact of support groups can be found in the case of U.S. military veterans who developed PTSD after seeing combat. Online support forums provide these patients with the chance to participate in discussions of such important themes as stigma and masculinity, which may not necessarily be discussed in traditional treatment modalities like prolonged exposure therapy. These veterans found online support groups most useful for discussing the stigma around PTSD, identifying with like members of the group, and learning to cope with and welcome conflict. The relative anonymity of online support groups also empowered these veterans to feel less inhibited by masculine gender roles, which ordinarily would discourage these men from frankly discussing their fears, emotions, and their desire to seek help.[84] The therapeutic value of peer support was demonstrated in studies of former child soldiers in Nepal. For these child soldiers, access to online support groups was not an option. However, researchers found that those individuals who were able to access social support in other ways, through friends, family, and community resources, were found to have a lower incidence of PTSD symptoms than those who did not.[85]

Healthcare providers also can refer patients to important resources like food or shelter which are available in his or her community after traumatic events. This intervention takes some of the burden of recovery off the individual and spreads it community-wide, increasing hope and encouragement and decreasing the individual's stress responses.[70]

Social support interventions also include debriefing and preventive psychoeducation exercises, which are increasingly being implemented at the level of work organizations and other social entities. In particular, debriefing protocols and other techniques, such as teaching stress management skills, are increasingly offered to first responders at high risk for trauma disorders, such as police officers and firefighters. A review of several decades of European studies demonstrated that generally, the most effective interventions were those which were designed to specifically reduce risk factors for poor overall mental health, for example by increasing physical exercise or teaching stress-reduction techniques. Debriefing alone following exposure to a dangerous event did not significantly reduce trauma symptom development in this population.

Another significant, community-wide intervention which increases growth and decreases distress in the aftermath of trauma involves the generation of a recovery narrative. A recovery narrative is a way of thinking about a traumatic experience that integrates the experience with the rest of the community's life and identity. While recovery narratives are traditionally thought of as being crafted with and by patients as individuals, they are also continuously formed and reformed by entire groups and communities, particularly in the aftermath of collective trauma. Collective trauma is trauma which affects an entire group, and over time it can be narratively transformed into an experience which provides meaning and resilience to members of the group. This kind of narrative emphasizes the group's resilience and ability to make meaning out of a dangerous event, rather than focusing on the destructive nature of the event itself. This engenders empowerment and strength from what was initially a traumatic and devastating experience.[60] The concept of a group or community recovery narrative can be thought of as a corollary to what in individual patients is termed "post-traumatic growth." This is the successful transformation of the internal experience of trauma, from one which causes distressing symptoms into one which has led to positive changes having overcome significant adversity. For larger groups, post-traumatic growth may take the form of the establishment of an identity which is greater than the sum of its individual members, one which spans generations and cannot be destroyed by single events. Group members who have experienced collective trauma become more tightly united and in turn more protected, after having worked through collective trauma.[60] The prototypical example of collective trauma, the Holocaust, also provides an example of how a social group creates a shared narrative around trauma. The Holocaust was a horrific event which impacted and cut short the lives of countless Jewish people. Over the years since, survivors and other Jewish people internationally have crafted out of this horrific trauma a narrative which crosses generations of group members and amplifies group connectedness and resilience. After facing such horror as a group, the Jewish people have continued to survive; this narrative of persistence in the face of threat and discrimination is one that provides meaning and a source of strength to individual group members.[60]

Of course, not all collective trauma is given the same level of recognition by society. Trauma narratives may turn from a source of strength to a source of further discrimination and disenfranchisement in what is termed "competitive victimhood." For example, a group of Sub-Saharan African people who immigrated to Belgium to escape devastation in their home region was noted to develop anti-Semitic views as a reaction to perceived differences in societal recognition. While the Holocaust is a well-recognized source of collective trauma in Europe, not as many of the immigrants' new community members were familiar with or sympathetic to the plight of Sub-Saharan African people. This lack of recognition contributed to the development of intergroup conflicts and discrimination. The group's collective recovery narrative became maladaptive, one which focused on continuing the cycle of persecution with another group, rather than emphasizing the group's own resilience and survivorship. Healthcare providers must thus take care to direct their patients toward those aspects of recovery narratives which promote resilience and symptom reduction, rather than those which may exacerbate intra- and intergroup divisions.[60]

Conclusion and Summary

The contemporary acknowledgment and recognition of the psychological effects of dangerous events have reduced suffering and have enabled many to receive help for PTSD and other psychiatric conditions. Not all dangerous events experienced by individuals result in the development of psychopathology, and sometimes events not directly experienced seem to produce this same symptomatology. As we move away from the direct experience of a dangerous event as a requirement for the psychiatric syndrome, some have felt a "conflation of distress with trauma." [2(p 96)] Our perception of trauma is ensconced in our sociological construction of the nature of the dangerous event, whether directly or indirectly experienced. Social identity modulates patients' responses to dangerous events, as a potential source of both resilience and vulnerability in the case of marginalized groups. Intersectionality further complicates the social identity factor. The nature of social support is an important key to ameliorating the effects of the traumatic experience.

References

1. Benjet C, Bromet E, Karam EG, Kessler RC, . . . Koenen K. The epidemiology of traumatic event exposure worldwide: results from the World Mental Health Survey Consortium. *Psychological Medicine.* 2015;46:1–17. doi:10.1017/S0033291715001981.
2. Summerfield D. The invention of PTSD and social usefulness of a psychiatric category. *British Medical Journal.* 2001;322(7278);95–98.
3. Snyder JA. *A sociology of trauma: violence and self-identity.* Dissertation University of Virginia. 2009.
4. Micale MS. Charcot and the idea of hysteria in the male: gender, mental science and medical diagnosis in late nineteenth century France. *Medical History.* 1990;34:363–411.
5. Janet P. Psychological healing: a historical and clinical study. *Print.* 1925.

6. Freud S. Beyond the pleasure principle. J Stratchey Ed., WW Norton & Co; 1920.

7. Freud S. Thoughts for the times on war and death. *Imago*. 1915;4(1-21):GW, 8, 324–355. https://www.panarchy.org/freud/war.1915.html

8. Jones E, Vermaas RH, McCartney H, Beech C, Palmer I, Hyams K, Wessely S. Flashbacks and post-traumatic stress disorder: the genesis of a 20th-century diagnosis. *British Journal of Psychiatry*. 2003 Feb;182:158–163. doi: 10.1192/bjp.182.2.158. PMID: 12562745.

9. Jones E, Wessely S. Psychological trauma: a historical perspective. *Psychiatry*. 2006;5(7):217–220. https://doi.org/10.1053/j.mppsy.2006.04.011.

10. Kardiner A. The traumatic neruroses of war. *National Research Council*. 1941; https://doi.org/10.1037/10581-000

11. Lifton RJ. *Home from the War: VIETNAM VETERANS Neither Victims nor Executioners*. Simon & Schuster: New York City; 1973.

12. Herman JL. *Trauma and Recovery*. Basic Books; 1992.

13. American Psychiatric Association. *Diagnostic and Statistical Manual of Mental Disorders*, 3rd ed. Washington DC; 1980.

14. Young A. Reasons and causes for post-traumatic stress disorder. *Transcultural Psychiatric Research Review*. 1995;32(3):287–298.

15. Freud S. Fixation to Traumas. Standard Edition; 16:235–254.

16. Jacobson E. Depersonalization. *Journal of the American Psychoanalytic Association*. 1959;7(4):581–610. https://doi-org.fgul.idm.oclc.org/10.1177/000306515900700401

17. Greenacre P. *Trauma, Growth, and Personality*. WW Norton and CO; 1952.

18. Garland C. *Understanding trauma—a psychoanalytical approach*. New York, Routledge; 1998.

19. Scharff JS, Scharff DE. *Object relations therapy of physical and sexual trauma*. Jason Aronson; 1994.

20. Kalsched D. *Trauma and the Soul: a psycho-spiritual approach to human development and its interruption*. Routledge, New York; 2013.

21. Kohut H. *The restoration of the self*. University of Chicago Press; 1977.

22. Young M. *Exploring the Meaning of Trauma in the South African Police Service*. PhD thesis, University of Pretoria; 2004. http://hdl.handle.net/2263/27855

23. Gerrity ET, Solomon S. The treatment of PTSD and related stress disorders: current research and clinical knowledge. In Marsella AJ, Friedman MJ, Gerrity ET, Scurfield RM, eds. *Ethnocultural aspects of posttraumatic stress disorder: issues, research, and clinical applications*. American Psychological Association; 1996:87–102. https://doi.org/10.1037/1055

24. Van der Kolk B. *Psychological Trauma*. American Psychiatric Press Inc; 1987.

25. McFarland W. Counselors Teaching Peaceful Conflict Resolution. *J Couns Dev*. 1992;71(1):18–21. doi:10.1002/j.1556-676.1992.tb02164.x

26. Horowitz MJ, Kaltreider NB. Brief treatment of post-traumatic stress disorders. *New Directions from Mental Health Services*. 1980;67–79. https://doi.org/10.1002/vd.23319800609

27. Ghafoori B, Hierholzer RW, Howsepian B, Boardman A. The Role of adult attachment, parental bonding, and spiritual love in the adjustment to military trauma. *Journal of Trauma & Dissociation*. 2008;9(1):85–106. https://doi.org/10.1080/15299730802073726

28. Okello J, Nakimuli-Mpungu E, Musisi S, Broekaert E, Derluyn I. The association between attachment and mental health symptoms among school-going adolescents in northern uganda: The moderating role of war-related trauma. *PLoS One*. 2014;9(3):e88494. doi: 10.1371/journal.pone.0088494. PMID: 24614005; PMCID: PMC3948618.

29. Winnicott DW. The use of an Object. *The International Journal of Psychoanlysis*. 1969;50(4):711–716.

30. Prager J. Danger and Deformation: A Social Theory of Trauma Part I: Contemporary Psychoanalysis, Contemporary Social Theory, and Healthy Selves. *American Imago*. 2011;68(3):425–448.

31. Freud S. Beyond the Pleasure Principle. J Stratchey Ed., WW Norton & Co; 1920.

32. American Psychiatric Association. *Diagnostic and Statistical Manual of Mental Disorders*, 5th Ed. Washington DC; 2013.

33. World Health Organization. *International Classification of Diseases for Mortality and Morbidity Statistics (11th Revision)*. 2018. https://icd.who.int/browse11/l-m/en

34. American Psychiatric Association. *Diagnostic and Statistical Manual of Mental Disorders*, 5th ed. Washington, DC: APA; 2013.

35. Hopwood TL, Schutte NS, Loi NM. Anticipatory traumatic reaction: outcomes arising from secondary exposure to disasters and large-scale threats. *Assessment.* 2019;26(8):1427–1443. https://doi.org/10.1177/1073191117731815.

36. Dunlop BW, Wong A. The hypothalamic-pituitary-adrenal axis in PTSD: Pathophysiology and treatment interventions. *Prog Neuro-Psychopharmacol Biol Psychiatry.* 2019;89:361–379. https://doi.org/10.1016/j.pnpbp.2018.10.010.

37. Yehuda R, Hoge CW, McFarlane AC, et al. Post-traumatic stress disorder. *Nat Rev Dis Primers.* 2015;1(1):15057. https://doi.org/10.1038/nrdp.2015.57

38. van der Hart O, Nijenhuis ERS, Solomon R. Dissociation of the personality in complex trauma-related disorders and EMDR: theoretical considerations. *J EMDR Pract Res.* 2010;4(2):76–92. https://doi.org/10.1891/1933-3196.4.2.76.

39. VanElzakker MB, Staples-Bradley LK, Shin LM. The neurocircuitry of fear and PTSD. In: Vermetten E, Germain A, Neylan TC, eds. *Sleep and Combat-Related Post Traumatic Stress Disorder.* New York: Springer; 2018:111–125. https://doi.org/10.1007/978-1-4939-7148-0_10.

40. Van Der Hart O, Nijenhuis E, Steele K, Brown D. Trauma-related dissociation: conceptual clarity lost and found. *Aust N Z J Psychiatry.* 2004;38(11–12):906–914. https://doi.org/10.1080/j.1440-1614.2004.01480.x.

41. Van der Hart O, Brom D. When the victim forgets. In: Shalev AY, Yehuda R, McFarlane AC, eds. *International Handbook of Human Response to Trauma.* New York: Springer; 2000:233–248. https://doi.org/10.1007/978-1-4615-4177-6_17.

42. DePrince AP, Freyd JJ. Trauma-induced dissociation. In Friedman MJ, Keane TM, Resick PA, eds. *Handbook of PTSD: Science and Practice.* New York: Guilford Press; 2007:135–150. https://dl.uswr.ac.ir/bitstream/Hannan/130962/1/2007%20-%20Handbook%20of%20PTSD%20-%20Friedman%2C%20Keane%2C%20Resick.pdf#page=151.

43. Armour C, Karstoft K-I, Richardson JD. The co-occurrence of PTSD and dissociation: differentiating severe PTSD from dissociative-PTSD. *Soc Psychiatry Psychiatr Epidemiol.* 2014;49(8):1297–1306. https://doi.org/10.1007/s00127-014-0819-y.

44. Meštrović SG. A sociological conceptualization of trauma. *Social Science & Medicine.* 1985;21(8):835–848. https://doi.org/10.1016/0277-9536(85)90139-X

45. Durkheim E. Individual and collective representations. In: Pocock DF, Trans, ed. *Sociology and philosophy.* New York, NY: The Free Press; 1974 [1898]:1–34.

46. Neria Y, Nandi A, Galea S. Post-traumatic stress disorder following disasters: A systematic review. *Psychol Med.* 2008;38(4):467–480. https://doi.org/10.1017/S0033291707001353.

47. Mohat NV, Thompson AB, Thai ND, Tebes JK. Historical trauma as public narrative: a conceptual review of how history impacts present-day health. *Soc Sci Med.* 2014;106:128–136. https://doi.org/10.1016/j.socscimed.2014.01.043.

48. O'Neill L, Fraser T, Kitchenham A, McDonald V. Hidden burdens: a review of intergenerational, historical and complex trauma, implications for indigenous families. *J Child Adolesc Trauma.* 2018;11(2):173–186. https://doi.org/10.1007/s40653-016-0117-9.

49. Yellow Horse Brave Heart M, Chase J, Elkins J, Altschul DB. Historical trauma among indigenous peoples of the americas: concepts, research, and clinical considerations. *J Psychoactive Drugs.* 2011;43(4):282–290. https://doi.org/10.1080/02791072.2011.628913.

50. Yalom I. *Staring at the Sun: Overcoming the Terror of Death.* Jossey-Bass: California, 2008.

51. Greenberg J. Terror management theory: From genesis to revelations. In: Shaver PR, Mikulincer M, eds. *Meaning, mortality, and choice: The social psychology of existential concerns.* American Psychological Association; 2012:17–35. https://doi.org/10.1037/13748-001

52. Cerulo KA. Identity construction: new issues, new directions. *Ann Rev Sociol.* 1997;23(1):385–409. https://doi.org/10.1146/annurev.soc.23.1.385.

53. Stets JE, Burke PJ. Identity theory and social identity theory. *Social Psychol Q.* 2000;63(3):224. https://doi.org/10.2307/2695870.

54. Muldoon OT, Haslam SA, Haslam C, Cruwys T, Kearns M, Jetten J. The social psychology of responses to trauma: social identity pathways associated with divergent traumatic responses. *Eur Rev Soc Psychol.* 2019;30(1):311–348. https://doi.org/10.1080/10463283.2020.1711628.

55. Hillman JL. The social psychology of trauma: what clinicians need to know. In: Stricker G, ed. *Crisis Intervention and Trauma.* Springer US; 2002:17–32. https://doi.org/10.1007/978-1-4615-0771-0_2

56. Başoğlu M, Paker M, Özmen E, Taşdemir Ö, Şahin D, Ceyhanli A, Incesu C, Sarimurat N. Appraisal of self, social environment, and state authority as a possible mediator of posttraumatic stress disorder in tortured political activists. *Journal of Abnormal Psychology.* 1996;105(2):232–236. https://doi.org/10.1037/0021-843X.105.2.232

57. Davis J. American Indian boarding school experiences: recent studies from Native perspectives. *OAH Magazine of History.* 2001;15(2):20–22. https://doi.org/10.1093/maghis/15.2.20.

58. Berckmoes L, Eichelsheim V, Rutayisire T, Annemiek R, Hola B. How legacies of genocide are transmitted in the family environment: a qualitative study of two generations in Rwanda. *Societies.* 2017;7:24. https://doi.org/10.3390/soc7030024.

59. Roth M, Neuner F, Elbert T. Transgenerational consequences of PTSD: risk factors for the mental health of children whose mothers have been exposed to the Rwandan genocide. 2014:12.

60. Hirschberger G. Collective trauma and the social construction of meaning. Front Psychol. 2018;9:1441. https://doi.org/10.3389/fpsyg.2018.01441.

61. Perrin PB, Sutter ME, Trujillo MA, Henry RS, Pugh M. The minority strengths model: development and initial path analytic validation in racially/ethnically diverse LGBTQ individuals. *J Clin Psychol.* 2020;76(1):118–136. https://doi.org/10.1002/jclp.22850.

62. Fattoracci ESM, Revels-Macalinao M, Huynh,Q-L. Greater than the sum of racism and heterosexism: intersectional microaggressions toward racial/ethnic and sexual minority group members. *Cult Divers Ethnic Minority Psychol.* 2020;27(2):176–188. https://doi.org/10.1037/cdp0000329.

63. Sadika B, Wiebe E, Morrison MA, Morrison TG. Intersectional microaggressions and social support for LGBTQ persons of color: a systematic review of the Canadian-based empirical literature. *J GLBT Fam Studies.* 2020;16(2):111–147. https://doi.org/10.1080/1550428X.2020.1724125.

64. Ghabrial MA. "Trying to figure out where we belong": narratives of racialized sexual minorities on community, identity, discrimination, and health. *Sex Res Soc Policy.* 2017;14(1):42–55. https://doi.org/10.1007/s13178-016-0229-x.

65. Bayrakli E, Hafez F. The State of Islamophobia in Europe. In: Enes Bayraklı, Farid Hafez, eds. *European Islamophobia Report 2018.* SETA, Istanbul: 2019;5–14. https://www.islamophobiaeurope.com/wp-content/uploads/2019/09/EIR_2018.pdf

66. Alessi EJ, Kahn S, Greenfield B, Woolner L, Manning D. A qualitative exploration of the integration experiences of LGBTQ refugees who fled from the Middle East, North Africa, and Central and South Asia to Austria and the Netherlands. *Sex Res Soc Policy.* 2020;17(1):13–26. https://doi.org/10.1007/s13178-018-0364-7.

67. UNHCR. *Putting People First: UNHCR Age, Gender and Diversity Accountability Report 2018–2019.* United Nations High Commissioner for Refugees; 2020. https://www.unhcr.org/5f04946d4.pdf.

68. House JS, Umberson D, Landis KR. Reviewed work(s): Structures and processes of social support. *Ann Rev Sociol.* 1988;14:293–318.

69. Schaefer C, Coyne JC, Lazarus RS. The health-related functions of social support. *J Behav Med.* 1981;4(4):381–406. https://doi.org/10.1007/BF00846149.

70. Benight CC, Bandura A. Social cognitive theory of posttraumatic recovery: the role of perceived self-efficacy. Behav Res Ther. 2004;42(10):1129–1148. https://doi.org/10.1016/j.brat.2003.08.008.

71. Pfefferbaum B, Seale T, Brandt E, Pfefferbaum R, Doughty D, Rainwater S. Media exposure in children one hundred miles from a terrorist bombing. *Ann Clin Psychiatry.* 2003;15(1):1–8. https://doi.org/10.3109/10401230309085664.

72. Charuvastra A, Cloitre M. Social bonds and posttraumatic stress disorder. *Ann Rev Psychol.* 2008;59(1), 301–328. https://doi.org/10.1146/annurev.psych.58.110405.085650.

73. Shang F, Kaniasty K, Cowlishaw S, Wade D, Ma H, Forbes D. Social support following a natural disaster: a longitudinal study of survivors of the 2013 Lushan earthquake in China. *Psychiatry Res.* 2019;273:641–646. https://doi.org/10.1016/j.psychres.2019.01.085.

74. Norris FH, Baker CK, Murphy AD, Kaniasty K. Social support mobilization and deterioration after Mexico's 1999 flood: effects of context, gender, and time. *Am J Commun Psychol.* 2005;36(1–2):15–28. https://doi.org/10.1007/s10464-005-6230-9.

75. Ben-Ezra M, Goodwin R, Palgi Y, et al. Concomitants of perceived trust in hospital and medical services following Hurricane Sandy. *Psychiatry Res.* 2014;220(3):1160–1162. https://doi.org/10.1016/j.psychres.2014.08.012.

76. Stanley IH, Hom MA, Chu C, et al. Perceptions of belongingness and social support attenuate PTSD symptom severity among firefighters: a multistudy investigation. *Psychol Serv.* 2019;16(4):543–555. https://doi.org/10.1037/ser0000240.

77. Lucero L. Safe spaces in online places: social media and LGBTQ youth. *Multicult Educ Rev.* 2017;9(2):117–128. https://doi.org/10.1080/2005615X.2017.1313482.

78. Djafarova E, Trofimenko O. Exploring the relationships between self-presentation and self-esteem of mothers in social media in Russia. *Comput Hum Behav.* 2017;73, 20–27. https://doi.org/10.1016/j.chb.2017.03.021

79. Craig W, Boniel-Nissim M, King N, et al. Social media use and cyber-bullying: a cross-national analysis of young people in 42 countries. *J Adolesc Health.* 2020;66(6):S100–S108. https://doi.org/10.1016/j.jadohealth.2020.03.006.

80. Jan M, Soomro SA, Ahmad N. Impact of social media on self-esteem. *Eur Scientific J.* 2017;13(23):329. https://doi.org/10.19044/esj.2017.v13n23p329.

81. Department of Veterans Affairs/Department of Defense. *Management of Posttraumatic Stress Disorder and Acute Stress Reaction 2017: VA/DoD Clinical Practice Guidelines* [General Information]. 2017. https://www.healthquality.va.gov/guidelines/MH/ptsd/.

82. Foa EB, Hembree E, Rothbaum B. *Prolonged Exposure Therapy for PTSD: Therapist Guide: Emotional Processing of Traumatic Experiences.* Oxford: Oxford University Press; 2007. https://doi.org/10.1093/med:psych/9780195308501.001.0001.

83. Kelmendi B, Adams TG, Yarnell S, Southwick S, Abdallah CG, Krystal JH. PTSD: From neurobiology to pharmacological treatments. *Eur J Psychotraumatol.* 2016;7(1):31858. https://doi.org/10.3402/ejpt.v7.31858.

84. Stana A, Flynn M, Almeida E. Battling the stigma: combat veterans' use of social support in an online PTSD forum. *Int J Mens Health.* 2017;16(1):20–36. https://doi.org/10.3149/jmh.1601.20.

85. Morley CA, Kohrt BA. Impact of peer support on PTSD, hope, and functional impairment: a mixed-methods study of child soldiers in Nepal. *J Aggress Maltreat Trauma.* 2013;22(7):714–734. https://doi.org/10.1080/10926771.2013.813882.

26

Social Psychiatry

Psychotic Disorders

Lakshmi Venkatraman, Greeshma Mohan,
Vijaya Raghavan, R. Padmavati, and R. Thara

Introduction

Psychosis, embedded in many psychiatric disorders, including schizophrenia and bipolar affective disorder, is traditionally considered to be a biopsychosocial disorder. While there is strong evidence for biological factors like hyperdopaminergia,[1] recent research has also identified a broad range of other psychosocial and environmental risk factors. While contemporary studies of psychosis typically encompass a wide range of variables, the relative influence of these domains has yet to be unequivocally established. It has become clear that there is not one specific factor that causes these disorders, but rather a complex interplay between biological and environmental factors. This chapter deals with the social factors contributing to the psychotic disorders and the social impact of these disorders on people's lives.

Historical Aspects of Social Concepts in Psychotic Disorders

Evidence for the social causation of schizophrenia and other psychoses was initially associated with family factors like marital schism, skew,[2] and schizogenic mothers.[3] However, scientific evidence did not support these theories and they were no longer considered.

Faris and Dunham[4] noted the higher incidence of psychosis in deprived neighborhoods with high poverty rates, marital instability, residential mobility, and ethnic heterogeneity. On the contrary, Goldberg and Morrison[5] and Silverton and Mednick[6] espoused a social selection perspective. They proposed that the social environment was more an outcome than a cause of psychosis. Exploration has continued whether these are causes or effects of psychosis. Social causation theories argue that chronic exposure to early adverse neighborhood in genetically vulnerable people predisposes to schizophrenia.

The social drift hypothesis, on the other hand, claims that people with schizophrenia end up in a downward socioeconomic trajectory, leading them to poverty and deprived neighborhoods. Goldberg and Morrison[5] conducted a survey among young men admitted for the first time with schizophrenia and found that the fathers' social classes were comparable to the general population and the young men themselves had careers before the onset of illness, similar to their home environment, and those with acute onset dropped in class just before admission.

Sariaslan[7] has made an argument for genetic liability as the common denominator for both schizophrenia and adult neighborhood deprivation, thus disputing the social drift hypothesis.

Social and Environmental Risk Factors

Our perusal of literature on risk and associated factors revealed that there were no striking differences in these in the groups of schizophrenia, first-episode psychosis, and bipolar disorders. Hence, we have decided to merge these disorders together in the context of the social risk factors. They have been broadly divided as prenatal and perinatal risk factors and postnatal and environmental risk factors (Box 26.1)

Prenatal Factors

Obstetric Complications

Interest in obstetric complications being a risk factor for schizophrenia goes back in time to the 1930s when Rosanoff and colleagues[8] mentioned "birth trauma" as one of the causal factors for schizophrenia and related psychosis. Recent focus has been on identifying specific obstetric complications affecting psychosis risk, and methodology has moved to population-based studies from case-control studies.

BOX 26.1 Risk Factors for Psychotic Disorders

Prenatal and Perinatal Risk Factors

Obstetric complications

Postnatal and Environmental Risk Factors

Childhood trauma and adversity

Adult life events

Social support

Substance use

Migrants and ethnic minorities

Urbanicity

Social deprivation

Mary Cannon and colleagues,[9] in their meta-analysis of obstetric complications and schizophrenia, grouped the risk factors as complications of pregnancy (bleeding, diabetes, rhesus, preeclampsia), abnormal fetal growth and development (low birthweight, congenital malformations, reduced head circumference), and complications of delivery (uterine atony, asphyxia, emergency caesarean section). Premature delivery (less than 32 weeks gestation) was found to be a significant risk factor for the development of bipolar disorder.

There is a possibility for mediating factors like hypoxia and gene-environment interaction that might explain how the obstetric complications increase the risk of psychosis.

Postnatal Social and Environmental Risk Factors

Childhood Trauma

Childhood maltreatment is one of the most studied postnatal environmental risk factors for later development of psychosis. Of these, emotional abuse or emotional neglect seems to be more significantly associated.

Higher rates of childhood adversity found in bipolar disorder are very similar to those for schizophrenia. In a recent meta-analysis, significant associations were observed between the development of bipolar disorder and childhood adversities such as prior physical, sexual, and emotional abuse, and physical and emotional neglect. Emotional abuse was found to be four times more likely in persons with bipolar disorder when compared with normal controls. Moreover, the risk of transition from a depressive episode to a bipolar disorder is higher in persons with a history of childhood adversities including abuse.

Similarly, significant association has been shown between schizophrenia and child physical abuse, exposure to domestic violence, and involvement in bullying.[10] A study from Belgium and Holland by Heins et al.[11] showed that childhood trauma increased the risk of psychotic disorder 4 times and showed a dose-response relationship. Dopaminergic hyperactivity and hypothalamic-pituitary-adrenal (HPA) dysregulation and genetic vulnerability have all been hypothesized to be the mediating factors for the increased risk.

There were significant associations between adversity and psychosis across all research designs; the integration of the case-control studies indicated that patients with psychosis were 2.72 times more likely to have been exposed to childhood adversity than controls. Similarly, the association between childhood adversity and psychosis was also significant in population-based cross-sectional studies, as well as prospective and quasi-prospective studies. While the risk is increased, it is unclear if this link is causative.

Migrants and Ethnic Minorities

Migration and ethnic minorities have been associated with increased incidence of psychoses. Craig Morgan et al.[12] have looked at several reviews from high-income countries and reported that the incidence of psychotic disorders in all minority ethnic populations combined is around 1.5 to 3.0 times the incidence in majority populations. The reported rates vary by population. For example, the rates are particularly high for the Black African and Black Caribbean population in the United Kingdom. The Netherlands reports particularly higher rates for the Surinamese and Moroccan population compared to the Turkish population.

In the same paper, Morgan and team[12] quote a study where Canada and Israel do not find increased rates of psychosis in their migrant population, suggesting that the host country of migration might also have a role to play. Studies have also explored factors mediating the increased incidence in ethnic minorities. Gender, ethnic density, refugee status, substance use, particularly of cannabis, and exposure to social adversities like discrimination have been associated with the increased risk. They proposed "a socio-developmental model, in which greater exposure to social risks across the life course accounts for the high rates of disorder in some groups, making the additional important point that these risks are socially structured."[12(p256)]

Concept of social capital and social cohesion have been considered as mediating the risk of schizophrenia in ethnic minorities, and Judith Allardyce and Jane Boydell[13] in their review state arguments for higher social cohesion being a protective factor against schizophrenia. Social capital is proposed to work as a "buffer" against stress through dopamine mechanism. An alternate view is that in vulnerable individuals, low social capital causes the individual to develop a persecutory attributional style leading to psychosis.

Urbanicity

Today, 55% of the world population lives in urban areas, and the next decade will probably see an increase. Risk of psychosis has been associated with urban birth, upbringing, and current city living. What are the characteristics of the urban environment that reflect social stressors and socioenvironmental adversity, which are increased by low social cohesion and high deprivation (e.g., low income, employment, and education), inequality, and social fragmentation?

Analyses by country revealed significant associations between urbanicity and higher psychosis risk in the United Kingdom and the Netherlands, but not in France, Italy, and Spain.[14] Interestingly, urbanicity was associated with higher positive and negative symptoms in the United Kingdom and lower positive and negative symptoms in Spain. No such associations were present in the Netherlands, France, or Italy.

A meta-analysis showed that the risk of developing schizophrenia and related disorders is approximately 2.37 times greater in urban compared with rural settings and is associated with the level of density of the urban environment and population density in a dose-response fashion that suggests the possibility of a causal effect.[15]

Another meta-analysis specifically focusing on low- and middle-income countries (LMIC) using the WHO World Health Survey of 42 countries from the LMIC region (215,682 respondents) did not find any difference between urban and rural setting in psychosis risk.[16] De Vylder and team used the data from individual LMIC and observed a higher risk for psychotic disorders (self-report) with urbanicity in Estonia, Mali, Laos, Morocco, and Mexico, but a lower psychosis risk with urbanicity in Nepal, Vietnam, Hungary, and South Africa. But the overall association was nonsignificant.

Several social and economic mechanisms might account for the urbanicity-psychosis link. Four studies showed that migrants/ethnic minorities have a higher psychosis incidence than native populations. Although migrant or ethnic minority status has been suggested as an underlying factor of urbanicity effects, the findings of Schofield et al.[17] implicate a more complicated relationship. Only after ethnic density (i.e., concentration of a particular group in an area) was included in the analysis, psychosis risk was elevated for European and Middle Eastern migrants, but not for Asian or African migrants. Thus, in some groups, urbanicity-psychosis associations appeared when ethnic density was low. In LMIC, lack of the urbanicity effect on psychosis risk could be due to reduced difference in economic factors, and family and social cohesion between rural and urban areas.

Kirkbride et al.[18] showed that regardless of urbanicity, Black Caribbean, African, and Pakistani, but not Arabic or Bangladeshi minorities, have a higher psychosis risk. Another investigation used the same data to disentangle effects of urbanicity, racial/ethnic diversity, density and fragmentation, economic deprivation, and social isolation on psychosis risk. Economic deprivation, social isolation, and urbanicity emerged as independent risk factors when ethnicity was accounted for.

In addition, lack of green space (in itself or as proxy for urban stress), environmental pollution, and toxin exposure have been suggested to increase risk. Urban factors may do most harm in individuals with a genetic liability for psychosis. Knowledge about urban risk factors is crucial to enable urban designs that mitigate risk.

Green space might reduce psychosis risk through stress reduction and reduced exposure to pollution. A Danish register study showed increased psychosis risk in those who during childhood (at age 10) lived in the least green compared to those who lived in the greenest areas. Risk decreased with accumulated green space exposure. The effects of green space were attenuated, but still significant when urbanicity and socioeconomic factors were taken into account. Evidence from the Netherlands showed that patients with psychotic disorders tend to reside in less green neighborhoods than the general population. Yet, greener living was unrelated to the duration of psychiatric admissions.

Cannabis and Tobacco

Evidence is mounting for substance use, especially cannabis use, as a risk factor for the development of psychosis. Daily substance use is associated with an increased risk of psychotic illness in both case-control and prospective studies.

Early use and daily use of high-potency cannabis and synthetic cannabinoids have the highest risk for subsequent development of schizophrenia.[19] Higher levels of cannabis use were associated with increased risk for psychosis in all studies. A logistic regression model gave an OR of 3.90 (95% CI 2.84 to 5.34) for the risk of schizophrenia and other psychosis-related outcomes among the heaviest cannabis users compared to nonusers.

The prevalence of smoking in patients presenting with their first episode of psychosis was 0.57 (95% CI 0.52–0.62; p <0.0001). Daily smokers developed psychotic illness at an earlier age than did nonsmokers (weighted mean difference −1.04 years, 95% CI −1.82 to −0.26). Those with psychosis started smoking at a nonsignificantly earlier age than did healthy controls (−0.44 years, 95% CI −1.21 to 0.34).

In causal terms, it seems to be a bidirectional association in affective psychosis. But this could not be ascertained due to the relative lack of prospective, longitudinal studies examining the relationship between them.

In a recent review, it was observed that cannabis use not only increased the risk of subsequent relapse of manic episodes, but also tripled the risk of new-onset subthreshold manic symptoms in vulnerable populations.[20] Similarly, cannabis use increased the risk by 5 times for first-episode bipolar disorders and demonstrated a dose-response relationship. Moreover, earlier age of cannabis use is associated with hypomania, when controlled for other confounding factors. Other substances of abuse are also important in the risk of bipolar disorders, such as opioids, alcohol, and stimulants. Opioid use increases the risk of developing bipolar disorder with age of onset of substance use before 25 years, in particular.

Therefore, although a causal link between substance use and psychosis cannot be unequivocally established, there is sufficient evidence to justify harm-reduction prevention programs.

Neighborhood-Level Social Deprivation

The level of social deprivation seems to be associated with the incidence of psychoses. However, when other neighborhood or individual factors were controlled for, the association became nonsignificant. There has been less research conducted on the association between social deprivation at the time of birth and the risk for developing a psychotic disorder or in those identified as having an at-risk mental state.[21] Understanding the relationship between social deprivation and psychotic disorders is critical to the understanding of the etiology of psychotic disorders and also the provision of clinical services.

A case-control study conducted by Harrison et al.[22] that included 82 individuals with a first episode of psychosis (FEP) and matched controls found that individuals who developed a psychotic disorder had over 6 times the odds of being born in an area of higher social deprivation (OR 6.3, 95% CI 2.7–15.2, p <0.001).

A number of studies in the United Kingdom were conducted by Kirkbride et al.,[23] the first of which included 295 individuals with psychosis and identified a higher rate of non-affective psychotic disorders in the most deprived neighborhoods. These findings were replicated in a further study, which found that wards with the highest level of social deprivation had a higher incidence of non-affective psychotic disorders (IRR 1.76, 95% CI 1.0–3.0). The study identified that 23% (95% CI 9.9–42.2) of the variance in the incidence of non-affective psychotic disorders could be attributed to neighborhood-level risk factors.[18]

In South Africa, Burns and Esterhuizen[24] found no association between the incidence of FEP and the level of poverty. In Canada, Anderson et al.[25] found that the incidence of first-episode schizophrenia spectrum disorder was significantly higher among people living in the most materially deprived areas (RR 1.75, 95% CI 1.3–2.3) and in the most socially deprived areas (RR 1.84, 95% CI 1.3–2.6) of Montreal.

Omer et al.[26] found an increased incidence of FEP in the more materially deprived neighborhoods of two rural counties in Ireland (IRR 1.13, 95% CI 1.0–1.2). In a subsequent study of O'Donoghue et al.,[27] in an urban and rural area of Ireland, a 3.4-fold increase in the incidence rate of FEP was observed in the most deprived neighborhood (IRR 3.4, 95% CI 1.2–7.8).

Lasalvia et al.[28] found a 2-fold increase in the incidence rate of all psychoses in the most deprived areas compared with the most affluent areas of Italy (IRR 2.09, 95% CI

1.5–2.9). Szöke et al.[29] found that the incidence of the first episode of psychosis was not associated with the level of social deprivation within an urban and rural area of France.

The vast majority of this research has been conducted in developed countries, and therefore the overall findings that there is a higher rate of psychotic disorders cannot be generalized to developing countries. If the incidence of psychotic disorders is indeed related to the level of social deprivation, then we would observe much higher rates of psychotic disorders in poorer countries with more socially deprived neighborhoods. Well-planned research is required to replicate this finding in LMIC.

Social Support

Research on expressed emotions (EE) was initiated in the 1990s in relation to relapses in schizophrenia.[30-32] This led to the development of interventions to address this aspect of family environment.

Family attitudes and interactional behaviors measured by EE and affective style (AS) were also found to be associated with relapse in bipolar disorder. It was also seen that persons with bipolar disorder with full inter-episode remission perceived social support better when compared with persons in partial remission. This perception of poor social support could lead to relapse.

Social and Environmental Risk Factors for Postpartum Psychosis

Previous Psychiatric Illness

Literature on the role of risk factors for postpartum psychosis is sparse. Personal or family history of bipolar disorder is seen in 40%–50% of women presenting with postpartum psychosis.[33] Similarly, postpartum psychosis in previous pregnancies is a risk factor for similar episodes in the current pregnancy. Postpartum psychosis might be associated with obstetric complications, including pre-eclampsia.[34]

Stressors and Social Factors

Other risk factors that could modulate postpartum psychosis include primiparity, maternal age, stress levels in the puerperium, and maternal sleep problems.[35] In contrast to postpartum depression, postpartum psychosis is not associated with social stressors experienced by the women during or after pregnancy. In one study, women from the poorest neighborhoods had higher chance of experiencing postpartum psychosis when compared with richest neighborhoods (OR = 1.49 (95% CI = 1.15–2.91, p = 0.002).[36]

Social Impact of Psychotic Disorders

Psychotic disorders such as schizophrenia and bipolar disorder are serious mental illnesses and have a significant impact on the social outcomes of those suffering from these disorders.

Employment, marriage, quality of life, and stigma are some of the social factors affected by psychotic disorders.

Employment

Unemployment is one of the major social deficits in many adults with psychotic disorders, especially schizophrenia. Employment rates in people with schizophrenia vary from 10% to 20%.[37] When compared with persons with chronic psychotic illness, people with FEP have a better employment rate. Chances of future employment are best predicted by previous work history. Studies have shown that people are more likely to take up jobs if they are not in receipt of welfare benefits, as in many developing countries.[38] A rural background appears to provide better chances for employment compared to urban areas. The individual nature of agricultural work, seasonality, flexibility, and family support could all be possible factors for better employment in rural areas for persons with psychotic disorders.

Marriage

Marriage rates in persons with psychoses appear to be different between Western world studies and those of other countries. While the former report lower marriage rates, the latter have found a 70% marriage rate in those with schizophrenia.[39] Shorter illness duration, onset of illness after marriage, and having children are associated with a better marital outcome. Unemployment, self-neglect, flat affect, and drop in socioeconomic status were related to poor marital outcome. Sociocultural aspects, such as the way marriages are still arranged in some parts of the world, the stigma attached to divorce/marital separation, and the lack of options for independent living for women in some countries may all be contributing to this, but require more detailed research.

Stigma

Psychotic disorders are probably one of the most stigmatized conditions. This remains a barrier to help-seeking and many other aspects of one's life.[40] Development and maintenance of psychotic symptoms are linked to stigma and the social meanings attached to experiences in psychosis.[41] Morrison goes on to state that the social norms of society defining types of beliefs which are removed from reality, and therefore delusional, make the interpretations made by people who are diagnosed as psychotic to be considered "culturally unacceptable." Major and O'Brien[42] opine that those who are stigmatized are viewed as deviating in some way from the social norm. So, stigma seems to define the norms and the deviations from these. The stigmatizing experience is not only limited to the patients but is also experienced by their close relatives.

Stigma results in (i) a lower priority for seeking help from mental health services; (ii) difficulty getting staff of good quality to work in these services; (iii) continuing problems in finding employment and housing for people who have had an episode of mental disorder; (iv) the social isolation of people who suffer from mental illness and their families; and (v) poorer quality of care for physical illnesses occurring in people diagnosed as having had psychiatric illnesses.[43] These effects of stigma are true for all mental disorders, and in particular for psychotic disorders.

BOX 26.2 Social Interventions for Psychotic Disorders

Family and Social Interventions
Family psychoeducation
Supported employment programs
Housing
Disability benefits

Despite the availability of evidence-based treatments for managing mental disorders, over 70% of individuals suffering from some form of mental disorder do not receive treatment.[44] Stigma attached to mental illness remains widely prevalent, and still poses formidable barriers in help-seeking by the mentally ill.

Quality of Life

Younger men, high level of education, unemployment, living alone, and homelessness are all associated with less favorable subjective quality of life. Depressive symptoms are associated with poor subjective quality of life.[45]

Social Interventions for Psychotic Disorders

A variety of social interventions exist to help persons with psychotic disorders recover from their illness (Box 26.2).

Family Psycho-education

Family psycho-education was developed 40 years ago as an intervention for schizophrenia and related disorders. Though its initial aim was to reduce the expressed emotions of the family members toward persons with psychoses in order to prevent relapse, psycho-education now encompasses many other aspects, such as social and role functioning, burden reduction, and general well-being. It is critical to engage the family members as equal partners in the treatment of the patients with psychosis by training them to use the required coping skills and complement professional intervention. There is emerging evidence that family psycho-education is one of the most effective interventions available.[46] For example, when compared to treatment as usual, family psycho-education intervention has shown to reduce relapse rate by 50%–60%. This effect has been more pronounced in FEP and in ultra-high-risk groups, where this intervention has shown to help in the substantial return of functioning.[47]

These sessions on family intervention should be offered to all persons with psychosis who live with their family, especially when the symptoms are florid with high risk of relapse. At least 10 sessions, spread over a period of 3 months, are to be planned to provide family interventions. This should include training in communication skills, problem-solving, and psycho-education.[48] It is also important that family interventions should enable families to better communicate their concerns to mental health professionals, especially in LMIC, where most people with psychotic disorders continue to live at home with their families.

Supported Employment Programs

Employment can provide financial benefits for an individual with psychotic disorders, for their symptom alleviation and psychological well-being. The extent of disability very often determines the readiness to work, the nature of work, and the extent of supervision required. Those who may not be ready right away to work will need prevocational training and sometimes have to work under sheltered conditions for varying periods of time. There will, however, be a group of severely disabled individuals who can work only under sheltered conditions.[37]

Mental health services should work in partnership with local stakeholders such as potential employers, locally available industry, and job coaches to enable people with psychosis to find work and to stay in it. Continuous monitoring of such persons who are placed in jobs is often essential.

Housing

One of the major milestones in the process of recovery among persons with psychotic disorders is independent living in their own homes. But this can be compromised due to the stigmatizing attitudes held by the general public toward persons with psychotic illness. At the same time, research has shown that many people with schizophrenia and related psychotic illness live in substandard and unstable accommodation, and this has an impact on the clinical and functional outcomes of the persons with psychotic illness. For example, in a study, one of the key determinants of relapse and high rates of readmission among persons with schizophrenia was the type of accommodation.[49]

In a comparative study among persons with schizophrenia, those who were living independently had a better outcome in both the psychotic and depressive symptoms, along with more motivation and better level of functioning.[50] Similarly, independent housing has shown to be associated with better social network and a better quality of life.[51]

In many LMIC, where persons with psychotic disorders continue to live with their families, housing may not be a critical area of intervention. For the homeless and wandering mentally ill, this does pose a challenge, even in many of these countries.

Disability Benefits

"Disability," according to the International Classification of Functioning (ICF) Disability and Health, is an umbrella term to include impairments, activity limitations, or participation restrictions According to the global burden of a disease study, schizophrenia is the sixth leading cause of years lived with disability. Recently, disability has been recognized as one of the outcome measures for chronic illnesses such as schizophrenia and other psychotic illness.

In the United States, under Social Security Administration (SSA) disability benefits, two major SSA disability programs are available for the persons with major mental illness: Social Security Disability Insurance (SSDI) and Supplemental Security Income (SSI). SSDI is an early retirement program for workers who have paid a portion of their earnings to Social Security. SSI, in contrast, is a program for people with low incomes who have not worked sufficiently to qualify for SSDI. In 2014, some 713,000 U.S. adults received SSDI or SSI for schizophrenia. Reliance on these programs is thus widespread among people with schizophrenia.[52]

In India, the Persons with Disabilities (Equal Opportunities, Protection of Rights and Full Participation) Act, which came into force in 1995, deals with the benefits for persons with disabilities in India. Even though the persons with mental retardation have been routinely included under this scheme and have been provided with benefits, persons with severe mental illness, such as schizophrenia and bipolar disorders, are not actively encouraged. The Rehabilitation Committee of the Indian Psychiatric Society introduced the Indian Disability Evaluation and Assessment Scale (IDEAS) in 2002 and gazetted in 2002 as the recommended instrument to measure psychiatric disability in India. The disabled are eligible for the following major welfare schemes: (i) disability pension/unemployment pension; (ii) insurance scheme for the mentally challenged; (iii) scheme helping to set up small shops; (iv) free legal aid; and (v) concessional railway and bus passes.[53,54]

Future Research Directions

To date, only a handful of studies have used an epidemiological approach to explore the association between social factors and specific psychosis symptoms or symptom clusters. Further empirical studies are needed to make sense of the mixed research findings, to understand the pathways through which they influence health, and to find out ways of reducing their magnitude.

Key Points

- Social factors are important in the genesis, course, and outcome of psychotic disorders.
- Pre- and peri-natal factors and early childhood factors are critical.
- Migration, urbanization, and globalization have an impact on the course.
- Social impact is seen in areas of employment, housing, disability, and stigma.
- Social and family interventions are key in reducing relapses and facilitating better functioning.

References

1. Howes OD, Kapur S. The dopamine hypothesis of schizophrenia: version III—the final common pathway. *Schizophr Bull.* 2009;35(3):549–562.
2. Lidz T, Cornelison AR, Fleck S, Terry D. The intrafamilial environment of schizophrenic patients: II. Marital schism and marital skew. *Am J Psychiatry.* 1957;114(3):241–248.

3. Heston LL. Psychiatric disorders in foster home reared children of schizophrenic mothers. *Br J Psychiatry*. 1966;112(489):819–825.

4. Faris REL, Dunham HW. *Mental Disorders in Urban Areas: An Ecological Study of Schizophrenia and Other Psychoses*. Univeristy Chicago Press; 1939.

5. Goldberg EM, Morrison SL. Schizophrenia and social class. *Br J Psychiatry*. 1963;109(463):785–802.

6. Silverton L, Mednick S. Class drift and schizophrenia. *Acta Psychiatr Scand*. 1984;70(4):304–309.

7. Sariaslan A, Fazel S, D'Onofrio BM, et al. Schizophrenia and subsequent neighborhood deprivation: re-visiting the social drift hypothesis using population, twin and molecular genetic data. *Transl Psychiatry*. 2016;6(5):e796.

8. Rosanoff AJ, Handy LM, Plesset IR, Brush S. The etiology of so-called schizophrenic psychoses: with special reference to their occurrence in twins. *Am J Psychiatry*. 1945;91(2):247–286.

9. Cannon M, Jones PB, Murray RM. Obstetric complications and schizophrenia: Historical and meta-analytic review. *Am J Psychiatry*. 2002;159(7):1080–1092.

10. Moffitt TE. Childhood exposure to violence and lifelong health: clinical intervention science and stress-biology research join forces. *Devel Psychopathol*. 2013;25(4pt2):1619–1634.

11. Heins M, Simons C, Lataster T, et al. Childhood trauma and psychosis: a case-control and case-sibling comparison across different levels of genetic liability, psychopathology, and type of trauma. *Am J Psychiatry*. 2011;168(12):1286–1294.

12. Morgan C, Knowles G, Hutchinson G. Migration, ethnicity and psychoses: evidence, models and future directions. *World Psychiatry*. 2019;18(3):247–258.

13. Allardyce J, Boydell J. Environment and schizophrenia: review: the wider social environment and schizophrenia. *Schizophr Bull*. 2006;32(4):592–598.

14. Fett A-KJ, Lemmers-Jansen IL, Krabbendam L. Psychosis and urbanicity: a review of the recent litera-ture from epidemiology to neurourbanism. *Curr Opin Psychiatry*. 2019;32(3):232.

15. Vassos E, Pedersen CB, Murray RM, Collier DA, Lewis CM. Meta-analysis of the association of urbanicity with schizophrenia. *Schizophr Bull*. 2012;38(6):1118–1123.

16. DeVylder JE, Kelleher I, Lalane M, Oh H, Link BG, Koyanagi A. Association of urbanicity with psy-chosis in low-and middle-income countries. *JAMA Psychiatry*. 2018;75(7):678–686. doi:10.1001/jamapsychiatry.2018.0577. Published online May 16, 2018.

17. Schofield P, Thygesen M, Das-Munshi J, et al. Ethnic density, urbanicity and psychosis risk for migrant groups: a population cohort study. *Schizophr Res*. 2017;190:82–87.

18. Kirkbride JB, Morgan C, Fearon P, Dazzan P, Murray RM, Jones PB. Neighbourhood-level effects on psychoses: re-examining the role of context. *Psychol Med*. 2007;37(10):1413–1425.

19. Murray RM, Quigley H. Quattrone D, Englund A, Di Forti M. Traditional marijuana, high-potency can-nabis and synthetic cannabinoids: Increasing risk for psychosis. *World Psychiatry*. 2016;15(3):195–204.

20. Gibbs M, Winsper C, Marwaha S, Gilbert E, Broome M, Singh SP. Cannabis use and mania symp-toms: a systematic review and meta-analysis. *J Affect Disord*. 2015;171:39–47.

21. Wickham S, Taylor P, Shevlin M, Bentall P. The impact of social deprivation on paranoia, hallucin-ations, mania and depression: the role of discrimination social support, stress and trust. *PloS One*, 2014;9(8):e105140.

22. Harrison G, Hopper, K, Craig T, et al. Recovery from psychotic illness: a 15-and 25-year international follow-up study. *Br J Psychiatry*. 2001;178(6):506–517.

23. Kirkbride JB, Hameed Y, Ioannidis K, et al. Ethnic minority status, age-at-immigration and psychosis risk in rural environments: evidence from the SEPEA study. *Schizophr Bull*. 2017;43(6):1251–1261.

24. Burns JK, Esterhuizen T. Poverty, inequality and the treated incidence of first-episode psychosis. *Soc Psychiatry Psychiatr Epidemiol*. 2008;43(4):331–335.

25. Anderson KK, Fuhrer R, Abrahamowicz M, Malla AK. The incidence of first-episode schizophrenia-spectrum psychosis in adolescents and young adults in Montreal: an estimate from an administrative claims database. *Canadian J Psychiatry*. 2012;57(10):626–633.

26. Omer S, Kirkbride JB, Pringle DG, Russell V, O'Callaghan E, Waddington JL. Neighbourhood-level socio-environmental factors and incidence of first episode psychosis by place at onset in rural Ireland: the Cavan–Monaghan First Episode Psychosis Study [CAMFEPS]. *Schizophr Res*. 2014;152(1):152–157.

27. O'Donoghue, B., Lyne, J. P., Renwick, L., et al. Neighbourhood characteristics and the incidence of first-episode psychosis and duration of untreated psychosis. *Psychol Med.* 2016;46(7):1367–1378.

28. LaSalvia A, Bonetto C, Tosato S, et al. First-contact incidence of psychosis in north-eastern Italy: influence of age, gender, immigration and socioeconomic deprivation. *Br J Psychiatry.* 2014;205(2):127–134.

29. Szoke A, Pignon B, Baudin G, et al. Small area-level variation in the incidence of psychotic disorders in an urban area in France: an ecological study. *Soc Psychiatry Psychiatr Epidemiol.* 2016;51(7):951–960.

30. Bebbington, P., & Kuipers, L. The predictive utility of expressed emotion in schizophrenia: an aggregate analysis. *Psychol Med.* 1994;24(3):707–718.

31. Brown GW. The discovery of expressed emotion: induction or deduction? In: Leff J, Vaughn C, eds. *Expressed Emotion in Families.* New York: Guilford Press; 1985:7–25.

32. Weintraub MJ, Hall DL, Carbonella JY, Weisman de Mamani A, Hooley JM. Integrity of literature on expressed emotion and relapse in patients with schizophrenia verified by ap-curve analysis. *Fam Process.* 2017;56(2):436–444.

33. Sit D, Rothschild AJ, Wisner KL. A review of postpartum psychosis. *J Women's Health.* 2006;15(4):352–368.

34. Upadhyaya SK, Sharma A, Raval CM. Postpartum psychosis: risk factors identification. *N Am J Med Sciences.* 2014;6(6):274.

35. Davies W. Understanding the pathophysiology of postpartum psychosis: challenges and new approaches. *World J Psychiatry.* 2017;7(2):77.

36. Nager A, Johansson L-M, Sundquist K. Neighborhood socioeconomic environment and risk of postpartum psychosis. *Arch Women's Mental Health.* 2006;9(2):81–86.

37. Marwaha S, Johnson S. Bebbington P, et al. Rates and correlates of employment in people with schizophrenia in the UK, France and Germany. *Br J Psychiatry.* 2007;191(1):30–37.

38. Srinivasan TN, Thara R. How do men with schizophrenia fare at work? A follow-up study from India. *Schizophr Res.* 1997;25(2):149–154. http://www.sciencedirect.com/science/article/pii/S092099649 7000169.

39. Thara R, Srinivasan TN. Outcome of marriage in schizophrenia. *Soc Psychiatry Psychiatr Epidemiol.* 1997;32(7):416–420.

40. Sartorius N. Iatrogenic Stigma of Mental Illness: Begins with Behaviour and Attitudes of Medical Professionals, Especially Psychiatrists. *BMJ.* 2002 Jun 22;324(7352):1470–1471. doi:10.1136/bmj.324.7352.1470

41. Morrison AP, Birchwood M, Pyle M, et al. Impact of cognitive therapy on internalised stigma in people with at-risk mental states. *British J Psychiatry.* 2013;203(2):140–145.

42. Major B, O'Brien LT. The social psychology of stigma. *Annu Rev Psychol.* 2005;56:393–421.

43. Knaak S, Mantler E, Szeto A. Mental illness-related stigma in healthcare: barriers to access and care and evidence-based solutions. *Healthc Manage Forum.* 2017;30:111–116.

44. Thornicroft G, Brohan E, Rose D, Sartorius N, Leese M, Group IS. Global pattern of experienced and anticipated discrimination against people with schizophrenia: a cross-sectional survey. *Lancet.* 2009;373(9661):408–415.

45. Priebe S, Roeder-Wanner U-U, Kaiser W. Quality of life in first-admitted schizophrenia patients: a follow-up study. *Psychol Med.* 2000;30(1):225–230.

46. Hogarty GE. Does family psychoeducation have a future? *World Psychiatry.* 2003;2(1):29.

47. Breitborde NJ, Woods SW, Srihari VH. Multifamily psychoeducation for first-episode psychosis: a cost-effectiveness analysis. *Psychiatr Serv.* 2009;60(11):1477–1483.

48. McFarlane WR. Family interventions for schizophrenia and the psychoses: a review. *Fam Process.* 2016;55(3):460–482.

49. Sfetcu R, Musat S, Haaramo P, et al. Overview of post-discharge predictors for psychiatric re-hospitalisations: a systematic review of the literature. *BMC Psychiatry.* 2017;17(1):227.

50. Juckel G, Morosini PL. The new approach: psychosocial functioning as a necessary outcome criterion for therapeutic success in schizophrenia. *Curr Opin Psychiatry.* 2008;21(6):630–639.

51. Hansson L, Middelboe T, Sørgaard KW, et al. Living situation, subjective quality of life and social network among individuals with schizophrenia living in community settings. *Acta Psychiatr Scand.* 2002;106(5):343–350.

52. Rosenheck RA, Estroff SE, Sint K, et al., RAISE-ETP Investigators. Incomes and outcomes: Social Security disability benefits in first-episode psychosis. *Am J Psychiatry*, 2017;*174*(9), 886–894. https://doi.org/10.1176/appi.ajp.2017.16111273.
53. Balhara YPS, Verma R, Deshpande SN. A study of profile of disability certificate seeking patients with schizophrenia over a 5 year period. *Indian J Psychol Med*. 2013;35(2):127–134. https://doi.org/10.4103/0253-7176.116235.
54. Kashyap K, Thunga R, Rao AK, Balamurali NP. Trends of utilization of government disability benefits among chronic mentally ill. *Indian J Psychiatry*. 2012;54(1):54–58. https://doi.org/10.4103/0019-5545.94648.

27

Social Psychiatry

Substance Use and Addictive Disorders

Rakesh K. Chadda and Roy Abraham Kallivalyalil

Every form of addiction is bad, no matter whether the narcotic be alcohol or morphine or idealism.
—Carl Jung

Introduction

Social psychiatry studies the role of social factors in genesis, clinical presentation, and management of mental disorders and includes interactions between mental disorders and society.[1] Substance use is often considered a social problem, a habit rather than an illness. The relationship between social psychiatry and substance use disorders (SUDs) is complex and includes social epidemiology of the SUDs, the associated burden and disability, myths and misconceptions, stigma, the role of social factors in the initiation and continuation of substance use, psychosocial management of substance use, prevention, rehabilitation, long-term social outcome, and the role of society and culture in substance use.[2]

Historical Development

Mankind has been using substances since time immemorial for recreational and ceremonial purposes. Such substances include alcohol, opium, cannabis, and stimulants like amphetamines, caffeine, and tobacco. Alcohol and tobacco come under the broad category of licit drugs, whereas cannabis, opioids, cocaine, stimulants, and many others come under the group of illicit drugs. A brief history of common substances of use is described here.

Alcohol has been used by human beings for at least 12,000 years. It has been described as a part of social ceremonies in Babylon, Greece, and the Roman Empire over 5,000 years ago. Reasons for its use included pleasure seeking, nutrition, and also for its medicinal properties.[3] Drunkenness and associated problems have been recognized in most of civilizations. Recreational and medicinal use of alcohol, opium, and cannabis has been seen since long in India as it is known Amanita muscaria had a religious significance in ancient India in 18th century and use of Soma, a sacred beverage in the Rigveda in ancient India. Mention of the consumption of alcohol by demons (*asuras*) and gods (*devas*) is also found in the ancient Indian mythological texts.[4] Use of alcohol was reduced during the Mughal period in India due to the influence of the Islamic traditions. However, during the Mughal period, recreational use of opioids increased and cultivation of opium was encouraged by the state.[5] Alcohol remains one of the prohibited drugs in most of the Islamic world.

Cannabis is the most commonly used illicit drug around the world. Cannabis preparations are obtained from the plant *cannabis sativa*, and are used for medicinal purposes. It was introduced to Europe in the early 19th century by Napoleon's army returning from Egypt. Recreational use of cannabis has been reported first by the Parisian bohemians in the late 19th century and later in Mexico and United States in the early 20th century.[6] In 1961, it was banned under the Single Convention on Narcotic Drugs. Recreational cannabis has been legalized by certain states in the United States, Canada, and certain other countries. Use of cannabis products for medicinal purposes is also well recognized.[7] Cannabis has also been used in India for thousands of years in the worship of the Lord Shiva, mostly as an orally administered form called *bhang*, which can consist of wet resinous leaves of the cannabis plant formed into pills, or added to a drink made of milk, cannabis, and various other spices, or by smoking the flowering buds of the cannabis plant. The practice is also mentioned in the ancient Vedas. In the past few decades, other forms of cannabis products, including *ganja* and *charas*, have been increasingly used, mostly smoked.[4]

Opioids, primarily a group of drugs that have the poppy plant as the primary source, have been one of the most dangerous drugs, but also have strong analgesic properties. Opium was probably first extracted by the Sumerians from the poppy plant around the end of the third millennium BC. It was brought to India and China by the Arab traders around the 8th century and traveled to Europe between the 10th and 13th centuries.[8] The opium poppy has been cultivated in India since the 10th century, and opium is listed as a remedy for a variety of ailments in "*Dhanvanatari Nighantu*," an ancient Indian medical treatise of the 10th century. Abuse and tolerance to opium have long been reported from Turkey, Egypt, Germany, England, and China. There were attempts by the Chinese to criminalize opium use, leading to conflict with the British and French powers. Morphine, the active ingredient, was isolated by Serturner in 1806, followed by codeine a few years later. The two compounds gradually replaced the crude opium in medicinal usage, though crude opium continued to be smoked in many parts of the world. Diacetylmorphine (heroin), the first semisynthetic opium derivative, was introduced to medicine in 1898, followed by meperidine in 1938 and methadone in the 1940s. Opioid addiction and withdrawal were first identified in the 19th century, have continued to the present, and have reached epidemic levels in the recent years.[8] In India, during the British era, opium farming and trade were regulated to increase the state revenue. There is a long-standing history of not only opioid addiction in India, but also managing this addiction through providing access to opioids in a regulated fashion, similar to the agonist maintenance treatment of today—the precursor to Opioid Substitution Therapy (OST) of current period. Use of opioids in agricultural labor in Punjab and certain other states to increase efficiency is well known.[2,4]

There is an interesting history of the rise in the abuse of drugs in India, especially in recent times, which has been attributed to a variety of geopolitical circumstances. India is located between the two major opium-growing regions of the world: the Golden Triangle (Laos, Myanmar, and Thailand) and the Golden Crescent (Afghanistan, Pakistan, and Iran). Large quantities of opioids are smuggled into India and trafficked onward. The geopolitical situation in this area since the late 1970s needs special mention, with Russian invasion followed by U.S. intervention in Afghanistan, the Indo-Pakistani conflict, Khalistan movement and terrorism in Punjab, and civil war in Sri Lanka. Opioids were used as a currency in the arms trade. The problem accentuated with raw opium being gradually replaced by heroin, which is easily transported, less bulky, more potent, and gives a greater rush when injected. India is the largest producer of licit opioids being utilized for medicinal purposes.[9] Opioid use has increased in India in the above background in Punjab, Rajasthan, and North-East India, and certain other states in the above background.[4,10]

Coca leaves, which are a source of cocaine, have been chewed in South America for about 15 centuries. The Spanish, following their intrusion to the continent, brought it to Europe. Cocaine, the active constituent of coca leaves, was extracted first by Friedrich Gaedecke in 1855 and also later by Albert Niemann, who gave it the name cocaine. [11] Cocaine use was quite popular across Europe and the Americas, and the users included the personalities like Sigmund Freud, who found it useful in their personal growth. Cocaine has also found its way into medicinal tonics and also in soft drinks including Coca Cola, though it was later removed in 1903.

Use of amphetamines, another group of stimulant drugs, can also be traced back many centuries. Ma-Huang, having similarities to ephedrine, has been used as a Chinese herbal remedy for thousands of years. Ephedrine, the active ingredient, was first isolated by Nagayoshi Nagia in 1887. Around the same time, amphetamine was synthesized by Lazar Edeleanu in Germany. Amphetamines were introduced in the West initially as bronchodilators in the 1930s. These were also used in the World War II to counter soldiers' fatigue. An increasing use was reported starting from 1960s following its abundant supply. In the current period, methamphetamine abuse is common across the United States and many other countries.[11]

Tobacco has been used by humankind since about 600 AD and was introduced to Europe in the 16th century. In the earlier period, it was smoked by pipes or cigars and used as smokeless tobacco. Cigarettes became common starting from the 1900s. The first reports of its adverse effects on health started appearing from 1950s, with an official recognition by the U.S. Surgeon General's Report on Smoking and Health in 1964. There have been strong anti-tobacco campaigns around the world, as well as a strong lobby by the tobacco companies for the earlier claims of safer filtered cigarettes and electronic controlled nicotine delivery (ECND) recently.[12] Tobacco has been used in India by chewing, and smoking bidis, hookah, and cigarettes. Though smoking has come down in the last 2 decades in India, its place has been taken by smokeless tobacco. Tobacco has often been a mode of socializing. In rural India, hookah is a part of rural culture and socializing in the community.[2,4]

Caffeine, a common ingredient of beverages, also has strong potential for abuse because of its unique stress-relieving properties. Caffeine-containing foods and beverages have been used by humans for thousands of years. Tea has been cultivated and used in China since 350 AD and coffee in Ethiopia since the 15th century. Coffee had become a popular beverage in Arabia in the 16th century and in Europe in 17th and 18th centuries. Similarly, tea also penetrated Europe and the Americas around the 16th–17th centuries. There was a shift from tea to coffee in the United States in late 18th century, following protests against the British taxes. Caffeine continues to be integral to the economic activity in many countries and is a part of many popular beverages and soft drinks.[13]

Extent of the Problem

SUDs can be designated as the most common mental disorders worldwide, and are associated with a huge global burden of disease and treatment gap for various reasons. Alcohol and tobacco remain the two commonest psychoactive substances of use/abuse, followed by cannabis, opioids, cocaine, stimulants, prescription drugs, inhalants, and others.

In the Global Burden of Disease (GBD) study, 2016, alcohol dependence has been recognized as the most prevalent SUD with 100.4 million estimated cases in 2016 (age-standardized prevalence 13.21 per 1000), followed by cannabis dependence with 22.1 million cases and age-standardized prevalence of 2.90 per 1000, and opioid dependence with 26.8 million cases and age-standardized prevalence of 3.53 per 1000.[14] Globally, in 2016, 99.2 million disability adjusted life years (DALYs) (95% uncertainty interval [UI] 88.3–111.2) and 4.2% of all DALYs (3.7–4.6) were attributable to alcohol use, and 31.8 M DALYs (27.4–36.6) and 1.3% of all DALYs (1.2–1.5) were attributable to drug use as a risk factor. Alcohol use has been identified as the 7th leading risk factor for both deaths and DALYs in 2016, accounting for 2.2% (95% uncertainty interval [UI] 1.5–3.0) of age-standardized female deaths and 6.8% (5.8–8.0) of age-standardized male deaths. GBD attributable to alcohol and drug use varies substantially across different geographical locations. A large proportion of this burden is due to the effect of substance use on other health outcomes. Thus, effective interventions are needed to prevent and reduce burden due to SUDs.

The prevalence of illicit drugs has shown an increase in the recent past. According to the World Drug Report, 2019, in 2017, 271 million people, or 5.5% of the global population age 15–64, had used drugs in the previous year.[15] Five percent of the global world population used (illicit) drugs at least once in 2015, 0.6% of the global population suffers drug use disorders, and 28 million health life-years are lost by premature death and disability due to drug use disorders. Less than 1 in 6 people with drug use disorders receives treatment. This number is 30% higher than in 2009, when 210 million had used drugs in the previous year. The increase was in part due to a 10% growth in the global population age 15–64, higher prevalence of opioid use in Africa, Asia, Europe, and North America, a higher prevalence of cannabis use in North and South America and Asia. Cannabis is the most widely used illicit drug worldwide, with an estimated 188 million people having used the drug in the previous year. In 2017, 53.4 million people worldwide had used opioids in the previous year, 56% higher than the estimate for 2016. North America continues to be the subregion with the highest annual prevalence of opioid use, with 4.0% of the population using opioids. The Near and Middle East and Southwest Asia are the subregion with the highest annual prevalence of opiate use (opium, morphine, and heroin) at 1.6% of the population. In terms of numbers of users, 35% of the global opioid users and almost half of all opiate users worldwide reside in South Asia. The magnitude of the problem is huge in South Asia, especially in the background of limited resources for treatment.

Recently, India completed a nationwide household survey on substance use, covering a population of 473,569 subjects in the age group of 10–75 and 72,642 subjects in respondent-driven sampling in its 36 states and union territories.[16] The findings of the Indian survey are compared here with those of the United States, as given by the Substance Abuse and Mental Health Services Administration,[17] two of the largest countries of the world, with one representing low and middle income and other representing the upper-income group. Life time prevalence of alcohol use as reported in the United States was 65.5%, with dependence seen in 5.4% of the population, whereas alcohol use was predominantly a male phenomenon in India in most of the states, with 14.6% of the population having used it in the previous year and 2.6% of the population meeting the criteria of dependence. Prevalence of marijuana use in the past year and dependence stood at 15.9% and 2.2%, respectively, for the United States and 2.8% and 0.25%, respectively, for India. Past-year heroin use and dependence were reported by 0.3% and 0.2% of the US population compared to 2.1% and 0.26% in India, respectively. Prevalence of inhalant use in the past year stood at 0.7% in both the United States and India. Two percent of the US population used cocaine in the past year, and the prevalence of dependence stood at 0.1%. Prevalence of tobacco dependence in India has been reported to be 20.9% by the National Mental Survey of India.[18] In the United States, past-year use of tobacco and cigarettes was reported to be 26.7% and 21.0%, respectively, and for lifetime use, 61.5% and 55.7%, respectively. The GBD 2016 study found some important regional differences. For example, Australasia has the highest age-standardized prevalence across all SUDS, with highest age-standardized prevalence of amphetamine dependence. Prevalence of cannabis, cocaine, and opioid dependence was highest in North America, and that of alcohol use disorders was highest in Eastern Europe.[14]

To summarize, cannabis remains the most commonly used illicit drug across the world. Tobacco and alcohol use are more extensively used than illicit drugs. Rates of prescription drug use have been a growing concern.

Physical Health Complications of Substance Use Disorders

It is important to briefly mention associated physical complications of the SUDs, which contribute to the GBD. Alcohol use is associated with gastrointestinal (liver damage, gastritis, pancreatitis, esophageal varices), neurological (Korsakoff syndrome, Wernicke encephalopathy, amnesic syndrome, dementia, delirium tremens, peripheral neuropathies, cerebellar degeneration), cardiovascular (hypertension, stroke, cardiomyopathy) complications and fetal alcohol syndrome. Use of tobacco has been implicated in chronic obstructive airway disease, lung cancer, and oral cancer.

Injection drug use is one of the most serious forms of substance use with its inherent health risks. As per the World Drug Report, 2019, more than 11 million people worldwide inject drugs.[15] One in 8 people who inject drugs lives with HIV, i.e., 1.4 million persons around the globe. The United Nations program on HIV/AIDS (UNAIDS) estimates that intravenous drug users (IDUs) are 22 times more likely than the general population to be infected with HIV. The prevalence of HIV among persons who inject drugs (PWID) is the highest by far in Southwest Asia and in Eastern and Southeastern Europe, with rates being 2.3 and 1.8 times the global average, respectively. Hepatitis C is highly prevalent among PWID, with almost one-half of PWID, or some 5.6 million people, living with hepatitis C. 585,000 people are estimated to have died as a result of drug use in 2017. More than half of these deaths were the result of untreated hepatitis C leading to liver cancer and cirrhosis, one-third of which were attributed to drug use disorders. Around two-thirds of the deaths attributed to drug use disorders were related to opioid use. It is estimated that around 42 million years of "healthy" life were lost (premature deaths and years lived with disability) as a result of drug use, mostly attributed to drug use disorders, especially from the use of opioids.

Psychosocial Consequences of the Substance Use Disorders

SUDs are associated with a range of adverse psychosocial consequences in personal life, family role, education and occupation, and in society, and also a high risk to develop co-morbid mental disorders. Social consequences begin with the initiation of drug use and keep adding up, as the drug use progresses. The user's life starts revolving around procuring and using the drug. Gradually, the severity of dependence increases and to control the withdrawal, one needs to take higher doses of the drug. In this progression, the person's life starts revolving around the substance use. The progression is faster in the case of opioids as compared to alcohol and other drugs.[2,15]

The drug addict starts neglecting his/her personal life, family, social circle, and job. The drug-related behaviors affect various areas of functioning, including education, job, and family. The person may start having financial problems due to money spent on drugs as well as loss of income due to irregularity at work. Over the period, the person may also lose his/her job, further adding to the financial hardships. In such a situation, he/she may indulge in criminal activities like stealing or other such behaviors and may also start getting involved in drug trafficking. The person may also resort to aggressive behavior, during intoxication as well as in withdrawal, to extract money from family members to get drugs. The family also gets neglected, and marriage may also end in divorce.[2]

Comorbidities

Psychiatric comorbidity is very common in patients with SUDs from all age groups, including adolescents as well as adults. Similarly, patients with most psychiatric disorders, including schizophrenia and related psychotic disorders, bipolar disorder, depression and anxiety disorders, personality disorders, and others, also report higher rates of SUDs, compared to that in the general population.[19,20] Strong associations have been reported between SUDs and mood and anxiety disorders, with strongest association being seen between illicit drug use disorders and major depression (pooled OR 3.80, 95% CI 3.02–4.78) and with anxiety disorders (OR 2.91, 95% CI 2.58–3.28). Similar associations exist between alcohol use disorders and major depression (OR 2.42, 95% CI 2.22–2.64) and anxiety disorders (OR 2.11, 95% CI 2.03–2.19).[19]

A study from South India of alcohol-dependent persons seeking care from a tertiary care hospital reported 67% of the subjects having a comorbid psychiatric disorder, out of which bipolar affective disorder was the commonest (20%) followed by unipolar depression (17%), phobia (9%), antisocial personality disorder (7%), and generalized anxiety disorder (7%).[21] A similar study from South Africa had a co-occurring psychiatric disorder in 62% of its subjects, the most common being major depressive (30%) and anxiety disorders (43%).[22]

Psychosocial Model of the Development of Substance Use and Dependence

A number of psychosocial factors are in the background of initiation of drug use and development of drug dependence. A wide range of social influences, including peer group pressures, immediate situational cues like availability of the drug, family influences, and internal cues like curiosity, mood states, and genetic endowment, may be in the background of initiation of the drug.[4] The first drug use may lead to deterrents or reinforcers for further seeking and using the drug, depending on the reinforcing or aversive experience. The behavior following the first use may receive disapproval and other negative responses or may get social approval from the peer group. A biological process of tolerance occurs with repeated use. Withdrawal symptoms and associated distress may be aversive, but its repeated relief by further drug taking sets up a conditioning process, further strengthening the development of dependence.[22]

Over the period, the environmental cues increase, since these are associated with the relief of withdrawal symptoms with drug intake. The user develops cues related to the drug intake and related experiences, and also to the specific locations or places associated with procuring and taking the drug. Such situations become potential stimuli for taking the drug again and again. For any kind of distress, the person stops looking into other avenues to relieve it, and resorts to taking the drug. Gradually the person needs increasing amounts of the drug due to tolerance, starts facing economic hardships since the drug use is also affecting his job, and psychological, physical, familial, and social consequences also start appearing.

It may be pointed out here that lack of reinforcement of behavior during the initial use, aversive consequences, and reduced availability with fewer cues are helpful in bringing back the sober state.[22] Competitive reinforcement, where behaviors other than drug taking are preferentially rewarded, is also helpful in stopping drug use.

Social Aspects of Substance Use Needing Intervention

There are a number of related social aspects of SUDs which need intervention. These include dealing with myths and misconceptions, stigma associated with substance use, role of media, role of the industry and the state, and the society in general.[24]

Myths and Misconceptions

There is a general misconception in laypeople that drug use is a habit and not an illness. Use of most psychoactive substances starts as a socialization or recreational activity. Both the patient as well as the family members often do not perceive the drug use as a problem and engage in denial. There is a belief that the user has control over his/her habit. Outside intervention is not perceived as needed, and it is perceived that greater willpower and greater efforts at control can restore tranquility.[25,26]

There are often many misconceptions about the use of drugs prevalent in the society. Alcohol is often perceived to relieve anxiety and stress and lead to mood elevation, and may also improve stage or sexual performance. Many users of opioids feel that they improve sexual performance. In rural India, bidi (an indigenous variant of cigarettes) is perceived to improve bowel movements and help in relieving constipation. Such beliefs further add to the use of drugs with an indirect social approval.[2,4]

A consistent message needs to be given to the community, using all media channels, that the scientific studies have shown that etiology of SUDs includes psychosocial and biological causes, with definite changes in the brain. Physical withdrawal and genetic loading further support the medical model. Thus, SUDs are a recognized illness entity and need to be treated.[2]

Stigma and Discrimination Due to Substance Use

Substance users experience stigma due to various reasons, such as their deplorable social conditions, including poverty and involvement in criminal activities, especially to procure the drug. Coexistence of other stigmatizing health conditions, such as HIV/AIDS, hepatitis C, and mental illness, further add to sigma and discrimination.[24] The subjects tend to indulge in potentially risky behaviors like rash driving, multiple sexual partners, and sharing of syringes, and are prone to impulsive and aggressive behavior. There is a general perception that the individuals have personal control over their drug use and thus are held responsible for their condition and are blamed. The society also holds a moralistic stance toward substance use which alienates the person. This has adverse impacts on multiple domains of life, such as employment, housing, and social relationships. The drug users also suffer poor physical and mental health, which further interferes in seeking proper medical treatment, adding to the existing treatment gap. Even when patients with SUDs seek treatment, they are often subjected to discrimination and devaluation from the treatment providers. This is associated with poor treatment outcomes and lower persistence in accessing health services.

Role of the Media

The media have an important role in dealing with the problem of SUDs. There is an utmost need for the media to be very responsible, especially in advertising, where direct as well as surrogate advertisements for substances of abuse like alcohol, tobacco, and others should not be published, broadcast, or telecast.[27] In the past, many movies have often glamorized certain characters smoking and drinking, where also the actors need to be responsible. In India, to sensitize the general population, a clipping "smoking and drinking are dangerous to health" has been added in all scenes showing smoking and drinking on movies/TV serials. Similarly, many sports events and beauty pageants are often promoted by industry under their brand name, which is similar across alcohol, tobacco, and other consumer products. Such endeavors need to be discouraged.[28]

Dual Standards of the State and Industry

The state and industry indirectly promote the sale of substances like tobacco and alcohol to generate revenue. The state also creates treatment facilities for alcohol- and tobacco-related illnesses. It has been estimated that the direct and indirect costs attributable to alcohol dependence are more than 3 times the profits of alcohol taxation and several times more than the annual state health budget.[27,29]

Industry comes with the concept of safe consumption like e-cigarettes, filtered cigarettes, surrogate advertisements, and supporting sporting events. There is a nexus between industry and those in power. The alcohol industry promotes and nurtures a concept called "responsible drinking." There is not enough evidence to promote drinking at so-called responsible levels, from a public health and policy perspective.[30]

Meeting the Challenge of Substance Use Disorders

Substance use is deeply ingrained in society since civilization started, and thus the principles of social psychiatry have an important role in dealing with this problem. SUDs have a high prevalence, often suffer non-recognition by the sufferers and their families, and tend to be chronic. There are many myths and misconceptions in society, which further delay the treatment. There is a huge treatment gap both due to lack of awareness and lack of adequate facilities. Internationally, only 1 out of 6 drug users seeks treatment. In low- and middle-income countries, the figure could be as low as 10%[31] SUDs pose a major challenge to healthcare professionals, policymakers, and society, considering their high prevalence and the huge burden of disease cause by them.

Conventionally, the problem of substance use is dealt with in 3 ways: supply reduction, demand reduction, and harm reduction.[32] Supply reduction is focused on reducing the availability of drugs by measures like illicit drug seizures, increasing costs, and restricting sale outlets. Demand reduction includes reducing the demand of the drug by raising community awareness and providing early treatment facilities, similar to the strategies of primary and secondary prevention. Harm reduction includes substitution therapies and can be subsumed under rehabilitation and tertiary prevention.[33]

The principles of social psychiatry can be effectively used in management of SUDs, since psychosocial factors have an important role in causation, and the social consequences of the SUDs are enormous. Steps at intervention could include preventive strategies, early identification, creating treatment facilities, bringing the untreated population into treatment, and rehabilitation of the treated subjects in the community.[2]

Preventive Approaches

Preventive approaches need to be implemented from the early period of life, since most SUDs begin in late childhood and adolescence. Preventive interventions focus on addressing the risk factors and strengthening the protective influences. The interventions should be age appropriate, begin at an early age, and continue throughout childhood and adolescence.[32,34]

Interventions in early childhood should focus on developing social and emotional competence and need not include education and awareness about substance use. Teachers need to be trained to provide strategies for developing social and emotional competence in children. Children with behavioral or academic difficulties should be given special attention and support. Life skills programs should be a part of school curriculum and be activity based. There is focus on development of an understanding of normative behavior (knowledge that substance use is not a common phenomenon and is not the usual behavior among the peers).[34] The children also need to be taught how to say no when offered any substance, and that the use of drugs is not an act of strength, but refusal is. The approaches should be participatory, based on peer learning, rather than didactic or prescriptive in nature. Teachers need to be trained to develop mentorship and supportive roles. The school environment should be positive, supportive, and inclusive in providing mentorship to all children irrespective of their academic performance. The school environment should be tobacco and alcohol free (teachers should also be encouraged to not use tobacco in school settings).

Children and adolescents with academic problems, learning disabilities, psychiatric conditions like attention deficit hyperactivity disorder, conduct disorder, oppositional defiant disorder, depression and anxiety disorders constitute a high-risk group and need to be identified and given extra attention. Teachers are to be sensitized and trained to identify the high-risk persons and refer them to school counselors. Schools also need to have the facility of counselors. There is also a need to focus on school dropouts, homeless children, street children, and children of drug users, who are also at high risk to develop substance use problems. Early identification of a substance use problem and referral to a suitable facility remain the standard approach.

Parents also need to be sensitized about substance use in parent-teacher meetings at the schools, especially to be watchful about the child's daily routines. Focus should be on adequate supervision, monitoring (being aware of how and with whom the child spends time). A positive healthy relationship and family environment act as a protection against substance use initiation.[34]

Families having any kind of conflict or with a history of substance use would need specific referral to counseling services in the community. Families can also be offered help by voluntary organizations in the community if they do not engage with school services.

Community-Based Interventions

Raising community awareness about substance use problems remains one of the important components of any prevention program. All channels of mass medica, including the print and audio-visual media, should be used for spreading the information. Community awareness camps, public rallies, poster competitions among the school and college students, and social events of a similar nature on the problem of substance use are some other strategies which can be used for sensitizing the community to the problem.[35,36] Mass media messages focusing on tobacco and alcohol use, especially among youth and women in the reproductive age group, should be evidence-based and not based on scare tactics. Preventive messages through different settings, such as health clubs, religious and spiritual organizations, youth programs, and workplace settings can be undertaken. Interventions in workplace settings can include workplace-based early identification and treatment. Referral to health services can be done for those requiring more intensive interventions. The World Health Organization has also come out with an intervention guide for the management of mental and substance use disorders in primary care settings.[37]

The focus of community-based interventions is also early identification and initiation of treatment for substance use, and engaging non-treatment-seekers to seek treatment. Special attention is required for high-risk populations like school dropouts, children of substance users, and children from disturbed family environments. Facilities for vocational guidance and training for school dropouts and other vulnerable populations can help in preventing the development of substance use problems in them.

Availability of Treatment Facilities in the Community

Most patients with SUDs can be treated on outpatient basis, but some may require more intensive inpatient care. Treatment should be easily available and accessible in the community. Suitable outpatient and inpatient facilities need to be created in the community. Inpatient facilities can be created in a general hospital setup. Drug abuse treatment clinics need to be established closer to the community, in hospitals or any other outpatient settings.[38] Patients requiring more intensive interventions may be referred to specialized settings. All patients visiting the healthcare settings should receive brief screening for use of tobacco and alcohol, since this would help in early identification and also sensitizes the community regarding the problem of substance use.

Messages about the availability of treatment in healthcare settings and the benefits of treatment should be publicized also. This will further the understanding of people about the medical model of substance dependence and thus reduce stigma as well.

Conclusion and Future Directions

Substance use disorders (SUDs) are common and contribute substantially to the global burden of disease. SUDs affect both physical as well as mental health. Psychosocial factors have an important role in the initiation and development of SUDs. There is a large treatment gap, with nearly 90% of the persons with SUDs remaining untreated, due to non-availability of treatment facilities in the community, as well as lack of awareness about the problem in the community. Stigma associated with SUDs also interferes with help-seeking. Social psychiatry needs to take a proactive role, by developing linkages with community leaders, media, policymakers, and caregiver and patient groups.

References

1. Chadda RK, Chawla N, Sarkar S. Concept of social psychiatry. In: Chadda RK, Kumar V, Sarkar S, eds. *Social Psychiatry: Principles and Clinical Perspectives.* Jaypee: New Delhi; 2018:45–58.
2. Chadda RK. Substance use disorders: need for public health initiatives. *Indian J Soc Psychiatry.* 2019;35:13–18.
3. Schuckit MA. Alcohol-related disorders. In: Sadock HI, Sadock VA, Ruiz P, eds. *Comprehensive Textbook of Psychiatry.* 10th ed. Baltimore, MD: Wolter Kluwer; 2017:1264–1279.
4. Basu D, Ghosh A, Patra B, Subodh B. Addiction research in India. In: Malhotra S, Chakrabarti S, eds. *Developments in Psychiatry in India.* New Delhi: Springer; 2015:367–404.
5. Murthy P. Culture and alcohol use in India. *World Cult Psychiatry Res Rev.* 2015;10:27–39.
6. Hall WD, Degenhardt L. Cannabis related disorders. In: Sadock HI, Sadock VA, Ruiz P, eds. *Comprehensive Textbook of Psychiatry.* 10th ed. Baltimore, MD: Wolter Kluwer; 2017:1303–1311.
7. Touw M. The religious and medicinal uses of Cannabis in China, India and Tibet. *J Psychoactive Drugs.* 1981;13:23–34.
8. Luo SX, Bisaga A. Opioid use and related disorders: from neurosciences to treatment. In: Sadock HI, Sadock VA, Ruiz P, eds. *Comprehensive Textbook of Psychiatry.* 10th ed. Baltimore, MD: Wolter Kluwer; 2017:1352–1373.
9. Paoli L1, Greenfield VA, Charles M, Reuter P. The global diversion of pharmaceutical drugs. India: the third largest illicit opium producer? *Addiction.* 2009 Mar;104(3):347–354. doi: 10.1111/j.1360-0443.2008.02511.x.
10. Murthy P1, Manjunatha N, Subodh BN, Chand PK, Benegal V. Substance use and addiction research in India. *Indian J Psychiatry.* 2010 Jan;52(Suppl 1):S189–199.
11. Lannucci RA, Weiss RD. Stimulant-related disorders. In: Sadock HI, Sadock VA, Ruiz P, eds. *Comprehensive Textbook of Psychiatry.* 10th ed. Baltimore, MD: Wolter Kluwer; 2017:1280–1290.
12. Ziedonis DM, Tonelli ME, Das S. Tobacco-related disorders. In: Sadock HI, Sadock VA, Ruiz P, eds. *Comprehensive Textbook of Psychiatry.* 10th ed. Baltimore, MD: Wolter Kluwer; 2017:1291–1302.
13. Juliano LM, Griffiths RB. Caffeine-related disorders. In: Sadock HI, Sadock VA, Ruiz P, eds. *Comprehensive Textbook of Psychiatry.* 10th ed. Baltimore, MD: Wolter Kluwer; 2017:1342–1351.
14. GBD 2016 Alcohol and Drug Use Collaborators. The global burden of disease attributable to alcohol and drug use in 195 countries and territories, 1990-2016: a systematic analysis for the Global Burden of Disease Study 2016. *Lancet Psychiatry.* 2018;5:987–1012.

15. United Nations Office on Drugs and Crime. *World Drug Report 2019*. Vienna: United Nations, 2019. https://wdr.unodc.org › wdr2019

16. Ambekar A, Agrawal A, Rao R, Mishra AK, Khandelwal SK, Chadda RK, on behalf of the group of investigators for the National Survey on Extent and Pattern of Substance Use in India. *Magnitude of Substance Use in India*. New Delhi: Ministry of Social Justice and Empowerment, Government of India; 2019.

17. Substance Abuse and Mental Health Services Administration (SAMHSA). National Survey on Drug Use and Health (NSDUH). 2018. https://www.samhsa.gov/data/report/ 2018-nsduh-detailed-tables. Accessed January 18, 2020.

18. Gururaj G, Varghese M, Benegal V, Rao GN, Pathak K, Singh LK; NMHS Collaborators Group, et al. *National Mental Health Survey of India, 2015–16: Prevalence, Patterns and Outcomes*. NIMHANS Publication No. 129. Bengaluru: National Institute of Mental Health and Neuro Sciences; 2016.

19. Lai HM, Cleary M, Sitharthan T, Hunt GE. Prevalence of comorbid substance use, anxiety and mood disorders in epidemiological surveys, 1990–2014: a systematic review and meta-analysis. *Drug Alcohol Depend*. 2015;154:1–13.

20. Colder CR, Scalco M, Trucco EM, Read JP, Lengua LJ, Wieczorek WF, Hawk LW Jr. Prospective associations of internalizing and externalizing problems and their co-occurrence with early adolescent substance use. *J Abnorm Child Psychol*. 2013 May; 41(4):667–677.

21. Kattukulathil S, Kallivayalil RA, George R, Kazhungil F. Psychiatric comorbidity in alcohol dependence: a cross-sectional study in a tertiary care setting. *Kerala J Psychiatry*. 2015; 28(2):156–160.

22. Gabriels CM, Macharia M, Weich L. Psychiatric comorbidity among alcohol-dependent individuals seeking treatment at the alcohol rehabilitation unit, Stikland Hospital. *S Afr J Psychiatry*. 2019;25:a1218. https://doi.org/10.4102/sajpsychiatry.v25i0.1218.

23. World Health Organization. Nomenclature and classification of drug- and alcohol-related problems: a WHO Memorandum. *Bull WHO*. 1981;59(2):225–242.

24. Barry CL, McGinty EE, Pescosolido BA, Goldman HH. Stigma, discrimination, treatment effectiveness, and policy: public views about drug addiction and mental illness. *Psychiatric Serv*. 2014;65(10):1269–1272.

25. Mattoo SK, Sarkar S, Gupta S, Nebhinani N, Parakh P, Basu D. Stigma towards substance use: comparing treatment seeking alcohol and opioid dependent men. *Int J Ment Health Addiction*. 2015;13(1):73–81.

26. Young M, Stuber J, Ahern J, Galea S. Interpersonal discrimination and the health of illicit drug users. *Am J Drug Alcohol Abuse*. 2005;31(3):371–391.

27. Gururaj G, Murthy P, Girish N, Benegal V. Alcohol related harm: Implications for public health and policy in India. Publication No. 73. Bangalore, India: National Institute of Mental Health And Neuro Science (NIMHANS), 2011.

28. The Parliament of India. The Cigarettes and Other Tobacco Products Act, COPTA. Prohibition of Advertisement and Regulation of Trade and Commerce, Production, Supply and Distribution. New Delhi: The Gazette of India; 2003.

29. World Health Organization. *Burden and Socio-Economic Impact of Alcohol: The Bangalore Study*. New Delhi: World Health Organization, Regional Office for South-East Asia; 2006.

30. Britton A, Bell S. The protective effects of moderate drinking: lies, damned lies, and . . . selection biases? *Addiction*. 2017;112:218–219.

31. United Nations Office on Drugs and Crime. *World Drug Report 2017*. Vienna: United Nations; May 2017.

32. American Public Health Association. *Defining and Implementing a Public Health Response to Drug Use and Misuse*. Policy Number: 201312; 2013. http://www.apha.org/advocacy/policy/policysearch/default.

33. Volkow ND, Poznyak V, Saxena S, Gerra G, and the UNODC-WHO Informal International Scientific Network. National Institute Drug use disorders: impact of a public health rather than a criminal justice approach. *World Psychiatry*. 2017;16:213–214.

34. Dhawan A, Pattanayak RD, Chopra A, Tikoo VK, Kumar R. Pattern and profile of children using substances in India: Insights and recommendations. *Natl Med J India*. 2017;30:224–229.

35. Alcohol Web India. Available from: https://www.alcoholwebindia.in/. Accessed on January 19, 2020.

36. Raj L, Chavan BS, Bala C. Community "de-addiction" camps: a follow-up study. *Indian J Psychiatry.* 2005;47:44–47.
37. World Health Organization. *mhGAP Intervention Guide for Mental, Neurological and Substance Use Disorders in Non-specialized Health Settings: Mental Health Gap Action Programme (mhGAP).* Geneva: World Health Organization; 2010.
38. Rao R. The journey of opioid substitution therapy in India: achievements and challenges. *Indian J Psychiatry.* 2017;59:39–45.

28

Suicide and Sociocultural Considerations

K. Sonu Gaind

Introduction

Life is a terminal condition, and for the vast majority of our lives we have the ability to end our lives earlier than death might otherwise occur, if we choose to do so. Despite this, even in societies with the most liberal attitudes toward death, suicide, or euthanasia, only a minority of people choose to end their lives prematurely. Reported suicide rates range from as low as below 1/100,000 (Antigua, Barbados) to as high as over 30/100,000 (Lithuania, Russian Federation).[1] This chapter examines the social and cultural considerations of suicide and seeking one's own death, including shifting societal contexts and implications for future policy setting.

What Is Suicide?

Multifactorial models of suicide accounting for social and environmental factors have long been proposed for low- and middle-income countries. For example, the sharp rise in suicide rates in Micronesia seen after the 1960s is often attributed to social disruptions driven by rapid modernization, rather than being a reflection of mental illness.[2] In high-income countries the biomedical model has traditionally predominated. In the medical model, suicide is traditionally considered to be linked to mental illnesses. Certainly there is strong evidence for this, especially in high-income countries, where over 90% of completed suicides occur concurrent with an active psychiatric diagnosis. The American Psychological

Association goes as far as attributing causation, describing suicide as "the act of killing yourself, most often *as a result* of depression or other mental illness" [*emphasis added*]. Suicide-prevention initiatives often properly include increasing access to services for diagnosing and treating mental illnesses.

In the medical model, in addition to a history of mental illness and past suicide attempts, and substance use or abuse, psychosocial factors such as relationship breakups or loss of loved ones, poverty, history of trauma, work or academic difficulties, and other nonmedical factors are acknowledged as risk factors for suicide; as are non-psychiatric medical factors such as continued suffering from chronic physical illness or chronic pain.

This raises a challenging question: Even when mental illness is present, is it the cause of suicidal ideation and action, or is it simply facilitating suicide in those for whom the social system has failed?

The question becomes even more challenging when we consider exactly what we mean when we talk of "suicide." Are we referring only to self-inflicted deaths we hope to prevent, for example for those individuals acting out of despair and hopelessness in the context of a severe but treatable clinical depression? Or do we also consider deaths that individuals seek for themselves that society sanctions and may even participate in? Euthanasia and assisted dying movements continue to build in countries around the world, challenging the notion that all suicidal wishes are undesirable problems needing correction.

Beyond abstract or academic distinctions, these questions have significant implications not just for our understanding of suicide, but for tangible resource allocation and policy setting, as well as ethical implications for what society considers a "good death" versus an unwanted and avoidable one. While the biological aspects of mental illness–related suicidality are important, the sociocultural elements of suicide play as big, if not a bigger, role in understanding suicide in the broader context. In terms of individual suicide prevention and mental healthcare, a shift away from a purely biomedical model, and toward a person-centered approach that accounts for the full spectrum of psychosocial issues in addition to biomedical needs, has been advocated.[3]

Variations in Suicide Rates

In addition to significant variation in suicide rates between different countries across the world, suicide rates within countries can vary tremendously. Among the most telling examples of this are suicide rates of Indigenous populations compared to general national suicide rates. For example, the First Nations suicide rate in Canada was 3 times higher than the rate for non-Indigenous Canadians, at 24.3 deaths per 100,000 versus 8 deaths per 100,000, respectively, between 2011 and 2016.[4] Even within this demographic, further striking differences emerge: the suicide rate for First Nations people living on a reserve was twice that of those living off reserve; and the suicide rate for Inuit was about 9 times higher than for non-Indigenous Canadians, at 72.3 per 100,000.

The medical model cannot account for these stark numbers. Even Statistics Canada acknowledges that these higher rates of Indigenous suicide are due to "socioeconomic characteristics" such as low income, poor labor-force status, level of education, and other socioeconomic factors. Even in 2020 in a country as well off as Canada, over 50 First Nation reserves continue to have long-term drinking water advisories (i.e., unclean water; though this number is admittedly lower than the over 100 communities in 2016 that had such advisories). Some communities have had continuous advisories in place for over two decades. Imagine an adolescent growing up their entire life without knowing clean drinking or bathing water, while neighboring non-Indigenous towns enjoy all the benefits of a "high-income" country. In this sense, the suicide rates reflect cultural disenfranchisement rather than medical illnesses. Thus while improving mental health services would be an important part of dealing with these challenges, especially considering that Indigenous communities and populations are also reported to have poor levels of access to health services, improved mental health services alone clearly cannot address the tragic suicide rates in these communities. Unless the underlying socioeconomic and cultural conditions fueling Indigenous suicide are addressed, it would be unrealistic to expect any meaningful reduction of these rates.

Canada is not unique in having disproportionately high suicide rates among Indigenous populations, and especially so in the Indigenous adolescent and even younger age group. Similar rate disparities and disproportionately high suicide rates are reported in other high-income countries, including among Aboriginal Australian and New Zealand populations, Native American populations in the United States, and Indigenous populations in Arctic nations, among others.[5] In understanding Indigenous suicide, solely focusing on suicide as a mental illness–related problem would not only be inappropriate, it could be harmful. It is clear that these suicide rates cannot be simply attributed to mental illness. It may even be a disservice to characterize sociocultural issues as "risk factors" rather than causative. Suicide in these populations is more often related to the legacies of colonization, resultant intergenerational trauma and discrimination, and continued socioeconomic and cultural marginalization. While important, focusing solely on improving mental health services in a medical model would fail to address the real issues driving suicide in these groups, while avoiding collective societal shame over historical and continued mistreatment of Indigenous populations.

Similarly, other groups have been shown to have disproportionately high suicide rates within their broader community. For example, LGBTQ2S+ (lesbian/gay/bisexual/transgender/queer/questioning/2-spirit) youth are found to have from 1.5 to 4 times the suicide rates of their heterosexual counterparts. Again, this is felt to be related to discrimination, stigma, and sociocultural stressors, including homelessness, rather than solely being linked to mental illness.

While the role of sociocultural stressors will naturally vary in individual circumstances of suicide—for example, they may have a relatively minor role in a situation where psychotic depression is fueling suicide—the examples of Indigenous suicide and LGBTQ2S+ youth suicide illustrate how important sociocultural factors are in understanding the driving forces behind suicide in all societies.

How Easy Is It?

In addition to potentially contributing to or protecting from individual suicidal thoughts and intent, sociocultural issues impact the likelihood and risk of suicide in other ways. Societal ease of access and availability of lethal means has been known for decades to potentially increase the risk of suicide.

Suicide by pesticide ingestion accounts for one-third of suicides worldwide, and in some regions of the world remains the most common method of suicide. In Sri Lanka, suicide rates peaked at 47/100,000 in 1995, and had halved by 2005. This decrease in overall suicide rates has been attributed to decreased availability of more toxic and lethal pesticides such as endosulfan, with significant reductions of suicide being seen after restrictions on import and sales of more toxic WHO Class I toxicity pesticides in 1995 and subsequently a ban on endosulfan in 1998.[6] Likewise in the United Kingdom, suicide rates fell dramatically between 1962–1963 and 1970–1971, from 28.7/100,000 to 19.0/100,000 for males and 19.6/100,000 to 13.3/100,000 for females, respectively. In the early 1960s, suicide by domestic carbon monoxide poisoning was a common method of suicide in the United Kingdom, and research has linked the above dramatic decreases in overall suicide rates to changes associated with domestic gas supplies from coal gas, which contained approximately 14% carbon monoxide, to natural gas, which is virtually free of carbon monoxide.[7] In each of the above examples, societal policy significantly changed availability and ease of access to a particularly common method of suicide, but of course could not eliminate every potential means of suicide, yet population-wide suicide rates fell. As Kreitman, the author of the UK paper, opines, "There is no shortage of exits from this life; it would seem that anyone bent on self-destruction must eventually succeed, yet it is also quite possible, given the ambivalence (or multivalence) of many suicides, that a failed attempt serves as a catharsis leading to profound psychological change. For others it may be that the scenario of suicide specifies the use of a particular method, and that if this is not available actual suicide is then less likely."

Policy setting for suicide prevention often needs to involve more than just providing mental health services. While the suicide rates in Japan remain relatively high, the country has also seen remarkable reductions in rates of suicide attempt by jumping at train stations not only where platform barriers have already been installed, but also at stations where blue light emitters have been installed in the interim. In a sociocultural context, this is an example of enlightened resource allocation (which also has an economic benefit, with reduced delays and avoidance of lost time and revenue) targeting known frequent methods of suicide.

Suicide-reduction strategies thus need to be sensitive to local sociocultural environments. Method of suicide continues to vary widely by country and region of the world, even among countries considered to have similar socioeconomic contexts. While drug overdose remains the most common method reported for suicide attempts, completed suicide by firearm is by far the most common method of suicide in the United States, accounting for just over 50% of completed suicides (with suffocation as the next most common, at over 25%, and poisoning at below 15%). This compares to under 25% of completed suicides by firearm in Canada, and under 10% in Australia. However, addressing firearm suicides in the United States (which exceed the number of firearm homicides in that country, despite firearm homicides typically being the spark of debate) touches on much more than resource allocation and mental health services; it touches on highly politicized issues of gun control and debates of individual versus collective rights under the Second Amendment to the U.S. Constitution. Once again, suicide-reduction strategies clearly need to address more than "mental illness"–related issues, and effective advocacy needs to address the full spectrum of sociocultural aspects of suicide.

Sociocultural Reactions to Suicide

Reactions to suicide are heavily influenced by societal norms. For example, historical past underreporting of death by suicide in Ireland has been widely noted, with suicide deaths instead being reported as deaths attributable to "undetermined" or "accidental" causes, and researchers citing stigma around suicide and religious implications as reasons for this underreporting. At the other end of the spectrum, suicide in certain situations has been historically associated with restoration of honor in some cultures, for example *seppuku* in Japan.

Notwithstanding the range of societal reactions, it is fair to say that on balance, reactions to suicide have traditionally tended to fall more on the stigmatizing side than the accepting side of the spectrum. Suicide and attempted suicide remain illegal in several countries, while in other countries where these acts were once illegal they have been decriminalized, though not necessarily destigmatized. Continued stigmatization can carry over to social policies that discriminate against those with mental illnesses, including for example denial of insurability if a history of past self-harm attempt is present, or inability to cross borders between jurisdictions.

Social stigma can not only make it difficult to come forward and reveal thoughts of suicide, but can impact reactions following suicide. Complicating completed suicides, surviving loved ones are left to deal not only with grief of loss, but also with confusion or lack of understanding regarding why their loved one took their own life, potential feelings of guilt or recrimination over actions taken or missed opportunities, a sense of shame, and even anger toward their loved one for taking their life. In this state of complex grieving, nuances conveyed by societal language and terminology can carry particular weight. For example, referencing that someone "committed suicide" conveys a judgment and resonates with a sense of the person having committed an immoral or illegal act.

Other language can likewise have unintended consequences, however well meaning. It is acknowledged that effective suicide-prevention strategies require comprehensive care in multiple settings, and an integrated team approach that avoids fragmentary care. The underlying components of such strategies have significant overlap, regardless of terminology used, and aim to overcome gaps in care that have historically existed when dealing with individuals at risk of suicide. However, despite the commonality of actual methods, controversy remains around appropriate language used to describe such efforts. Some advocate for a "zero suicide" approach, arguing that an aspirational goal of zero suicide is warranted.

Others counter that, especially given the complex reactions to suicide and grief, the terminology of "zero suicide" is counterproductive, as it feeds into the notion that every suicide reflects a failure of the system and that someone is "at fault" for every suicide, thereby fostering projection of blame during a time of complicated grieving.

Striking the right balance between destigmatizing suicide, while also not encouraging unwanted suicides, presents another challenge. While societal responses to suicide and suicide attempts should not foster shame and blame, they likewise should not glorify or romanticize suicide. Suicidologists have long described the risks of suicide contagion, and clusters of increased suicide rates, in response to media reporting of suicides. Many organizations and jurisdictions have developed media guidelines for how to responsibly report on suicides, including avoiding graphic or sensational depictions, excessive detail, prominent photos, inappropriate language, simplistic or superficial reasons for the suicide, or portraying suicide as solving problems.[8]

In addition to increased risk associated with certain types of media reporting, other social factors can impact the risk of suicide and suicide rates. Suicide contagion and cluster effects of increased suicide rates following celebrity suicides have been shown in countries across the world. Even fictionalized accounts of suicide have been potentially implicated in leading to increased suicidal thoughts and actions. Significant controversy surrounded the release of the Netflix show "13 Reasons Why," which depicted in graphic detail the suicide of a 16-year-old girl who left behind a series of tapes outlining why she chose to end her life. The series drew heavy criticism from suicide-prevention groups, who voiced concern that the series failed to adhere to responsible media guidelines regarding suicide and could lead to suicide contagion effects. Some subsequent research has shown increases in rates of youth suicide in the months following the release of the series.[9,10]

Cultural Concepts of Death

There is a potential tension between suicide prevention, and deaths that society would like to avoid, and deaths that might be considered "good deaths" in the context of "dying with dignity" movements. Where is the boundary between undesirable versus acceptable deaths? Broader cultural concepts of death need to be considered to appreciate the nuances of this.

Death is naturally associated with a complex range of reactions, including grieving and loss, fear, avoidance, and at times denial. All cultures have rituals, whether religious or secular, that provide individuals the opportunity to grieve communally to varying degrees, and death is also seen as a part of the life cycle and renewal.

When premature death, or bringing about death sooner than it would otherwise naturally occur, is involved, things get more complicated. On one hand, suicide-prevention initiatives have focused on trying to assist in avoiding premature and avoidable deaths. On the other hand, various forms of dying with dignity movements have been advocating since at least the 1930s for increased autonomy for individuals to have more control over how and when they die, including getting societal assistance with dying. While sometimes the debate over assisted dying focuses on aiming to alleviate suffering from illness, some have gone as far as to advocate for the right for assisted dying above a certain age if one is "tired of life," even in the absence of illness (Out of Free Will, *Uit Vrije Wil*, in the Netherlands, which has advocated that those above 70 years of age should have the right to assisted dying if they are tired of living).

While these debates are often framed as issues of individual autonomy and rights, broader social concepts of death need to be understood when considering what may lead individuals to consider or seek their own deaths. Individual decisions and thoughts of death are not isolated and removed from the social context, but rather reflect an individual's sense of the value of their life in the world. For an individual with an active depressive disorder, this could reflect illness-driven cognitive distortions of self, the world, and the future being terrible, fueling hopelessness, despair, and suicidality. For an otherwise healthy adolescent on a Native reserve, it could reflect cultural disenfranchisement and social despair, and their conviction that suicide was their only option. For an 80-year-old isolated widower with no mental illness and moderate loss of functioning from arthritis and age-related frailty, it could reflect a sense of their life not having value, fueled by an internalized sense of societal ageism.

Acknowledging fictional literature and popular media references for what they are, entertainment, it can still be informative to consider the themes reflected in popular culture. Dystopian futures where less useful citizens free up resources to make way for younger, more useful ones are common, from the Death Conditioning in Brave New World, to formal killing of those above the age of 30 in the film *Logan's Run* (or above the age of 20 in the book). While not always based on age, modern storytelling continues to reprise these themes of death for the purposes of resource reallocation, for example Thanos's plan in Marvel's *Infinity War* to eliminate 50% of life so that the remaining 50% can thrive.

Back in our real world, we do know that healthcare costs rise sharply with age, and so are drivers of resource utilization. While providing ongoing healthcare for chronic conditions is costly, providing assisted dying in jurisdictions that permit it is much less costly and reduces costs compared to regular ongoing care. For example, early estimates of the Canadian experience with assisted dying have suggested annual savings of between approximately $35 million to $139 million Cdn likely to accrue annually as a result of providing assisted dying compared to ongoing health care.[11] This is, of course, not to suggest that policy would deliberately be set with such cost-saving goals in mind, but it is important to recognize the different societal gears that could turn if society is considering that the 80-year-old widower above should be able to apply for assisted dying because he is "tired of life."

The Pathway to Death—When Is It Suicide?

At one end of the spectrum, the term "suicide" is used to refer to avoidable and unwanted self-initiated deaths that occur in the context of mental illness or acute psychosocial stressors. These suicides are typically acts conducted in isolation (or even when others are present, for example in cases of jumping in front of a train or off a bridge, the suicide act is initiated by the individual without the awareness or assistance of others), and often of violent means (though this largely reflects the fact that violent means are more lethal, hence more likely to lead to completed suicide). At the other end, in some jurisdictions assisted dying is referred to as "assisted suicide," and involves communication with others, team planning and coordination, and what is often perceived as a peaceful death, sometimes surrounded by loved ones. Other jurisdictions avoid the word "suicide" entirely, and associated connotations, and instead use terms such as "assistance in dying" or "voluntary euthanasia" in describing their assisted-dying frameworks.

While assisted dying remains illegal in most countries in the world, in recent years an increasing number of countries have introduced some form of medically assisted dying legislation or policies, and some form of medically assisted dying is now allowed in certain situations in over a dozen jurisdictions around the world, with several other jurisdictions considering implementing such policies. Most of the jurisdictions currently allowing for medically assisted dying only allow for it in circumstances of suffering from severe medical illness anticipated to eventually lead to death; however, a small minority allow for assisted dying for the sole criterion of mental illness, even in the absence of any condition foreshortening anticipated life span.[12]

Notwithstanding the nuances of whether the act is carried out by others (i.e., euthanasia) or the individual themselves (i.e., suicide) (and this difference can have significant implications for assisted dying frameworks), for purposes of this chapter, wishes or intent of the individual seeking their own death are considered "suicidal" wishes, regardless of who actually performs the actions leading to death. In terms of several of the other features cited above that differ between traditional "suicide" and "assisted suicide" or "assisted dying," such as planning and the presence of others, those are operational or process-related issues; they do not obviate the individual's intent in seeking their own death. While it is important to recognize the connotations associated with the word "suicide," it is also important to recognize that wishes for one's own death do literally reflect suicidal thoughts, and not attempt to sanitize language by pretending otherwise.

When Is Suicide Acceptable?

Regarding terminology, the concept discussed in the literature of "rational suicide" most aligns with what advocates would describe as the difference between traditional suicides that society wishes to prevent, and assisted deaths that society facilitates.[13] Rational suicide implies that, in the individual's particular circumstances, the person's wish for suicide can be well reasoned and rational, rather than the result of emotional or psychological problems, or mental illness. However, while the concept of rational suicide aims to empower the individual and support autonomy in decision-making, it too requires an external judgment—who determines whether the person's wish for death is well reasoned?

Societal views on this have shifted significantly over the past few decades, most notably in jurisdictions that have in that time introduced some form of assisted dying policy. As an example, in a 1993 Canadian Supreme Court decision, *Rodriguez v. British Columbia*, in a split decision the Supreme Court upheld Canada's legal prohibition against any form of assisted dying.[14] This meant that anyone who assisted a person in ending their life, under any circumstances, could be charged under the Criminal Code of Canada with a criminal act. Just over two decades later, in 2015, a similar challenge in *Carter v. Canada* had the opposite outcome and led to a unanimous Supreme Court decision overturning the same prohibition, and mandating policy that allowed for medically assisted dying in cases of intolerable and enduring suffering and a grievous and irremediable medical condition.[15]

In addition to representing a significant legal shift, this paralleled societal views in Canada. By 2015, most people in Canada, including physicians, agreed that some form of assisted dying should be available under certain circumstances, for example for those suffering from terminal cancer. In this sense, these views reflect an acceptance of "rational suicide" under these circumstances. However, significant debate continues regarding which circumstances should be eligible for consideration of assisted dying, even among those who agree that assisted dying, or suicide, can be "rational" in some cases. For example, the same surveys that show the majority of psychiatrists support some form of assisted dying also show that the majority of psychiatrists do not support assisted dying if the sole condition is mental illness and no other medical condition contributing to suffering or foreshortened life span is present.

These nuances show the risks of having policy driven by legal outcomes, as is happening in Canada. Legal cases necessarily focus on the particular aspects of each specific case. For example, in both *Carter v. Canada*, and *Rodriguez v. British Columbia* before it, the plaintiffs were suffering from neurodegenerative conditions (degenerative spinal stenosis, and amyotrophic lateral sclerosis); no mental illness was present. The facts before the Court did not deal with issues related to mental illness, yet subsequent policy in response to legal rulings has the potential to impact situations far beyond individuals with neurodegenerative conditions, including affecting those with mental disorders.

This is why it is advisable to have robust policy discussion and formation on these issues, including whether society believes any situations could be considered a "rational suicide," since if policy is instead driven by court rulings, issues that may be relevant for just a specific set of circumstances risk being inappropriately generalized more broadly, and setting policy with unforeseen consequences.

Assisted Dying and Mental Disorders

Considerable controversy exists regarding whether assisted dying policies should allow individuals to seek medically assisted dying for the sole underlying condition of a mental disorder. Some have argued that allowing this would risk assisting individuals to die who are suicidal due to their mental illness, when traditionally we have worked to avoid their deaths: the same person presenting to the emergency room might be prevented from harming themselves, while going to a different clinic they might be assisted in taking their life. Others argue that it would be discriminatory to allow assisted dying for certain conditions, like cancer or spinal stenosis, but not for mental illnesses.

In an attempt to address these issues, following the 2015 *Carter v. Canada* ruling, the Canadian government commissioned an Expert Panel report from the Council of Canadian Academies to review the experience and evidence regarding medical assistance in dying where a mental disorder is the sole underlying medical condition. Our 15-member Expert Panel met over a period of 15 months, reviewed the worldwide literature and experience, and produced a 247-page report with 25 key findings, which was tabled in the Canadian Parliament in December 2018.[16] By the end of this exhaustive process, perhaps more telling than the Key Findings were the remaining 5 highlighted areas of Disagreement we had on Fundamental Issues. As noted in the report, "In some situations, even after consideration of available data and Panel discussions, agreement could not be achieved and significant differences of opinion remained, reflecting the complex and conflicted nature of the issues being reviewed."[16]

One of our fundamental disagreements was whether it was possible to distinguish between suicide, in the traditional sense, and medically assisted dying sought for a mental disorder. While some panel members had the opinion it was possible to make this distinction, the available evidence did raise concerns that "some people who have sought psychiatric euthanasia and assisted suicide in jurisdictions that permit it share certain characteristics with people who attempt suicide" (Section 4.2), including ambivalence, demoralization, and hopelessness regarding life being unbearable, and social isolation and loneliness.[17,18]

This also serves to again highlight how unresolved psychosocial issues can fuel suicidal wishes. In the context of assisted dying requests, the challenges associated with the cumulative suffering from psychosocial stressors that are often prevalent when mental illness is present cannot easily (or even possibly) be separated from suffering due to mental illness. Similar to the concept of total pain in palliative care as described by Dame Cicely Saunders,[19] it is total life suffering that forms the person's experience and can drive a wish for death, not just illness suffering.

It is essential to understand the impact of total life suffering, as this has potential significant implications for what society might consider a "rational suicide." Would it be rational suicide if a competent individual was suffering from moderate non-psychotic depression, and had significant suffering from unresolved loneliness, poverty, and homelessness? In an assisted dying framework allowing for applications for mental disorders as the sole underlying medical condition, if individual autonomy was valued above all else, then such a request for assisted dying could likely be granted.

Complicating matters further, when mental illness is present, are the potential cognitive distortions and loss of emotional resilience that mental illness can bring, even when the person remains formally and legally competent. And perhaps most difficult if not impossible to reconcile is the reality that even in 2020, we simply cannot predict with any certainty the future course or irremediability of mental illness in any particular individual. Keeping in mind that typically professional associations like to cite expertise of what they do know, as the Canadian Psychiatric Association (CPA) has explicitly acknowledged, "there is no established standard of care in Canada, or as far as CPA is aware of in the world, for defining the threshold when typical psychiatric conditions should be considered irremediable."[20] This has been echoed by other expert bodies, including the Centre for Addiction and Mental Health and others, citing that it is not currently possible to prognostically identify irremediability in any individual case of mental illness.[21]

Finally, in terms of irremediability of suffering, given the frequent association of psychosocial stressors with mental illnesses, the question of what is irremediable, be it illness symptoms or psychosocial suffering, becomes a challenging question for society.

With all that in mind, would it be considered a "rational suicide" if a competent individual sought death in the context of suffering from a clinical depression, with significant unresolved psychosocial stressors, negative cognitive distortions, and loss of emotional resilience due to mental illness symptoms, and inability to predict whether their suffering was irremediable (though in a state of hopelessness and despair they were convinced it was)? The total life suffering of this individual could well lead them to attempt suicide, or to seek assisted dying were it available. Challenging as these issues are to deal with, society would need to consider whether such circumstances constituted a wish for "rational suicide," or whether a response other than individually sought or state-sanctioned death was the appropriate solution.

Concluding Remarks

Suicide is a complex phenomenon that must be understood by taking into account a person's complete biopsychosocial and cultural experience, and the societal context, and cannot be properly understood by only considering suicide as a function of mental illness. A person's total life suffering contributes to their wish to die, and must be considered and addressed if suicide-prevention strategies are to succeed in fostering a will to live. As assisted dying frameworks expand in various jurisdictions globally, these issues, and consideration of what may or may not constitute a "rational suicide," need to be openly discussed to ensure that suicide-prevention initiatives align with societal priorities, and to avoid policy being driven by reactions to court proceedings, rather than deliberate and thoughtful policy setting.

References

1. World Health Organization. Suicide rates. 2016. https://www.who.int/gho/mental_health/suicide_rates_crude/en/.
2. Rubinstein D. Epidemic suicide among Micronesian adolescents. *Soc Sci Med.* 1983;17(10):657–665.
3. Rutz W, Fernandez M, Trivedi J. Social perspectives on psychiatry for the person. *Int J Person Centered Med.* 2011;1(1):140–142. doi: 10.5750/ijpcm.v1i1.36
4. Kumar M, Tjepkema M. Suicide among First Nations people, Métis and Inuit (2011–2016): findings from the 2011 Canadian Census Health and Environment Cohort (CanCHEC). *Statistics Canada.* 2019. ISBN 978-0-660-31402-0. https://publications.gc.ca/site/eng/9.874824/publication.html. Last accessed December 17, 2022.
5. Pollock NJ, Naicker K, Loro A, et al. Global incidence of suicide among Indigenous peoples: a systematic review. *BMC Med.* 2018;16:145. doi: 10.1186/s12916-018-1115-6.
6. Gunnell D, et al. The impact of pesticide regulations on suicide in Sri Lanka. *Int J Epidemiol.* 2007;36(6):1235–1242.
7. Kreitman N. The coal gas story: United Kingdom suicide rates, 1960–71. *Br J Prevent Soc Med.* 1976;30(2):86–93.

8. Sinyor M, Schaffer A, Heisel M, et al. Media guidelines for reporting on suicide. *Can J Psychiatry*. 2018 Mar;63(3):182–196. doi: 10.1177/0706743717753147.

9. Niederkrotenthaler T, Stack S, Till B. Association of increased youth suicides in the United States with the release of 13 Reasons Why. *JAMA Psychiatry*. 2019;76(9):933–940. doi: 10.1001/jamapsychiatry.2019.0922.

10. Bridge JA, Greenhouse JB, Ruch D, Stevens J, Ackerman J, Sheftall AH, Horowitz LM, Kelleher KJ, Campo JV. Association between the release of Netflix's 13 reasons why and suicide rates in the United States: an interrupted time series analysis. *J Am Acad Child Adolesc Psychiatry*. 2020 Feb;59(2):236–243. doi: 10.1016/j.jaac.2019.04.020. Epub 2019 Apr 28. PMID: 31042568; PMCID: PMC6817407.

11. Trachtenberg AJ, Manns B. Cost analysis of medical assistance in dying in Canada. *CMAJ*. 2017 Jan 23;189(3):E101–E105. doi: 10.1503/cmaj.160650. PMID: 28246154; PMCID: PMC5250515.

12. Sheehan K, Gaind KS, Downar J. Medical assistance in dying: special issues for patients with mental illness. *Curr Opin Psychiatry*. 2017;30(1):26–30.

13. Werth J. *Rational Suicide? Implications for Mental Health Professionals*. London: Routledge, 1996.

14. Melvin J. Rodriguez vs. Attorney General of Canada (trial court opinion). *Law Med*. 1993 Winter;9(3):309–321.

15. Downie J. SJD Carter v. Canada: What's next for physicians? *CMAJ*. 2015 Apr 21;187(7):481–482. doi:10.1503/cmaj.150202. PMCID: PMC4401588, PMID: 25754706.

16. Council of Canadian Academies. *The State of Knowledge on Medical Assistance in Dying Where a Mental Disorder Is the Sole Underlying Medical Condition*. Ottawa, ON: The Expert Panel Working Group on MAID Where a Mental Disorder Is the Sole Underlying Medical Condition; 2018.

17. Thienpont L, Verhofstadt M, Van Loon T, Distelmans W, Audenaert K, De Deyn P. Euthanasia requests, procedures and outcomes for 100 Belgian patients suffering from psychiatric disorders: a retrospective, descriptive study. *BMJ Open*. 2015;5(7):e007454.

18. Kim SYH, De Vries RG, Peteet JR. Euthanasia and assisted suicide of patients with psychiatric disorders in the Netherlands 2011 to 2014. *JAMA Psychiatry*. 2016;73(4):362–368.

19. Saunders CM. *The Management of Terminal Malignant Disease*. 1st ed. London: Edward Arnold; 1978.

20. Gaind KS. Canadian Psychiatric Association interim response to Report of the Special Joint Committee on physician assisted dying. *Can J Psychiatry*. 2020 Sep;65(9):604–606.

21. Centre for Addiction and Mental Health (CAMH). *Policy Advice on Medical Assistance in Dying for Mental Illness*. Toronto, ON: CAMH; 2017.

29

Medical Illness in Psychiatry

Joseph E. Thornton

Introduction

Illness in an individual has an impact on social function. This is a reciprocating relationship, as the response of the social network has an impact on the expression and course of illness. Medical illnesses in psychiatry can be explored in the framework of somatic symptoms and function in a social network. The complexity of this interplay of symptoms and illness makes it difficult for physicians to analyze each patient presentation consistently and comprehensively. In general, physicians and other healthcare providers simplify this complexity by beginning with cognitive biases; e.g., somatic symptoms represent medical illness and psychological symptoms represent psychiatric illness. These cognitive biases often are in error and lead not only to unproductive interventions but also to maladaptive interventions from healthcare providers and maladaptive behavioral responses from the identified patient. This chapter aims to provide a simplified yet systematic and comprehensive strategy to care for patients presenting with medical illness.

The Examination

For comprehensive examination of medical illness and social psychiatry, we present here a person-centric view of symptoms confronting the psychiatrist and will focus on the role of medical illnesses as the cause of the symptoms. In the course of this discussion we will also note the psychiatric illnesses or psychological circumstances that can present as somatic symptoms that may be covered elsewhere in this book. It is also necessary in discussion of medical illnesses to describe the psychiatric symptoms that can be caused by medical illnesses, medical interventions, medications, and substances of abuse. Since epidemics are the quintessential manifestation of social illnesses, in the final sections of this chapter we

TABLE 29.1 Psychiatric Syndromes Based on Mental Status Findings

Psychiatric Syndrome by Symptom Cluster on Mental Status Examination	Mood and Affect	Sensorium (Levels of Consciousness, Attention, Orientation)	Intellectual Functioning (Language, Fund of Information, Memory, etc.)	Thought Processes and Content	Executive Control Functions
Delirium	+	+++	++	+	+
Major Neurocognitive	+	++	+++	+	+
Psychosis	+/-	+/-	+/-	+++	+/-
Affective	+++	+/-	+/-	+/-	+/-
Other					

will also take a look at the role of social behaviors in initiating and maintaining epidemics. We conclude with a new imperative for ethical engagement in society for health.

Clinical Examination

The process of generating the differential diagnosis entails the skills of clinical examination of the person to identify the clinical syndrome and then to use clinical reasoning with our fund of information to best identify the etiological causes of the syndrome. This is best done with the idea of hypothesis generation to stimulate a treatment plan to verify and test the hypothesis, rather than a final diagnosis to which the treatment plan is rigidly adhered. As shown in Table 29.1, we find it useful to conceptualize syndromes that are identified as the predominant symptoms from the clinical examination. Although the DSM-5 does not use a hierarchical diagnostic system, it is heuristically useful to use the formerly accepted hierarchical system of dementia, psychosis, affective, and other syndromes in our formulation. Next we analyze the syndromes according to the 4 domains of diagnosis, as taught by my colleague Dr. Robert Averbuch (personal communication). These domains are to be considered in every diagnostic case and consist of general medical condition, substance-related including medications, psychiatric syndromes, and stress-related or trauma-related syndromes. For the purposes of this chapter we will subsequently go in detail only for the first domain of general medical conditions.

The Mental Status Examination and Psychiatric Syndromes

Let us briefly describe the clinical syndromes and how we identify them. In the DSM-5, delirium is defined as an alteration in cognitive function with decrease in attention fluctuations and levels of alertness that occur over a relatively short period of time. Any psychiatric or somatic symptom can be present in delirium, but the hallmark clinical feature is a relatively brief onset in the context of medical versus substance conditions and a predominant impairment of attention. Dementia, which is now called major or minor neurocognitive disorder, is characterized by impairment in memory and other cognitive functions, which may be insidious as in Alzheimer's disease or acute as in physical trauma or multi-infarct dementia. The difference in major and minor categorizations is the level of functional impairment. Psychosis is generally defined as a syndrome with impaired reality testing, manifested by hallucinations, delusions, or disorganization of the speech and behavior. There may be some cognitive and affective dysfunction present, but the predominant impairment is in reality testing. The category of affective syndromes is defined as a disturbance and mood; this can be either elevated as in mania, or depressed as in depression, or mixed. Psychotic symptoms may be present, but the predominant focus of attention is the disturbance in mood. Anxiety syndrome is characterized by excessive worry, but absent significant impairment from cognition, psychosis, or affective disturbances.

In consideration of general medical conditions which can cause a syndrome, it is heuristically useful to think of the variety of syndromes associated with just a few conditions. For example, autoimmune disease, HIV disease, syphilis, and thyroid dysfunction are associated with each of the major syndromes of delirium, neurocognitive disorder, psychosis, affective disorder or[i] anxiety disorder in any mix of predominance.[1] Delirium must be in the context of a physiological disturbance. Other conditions classically have a more specific association, for example psychosis associated with anti-NMDA receptor encephalitis, depression associated with pancreatic cancer, or anxiety associated with pheochromocytoma. See Table 29.2 for listing of additional medical disorders.

Substances and medications may also be associated either with all the syndromes or more classically associated with a specific syndrome. For example, alcohol misuse has 16 different DSM-5 diagnoses, ranging from delirium from intoxication or withdrawal to alcoholic dementia, alcohol-related sleep disorder, alcohol colic hallucinosis, or the anxiety associated with alcohol craving; whereas amphetamines are classically associated with paranoid psychotic syndromes and may be associated with anxiety or disturbances in mood.

TABLE 29.2 A Comprehensive, Systematic Differential Diagnosis for Psychiatric Syndromes

Psychiatric Syndrome	General Medical Illnesses	Substance Related	Psychiatric	Stress/Trauma
Delirium Neurocognitive		Alcohol Ecstasy	n/a	Amnestic fugue
Psychosis	AntiNMDA receptor encephalitis HIV encephalitis Thyroid disease	Alcoholic hallucinosis Amphetamine paranoia Beta blocker depression	Schizophreniform Schizophrenia Schizoaffective	Brief psychotic disorder
Affective	Pancreatic cancer Hypothyroidism GI dysfunction Thyroid disease	Alcohol Cocaine Amphetamine Beta blockers Interferon Retinoic acid	Major depression Dysthymia	Adjustment disorder with depressed mood
Other				

More specific effects of medications include the example of beta-blockers associated with depression. Additional medication and substance related specifics are noted in Table 29.2.

Medical Review of Systems in Relation to Psychiatric Syndromes

Just as we did a comprehensive examination of psychiatric syndromes, we now examine somatic symptoms that may have their origins in psychiatric illnesses.[2] In this exercise the left-hand column represents the somatic symptom systems that are organized in the standard 14 systems as defined by the U.S. Center for Medical Services. For heuristic purposes, the other columns are organized according to the psychiatric syndromes that we identified in the clinical examination of the patient. Let us begin with the first column of the delirium syndrome; as noted earlier, any psychiatric or somatic symptom may be present in a delirium syndrome. The hallmark symptom of delirium is impaired attention in the context of a physiological disturbance; therefore no single somatic symptom stands out. rather you will get disturbances in general function such as impaired sleep or disrupted sleep or impaired appetite or activity. Dementias such as Alzheimer's disease are often striking by the absence of somatic symptoms other than sleep disturbance. Psychotic disorders are defined as impairment of reality testing or distortions of reality, and somatic symptoms, particularly bizarre symptoms, are common in these disorders. Patients with schizophrenia may complain about eye pain, genital pain, or back pain. They may also have sexual complaints. Patients with affective disorders such as mania will most often deny any impairment or symptom despite evidence to the contrary. However, some patients with depression are focused almost entirely on their somatic symptoms. Classically depression is associated with poor sleep, poor appetite, impaired bowel function, decreased energy, decreased psychomotor activity, impaired sexual function, and orthostatic hypotension. They may also complain of shortness of breath and chest pain, generalized body pain, or localized body pain. Gastrointestinal symptoms are very common and dramatic and at times of delusional proportions. Patients diagnosed with conversion disorder or factitious disorders often have an underlying depressive syndrome that can be treated. Anxiety disorders actually are defined by somatic symptoms such as increased sweaty palms and palpitations and often shortness of breath. Additionally, patients may complain of headaches, ringing in the years, dry mouth, tingling and numbness, and periods of weakness.

See Table 29.3 for additional examples.

Psychotherapeutic Medications That May Present with Somatic Syndromes and Symptoms

In consideration of medical illnesses in psychiatry, we must also consider medical symptoms (side effects) that are caused by psychotherapeutic medications (Table 29.4). These symptoms may manifest as specific clinical syndromes or as isolated somatic side effects.[3] Most psychotherapeutic medications will have some impact on sleep, either disturbance or excessive sedation. Antipsychotics are associated in varying degrees with blurred vision, dry mouth, constipation, and sedation generally related to anticholinergic side effects of the medication. Quetiapine is often used as a sedating agent; even though it has relatively weak

TABLE 29.3 Medical Review of Systems in Relation to Psychiatric Syndromes

Somatic Syndrome	Delirium/ Neurocognitive	Psychosis	Affective	Anxiety	Other
General	Poor sleep Malaise Appetite changes	Poor sleep	Poor sleep Malaise Appetite changes	Poor sleep	Poor sleep
EYE		Pain Sensory misperceptions		Blurred vision	
ENT		Sensory misperceptions			
PULM				SOB	
CARD			Chest pain	palpitations	
GI		Sensory misperceptions			
GU					
Muscl-Skl					
Neuro		Sensory misperceptions		Tingling, numbness	
Psych	See Table 29.1	See Table 29.1	See Table 29.1	See Table 29.1	See Table 29.1
Skin		Flushing			
Endo					
Heme					
Immune			Decreased function		

anticholinergic activity, it is important to note that quetiapine has a black box warning for the development of cataracts, and healthcare providers are expected to periodically monitor the development of cataracts when prescribing quetiapine. The classes of antidepressants vary widely in side effects and they will be discussed separately here. Selective serotonin reuptake inhibitors (SSRIs) are associated with initial insomnia, jitteriness and then later on may cause anorgasmia, and weight gain. The greater clinical concern is the abrupt withdrawal of this class of medications, which is associated with nausea, vomiting, and diarrhea, often called the SSRI withdrawal syndrome. Serotonin-norepinephrine reuptake inhibitors (SNRIs) at higher doses have the same side effects. Venlafaxine is specifically associated with an increase in blood pressure, typically minor but measurable at 7–10 mmHg.[4] Bupropion is its own class of antidepressants and does not have the reported sexual side effects, but is associated with increased risk of seizures, particularly at higher doses or with an increase in dosing, and may have higher incidence of episodes of confusion. Since bupropion is also used for smoking cessation and primary care, it is important that the clinicians track all the medications that patients are taking and avoid untoward drug-drug interactions or additive effects of drugs. Mirtazapine and trazodone are distinctly different antidepressants, but are both used most commonly for their excessive sedation effect, so they are used for sedative hypnotics. Mirtazapine is associated with weight gain. Trazodone, on the other hand, is

TABLE 29.4 Medical Review of Systems in Terms of Psychotherapeutic Medications

Somatic Systems	Antipsychotics	Antidepressants	Anxiolytics benzodiazepines	Anticonvulsants	Lithium	Stimulants
General	Poor sleep Malaise Appetite changes Weight gain	Poor sleep Weight gain	Poor sleep Poor memory Confusion Weight gain	Poor sleep Weight gain Or weight loss	Poor sleep Poor memory Confusion Weight gain	Weight loss
EYE	Cataracts, glaucoma	glaucoma		Cataracts		
ENT						
PULM						
CARD	Irregular heart beats, tachycardia	Tachycardia, Irregular heart beats		—	Irregular heart beats	Tachycardia hypertension
GI	Toxic megacolon (clozapine)	Constipation from tricyclics,			Diarrhea, nausea, vomiting	
GU	Urinary retention	Urinary retention from tricyclics				
Muscl-Skl	Dystonia,					
Neuro	Tremor	Myoclonus	Ataxia	Ataxia	Tremor	Jitteriness
Psych	Decreased alertness, apathy					
Skin	Photosensitive rash			Steven Johnson Syndrome		
Endo	diabetes				Hypothyroidism	
Heme		Bleeding dyscrasia		Bleeding dyscrasia	Increased WBC	
Immune						

associated at high doses with headaches, orthostatic hypotension and on an idiosyncratic basis, with priapism. Tricyclic antidepressants are still used despite the fact that other medications are just as efficacious, and tricyclics have almost universal side effects of dry mouth, constipation, blurred vision and dizziness. Due to the risk of fatal arrhytmias in the event of an overdose, prescribers may often dispense only a 2 week supply of tricyclic medications. Monoamine oxidase inhibitors continue to have a special role for refractory depression, anxiety, or panic disorders, but are complicated to use due to dietary restrictions, crises, and drug-drug interactions which may present as hypertensive crisis.

Anticonvulsant medications are also a diverse group with potentially diverse side effects in psychiatry. Divalproex is the most widely used anticonvulsant. Divalproex has related side effects of nausea, vomiting, diarrhea, and associations of hepatotoxicity, particularly when used in polypharmacy. Lamotrigine is widely used for bipolar disorder, particularly bipolar depression, and is generally well tolerated, but unfortunately is associated with the development of skin rash and even Stevens-Johnson syndrome which must be mitigated by slow upward titration of the drug and special caution when reinitiating the drug after discontinuation of even just 48 hours. Topiramate is little less widely used, although it has a favorable side effect of weight loss, but this is most often offset by the frequent occurrence of muscle pain and reports of cognitive confusion, particularly word-finding difficulties. Gabapentin may be the most widely used anticonvulsant for non-epileptic reasons; it is customarily used for mood stabilization, anxiety disorders, alcohol withdrawal, alcohol craving, and pain syndromes, specifically neuropathic pain. Gabapentin is renally excreted and is generally safe in context of hepatic impairment, but it does have the related side effects of sedation, ataxia, and falls; there are some indications that gabapentin may have addictive properties.

Lithium is a class of its own. Lithium has physiological impairment on renal function and thyroid function, specifically diabetes insipidus and hypothyroidism from blocking the uptake of T3. There is a very narrow therapeutic window for lithium, so that toxic levels that are just 50% greater than therapeutic and may be associated with altered mental status, convulsions, and death. Lithium also has a physiologic function to increase white blood cell count and has a use described in the literature to help mitigate the leukopenia properties of clozapine.

Stimulants have shown marked resurgence in use and widespread distribution, particularly in the United States. This increasing use is driven not only by suspected misuse by high school students who want a competitive edge, but more so by the acceptance of a diagnosis of adult attention deficit hyperactivity disorder (ADHD). In children, the major concern of the use of stimulants is growth retardation. Use of growth charts is recommended. In adults, the major concerns with the use of stimulants revolve around misuse, development of addiction, and/or potential cardiac side effects. As described in Table 29.4 this is associated with paranoid syndromes, panic, and anxiety.

Table 29.5 describes common physical syndromes and the associated psychotherapeutic medications. Neuroleptic malignant syndrome is characterized by confusion, physical rigidity, and fever in the context of antipsychotic medication use.[5] Classically all three symptoms must be present and most often in the context of doses of antipsychotics in excess of what is now maximum use in the United States. However, the literature is replete with case report descriptions of what may be better described as benign malignant neuroleptic syndrome and in very low dose or absence of antipsychotic medication use. Serotonin syndrome is similar to neuroleptic malignant syndrome and it is associated with confusion and fever, but has a more pronounced presentation of fluctuating fevers, blood pressure, and changes in motor function.[6] Serotonin syndrome is associated with antidepressants such as the SSRIs, but can be found in any medications with seroteonergic activities, such as quetiapine and risperidone, or with combinations of medications for the additive effects.[7] Parkinson's syndrome is not only well characterized with antipsychotics, but is an expected side effect of high doses of the first-generation antipsychotics. Parkinsonian symptoms of psychomotor retardation, bradykinesia, and tremor are reversible with anticholinergic treatment, or best by reduction or switch from the offending antipsychotic agent. On the other hand, as implied in its name, tardive dyskinesia is a later onset of dyskinetic movements that

TABLE 29.5 Somatic Syndromes associated with Psychotherapeutic Medications

Syndrome	Symptoms	Associated Medications
Neuroleptic malignant syndrome	Fever, confusion, rigidity	Antipsychotics
Serotonin syndrome	Fever confusion, autonomic instability, myoclonus	Antidepressants, some antipsychotics
Parkinsonism	Bradykinesia, resting tremors, hypothermia,	Antipsychotics
Tardive dyskinesia	Choreiform movements, dyskinesia, dystonia, altered gait	Antipsychotics
Metabolic syndrome	Obesity, diabetes Dyslipidemia,	Antipsychotics, especially second generation
Prolonged QT syndrome	Weakness, syncope, sudden death	Antipsychotics, especially thioridazine, zisprazadone ziprasidone, haloperidol,
Memory impairment	Anterograde memory impairment, decreased attention	Benzodiazepines, anticholinergics

are attributed to long-term, high-dose treatment with antipsychotics. There is substantial data to suggest that the occurrence of parkinsonism with antipsychotic use is a harbinger of vulnerability to the development of tardive dyskinesia. The most significant syndrome associated with psychotropic medication use and associated with the majority of the premature mortality associated with psychiatric illnesses is the development of metabolic syndrome. Metabolic syndrome is characterized by obesity, diabetes, and dyslipidemia, and can begin within 6 months of use of antipsychotics, most often associated with the second-generation antipsychotics. Smoking magnifies the risk of mortality associated with metabolic syndrome. For decades, psychiatrists and other providers either did not recognize the metabolic syndrome or when it was recognized felt that it was less important than treating the psychiatric illness. There was a general belief that it was fruitless to try to intervene with patients with schizophrenia to modify their behaviors to mitigate against metabolic syndrome. This is proven to be a false bias, and with standard behavioral interventions such as education and feedback, patients with schizophrenia can modify their lifestyle and make significant improvements in terms of weight gain and management of hypertension and diabetes. Prolongation of the QT interval on the electrocardiogram has received greater recognition of its importance in the past decade as a potential contributor to premature mortality in patients treated with psychotropic medications. Table 29.5 lists antipsychotics and other medications with relative associations and impact on electrocardiogram QTC interval. Recent research shows that the vulnerability to the development of prolonged QTC is significantly related to the genotype of the person as much or more so than the prescribed medications. There is optimism that with the use of precision medicine (genetic testing) that we will soon be able to mitigate the occurrence and tasks associated with prolonged QTC. Anterograde memory impairment has long been recognized as a complication of benzodiazepine use. There are disturbing new data suggesting that chronic benzodiazepine use may not only be associated with memory impairment, but may actually accelerate the pathophysiology of the development of Alzheimer's disease.

Formulating Holistic Interventions

Social Behavioral Responses to Stress and Medical Illness

Over the past three decades, data clearly show that the root causes of most of the medical, psychiatric, and substance use disorders are due to social determinants of health that result from maladaptive behavioral responses to trauma experienced in childhood and the stressors in everyday life.[8] Less recognized is that these behavioral responses to stress are mediated by the social context of the experiences and of the interventions. The remaining sections of this chapter present the basic association of stress and behavior, plus the impact of the social context of the experience and response. These social contexts are now evident in global attention due to COVID-19 pandemic and the shocking magnification of structural racism.[9]

Stress begets stress. A cascade of maladaptive behaviors often follow physical trauma or serious illness. Persons with consistent maladaptive behavioral responses to stressors and further consequences may be diagnosed with having a personality disorder, which complicate healthcare provider efforts to provide medical treatments for their medical conditions.[10] This is particularly evident when we look at outlier utilizers of emergency departments and hospital services.

At each level of care, the healthcare provider targets health behaviors. The top 6 problematic health behaviors are: (1) sedentary lifestyle, (2) alcohol and other drug use, (3) sexual activity, (4) behaviors associated with injuries, (5) tobacco use, and (6) poor eating habits (see Table 29.6).

Mental health providers are often called in to provide consults to hospital teams caring for angry noncompliant patients or to assess the patient's medical decision-making capacity.[11] Capacity determinations are particularly challenging in patients with long-established patterns of medical noncompliance and destructive habits such as smoking, cocaine use, etc. How is the mental health provider to determine if the current bad decision is substantially different from the lifelong pattern of ill-advised decisions? Even if the pattern is consistent, this is within the patient's free will.

Whole Health Integration

Up to now the discussion has focused on the dyad of the person with illness and the healthcare provider. As we note in the premise of this book, the basic unit of a person is their social system; i.e., no one exists on his/her own. As we see that much of what we recognize in conventional medicine are missed diagnoses or adverse reactions to medical interventions. We can see these medical errors are often the result of the biases that we use to simplify our work, i.e., the artificial division of medical illness from psychiatric illness. We can use an integrated whole healthcare schema to avoid these medical errors and yet still maintain the ability to function efficiently. A description for the cognitive paradigm of integrated whole health is shown in Figure 29.2.

TABLE 29.6 Behavioral Responses to Stress and Medical Illness

Behaviors	Medical Consequences	Psychiatric Consequences	Social Consequences
Sedentary	Obesity heart disease diabetes; disability	Depression, anxiety	
Alcohol and other drug use	Liver disease, heart disease, infectious disease	Depression, impaired cognition, insomnia	Poverty, incarceration
Sexual activity	STD, HIV, HPV cancer	Anxiety depression	Superficial relationships
Risk taking	Physical trauma, disability		Poverty incarceration
Smoking	Heart disease, cancer	Anxiety	Ostracization in work and social environments
Overeating	Obesity heart disease diabetes	Depression	Social isolation

The ACE Pyramid   –

The ACE Pyramid represents the conceptual framework for the ACE Study. The ACE Study has uncovered how ACEs are strongly related to development of risk factors for disease, and well-being throughout the life course.

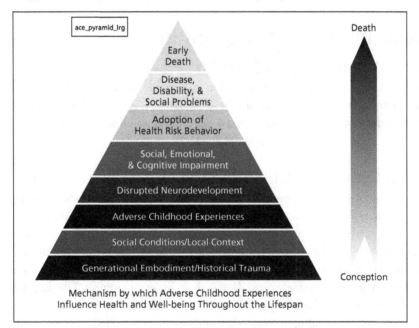

FIGURE 29.1. The ACE Pyramid. From https://www.cdc.gov/violenceprevention/acestudy/about.html?CDC_AA_refVal=https%3A%2F%2Fwww.cdc.gov%2Fviolenceprevention%2Fchildabuseandneglect%2Facestudy%2Findex.html.

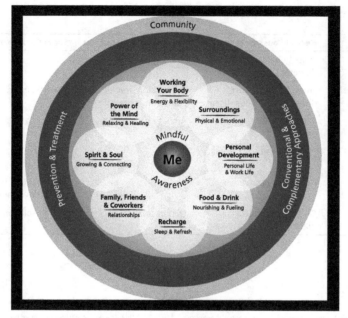

FIGURE 29.2. The Whole Health Circle.

Social Targets for Intervention

Social Determinants of Health

As we move towards the big picture of health, we observe that traditional medical care contributes only a small percentage towards health outcome (Figure 29.3). However, we are not victims of destiny. By examination of the social contributors (not determinants) to health, we can alter those factors for different outcomes.[12]

Global Whole Health Integration: Social Psychiatry

Now we build toward the completion of the health model by adding the social context of the experiences and expressions of experience. The interplay of social forces can be viewed under perspective of the patient within a culture. For example, in the United States we commonly see alcohol abuse as a response to symptoms of stress, but in cultures where alcohol use is prohibited those medial consequences would not be seen. We can also examine how the same presentation is viewed differently in different cultures. Likewise, healthcare delivery can be viewed from the perspective of the healthcare provider's encounter with patients from dissimilar cultures, which then adds to the group effect of cultures attempting acculturation.[13] Ultimately with large groups of people in mass migration or economic exchanges, we describe this as the globalization of healthcare.

The rapid changes in the globalization of healthcare have required our academic health systems to develop new methodologies for establishing a knowledge base and competencies to deal with hundreds, if not thousands, of unique cross-cultural encounters. Discussed elsewhere in this book are the activities of other professional groups, such as the World Association for Social Psychiatry, dedicated

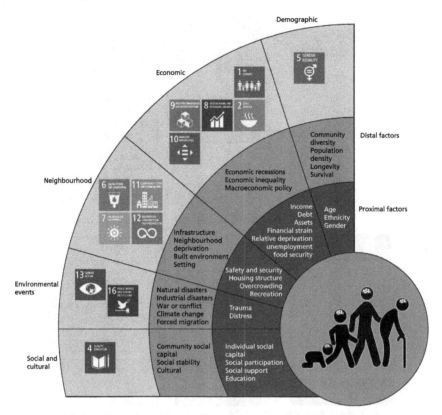

FIGURE 29.3. Global Health Goals and Targets.[20]

to promote greater understanding of the interactions between individuals and their physical and human environment (including their society and culture), and the impact of these interactions on the clinical expression, treatment of mental and behavioral problems and disorders and their prevention.
(http://www.worldsocpsychiatry.org/aboutus.asp#about_society_tag)

Although we have a rich catalog of culture-associated syndromes in medicine and psychiatry (see Culture Bound Syndromes in DSM-IV TR), we know this is no longer sufficient, shifting instead toward concepts of cultural influences on behaviors and cultural competencies for assessment with the Cultural Formulation Interview.[14] Universities now focus on tools and methodologies to aid practitioners and researchers in approaching cultural competence in context.[15]

There is a danger in the global health field that efforts to improve global health (originating in well-developed countries and applied to less-developed countries; see Figure 29.3) become another platform for ethical imperialism.[16] For practicing clinicians, Trihn et al.[17] present a model called cultural humility to aid the clinician's understanding of illness from the patient's perspective by building on their relationship rather than presupposed knowledge. Thus there is a new paradigm structuring ethical interactions from principalism and the 4 principles of Western ethics toward a transactional ethics based on human dignity, such as seen in the UNESCO Declaration on Bioethics and Human Rights (UDBHR).[18,19]

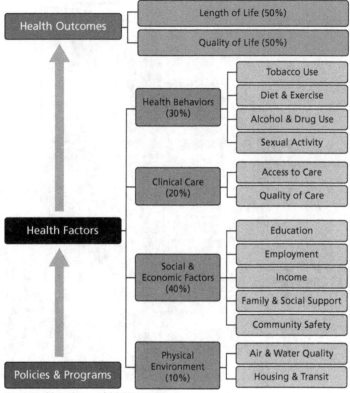

County Health Ranking model © 2016 UWPHI

FIGURE 29.4. UNESCO Bioethics.
Article 3—Human dignity and human rights.
Article 4—Benefit and harm.
Article 5—Autonomy and individual responsibility.
Article 6—Consent.
Article 7—Persons without the capacity to consent.
Article 8—Respect for human vulnerability and personal integrity.
Article 9—Privacy and confidentiality.
Article 10—Equality, justice and equity.
Article 11—Non-discrimination and non-stigmatization.
Article 12—Respect for cultural diversity and pluralism.
Article 13—Solidarity and cooperation.
Article 14—Social responsibility and health.
Article 15—Sharing of benefits.
Article 16—Protecting future generations.
Article 17—Protection of the environment, the biosphere and biodiversity.

Social Behavioral Aspects of Epidemics

All epidemics are social behaviors. This statement is based on the behaviors of (1) transmission, (2) health professions response, (3) public response, and (4) government response. Knowing the means of transmission theoretically allows people the option to avoid transmitted disease. This could be from a simple matter of avoiding eating uncooked meat or unwashed vegetables, avoiding sex with multiple partners, or as simple as washing hands and wearing a mask. When some segments of the population find that the transmission of illness occurs during parts of their usual activities that are important individual or cultural activities, such as attending sporting events or funerals, we find that the behaviors are not altered.

The public response to instructions on avoiding illness during epidemic is most similar to response to illness in general. Behavior fundamentals apply even in epidemics, and the behaviors are still driven by proximal and distal temporal factors of pleasure and pain. In the current COVID-19 pandemic, hundreds of millions of people are asked to experience the immediate pain of social isolation and economic hardship for the distal pleasure of avoiding transmitting illness to vulnerable society members or themselves. To change behaviors that place members of the public at risk, health providers and social leaders must present a credible message to motivate behavior change. Conveying such a message is extremely difficult when the facts are uncertain, the experts not familiar, and the counter messages are more appealing.

Government response to epidemics is driven by the balance of power. For example, is a government to devote a marked share of its resources and inflict economic harm on most of the population to protect marginalized members of that society? At times the interests of the government leaders or business leaders may be at odds with the altruistic interest of some but not all healthcare providers. There are disparate examples of situations where healthcare providers have fled an area that saw the development of plague (Surratt, India) and other examples of courage and perseverance, as with Dr. Carlo Urban in the SARS epidemic in Vietnam,[21] or Dr. Li Wenliang in China for the COVID-19 outbreak.[22]

Principles
Global Bioethics, Health, and Social Psychiatry

> The first step in the evolution of ethics is a sense of solidarity with other human beings.
> —Albert Schweitzer

Pandemics are the ultimate medical illness associated with social behaviors. Each pandemic has its own social challenges. Tuberculosis is viewed as a problem for poor people, Ebola for poor countries; AIDS has been viewed in moralistic terms, and in many countries COVID-19 is viewed in political terms. Core to any of these viewpoints are the ethical challenges. The ethical dilemmas have been extensively described and cover among many other areas: the duties to plan, safeguard and guide; allocation of resources for research into effective treatments, resources for data collection, managing the use of social media for case tracking, constraints on human rights for freedom of movement, freedom of association, and constraints on international trade due to protectionist impulses.[23]

The acutely challenging and socially transformative COVID-19 pandemic has even unveiled deeper strains in our societies resulting from social structure of racism and other forms of discriminations.[9] The pandemic has proven that the disease-focused model of care is insufficient to save lives and to protect the health of communities.

A relatively new ethical framework can provide the tools for that leadership role. By engaging stakeholders in problem-solving under the 15 principles (Figure 29.1) of the UNESCO Declaration on Bioethics and Human Rights, we can progress toward agreement for action. In the United States we have a saying, "If you are in healthcare you are in politics," and nowhere has that been more evident that the COVID-19 pandemic. In advocacy for prevention of global genocide, David Hamburg wrote, "leadership matters." Hamburg and colleagues[24] outline a pathway for social psychiatrists to contribute to improving local and global leadership. The core dysfunction was the lack of political will to take necessary action to protect vulnerable populations. They describe very psychological pitfalls in decision-making: group think, mirror imaging, and risk aversion. Structural factors that lead to these stylistic errors are rigid hierarchal intelligence gathering and shrinkage of the advisory group to like-minded persons. Limited data, among limited decision-makers, lead to limited options. As clinicians we change our advice to patients based on evolving science; likewise in our professional roles we have to change the way we communicate to leadership as circumstances require. The circumstances of the COVID-19 pandemic and structural racism require committed actions by professional organizations. We must also look within our own organizations to expand diversity and inclusiveness. Collectively clinicians have to cooperate, acquire more data, and present effectively to leadership and the public. Our professional groups must also provide an analysis of the data and propose viable solutions. Professionally we can challenge binary and sensationalist policies with concise, clear, thoughtful, evidence framed within a value system.

Lack of a common ground for a value system has been a significant barrier to reaching consensus for action. Too often we are offered a binary view of safety versus freedom. The UNESCO Bioethics framework requires a more comprehensive discussion and engagement.

With COVID-19, society has to change the behavior of the many initially to protect the few and the vulnerable. Also, with COVID-19 we are experiencing millions losing jobs, income, and resources during quarantine with the perception of saving the lives of thousands of people already dependent on society at large in nursing homes, prisons, or chronic healthcare. The field of social psychiatry has subject matter responsibility for assuming a leadership role on addressing behaviors associated with pandemics.

Concluding Comments

Think globally, act locally. This adage from environmentalism is applicable to clinical practice. The clinician has a caring relationship with individual patients who are within a larger social context. We conclude where we began—that is, with the person. Change is hard. We see the complex interdependent relationships of the person and their social environment. In a world where our social paradigms are failing, our social institutions are ill from their own behaviors and decisions. As clinicians, we guide our patients to behavior change; now we must do the same with ourselves. We are accustomed to being in a position of power, guiding others to change. But in the current context, where we are subject to powerful external forces, we must act as individuals to collectively change global and local social determinants of health. As individuals, we must act on our social environment, which includes our professional and governmental environments, to make changes in social behavior that are more compatible with long-term survival and prosperity for all. We may not have the answers, but we do have the means. We have a lot of work to do.

Key Points

- The clinician
  - Examines the patient,
  - Formulates a diagnosis as a hypothesis,
  - Initiates interventions
  - Monitors progress.
- The diagnostic formulation must include the assessment of the social-cultural context.
- Social analysis includes ethical analysis of social functioning.
- Interventions are directed with the patient and the social context.

References

1. Castro J, Billick S. Psychiatric presentations/manifestations of medical illnesses. *Psychiatr Q.* 2013;84:351–362.
2. Stoudemire A. Integrating medical and psychiatric treatment in an inpatient medical setting. *Psychosomatics.* 2000;41:366–369.
3. Grover S, Kate N. Somatic symptoms in consultation-liaison psychiatry. *Int Rev Psychiatry.* 2013;25:52–64.
4. Thase ME. Effects of venlafaxine on blood pressure: a meta-analysis of original data from 3744 depressed patients. *J Clin Psychiatry.* 1998;59:502–508.
5. Christensen RC. Recognizing early signs of neuroleptic malignant syndrome. *Am J Emerg Med.* 1998;16:95–96.
6. Christensen RC. Identifying serotonin syndrome in the emergency department. *Am J Emerg Med.* 2005;23:406–408.
7. Mazhar F, Akram S, Haider N, Ahmed R. Overlapping of Serotonin Syndrome with Neuroleptic Malignant Syndrome due to Linezolid-Fluoxetine and Olanzapine-Metoclopramide Interactions: A Case Report of Two Serious Adverse Drug Effects Caused by Medication Reconciliation Failure on Hospital Admission. *Case Reports in Medicine.* 2016;2016:7128909.
8. Chiang M, Chang J, Nakash O, Cruz-Gonzalez M, Fillbrunn MK, Alegría M. Change in patient activation and mental illness symptoms after communication training: a multisite study with a diverse patient sample. *Psychiatr Serv.* 2019;70:696–702.
9. Bailey ZD, Krieger N, Agénor M, Graves J, Linos N, Bassett MT. Structural racism and health inequities in the USA: evidence and interventions. *Lancet.* 2017;389:1453–1463.
10. Kornfeld DS, Muskin PR, Tahil FA. Psychiatric evaluation of mental capacity in the general hospital: a significant teaching opportunity. *Psychosomatics.* 2009;50:468–473.
11. Nash SS, Kent LK, Muskin PR. Psychodynamics in medically ill patients. *Harv Rev Psychiatry.* 2009;17:389–397.
12. Magnan S. Social determinants of health 101 for health care: five plus five. *NAM Perspectives.* Discussion Paper, National Academy of Medicine, Washington, DC.
13. Rothe EM, Tzuang D, Pumariega AJ. Acculturation, development, and adaptation. *Child Adolesc Psychiatr Clin N Am.* 2010;19:681–696.

14. Jarvis GE, Kirmayer LJ, Gómez-Carrillo A, Aggarwal NK, Lewis-Fernández R. Update on the Cultural Formulation Interview. *Focus (Am Psychiatr Publ).* 2020;18:40–46.

15. Mews C, Schuster S, Vajda C, et al. Cultural competence and global health: perspectives for medical education—position paper of the GMA Committee on Cultural Competence and Global Health. *GMS J Med Educ.* 2018;35:Doc28.

16. Barugahare J. African bioethics: methodological doubts and insights. *BMC Med Ethics.* 2018;19:98.

17. Trinh NH, Tuchman S, Chen J, Chang T, Yeung A. Cultural humility and the practice of consultation-liaison psychiatry. *Psychosomatics.* 2020;61:313–320.

18. Andorno R. Global bioethics at UNESCO: in defence of the Universal Declaration on Bioethics and Human Rights. *J Med Ethics.* 2007;33:150–154.

19. Langlois A. The UNESCO Bioethics Programme: a review. *New Bioeth.* 2014;20:3–11.

20. Lund C, Brooke-Sumner C, Baingana F, et al. Social determinants of mental disorders and the Sustainable Development Goals: a systematic review of reviews. *Lancet Psychiatry.* 2018;5:357–369.

21. Fleck F. How SARS changed the world in less than six months. *Bull World Health Organ.* 2003;81:625–626.

22. Petersen E, Hui D, Hamer DH, et al. Li Wenliang, a face to the frontline healthcare worker: the first doctor to notify the emergence of the SARS-CoV-2 (COVID-19), outbreak. *Int J Infect Dis.* 2020;93:205–207.

23. Garrett JR, McNolty LA, Wolfe ID, Lantos JD. Our next pandemic ethics challenge? Allocating "normal" health care services. *Hastings Cent Rep.* 2020;50:79–80.

24. Hamburg DA, George A, Ballentine K. Preventing deadly conflict: the critical role of leadership. *Arch Gen Psychiatry.* 1999;56:971–976.

30

Social Psychiatry in Major Neurocognitive Disorders

Brian Harlan and Joseph E. Thornton

Background/History

The social burden of dementing illnesses is immense. The direct economic impact of neurocognitive disorders was estimated to be over $600 billion worldwide for 2010, and cost growth disproportionate to population growth continues to occur due to increasing life expectancies.[1] Over 10% of the population over the age of 65 have dementia, and as much as 45% of the population over the age of 85 have dementia.[2] Despite resource allocation for research, increases in caregiver training, and the development of specialty care, clinicians and patients find that adequate treatment and access to care is lacking.

Implications for the social supports of a patient with dementia add to the overall disease burden and are difficult to quantify. For caregivers, development of depression, along with resentment, guilt, and productivity loss, contribute.[3]

In this chapter, we will describe the social aspects of progressive neurocognitive disease, focusing on frequent challenges encountered by families, communities, and clinicians. Difficulties associated with various cultural differences, economic class, and barriers to access for dementia care and caregiver support will also be addressed.

Initial Diagnosis and Communication with Patients and Families

Initial diagnosis and treatment are stressful for patients and their families. Collaboration with families is essential to the establishment of a diagnosis and treatment plan. Though advances in diagnostic accuracy have occurred, definitive diagnostic testing for dementia remains elusive. Uncertainty regarding the differential diagnoses often creates confusion that is disruptive to a therapeutic alliance.[4]

Patients and families present to physicians and mental health professionals with different levels of distress. Often, a cognitive decline has been noticed, but has been minimized or dismissed as normal aging. As a result, patients may present only after concerning events, such as activation of a "Silver Alert" for a missing adult. In these instances, a dementia diagnosis may be a confirmation of previous suspicions. Other patients' neurocognitive problems may be discovered incidental to presentation for other medical problems. Clinicians need to be sensitive to the multitude of needs of the patients and families who will be informed of the suspected presence of a dementing illness and assess for the most appropriate time and manner in which to communicate the diagnosis.

Unfortunately, many dementing illnesses are diagnosed at a relatively advanced stage, when treatments that may slow the course of the disease may be less effective. Distinctions between dementing illnesses have prognostic value, but specificity of diagnostic testing is poor.[4]

Questions regarding care and prognosis are expected. Families may feel helpless or overwhelmed when they cannot predict the course of dementia and cannot control the symptoms of illness. Psychiatrists must assess the limits of the patients' primary supports based on multiple factors, including psychiatric consequences of caregiver stress.

Specific Stressors Related to Caregiving

Dementia caregivers average 21.9 unpaid hours per week providing care.[5] Negative impacts occur for caregivers' mental and social health. Psychiatrists treating dementia patients may expect to address vulnerable family members and will encounter disruptions and conflict within family relationships.[6,7]

Differing expectations among close and distant family members often create or exacerbate conflict. Additional strain occurs with more than one family member requires care at the same time. Encouraging family members to create a plan to manage foreseeable developments should be an important part of treatment planning. For example, when patients increasing rely on caregivers to provide support for activities of daily living such as bathing, toileting, and dressing, a previously defined threshold for supplementing family support or for placement in a nursing facility may ease distress and guilt. Identifying appropriate facilities and resources before they become necessary reduces the sense of urgency and allows for more exploration of suitable choices for care.

Unforeseeable problems, such as the illness of another family member, may be more difficult to manage. Each family will negotiate solutions to unpredictable challenges differently. Psychiatrists should attend to evidence of caregiver stress, including anxiety, self-neglect, depression, and suicidal thoughts, as well as monitor the patient for evidence of abuse or neglect. Successful families gather information, take action when possible, and adjust expectations. Caregivers anticipating their own reactions to stress or lack of control may access appropriate resources more efficiently. Psychiatrists may assist by assessing the caregivers' adaptation to stress and encouraging the use of appropriate resources such as referrals for mental healthcare for the family.

Social Systems in Dementia

Extended communities having shared values in the care of their patients with dementia may influence the course of the disease. Research suggests that individual and family counseling with caregivers can result in additional support from the community and additional family members, reducing negative consequences for the primary caregiver by providing respite care and encouraging socialization.[8]

Social Challenges by Dementia Subtypes

Dementia of the Alzheimer's Type (DAT)

The most common dementing illness is dementia of the Alzheimer's type with late onset. Onset is insidious and often unappreciated for several months or years prior to diagnosis. Gradual social changes may include social withdrawal and personality changes that can create family conflict, which delays diagnosis.

Though dementia of the Alzheimer's type with early onset typically has disease course similar to late onset, with median survival from the time of diagnosis being from 4.2 years (males) to 5.7 years (females),[9] the age of the patient with early onset Alzheimer's may complicate placement due to incongruence with the ages typical of patients on memory care units. The relatively lower rate of comorbid medical conditions common in older patients (e.g., sarcopenia) may pose an increase in risk to caregivers, other residents, or staff when a younger patient experiences behavioral dyscontrol.

Dementia with Lewy Bodies (DLB)

Dementia with Lewy bodies shares many histopathologic and behavioral characteristics with Alzheimer's. The diagnosis of DLB is usually made when a patient exhibits more pronounced Parkinsonian traits, such as shuffling gait, rigidity, decreased arm swing, etc. One particularly distinctive characteristic of DLB is the presence of crepuscular agitation, often with hallucinations. In DLB, patients may have markedly worsening cognitive and behavioral symptoms each afternoon and evening. The timing of appointments may influence the diagnosis and evaluation of severity. Families may have difficulty managing the patient in the evening, so morning appointments are preferable, but clinicians may underestimate the actual disease burden in these instances. Behavior logs and videographic documentation may be helpful in assessing a patient's actual functional status.

Vascular Dementia

Chronic neurovascular disease leads to progressive cognitive decline in a pattern similar to DAT, and indeed, DAT may be a complication of neurovascular disease.[10] Classically, however, vascular dementia is associated with acute worsening of cognitive or behavioral problems, followed by periods of relatively slower functional decline. Vascular disease superimposed upon other dementing illnesses may lead to unpredictable or abrupt decline, complicating care planning and requiring adaptation to new problems.

Frontotemporal Dementias (FTD)

In recent years, frontotemporal dementias have been increasingly recognized as a reason for behavioral changes in patients without preexisting psychiatric problems, particularly behavioral variant frontotemporal dementia (bvFTD). These diseases are poorly character-ized and perhaps inappropriately categorized as a single entity despite wide variations in etiology and manifestations. The course of illness may be malignantly rapid, and the rela-tively young age of onset may create difficulties with care access due to other health factors, including preserved physical strength, unpredictable disease course that may even include the arrest of disease progression, and maintenance of functioning in some cognitive do-mains while experiencing profound worsening in other areas.

Psychiatrists and neuropsychologists may need to work closely with several other dis-ciplines, including social work and occupational therapy, to optimize patient care and help to manage caregiver burden, as FTD tends to have increased levels of caregiver burden rel-ative to other dementing illnesses.[11]

Alcoholic Dementia

Alcohol-related dementia is complicated by other alcohol-related medical problems, as well as the psychosocial problems stemming from years of alcohol use disorder. An increased in-cidence of alcohol-related health problems such as cirrhosis may limit pharmacologic treat-ment options, and the variant of alcohol-related dementia known as Wernicke-Korsakoff's syndrome impairs behavioral interventions due to the volatility of memory and the fre-quent confabulation exhibited by patients.

Chronic Traumatic Encephalopathy (CTE)

Chronic traumatic encephalopathy, or major neurocognitive disorder due to brain injury, has become an area of increasing concern and visibility over the past few years, partially due to high-profile court cases, such as those involving American football players and the increasing body of literature describing histopathologic changes attributable to repetitive or severe traumatic neuronal injury. As with other dementias that are prevalent in a younger population, unique social difficulties may emerge when the patient retains physical health and strength that make the management of behavioral problems more difficult or dan-gerous for caregivers.

Suicidality in Dementia

Dementia increases the risk for suicidal behavior. This is not surprising because dementia afflicts a population already at increased risk for suicide (the elderly) and adds to that risk by increasing impulsivity, decreasing judgment, decreasing problem-solving, and comorbid depression and psychoses. An additional risk, particularly with male caregivers, is the depressed male caregiver who in despair may feel that there is no one who can take care of the afflicted spouse, thus leading to murder-suicide.

Suicide-prevention interventions include screening for suicide history, suicide ideation screening, treatment for depression, safely securing firearms, and screening and intervention for substance abuse. A validated method for suicide risk assessment is the use of the Columbia suicide risk assessment scale.

Delirium

Delirium may be described as a cognitive impairment that affects the sensorium that waxes and wanes. It is often mistaken for dementia, and it is much more common in patients with dementia than other populations. Delirium can be mitigated by risk reduction, early recognition, and intervention. The main activities for delirium risk reduction are to maintain healthy behaviors and to minimize polypharmacy. Any relatively sudden changes in behavior should prompt the search for medical causes and correction. Patients who are hospitalized should be screened for a history of delirium and should have a screen for cognitive impairment. To mitigate the risk of delirium: minimize polypharmacy, maintain the day night cycle, and support physical activity. Including familiar items in the patient's room, such as family photos and favorite objects, can be helpful. Whenever possible, family presence is helpful. Physical restraints are harmful to patients and should be avoided. The most common validated screening for delirium is the confusion assessment method (CAM).[12]

Interventions for Families

Because effect size of individual interventions may be small,[13] multidisciplinary interventions for families and caregivers are needed to improve the burden of care, decrease disruptive behaviors, and increase subjective well-being.[14] Effective interventions will be flexible and will account for individual needs. Support and intervention during transitional periods and events leading to increased stress on the patient and caregiver are keys to success. Support groups may be beneficial for some families, but others may not feel the need to talk about family problems with strangers. Families may obtain support from other groups to which they already belong, such as religious organizations or fraternal groups. As with other interventions, repetition may be needed for optimal effect. Services not utilized at one point in the disease process may be invaluable at another point in time.

Resources

Alzheimer's Association: www.alz.org.
National Institute on Aging: www.nia.nih.gov.
Family Caregiver Alliance: www.caregiver.org.
The Broyles Foundation: www.broylesfoundation.org.

Future Directions and Needs

Drug treatment for dementia is most promising since the 1990s with the introduction of cholinergic enhancers. Newer treatments targeting the production of amyloid plaques offer not only the promise to arrest progression of the illness but actually some reversal. Two phase III drugs in the United States address plaque formation directly (tamiprosate [aka homotaurine], available in oral form, and the intravenous drug aducanumab). A new Chinese drug, oligomannate, is believed to act by killing bacteria within the gastrointestinal tract that are associated with byproducts that facilitate plaque formation in the central nervous system (CNS).

Digital health tools and artificial intelligence technology also are in development to assist caregiver supervision for patients, cognitive aids for patients, and early recognition of concurrent illnesses.

The greatest need is for early biomarkers and prevention for all the other dementias, including dementia associated with head trauma.

Key Points

- Dementia refers to a diverse group of disorders characterized by memory impairment and cognitive impairment.
- There is significant diversity in the rate and progression of dementias.
- Dementias are commonly complicated by depression, psychosis, anxiety, insomnia, and behavioral disturbances.
- Current medication treatments offer minimal benefit in terms of slowing the rate of progression.
- Efforts to mange behavioral disturbances often focus on treating co-occurring conditions such as depression or underlying medical illness such as a urinary tract infection.
- Caregiver support is important for the health and welfare of the patient.
- Delirium is an acute disturbance of attention, consciousness, and cognition, generally precipitated by medical illness, trauma, or other stressors. Delirium is treated by treating the underlying cause.
- Even after recovery from delirium, residual deficits and worsening of prognosis are common.

References

1. Wimo A, et al. The worldwide economic impact of dementia 2010. *Alzheimers Dement.* 2018;9:1–11.
2. Hudomiet P, et al. Dementia prevalence in the United States in 2000 and 2012: estimates based on a nationally representative study. *J Gerontol: Series B.* 2018 May;73(suppl 1):S10–S19.
3. Goren A, Montgomery W, Kahle-Wrobleski K, et al. Impact of caring for persons with Alzheimer's disease or dementia on caregivers' health outcomes: findings from a community based survey in Japan. *BMC Geriatr.* 2016;16:122
4. Shinagawa S, Catindig JA, Block NR, Miller BL, Rankin KP. When a little knowledge can be dangerous: false-positive diagnosis of behavioral variant frontotemporal dementia among community clinicians. *Dement Geriatr Cogn Disord.* 2016;41:99–10.8

5. Family Caregiver Alliance (www.caregiver.org). April 17, 2019.
6. Brodaty H, Donkin M. Family caregivers of people with dementia. *Dialogues Clin Neurosci.* 2009;11(2):217–228.
7. Vernooij-Dassen M, Jeon YH. Social health and dementia: the power of human capabilities. *Int Psychogeriatr.* 2016 May;28(5):701–703.
8. Yates MD, Tennstedt S, Chang BH. Contributors to and mediators of psychological well-being for informal caregivers. *J Gerontol B Psychol Sci Soc Sci.* 1999;54:P12–P22.
9. Larson EB, Shadlen M, Wang L, et al. Survival after initial diagnosis of Alzheimer disease. *Ann Intern Med.* 2004;140:501–509.
10. Arvanitakis Z, Capuano AW, Leurgans SE, Bennett DA, Schneider JA. Relation of cerebral vessel disease to Alzheimer's disease dementia and cognitive function in elderly people: a cross-sectional study. *Lancet Neurol.* 2016;15(9):934–943.
11. Uflacker A, Edmondson M, Onyike C, Appleby B. Caregiver burden in atypical dementias: comparing frontotemporal dementia, Creutzfeldt-Jakob disease, and Alzheimer's disease. *Int Psychogeriatr.* 2016;28(2):269–273.
12. Brefka S, Eschweiler GW, Dallmeier D, Denkinger M, Leinert C. Comparison of delirium detection tools in acute care: a rapid review. *Z Gerontol Geriatr.* 2022 Mar;55(2):105–115.
13. McCurry SM, Logsdon R, Gibbons LE. Training community consultants to help family members improve dementia care: a randomized controlled trial. *Gerontologist.* 2005;45:802–811.
14. Sorensen S, Pinquart M, Duberstein P, et al. How effective are interventions with caregivers? An updated meta-analysis. *Gerontologist.* 2002;42:356–372.

31

Culture, Ethnicity, and Sleep Patterns and Disorders

Abram Estafanous and Karim Sedky

Introduction

Sleep is controlled through the interaction between biological, psychological, and socio-cultural factors. Biological factors include homeostatic drive and zeitgebers/chronological factors (i.e., factors that regulate circadian rhythm including food intake times, exercises, etc.). Psychological factors include any trauma or stress, while social factors include school and/or work schedule. An example of the effect of these factors on sleep can be seen in children. Parental perceptions and beliefs about sleep can affect a child's training to sleep by specifically affecting sleep pattern, sleep environment, and napping. While it is important to note that sleep pattern in children can be strongly affected by this social factor, it is also important to note the dynamic and changing face of culture; some changes are gradual, while others are rapid.

Sleep can be affected by an individual's age, and the effects of age can be significantly affected by culture and country location. While children's sleep is commonly controlled by parental behavior and their perception about sleep, adult sleep might be related to traditions and work schedule. Sleep time and duration, napping, sleep setting, and bed partners can significantly vary by location. While Western countries display the characteristics of sleeping on a bed, with bed partners (if they are adults, but alone if they are children) and in separate rooms, many cultures differ from these trends by, for example, promoting sleeping with the family. This chapter will offer an introduction of the effects of culture and ethnicity on adult sleep, as well as highlighting the phenomena of culture-bound sleep disorders and how culture and ethnicity affect sleep disorders.

Sleep and Culture in Adults

Sleep Duration and Culture

The past several decades have demonstrated an increase in the quantity of adult sleep research. Despite the growth, little is known about trends found in adult sleep. Yet, the present research makes it clear that the factors that affect sleep are multifaceted and likely include influences by ethnicity and culture. The susceptibility of sleep to cultural modifiers can be seen in perhaps the most objective aspect of sleep—that of sleep duration. One recent systematic review of 15 countries revealed that 7 showed an increase in average sleep duration: Bulgaria, Poland, Canada, France, Britain, Korea, and the Netherlands. However, 6 countries showed a decrease: Japan, Russia, Finland, Germany, Belgium, and Austria. Inconsistency in studies for sleep duration was found for the United States and Sweden.[1] These differences in average sleep duration cannot be explained by one aspect of a country's makeup. The study made the point that an aging population is found in Japan (a country that demonstrated a decreased average sleep duration) but is also found in Britain, France, and Canada (countries that demonstrated an increased average sleep duration). This comparison demonstrates that no single aspect of these countries likely has a sole influence on sleep duration. Rather, it is an intersection of a variety of factors, including the various ethnicities and cultures found in these countries, in addition to the demographic phenomenon of an aging population, that is causing variations in sleep duration.

Types of Sleep Patterns, Naps, and Culture

Several types of sleep patterns exist—monophasic, in which people sleep only at night; biphasic, in which people sleep mostly at night but also have one nap during the day; and polyphasic, in which people have multiple daytime naps but their primary sleep continues to be at night. Segmental sleep occurs when individuals have a split sleep time, with half the time occurring after sunset and a second period before dawn, and an in-between duration where they are awake. Weather has at times been attributed to the different sleep patterns, but this notion has also been questioned. While monophasic sleep has been common in many Western countries, biphasic and even polyphasic sleep have been reported in many cultures.

Monophasic Sleep

This type of sleep occurs mostly in Western (non-Hispanic) countries. People in this group have all their sleep consolidated at night, with no daytime naps. We continue to encourage this pattern of sleep while we are reviewing sleep hygiene with patients.

Biphasic Sleep

Naps are common in many African countries, the Mediterranean region (e.g., Greece), Spain, former Spanish colonies (e.g., Mexico), and China. Biphasic sleep usually includes one nap in the early afternoon, but most of the sleep is still at night. This afternoon nap is called the siesta. Some researchers have attributed this napping to hot climates, mainly those living close to the equator (or seasonally in non-equatorial counties). Thus, it is viewed as advantageous for energy conservation and adaptation to hot weather due to the weather's interference with afternoon activities. Others have attributed the siesta to decreased awareness and appreciation of time value—for example, increased naps occurred in the Peruvian population compared to the Belgian population. It is important to note the higher prevalence of the siesta in rural agricultural or non-industrial areas and the decreased prevalence of the siesta as these communities shift to an urbanized lifestyle.

Some researchers have observed a decrease in siestas with modernization. Higher professional levels and urbanization were linked to a decrease in siestas. Similarly, a decrease in the siesta is found in Spain with its modernization, while in Chile it occurred after political decree to avoid the siesta as a way to demonstrate appreciation of the usage of time. Other studies did not find a change in siestas among their college students and attributed this to modernization. However, others argue that this relationship cannot be established given the lack of baseline assessment longitudinally to establish this decrease in siestas.

Polyphasic Sleep

This type of sleep is characterized by multiple short naps during the day, with primarily nocturnal sleep duration. A specific example can be observed in Japan. The Japanese are encouraged to take *inemuri*, or naps during work or while on public transportation, which would increase productivity. *Inemuri* is derived from the Japanese characters *iru* (meaning to be present) and *nemuri* which means to be asleep (i.e., people are present in the workplace or on transportation but sleeping). While in Western countries sleeping on the job or in different places (such as public transportation) may be considered a sign of laziness, the Japanese consider it a sign of devotion to their job.[2] Both Confucian and Buddhist teachings encourage a decrease in nighttime sleep: the former emphasizes the need for late nighttime sleep and early morning awakening as a basic requirement for rulers and devoted wives, while the latter urges control of sleep. A significant decrease in nighttime sleep duration is consistently observed as leading to compensation by daytime napping in different places. In a study, 65% of males and 71% of females reported sleeping while on public transportation.

Similarly, polyphasic sleep can be observed as a function of other cultural traits. For example, it is usually acceptable for Muslims to sleep during the day, having frequent naps as they fast during the month of Ramadan. Thus, during the day they are fasting and tired, and this is followed by feasting in the evenings and nights after breaking their fast. This usually causes circadian rhythm phase delay during that time.

Co-Sleeping Among Adults and Culture

Historically, families sleeping in the same common area was common due to a lack of space, extreme temperatures, and/or a belief that one would be protected in a group. Even in Western cultures a few centuries ago, several people slept on the same bed. In the 19th century, there was an increased awareness of privacy and sleeping individually or with a significant other. Yet, until this day, Appalachian communities continue the co-sleeping tradition, especially parents sleeping with younger children.

Sleeping Beds, Sleeping Place, and Culture

Beds

Throughout history, the design, types, shapes, and constituents of beds have differed. The wealthy class of ancient Egyptians slept elevated from the floor on bedding that was made of different materials, such as wood, metal, and leather. Ancient Greeks and Romans used wooden couches that were also used for eating, with the Romans using mattresses made from plants, wool, or feathers. Nets were added for protection against mosquitoes. The Tudor period in England introduced beds that were decorated with carvings and the presence of curtains.[3]

Elevation from the Floor

While some cultures have bedding that is elevated from the floor, others have used matts or hammocks. Weather and safety, in addition to culture, have played a factor in this choice. For example, Inuit individuals used above-ground beds covered with animal fur to provide warmth. In environments having pests, hammocks (a sling type of bed hung from both ends on trees) provide distance from ground insects and animals and therefore increased safety. The Japanese have used tatami mats which are made with a mix of rice straw, paper, grass, and cloth. These futons at times had seaweed filling instead of cotton, especially in coastal areas.[3]

Mattresses

The use of mattresses started in the 18th century, where they were stuffed with wool, cotton, or feathers. The use of springs started after the industrial revolution later in that century, and developed over the years to include water mattresses and mattresses that were adjusted to firmness. While mattresses are common in Western countries, some cultures avoid using them due to the cost or space needed to store them. The use of futons in the Japanese culture is an example; these futons are rolled up and stored after each night. In Central and South America, locals often use hammocks by tying them between trees, especially for siestas.[3]

Pillows

Pillows have also varied among cultures and have gone through development over the years. In some African cultures, a wooden headrest was used. The Japanese have used the *takamakura*, a cylindrical pillow made of cotton or silk, wrapped in paper, and tied to a wooden base. This was thought to work by elevating the head of the person and thus protected their hairstyle.[3]

Sleeping Rooms

While rooms are commonly used now in many parts of the world, some cultures continue to have a common area for sleeping for the family. Especially in wealthy communities, sleeping rooms were considered private and offered warmth and a safe environment from insects.

Culture-Bound Sleep Syndromes

Culture-Bound Sleep Syndromes Involving Sleep Paralysis

Culture-bound syndromes describe conditions that are perceptible only within a specific culture. Several culture-bound sleep syndromes have been identified. The most studied of these involves the symptom of sleep paralysis, a condition that occurs while an individual awakens from sleep but is unable to move their limbs and has accompanying dreaming and/or hallucinations. Sleep paralysis has been interpreted across a variety of cultures. The peoples of Alaska, Newfoundland, Japan, and Hong Kong, as well as African Americans from Chicago, each offer different interpretations of the symptoms of sleep paralysis. For example, among the Inuit people, sleep paralysis was interpreted as the individual being attacked by evil spirits, and the condition had a specific name depending on the geographic region of the Inuit population. It was called *uqumangirniq* among those from the Baffin region and *aqtuqsinniq* among those from the Kivalliq region. However, the sleep paralysis experienced by the Inuit population in these two regions represents a distinct culture-bound syndrome as opposed to a diagnosis of sleep paralysis. The populations studied displayed unique experiences of anxiety and depersonalization upon awakening, in addition to the sleep paralysis. Thus, the conditions of *uqumangirniq* and *aqtuqsinniq* represent culture-bound syndromes identifiable only in the Inuit population of Baffin and Kivalliq, respectively. In addition, the effect of culture on the interpretation of sleep paralysis symptoms can also be observed within a single culture. Specifically, the younger members of the Inuit population have incorporated a blend of personal, medical, and traditional explanations of sleep paralysis symptoms.[4]

In Nigeria, a condition with symptoms that overlap with sleep paralysis is referred to as *ogun oru*, which has a literal translation of "nocturnal warfare." *Ogun oru* has been identified as demonic possession while the individual is asleep. Thus, while asleep, the individual is attacked or poisoned by an enemy through eating in a dream. The physical manifestations of *ogun oru* have been identified as the individual awakening from sleep, being unable to return back to sleep, and subsequently behaving in an agitated manner or crying out like a goat.[5] One modern study suggested a differential diagnosis that mainly included parasomnias, such as sleep paralysis. Sleep paralysis was likely included in the differential due to the presence of hallucinations upon awakening. Nevertheless, *ogun oru* stands on its own as a specific culture-bound syndrome because many of its associated symptoms do not allow it to strictly fit into any of the parasomnias. Based on three case studies that illustrated a variety of symptoms that are usually not found in sleep paralysis (e.g., foaming at the mouth, or urinary incontinence), the study hypothesized that *ogun oru* is a clinical state that can stand on its own as a culture-bound syndrome that is identifiable only in Nigeria.[6]

Culture-Bound Sleep Syndromes Involving Insomnia

Similar to sleep paralysis, insomnia has been identified as a common symptom in several culture-bound syndromes. In Korean culture, *hwa-byung* is a culture-bound sleep phenomenon that translates to "anger sickness" and describes a condition where patients suppress anger and other negative emotions during times of stress, such as relationship strains.

In addition to anger, other emotional symptoms that characterize this condition include feelings of hopelessness, resentment, and fear. A variety of physical symptoms have also been associated with *hwa-byung*, including chest pain, difficulty breathing, and insomnia. Traditional healers note an "excessive fire" in patients, as well as epigastric pain, that patients initially fear might lead to their death. While this condition includes the symptom of insomnia, the presence of other emotional symptoms and a variety of physical symptoms preclude a diagnosis of insomnia as defined by the DSM-5. The condition represents a culture-bound disorder that is recognizable only in Korean culture.

Among Mexican Americans, the culture-bound phenomenon of *susto* describes the belief that the spirit leaves the body and wanders while the person is dreaming. If the spirit is not close enough to the body, insomnia, anorexia, anxiety, and irritability will develop. Another Mexican American culture-bound phenomenon is *espanto*, which can occur when the person is awakened by a frightening experience. The spirit is described to be far away, wandering, and unable to return to the body when required to come back, such as when the individual is suddenly awakened by something frightening, such as a burglary. Both *susto* and *espanto* include the symptom of insomnia, but also a host of other symptoms that puts them outside a diagnosis of insomnia. This makes them culture-bound sleep syndromes that are identifiable only in Mexican American culture.

Sleep Disorders and Ethnicity

Sleep disorders are diverse types of sleep—they are grouped into 6 major groups: insomnia (problems with going to sleep, frequent arousals, or early morning awakening); hypersomnia (requiring increased hours of sleep); circadian rhythm disorders; sleep-related breathing disorders (including obstructive sleep apnea); movement disorders (including restless leg and seizures); and parasomnias. While factors other than ethnicity and genetics might contribute to the link of some of these disorders to certain ethnicities (such as low socioeconomic status among immigrants compared to non-immigrant Caucasians), genetic links have been proposed in certain disorders. This section reviews the relationship of ethnicity and possible contributing cultural and genetic factors that might increase the risk.

Insomnia

Some studies, as previously described, suggest a normal total sleep duration among ethnicities, although more naps occurred among African Americans as compared to Caucasians. Some researchers suggested that genetic and homeostatic differences in ethnicities, as well as cultural beliefs and traditions, have led to more acceptance of naps. When compared to Caucasian Americans, Hispanic Americans, and African Americans, Chinese American adults reported less signs of insomnia as defined by the Women's Health Initiative Insomnia Rating Scale (e.g., longer sleep maintenance, less early morning awakenings, and higher sleep quality) However, the same study also demonstrated that Chinese American men and women had higher odds of short sleep and poor sleep quality (based on actigraphy-measured) as well as daytime sleepiness (based on the Epworth Sleepiness Scale) as compared to their Caucasian counterparts. This was still the case after adjusting for body mass index (BMI).[7]

This discrepancy between Chinese American adults reporting less signs of insomnia and the elevated odds ratio of symptoms suggesting insomnia may be reflective of decreased reporting of symptoms by Asian Americans during doctor visits. Indeed, one study found that Asian Americans were less likely to receive lifestyle counseling by their doctors as compared to their Caucasian counterparts. The study also found that Asian Americans were more likely to report not receiving as much time with the doctor as they wanted and being less involved in decision-making about their care This difference may be explained by cultural variations in communication between doctors and their Asian American patients. The same study noted that Asians may often use the cultural mannerism of smiling and nodding to portray respect toward the doctor, rather than agreement. This indirect method of communication may be misinterpreted by healthcare providers as the patient agreeing with the suggested treatment plan and not conveying any complaints or disagreements. Therefore, if doctors do not specifically ask patients if they have disagreements, medical issues may go unacknowledged.[8]

Hypersomnia

Kleine-Levin syndrome (KLS) is a sleep disorder that is characterized by recurring episodes of excessive sleepiness and sleep duration. The condition is mostly found in adolescents and young adults, and the hypersomnia episodes include intermittent periods of normal somnolence. One study indicated that a larger percentage of patients from Saudi Arabia reported poor sleep between KLS episodes as compared to Caucasian American, French, and Chinese cohorts of other studies. One plausible explanation for this marked difference that characterizes Saudi Arabian KLS patients may be the culture of Saudi Arabia versus the societies of the other cohorts. Specifically, one study that examined over 1000 high school students age 14–23 years in Jeddah, Saudi Arabia, demonstrated that while 65% of students had a Pittsburgh Sleep Quality Index (PSQI) >5 (which indicates disturbed sleep), female students specifically were more likely to have higher PSQI scores. This may be explained by the fact that females in Saudi Arabia in 2014 were not allowed to drive. Thus, female students were more likely to take a school bus or be dropped off by a male driver. Both of these scenarios demonstrate instances where female students may have to wake up earlier to arrive at school on time as compared to male students who drive themselves.[9] This represents one example of how individual culture may disrupt sleep.

Sleep-Related Breathing Disorders

While this group of disorders includes obstructive sleep apnea (OSA) and different types of central apneas and obstructive hypoventilation syndrome, OSA is the most studied and will be the focus here. In children, OSA was up to 4 times more prevalent among African Americans compared to Caucasians, partially attributed to oropharyngeal narrowing.[10] In addition, some studies have linked obesity in African Americans and Asians to OSA in children. Similarly in adults, a higher prevalence of OSA has been found in African Americans compared to other groups. While OSA was linked to obesity in children, Asian adults with

OSA tend to be normal in weight compared to other groups, possibly related to craniofacial abnormalities (compared to obesity in other ethnicities). In addition, some disorders that are associated with an increased risk of OSA are more common in certain ethnicities. For example, sickle cell disease is more common in African Americans, the Mediterranean population, and Asians, thus increasing the risk of OSA in these groups.[11]

Circadian Rhythm Disorders

The circadian rhythm may differ among ethnic groups due to a variety of factors. Several studies have examined the effect of fasting during the Muslim month of Ramadan and have demonstrated fluctuations in the circadian rhythm, indicating that the cultural practice of fasting for Ramadan may affect circadian rhythm. Some have suggested that due to the hot weather in the Arabian Peninsula, especially laborers start their day earlier to avoid the heat. As such, they end up having circadian rhythm phase advance. Conversely, some societies, such as Brazil, include a late-night dinner (sometimes at 11 PM), leading to circadian rhythm phase delay. In addition, other studies have demonstrated the effect of lifestyle of genetics. Namely, one study reported circadian rhythm dysregulation during Ramadan and found that *Clock* gene expression was significantly higher during Ramadan.[12]

Indeed, several studies have shown that there are intrinsic ethnic differences of baseline circadian rhythm length, as well as ethnic differences of the response to circadian rhythm phase advance and delay. One study revealed that its African American participants had a significantly shorter circadian rhythm length as compared to their European American cohorts.[13] The study induced artificial phase advance by slowly advancing the participants' sleep schedule and incorporating bright light in the morning on awakening. The phase advance study revealed that the African American subjects had larger phase advances. The same study also induced artificial phase delay, which revealed that its African American participants had smaller phase delays. The proposed theory is that human migration out of Africa and into greater latitudes resulted in the racial differences of circadian rhythm. Specifically, higher latitudes possess more significant changes in light across the different seasons, as opposed to closer to the equator where the photoperiod is more constant.

Restless Leg Syndrome/Periodic Limb Movements

Several studies have demonstrated that the *prevalence* of RLS differs between ethnic groups. Differences in cultural factors have been hypothesized to play a role in the prevalence of RLS. One study found that highly acculturated Hispanics of Mexican descent (measured by the Short Acculturation Scale for Hispanics that assesses language use and media and ethnic social relations) had a higher prevalence of RLS. The intersection of RLS and anxiety is a possible explanation. Several studies have shown that RLS is associated with stress. A study of Korean adults indicated that RLS was associated with anxiety disorders. Another study, which examined cancer patients, found that cancer patients with RLS had higher levels of anxiety as compared to their cohorts without RLS.[14] Acculturation has been associated with changes in the health of the Hispanic population, which includes increases in cardiovascular disease, psychiatric disorders, and social status. The phenomenon of acculturation in

Hispanics of Mexican descent may be associated with stress due to change in social status, culture, and health status, thus making these individuals susceptible to RLS.

Parasomnias

One study discussed the possible influence of Turkish family structures on the prevalence of parasomnias in children. The relatively larger size of Turkish families living under one roof, as compared to the classic nuclear family, may negatively impact sleep hygiene. Sleep disorders, including parasomnias, were shown to have a decreased prevalence in children who had bedrooms that were used by a single child and that facilitated good sleep hygiene (i.e., bedrooms that are silent and at an appropriate temperature and lighting).[15] Indeed, children who do not have access to bedrooms appropriate for good sleep hygiene were shown to have a higher prevalence of parasomnias. Specifically, insomnia frequency was statistically significantly increased in Turkish households where 7 or more people were living together and also in individuals who shared a bed or a bedroom.[16] These factors may all be magnified in cultures with larger family structures residing in a single household. The study demonstrated that 41.9% of the students surveyed shared a room, while 15% shared a bed. It was these students who had a considerably greater prevalence of insomnia. Furthermore, these percentages of students sharing a room and sharing a bed were greater than their cohorts in the United States and Europe. This comparison may warrant further studies to examine the prevalence of insomnia in Turkish, American, and European populations.

Conclusion and Social Psychiatry

This chapter has presented a survey of the relationship between culture, ethnicity, and sleep, specifically how cultural factors and ethnic differences affect sleep patterns and the prevalence and manifestations of sleep disorders. An application of this relationship to the clinical setting necessitates a framework that integrates a consideration of cultural and ethnic factors with sleep management. Specifically, social psychiatry provides an approach to psychiatric care that recognizes the interaction of social factors and psychological well-being. For example, regarding the decreased reporting of insomnia symptoms by Asian Americans despite higher odds of poor sleep, a social psychiatry approach would provide an approach that would optimize patient care because it would consider the social idiosyncrasies that would produce this phenomenon. Ultimately, understanding the intersection of culture, ethnicity, and sleep will enable clinicians to optimize patient sleep care and management.

References

1. Bin YS, Marshall NS, Glozier N. Secular trends in adult sleep duration: a systematic review. *Sleep Med Rev.* 2012;16:223–230.
2. Steger B. Getting away with sleep: social and cultural aspects of dozing in Parliament. *Soc Sci Japan J.* 2003;6(2):181–197.
3. Krahn LE, Silber MH, Morgenthaler TI. *Atlas of Sleep Medicine.* Boca Raton, Fl: CRC Press; 2010.
4. Law S, Kirmayer LJ. Inuit interpretations of sleep paralysis. *Transcult Psychiatry.* 2005;42:93–112.

5. Simpson GE. Traditional medicine: diagnoses, causes and treatment of illnesses. In: Simpson GE, ed. *Yoruba Religion and Medicine in Ibadan.* Ibadan, Nigeria: Ibadan University Press; 1980:93–113.

6. Aina OF, Famuyiwa OO. Ogun oru: a traditional explanation for nocturnal neuropsychiatric disturbances among the Yoruba of Southwest Nigeria. *Transcult Psychiatry.* 2007;44:44–54.

7. Chen X, Wang R, Zee P, et al. Racial/ethnic differences in sleep disturbances: the Multi-Ethnic Study of Atherosclerosis (MESA). *Sleep.* 2015;38(6):877–888D.

8. Ngo-Metzger Q, Legedza ATR, Phillips RS. Asian Americans' reports of their health care experiences. *J Gen Intern Med.* 2004;19:111–119.

9. Merdad RA, Merdad LA, Nassif RA, El-Derwi D, Wali SO. Sleep habits in adolescents of Saudi Arabia; distinct patterns and extreme sleep schedules. *Sleep Med.* 2014;15:1370–1378.

10. Redline S, Tishler PV, Schluchter M, Aylor J, Clark K, Graham G. Risk factors for sleep-disordered breathing in children: associations with obesity, race and respiratory problems. *J Resp Crit Care.* 1999;159:1527–1732.

11. Kirkham FJ, Datta AK. Hypoxic adaptation during development: relation to pattern of neurological presentation and cognitive disability. *Devel Sci.* 2006;9(4):411–427.

12. Ajabnoor GMA, Bahijri S, Shaik NA, et al. Ramadan fasting in Saudi Arabia is associated with altered expression of CLOCK, DUSP and IL-1alpha genes, as well as changes in cardiometabolic risk factors. *PLoS ONE.* 2017;6:12.

13. Smith MR, Burgess HJ, Fogg LF, Eastman CI. Racial differences in the human endogenous circadian period. *PLoS One.* 2009; 4(6):e6014

14. Ostacoli L, Saini A, Ferini-Strambi L, et al. Restless legs syndrome and its relationship with anxiety, depression, and quality of life in cancer patients undergoing chemotherapy. *Qual Life Res.* 2010;19:531–537.

15. Kahn A, Van de Merckt C, Rebuffat E, et al. Sleep problems in healthy preadolescents. *Pediatrics.* 1989;84:542–546.

16. Ozgun N, Sonmez FM, Topbas M, Can G, Goker Z. Insomnia, parasomnia, and predisposing factors in Turkish school children. *Ped Int.* 2016;58:1014–1022.

32

Child Maltreatment from a Sociocultural Perspective

Then and Now

Michael Shapiro

Introduction

The World Health Organization (WHO) defines "child maltreatment" as abuse or neglect which causes actual or potential harm to children under 18 years of age.[1,2] Most cases of abuse and neglect, including cases that result in death, occur in children age 5 years or younger.[3] Child maltreatment includes all forms of abuse and neglect, primarily physical abuse, sexual abuse and exploitation, emotional/psychological abuse, and neglect. Almost 1 in 4 adults worldwide report having been physically abused as children,[1] with physical abuse being just one form of child maltreatment. It is estimated that between 500 million and 1.5 billion children experience some form of violent victimization annually, but emotional and psychological abuse rates are more difficult to estimate and have received less global attention than physical and sexual abuse.[4] Consequences of child maltreatment include impaired lifelong physical and mental health; the global impact can lead to shortened life spans, a diminished workforce, increased healthcare costs, and ultimately slow the economic and social development of a society.[1]

Physical abuse is defined as non-accidental injury from a caregiver to a child that causes harm. It is often associated with punishment administered by an angry or frustrated caregiver or caregiver's partner.[5] Most societies have at one time or another permitted severe physical punishment of children by parents, teachers, and other authority figures acting *in loco parentis.* Historically such action has been considered necessary to maintain discipline. "Spare the rod and spoil the child" is a biblical warning of the dangers of parental leniency. Physical punishment was also doled out with healing intent, such as to drive out evil spirits thought to possess them.

Child sexual abuse includes non-consensual completed or attempted sexual contact, acts of sexual trafficking committed against someone who is unable to consent or refuse, and online exploitation.[2] In recent years, there has been a concerted effort to focus on sexual trafficking and exploitation of minors. Childhood sexual abuse is perhaps the form of child maltreatment taken most seriously by the public and child protective services.[4]

Although WHO defines maltreatment to include harm to the child's "development or dignity in the context of a relationship of responsibility, trust, or power,"[1] there is otherwise a lack of a clear definition of emotional abuse. This lack, combined with the fact that the harm produced is often not visible to the naked eye, has often failed children. Child protection organizations have often not intervened in cases of emotional abuse because this kind of abuse is difficult to detect. One could argue that all forms of child maltreatment can be classified as psychological maltreatment, psychological abuse, or emotional abuse,[6] particularly when taking into account the deleterious effects to attachment when abuse occurs in an early relationship with a trusted authority figure. It can also be argued that neglect is at the core of maltreatment, and neglect is by far the most prevalent type of maltreatment identified by child protective services.[3] Neglect is defined as the failure or inattention to meet a child's basic physical and emotional needs, including housing, food, clothing, education, and access to medical care.[7] Neglected children are at risk of deterioration in their developing health and emotional well-being, with the effects of neglected emotional needs being evident in the Romanian orphanage studies.[8] However, co-occurrence of different types of maltreatment is the rule rather than the exception.[3]

It has been postulated that the best working definition of "child maltreatment" includes the context of contemporary community values, professional expertise, and/or scientific evidence of what is considered inappropriate and damaging.[6] Doing so acknowledges that the declaration of what constitutes maltreatment is not static, but rather a continuous ongoing effort to raise the standards for how children across the globe are treated; thus the definition at any particular time and place may change based on what institutions and communities come to understand regarding what the minimum standards of childcare should be, and the many ways that such standards can be violated.[6] However, while there is explicit understanding that child maltreatment is a global problem, much of the published research is from Western or developed countries. Although evidence from non-Western countries is emerging, this highlights the considerable variation over time and between cultures about what is deemed abusive to children.[9] This shifting scope of the definition, which can differ across cultures and throughout time, makes it difficult to accurately identify, report, handle, treat, and research child maltreatment. This chapter provides a sociocultural overview of the history of child maltreatment, followed by current cultural influences on child maltreatment.

Sociocultural Development of "Childhood" and Children's Rights

In the aftermath of World War II and the Holocaust, the United Nations drafted the Universal Declaration of Human Rights in 1948 as a set of fundamental human rights to be universally protected, a common standard for all peoples and nations.[10] In this milestone document, the United Nations declared that childhood was "entitled to special care and assistance." This statement and document were later referenced in the United Nations Convention on the Rights of the Child,[11] which reiterated the conviction that particularly children, "should be afforded the necessary protection and assistance," and "the child, for the full and harmonious development of his or her personality, should grow up in a family environment, in an atmosphere of happiness, love and understanding." This "necessary protection" is required because children are vulnerable, generally being totally dependent on adults, emotionally and materially. This very vulnerability is what allows children's qualities, needs, roles, and purpose to be almost entirely determined by adults, not by children themselves. The concept of "childhood" itself is a relatively new social construct by historical standards in which the young are afforded a unique time and space in which to grow.[5] Childhood is no different than other social constructs, the views of which and treatment of depend on attitudes and beliefs which vary with changes in the unique time and space that the society exists.[5] A longitudinal view of child maltreatment may be viewed merely as reflective of child-rearing practices of a given time and culture, practices that were descended from the society's view of children in general.

A review of the historical treatment of children traces its roots to ancient cultures which routinely practiced infanticide, child sacrifice, ritualistic mutilation, and willful abandonment, with such practices being officially sanctioned by societal or religious doctrine.[12] Infanticide was a commonly practiced form of child-rearing through the 4th century,[5] with Ancient Greek and Roman societies declaring children to be the absolute property of the father, who could keep or dispose of such property as he wished.[12] Discretion was given to fathers and families to determine whether they had the resources to care for children, and if not, disposition of such children. Change was slow, with heavy influences from religion moving the needle of general treatment of children from murderous, to negligent, to merely indifferent through most of the Middle Ages.[5]

The emergence of the Renaissance, with a focus on education and academia, shifted the emphasis of children's roles to be educated and employed beginning in the 13th century,[5] although formal education was merely an extension of parental authority and obedience, with teachers having the right to dole out punishment with harshness that lasted through the 18th century.[12] Children had been viewed as being "imbued with original sin," needing to be subdued and controlled to produce individuals who would become productive members of society while maintaining subservience to authoritarian leaders.[5] Such views would understandably be associated with harsh discipline practices, lack of emotional warmth, and use of shame, blame, and extreme corporal punishment. Early English common law dictated that the father of the household had legal custody over his children as if property, which was interrelated with the father's role in providing financial support to the family; it was not that long ago in human history that father's custody rights were considered superior to the rights of mothers.

There is perhaps no greater proof of the pervasive historical acceptance of childhood abuse than sexual abuse, particularly incest. The condemnation of incest has been viewed by social scientists as "the only universal trait that has been found in every culture" and that the prohibition of incest "must have occurred at the very beginning of civilization".[13(p7)] In fact, incest was quite frequent and widespread among the general population and even the royal courts of ancient Greece, Rome, and Egypt.[13] Even through the late Renaissance, young girls were killed for attempting to "seduce" innocent men, in a continuation of long-standing practice of men projecting their own sexual feelings onto women.[13] Incest continued to be a common practice in Western cultures into the late 1800s, whereas in Eastern cultures it continued for much longer. Demause has identified the attitude that children are used to meet the emotional needs of adults to be more pervasive in Eastern cultures, which predisposes to incest and child abuse.[13]

The evolution of human rights—particularly women's rights—coincided with evolution in child-rearing practices. This in turn shapes the concept of what treatment toward children is considered proper or improper. Beginning in the later 20th century following World War II, there was an increase in psychological research of human dynamics, including mother-child relationships, which advanced our understanding of children's emotional and cognitive development, and how they are shaped by the environment. This slowly led to a paradigm shift in developmental theories concerning children's emotional and psychological development, along with the realization that rather than projecting the wishes of an adult or society onto a child, it is imperative to mirror children's innate value and potential.[5] Women and children historically had been without power or authority within most societies due to financial dependency and society's norms; this led inevitably to maltreatment.[5]

The industrial revolution and urbanization created different forms of child maltreatment in the 18th and 19th centuries through the exploitation of child labor. In England, children as young as 5 worked up to 16 hours per day, sometimes with weights tied to their ankles to keep them from running away. Child laborers were often starved or beaten, and some died from occupational hazards. When parents eventually rallied against such conditions, orphaned or abandoned children were put to work. The increasing use of "apprenticeships" for orphaned or abandoned children was on some level merely a way to make these children more financially appetizing so a family would take their charge off the hands of the government. Those children who could not find work were kept in poor houses or insane asylums with adults.

In the early 1800s, it became gradually understood that states had a responsibility to intervene in cases of parental neglect; such efforts were primarily aimed at preventing neglected children from having a life of destitution and becoming a threat to the state by criminal means or using state financial resources.[12] The 19th-century philosophy was driven by the belief that society should identify conditions in childhood which would lead to future deleterious effects on communities and governments, such as crime, poverty, child abandonment, and others. Thus, children exposed to such conditions should be committed to institutions—orphanages or industrial schools—where techniques and resources were available to teach children to work and receive "moral training," thus preventing future crime and need for state welfare.[12]

The concept of protecting children didn't take hold until the later 19th century; a British lawsuit in 1875 on the case of Mary Ellen alleged that children deserved at least the same rights as animals, as animal cruelty prevention groups had formed first.[12] Once this cause was furthered, deaths of children became the earliest and easiest cases prosecuted. Physical abuse that did not result in death often continued, perhaps as there became increasing stigma toward parents who exposed their children to conditions that would result in commitment. This changed with the publication of Kempe's seminal 1962 article, "Battered Child Syndrome," which described from a medical perspective the toll that physical abuse takes on children's bodies.[12] At this point, the health professions, governments, and general public caught up on the severity of abuse of children in families.

Cultural Influences on Child-Rearing and Child Maltreatment

The distinction between proper and improper parenting practices cannot be made without cultural consideration.[14] When individuals experience harsh punishment in childhood, they are less likely to consider such behaviors to be abusive when they are adults. In cultures dominated by conservative ideologies, deviations from these social norms may be viewed as an unacceptable challenge to authority or status quo, jeopardizing the household's place in the culture or community.[15] Cultural sociology suggests that economic development and political stability influence attitudes regarding social values. Nations with greater economic and political stability typically tend to tolerate more self-expressive values which focus on an individual's autonomy and enhancing the quality of life. Nations with a survivalist orientation, often characterized by greater economic uncertainty, are less supportive of behaviors that may result in further instability, and thus rely on authoritarian principles to ensure obedience and control.[4]

The concept of child abuse necessitates that a given society be willing to sanction societal intrusion into child-rearing within individual families.[5] Previous research has suggested that agency is socioculturally conditioned, meaning that children in certain environments might be more restricted in how they are permitted to show agency.[5] Throughout most of human history, children had little if any agency. Regarding child maltreatment, parents could not be held liable in civil suit for excessive or brutal punishment, as a minor child could not sue their parents in tort. Prior to the late 19th century, courts reasoned that "an orderly society depended on parents having discretion in disciplining within the home in order to maintain domestic harmony and family government".[12] An actual court case from the mid-19th century reveals the prevailing doctrine that "[t]he right of parents to chastise their refractory and disobedient children is so necessary to the government of families, to the good order of society, that no moralist or lawgiver has ever thought of interfering with its existence, or of calling upon them to account for the manner of its exercise, upon light or frivolous pretenses [sic]."[12(p305)] Current issues in children's agency have expanded not merely to prevent abuse or neglect, but to consider whether children have rights to make active choices for themselves outside the sphere of influence of their parents, such as in receiving childhood vaccinations despite parental objections, refusing conversion therapy for sexual minority youth, and accepting medical treatment of gender nonconformity. These issues await further decisions on whether youth will be given agency and self-determination in a way never before bestowed on this age group. What follows are specific cultural factors that continue to influence the perception of children's agency and parental authority in relation to child maltreatment.

Religious Influences

Authoritarian ideology, including religious conservativism, endorses obedience to authority and physical punishment of children.[15] The Bible contains many references to infanticide: from the Old Testament, the story of Abraham, whose loyalty to God was tested when he was instructed to sacrifice his son, Isaac; Moses being sent down the river is infant abandonment; the Semitic religions include various episodes of authoritarian commandments to kill children, usually first-born males.[12] Rigid standards of conduct and power in a higher authority can be based on religious views of deities, religious leaders, and finally religious parents. Religiously based authoritarian Christian ideology has been associated with the use of corporal punishment.[15] Evangelicalism defends parents' rights to be in control of their household, and if necessary, to use physical punishment to curb children's misbehavior and ensure their obedience. Conservative, traditional views in other religions, such as ultra-Orthodox Jewish and Arab societies, are not as consistently associated with endorsement of obedience or spanking and have lower rates of child maltreatment.[15] Islam is diverse in culture and has complex views of children, yet Islamic parents generally value the protection of children, and are encouraged to be affectionate and compassionate with their offspring; views of corporal punishment differ but may be viewed as consistent with Islamic law.

Mere religious affiliation itself has not been linked to child abuse. Rather, it is more likely that specific aspects of conservative doctrine, namely biblical literalism and belief in hell, predict parental support for harsh punishment. In addition, sociopolitical conservativism predicted attitudes toward punishment more significantly than affiliation with any specific political party. Conservative sociopolitical ideology, highlighted by biblical literalism and social conformity, are associated with attitudes that devalue children, value obedience, endorse the use of physical punishment, and have higher potential for child abuse.[15] However, there may also be several confounders in such research; communities in the United States that are predominantly religiously and politically conservative also tend to be less educated, have lower income, and be more rural, each of which is a risk factor for child abuse.[15]

Community Influences

As mentioned above, community and socioeconomic factors have been correlated with child abuse rates. The most consistent variables associated with rates of child maltreatment and indicators of the economic status or resources of a community include income level, median residential housing/property value, unemployment rate, and poverty rate.[16] In a harken back to the views of children in Ancient Rome or Greece, there is likely a link between family perceived resources, stress level, and view of children as being expenditures of limited resources.

Two theories that may explain this association are social disorganization, which is the tendency for social problems to be concentrated in geographic regions marked by poverty and social isolation, and ecological-transactional development, which refers to how child development and parenting are influenced by neighborhood development and the greater social system.[16] A large meta-analysis looking at U.S. neighborhoods and maltreatment rates show that neighborhoods with high rates of maltreatment also experience social and economic deprivation, high resident turnover, and high unemployment (particularly male unemployment). There is some limited evidence to link certain types of maltreatment with environmental factors, with a tentative conclusion that neglect, compared to other types of maltreatment, may be more strongly associated with geographic and structural characteristics of neighborhoods.[16] Relatedly, urban community members may also differ in their perceptions of maltreatment and willingness to report it.[15]

Immigrant and Refugee Experiences

The issue of refugees has been of great importance throughout the world in the early part of the 21st century, with estimates of over 25 million global refugees as a result of war, persecution, violence, or human rights concerns, over half of whom are under the age of 18.[17] Research on family-related violence among refugees is scarce, although a few existing studies concerning such violence have found the prevalence rate to be as high as 30%–50%.[17] One plausible theory for such high rates is that refugee parents may perceive their pre-migration experiences to be traumatic, and thus react by holding on more firmly to culturally determined child physical discipline practices, or by exerting an overprotective, restrictive, and controlling behavior toward their children as a reaction to the trauma.[18] Unfortunately, most studies of intra-familial violence in refugees do not account for individual trauma or symptoms of post-traumatic stress disorder (PTSD). In one study of Liberian refugees, many of the women indicated that the war, migration, and refugee camp experiences prevented them from performing their usual roles in protecting their children.[19] From a perspective of attachment, it is possible, or likely, that such experiences lead to disrupted attachment in both the children and the mothers, and only further contribute to decreased parental emotional availability, resulting in behavioral disorders in children and repeated re-traumatizations and broken attachments, with perhaps physical abuse to control the behaviors.[18] Other factors placing refugee families at risk for child maltreatment include single parenthood, large family size, parental separation, low socioeconomic status, and unemployment,[18] all of which are risk factors in non-refugee families, but perhaps more prevalent among refugees. Risk factors specific to immigrants include acculturation stress and length of residence, as new immigrants with shorter residences in the host country were correlated with more frequent and more severe abuse and maltreatment.[18] Another factor may be lack of familiarity with new child protection laws in the host country, or at least lack of awareness that culturally sanctioned parenting practices may significantly differ in the host country. In evidence of this, families who have resided in their new host country for less sustained time are more likely to perpetrate family violence, possibly for these reasons, coupled with increased acculturation stress.[18] In general, greater parental acculturation, ease of resettlement, and longer time of resettlement are associated with decreased risk in child abuse. However, there seems to be an exception for when acculturation alters traditional family roles and power dynamics, such as increased education or employment by women, leading to exacerbation of men's patriarchal beliefs and attempts to regain control over women and children.[18]

Race and Ethnicity

Past research has hinted at ethnic differences in the prevalence and severity of different types of abuse and neglect, particularly in the United States.[3] However, disagreement exists whether such results are independent of biases in reporting procedures and confounders such as historical systemic oppression of minorities in regard to education level and socioeconomic status.[20] One study asking parents of different ethnicities their opinions on parenting practices did not find any differences in ratings of how serious child abuse or neglect was between African Americans, Hispanic Americans, or white Americans,[20] although white Americans were slightly more tolerant of parental behaviors depicting abuse or neglect. This contradicts factual reporting data, as a higher proportion of ethnic-minority families are reported to child protective services; thus this likely has more to do with biases in reporting.[20] Indeed, studies of medical professionals' attitudes in the United States reveal biases that conflate race with child maltreatment.[21] Although African American parents reported using more physical and verbal punishment, they also rated highly on nurturing behaviors, particularly mothers. Therefore, high levels of nurturance may counteract the potential deleterious effects of authoritarian control. Rather than ethnicity, specific individual/family values may be associated with child maltreatment, including high levels of machismo, low levels of familism, and parental history of childhood maltreatment.[20] Another U.S. study found that higher rates of reported maltreatment in ethnic minorities were more likely explained by disparities in poverty level, and this disparity was most evident in population-dense metropolitan areas and the most sparsely populated areas.[22]

National Influences and Policy

Childhood sexual abuse is perhaps the mode of maltreatment that has the most worldwide agreement on its negative consequences and efforts to reduce it, and it is certainly a global problem.[9] A report issued by the United Nations Office on Drugs and Crime found that one-third of all human trafficking victims across 148 counties were children.[23] Despite the almost universal consensus on condemning sexual abuse, different regions around the globe have different perspectives on what constitutes these acts. Sexual acts involving a parent or caregiver are almost universally determined to constitute sexual abuse. However, depending on the survey, other social situations are more mixed; for example, child marriage is considered by 35% in America and 85% in Africa/Asia to be child abuse.[24] This may also be an artifact in that perhaps only incidents common to those regions were rated highly, as if infrequent events were perceived to be less problematic. What is problematic is that unless there are national laws against child marriage, the custom may not legally qualify as sexual abuse. High-income countries generally have the most liberal view of circumstances that qualify as abuse or exploitation, compared to middle- and low-income ones, which did not differ substantially.[24] Most countries had clear definitions of child sexual abuse, and most countries' laws allowed the removal of maltreated children from their home (although less so for removing alleged perpetrators). Almost three-quarters of countries had made an arrest in the prior year for child sexual exploitation or child pornography; this was most common in Europe and Oceania, and least common in Asia. Less than half of victims regularly received mental healthcare, with victims in high-income countries receiving more than those from middle- and low-income ones. In about one-quarter of countries, the involved children themselves were arrested, more commonly in Africa and Asia. Mandatory reporting laws also strikingly differ between counties; high- and middle-income countries generally favor mandated reporting, whereas low-income countries appear to have a higher threshold for considering certain experiences reportable. However, this may reflect less resources devoted to developing child welfare, with limited resources being focused on other priorities.[24]

There is much more variability in national responses to child maltreatment as a whole, and specifically physical abuse and the use of violence.[4] The use of violence, such as in intimate partner violence (IPV), is a well-established risk factor for child maltreatment; countries or regions that tolerate one would likely tolerate the other. A study in Egypt showed that there were elevated odds of child maltreatment by the mother if the mother was a victim of IPV and if the mother justified the violence perpetuated against herself.[25] As mentioned earlier, nations with more self-expressive values tend to have greater economic and political stability, whereas nations with a survivalist orientation are often characterized by greater political and economic uncertainty and rely on authoritarian principles to ensure obedience and control.[4] Individuals living in nations that favor a survivalist orientation are more likely to have views consistent with child maltreatment. Likewise, persons living in countries that espouse greater support for use of violence were also more likely to tolerate child maltreatment. A review of almost 30 developing and transitional countries revealed that in developing African countries, 83% of children experienced psychological abuse, 64% experienced moderate physical abuse, and 43% experienced severe physical abuse. A considerably lower percentage of children in transitional Eastern European countries experienced these forms of maltreatment (56%, 46%, and 9%, respectively). As before, this study identified parental attitude toward corporal punishment as the strongest variable associated with all forms of child abuse. The risk of all forms of child abuse was also higher for male children, those living with many household members, and those living in poorer families.[26]

Suggestions for Future Research

More research regarding factors related to the proliferation and prevention of child maltreatment is needed. In regard to community factors, it would be important to delineate whether perceived environmental stress and social support are the initiating triggers of neglectful or abusive parental behavior.[16] On health disparities, systematic data collection on community-level resources devoted to child protection and family support would address this issue. Regarding individual risk factors, the confounding of multiple risk factors that tend to occur along with child maltreatment needs to be delineated. These other risk factors include poverty, parental mental illness, absence of a parent, low parental educational attainment, large number of children in the family, exposure to racism, and substance abuse in a parent. Therefore, whether child maltreatment is what "causes" bad outcomes significantly depends upon the context and other variables.[6] In regard to immigrants and refugees, there is an increasing number of internally and externally displaced children and families, such as those living inside Syria during the conflict, among Palestinians in refugee camps under Israeli occupation, and large numbers of immigrants and refugees entering the United States and Europe. More research regarding risk and protective factors for displaced individuals living closer to their homes are needed.[18] Although already deemed by several medical and advocacy organizations as a practice that should at best be avoided, corporal punishment remains widespread.[4] Moreover, the majority of substantiated physical child abuse cases result from the apparent misuse of corporal punishment.[4] Additionally, there is little evidence to support that national bans on corporal punishment are associated with any changes in personal attitudes or views toward child maltreatment.[4] Further research on attitudes toward corporal punishment can inform our understanding regarding attitudes toward and prevention of child maltreatment. Children who grow up in nations with greater support for violence may interpret the behavior as normative, and individuals within these nations may express greater support for other forms of violence. Therefore, further research on global efforts that work to alter cultural and social norms that support violence would have many benefits even beyond that of the prevention of child maltreatment.[3] Although there is some evidence for parenting programs that prevent or reduce child maltreatment, there is a dearth of knowledge regarding what specific components of such programs make them effective, particularly in a variety of cultures.[27] A meta-analysis published in 2018 of 121 sample populations revealed that home visitation and parent training were effective, although effect sizes were larger for short-term interventions, and effect sizes were lowered when studies had longer duration of follow-up periods. Additionally, these studies do not represent a wide variety of cultural practices, as almost 82% were from North America.[27]

Limitations include research that looks at sociocultural views toward child maltreatment that may or may not be related to the actual incidence or prevalence of events of child maltreatment. An inherent limitation in most of this research is the reliance on child maltreatment that is reported, compared to what proportion of cases or incidents go unreported.

Conclusion

It seems impossible to have a global view of child maltreatment without an understanding of culture. In developing culturally responsive definitions of child maltreatment, it has been suggested to acknowledge cultural differences in child-rearing practices, to recognize that deviations from the culturally appropriate child-rearing practices of any specific cultural group are considered by that cultural group to be abusive, and to understand circumstances that exist—poverty, war—where societal harm undermines children's well-being beyond the control of a caregiver.[28] In countries with increased recognition of and societal response to child maltreatment, the prevalence of reported incidents has decreased; it is fundamentally important to include culture in the discussion of child maltreatment.[14] A cross-cultural perspective on what is "good" or "bad" for children, incorporating the latest research advances, forces a continual re-examination of commonly held beliefs about children, parents, child-rearing, and child maltreatment.[9] This process must emphasize a "child rights–based approach"[11] and focus on efforts addressing education and resources, in addition to supporting the protective aspects of cultures, as any delivery of such education and resources necessarily must occur within the culture in which the maltreatment grew.

Key Points for Social Psychiatrists

- Child maltreatment is a global problem with devastating individual and generational consequences, including multigenerational transmission of mental health problems.
- Rather than specific religions, nations, or ethnicities, there are several risk factors related to cultural attitudes or beliefs that contribute to the tolerance of child maltreatment.
- There are many risk factors—of which families have no control—that also contribute to environments that foster the development of child maltreatment.
- Medical professionals would be advantaged by understanding these risk factors, as otherwise they would be subjected to their own biases about specific groups.
- Education and resources to combat and prevent child maltreatment must be delivered with cultural humility and within the culture in which the maltreatment grew out of.
- A growing push toward "children's rights" is necessary but may paradoxically lead to more maltreatment if individuals and communities feel their parenting authority, as defined by their traditional cultures, is being threatened.

References

1. World Health Organization (WHO). *Child Maltreatment Fact Sheet*. 2016. Retrieved from https://www.who.int/en/news-room/fact-sheets/detail/child-maltreatment
2. World Health Organization (WHO). *Violence Against Children Fact Sheet*. 2020. Retrieved from https://www.who.int/en/news-room/fact-sheets/detail/violence-against-children
3. Zeanah CH, Humphreys KL. Child abuse and neglect. *J Am Acad Child Adolesc Psychiatry*. 2018 Sept;57(9):637–644. doi: 10.1016/j.jaac.2018.06.007.
4. Hayes BE, O'Neal EN. The effects of individual- and national-level factors on attitudes toward child maltreatment. *Child Abuse Negl*. 2018;83:83–93.
5. Haring U, Sorin R, Caltabiano NJ. Reflecting on childhood and child agency in history. *Palgrave Communications*. 2019;5:52. https://doi.org/10.1057/s41599-019-0259-0.
6. Garbarino J. Not all bad treatment is psychological maltreatment. *Child Abuse Negl*. 2011;35:798–801.

7. Fortson BL, Klevens J, Merrick MT, Gilbert LK, Alexander SP. *Preventing Child Abuse and Neglect: A Technical Package for Policy, Norm, and Programmatic Activities.* 2016. Atlanta, GA: National Center for Injury Prevention and Control, Centers for Disease Control and Prevention; 2016. Accessed from https://www.cdc.gov/violenceprevention/pdf/can-prevention-technical-package.pdf.

8. Nelson CA, Fox NA, Zeanah CH. *Romania's Abandoned Children: Deprivation, Brain Development, and the Struggle for Recovery.* Cambridge, MA, and London: Harvard University Press; 2014.

9. Raman S, Hodes D. Cultural issues in child maltreatment. *J Paediatr Child Health.* 2012;48:30–37. doi: 10.1111/j.1440-1754.2011.02184.x.

10. United Nations. Universal Declaration of Human Rights. 1948. Retrieved from https://www.un.org/en/universal-declaration-human-rights/.

11. United Nations. Convention on the Rights of the Child. 1989. Retrieved from https://www.ohchr.org/en/professionalinterest/pages/crc.aspx

12. Thomas MP Jr. Child abuse and neglect. Part I: historical overview, legal matrix, and social perspectives. *N Carolina Law Rev.*1972;50(2):293. Available at: http://scholarship.law.unc.edu/nclr/vol50/iss2/3.

13. Martin EJ. Incest/child sexual abuse: historical perspectives. *J Holistic Nursing.* 1995;13(1):7–18.

14. Kolhatkar G, Berkowitz C. Cultural consideration in child maltreatment: in search of universal principles. *Pediatr Clin N Am.* 2014;61:1007–1022.

15. Breyer RJ, MacPhee D. Community characteristics, conservative ideology, and child abuse rates. *Child Abuse Negl.* 2015;41:126–135.

16. Coulton CJ, Crampton DS, Irwin M, Spilsbury JC, Korbin JE. How neighborhoods influence child maltreatment: a review of the literature and alternative pathways. *Child Abuse Negl.* 2007;31:1117–1142.

17. The UN Refugee Agency. 2019. *Figures at a glance.* https://www.unhcr.org/en-us/figures-at-a-glance.html; accessed Dec 8, 2019.

18. Timshel I, Montgomery E, Dalgaard NT. A systematic review of risk and protective factors associated with family related violence in refugee families. *Child Abuse Negl.* 2017;70:315–330.

19. Zannettino, L. ". . . There is no war here; it is only the relationship that makes us scared": factors having an impact on domestic violence in Liberian refugee communities in South Australia. *Violence Against Women.* 2012;18(7):807–828.

20. Ferrari AM. The impact of culture upon child rearing practices and definitions of maltreatment. *Child Abuse Negl.* 2002;26:793–813.

21. Najdowski CJ, Bernstein KM. Race, social class, and child abuse: content and strength of medical professionals' stereotypes. *Child Abuse Negl.* 2018;86:217–222.

22. Maguire-Jack K, Lanier P, Johnson-Motoyama M, Welch H, Dineen M. Geographic variation in racial disparities in child maltreatment: the influence of county poverty and population density. *Child Abuse Negl.* 2015;47:1–13.

23. United Nations Office of Drugs and Crime. *Global Report on Trafficking in Persons 2020.* 2021. United Nations publication, Sales No. E.20.IV.3. Accessed from: https://www.unodc.org/documents/data-and-analysis/tip/2021/GLOTiP_2020_15jan_web.pdf

24. Dubowitz H. Child sexual abuse and exploitation: a global glimpse. *Child Abuse Negl.* 2017;66:2–8.

25. Antai D, Braithwaite P, Clerk G. Social determinants of child abuse: evidence of factors associated with maternal abuse from the Egypt demographic and health survey. *J Inj Violence Res.* 2016 Jan;8(1):25–34.

26. Akmatov MK. Child abuse in 28 developing and transitional countries: results from the multiple indicator cluster surveys. *Int J Epidemiol.* 2011;40:219–227.

27. Van der Put CE, Assink M, Gubbels J, Boekhout van Solinge NF. Identifying effective components of child maltreatment interventions. *Clin Child Fam Psychol Rev.* 2018;21:171–202.

28. Korbin JE. Culture and child maltreatment: cultural competence and beyond. *Child Abuse Negl.* 2002;26:637–44.

33

The Mental Health of Prisoners

An International Overview

Angus McLellan and Andrew Molodynski

Background

Prisons have existed since the birth of organized society and have been used as places of legal detention for those judged to have violated the law. The first recorded prisons were as far back as 1750 BC, and prisons were first used as a punishment by the Romans. Plato was among the first to suggest that prisons could be used as both punishment and to reform convicts, rather than simply to exact revenge. Prisons have also been used over time by political regimes to imprison those who oppose their views and who speak out against those in power. Such practices continue to this day, as evidenced in China and North Korea, among other countries. Prison restricts a citizen's access to their family and friends, their social environment, and their occupational roles and responsibilities. It also significantly changes the way they are viewed by society.

Prisons remain an integral part of penal systems internationally with imprisonment being used for a variety of crimes—some serious, some less so. The most recent update of the World Prison Population List reports that just over 11 million people are currently in prison worldwide; approximately 93% are males and 7% females.[1] Most inmates are between the ages of 26 and 50. Immigrants, those from ethnic minority populations, and those of lower socioeconomic status are all overrepresented.[2]

The global prison population rate is 145 per 100,000 people, but there is great variation in total prison populations and (crucially) rates of incarceration between countries and continents. Asia has the highest total prison population (4,150,000) and the Americas have the highest incarceration rate (376 per 100,000). The total prison population is highest in the United States (2,100,000), followed by China (1,600,000), Brazil (700,000), Russia (500,000), and India (400,000). Lowest overall prison populations are unsurprisingly usually in the smallest countries. However, rates of incarceration per 100,000 population contrast; while the United States retains the highest rate (655 per 100,000), the other top 5 countries are El Salvador, Turkmenistan, Virgin Islands, and Thailand.[1]

Country	Rate of Incarceration per 100,000 Population
United States	655
El Salvador	604
Turkmenistan	552
Virgin Islands	542
Thailand	526

Incarceration rates vary significantly over time and are affected by a number of factors. The rate of incarceration has fallen by 22% in Europe since 2000, which is thought to be related to decreased rates of detention in Russia and other Eastern European countries. Throughout history, political agendas and legal reforms have increased incarceration rates, with one example being the vastly increased imprisonment rate in Rwanda following the genocide there.[3] Globally, changes in recent years have been mostly in keeping with the increasing size of the general population (24.2% increase in global population since 2000 vs. 24.0% increase in prison population) but this varies significantly between continents, with Europe seeing a 22.0% decrease and Oceania experiencing an 86.5% increase in prisoners.[1]

Conditions in which people are held are crucially important when considering prisoners' well-being, particularly with regard to mental health. A key factor relating to the likely quality of the conditions in prison is the occupancy rate.[2] The number of current prisoners exceeds the official capacity in 123 countries globally, with 52 countries reporting occupancy rates of greater than 150%. The Philippines reports the highest occupancy level at 464%.[4] The use of solitary confinement is also thought to have a significant negative impact on prisoner well-being. There is little high-quality data available for this, but estimates suggested that up to 100,000 people are being kept in solitary confinement at any given time in the United States alone.[5](4)

There have been several occasions throughout history whereby a diagnosis of mental illness has been used to detain people in either hospital or prison. Drapetomania was proposed as a mental illness in slaves in 1851[6]; the main symptom was attempting to flee captivity and a diagnosis allowed for detention in prison or hospital. Another example is the diagnosis of sluggish schizophrenia, which was used in the Soviet Union[7] to discredit and allow the detention of people who disagreed with the leaders' political views.

The provision of healthcare in prison, including mental healthcare, is often poor, certainly when compared to that provided for the general population. The "Nelson Mandela Rules," revised and adopted in 2015 by the United Nations, relate to the treatment of prisoners and state that all prisoners have the right to access the same level of healthcare as they would if they were not in prison.[8] However, this is not the case in many (if not most) prisons, and this has a significant impact on the well-being, health, and mortality of prisoners in both the short term and the long term.

Mental Health Problems in Prisons

It has been established that there is a higher prevalence of mental health problems in prison compared to the general population.[2] Rates of mental illness are highest during the first few weeks after a person is imprisoned.[9] There is variable evidence with regard to different diagnoses in prison, but there is good evidence to show that there are increased rates of major depression and psychosis, with 1 in 7 prisoners experiencing one or both illnesses.[9] Studies also report increased use of illegal substances in prisoners; we know this worsens outcomes in mental healthcare.[10] Depression and substance misuse are particularly prevalent among the female population in prisons. The rate of self-harm and suicide in prisons is significantly elevated, with death by suicide occurring 3–6 times more frequently in prisoners than in their peers. A recent study also showed that 5%–6% of male prisoners and 20%–24% of female prisoners had intentionally harmed themselves in the last 12 months.[11] It is well established that untreated mental illness contributes to significantly worse health and social outcomes and leads to longer periods of ill health and social isolation. The stigma associated with mental illness continues to be a problem in and out of prison.

General Rates

The World Health Organization (WHO) estimates that up to 40% of prisoners suffer from a mental illness and a relatively comprehensive study conducted in the United Kingdom reported that around 90% of prisoners had a mental disorder, including addiction or personality disorder, and 70% had two or more diagnosable disorders.[12] Within this, it is believed that 10%–15% of the prison population have a severe and enduring mental illness (schizophrenia, bipolar disorder, or autism spectrum disorder). The authors also reported that the majority of those with a mental disorder had significant impairment in one or more areas of social functioning. Another recent paper looking at systematic reviews reported the rates of different mental illnesses in the global prison population as follows:[11]

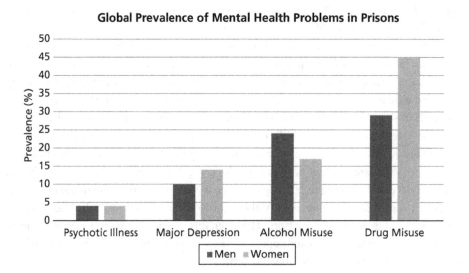

A paper published in 2019 showed that prisoners in low- and middle-income countries (LMIC) have a significantly higher rate of psychosis and major depression than those in higher income group (HIG) countries but have lower rates of alcohol and drug misuse.[13] A systematic review published in 2019 looked specifically at the rates of mental illness in prisoners in Africa. This study showed an even more troubling picture, with particularly high levels of psychosis and substance misuse:[14]

	Prevalence in LMICs	Prevalence in Africa
Psychosis	6.2%	33%
Major Depression/Mood disorder	16%	22%
Alcohol misuse	3.8%	-
Drug/Substance misuse	5.1%	38%

One of the difficulties in tackling these problems is the question of who provides the services needed to get better outcomes for prisoners. It is worth considering which interventions fall under the scope of a mental health service in prisons. While it is appropriate for a mental health service to provide pharmacological and psychological treatment and support for those with a mental disorder, it is appropriate to ask whether social interventions such as support for employment, ensuring privacy, and facilitating engagement with friends/family would fall within this scope. In places where it does not, there is often a void, with no clear service fulfilling these roles, and it is well established that without adequate social engagement, the risk of mental illness is increased, and existing conditions are prolonged and/or exacerbated.

Suicide and Reporting

Rates of suicide and self-harm among prisoners vary widely according to official statistics. Several risk factors for suicide in prison have been identified, including single cell occupancy, being married prior to imprisonment, and being held on remand (i.e., non-convicted and awaiting trial).[15] These three factors suggest a social element relating to the risk of suicide. Risk related to single cell occupancy may be due to others not being able to alert staff to dangerous behavior. It could also be that reduced regular social contact with a cell mate(s) has a negative impact. For those who are married before being imprisoned, they will often have a more developed social system, which should be protective, but being in prison often causes relationship breakdowns and/or feelings of guilt, particularly if the wider family are involved. Being held on remand brings the added stress and uncertainty of an upcoming trial and what might happen, turning lives upside down.

A further factor to consider when looking at rates of suicide and self-harm among prisoners is reporting bias. It has been suggested that while some countries clearly and reliably record suicide as a cause of death, many do not and will record alternative causes of death. Socially, this is of interest when considering attitudes toward mental health. It may be that suicide is not recorded as a cause of death because it is illegal or socially unacceptable and could have effects on how the deceased and their relatives are viewed by their communities. In other examples it could be a product of officials not wanting to highlight high rates of suicide in their penal systems. Either way, reduced reporting may mean that resources are not correctly allocated to the prevention of suicide and management of mental health conditions.

Variation During Imprisonment

A recent study looked at changes in the rates and presentation of mental illness during periods of incarceration.[9] It found that the first few weeks after incarceration are when prisoners are at the highest risk of developing a mental illness. As time passes, this risk reduces, except for prisoners who are kept in isolation, where the risk continues. This information is important as it allows services to plan where assessment and management of people are most necessary to reduce harm, certainly during the early period of imprisonment.

Substance Misuse in Prisons

Alcohol and/or drug misuse is a relatively common issue in society, with 1.4% of the global population (107 million people) having an alcohol use disorder and 0.9% (71 million people) having a drug use disorder.[16] It was estimated that 166,000 deaths were attributable to a drug use disorder in 2017.[16] Few studies have looked at the global rate of the use of drugs in prison. The use of alcohol and drugs can have a significantly negative impact on both the quality and the length of a person's life. Alongside the health issues that drug misuse can cause, it can also have significant effects on an individual's social life. Drugs are often viewed negatively in society, and there are multiple knock-on effects from this, including: isolation from friends and family, reduced employment rates or loss of employment, police involvement, and financial difficulties. The rate of drug misuse is higher in prison than in the general population, and this is a concern as drug misuse will contribute to perpetuating the difficulties that led to a person coming to prison in the first place. It may also make it more likely that those who have not used drugs before take them up in prison.

In the United Kingdom, 34.2% of the population report having used an illicit substance on at least one occasion, with 8.5% reporting use in the last year and 4.0% in the last month.[17] Among prisoners, these numbers are significantly higher, with 40% reporting use of cannabis alone in the 2 months before arriving in prison. In Scotland, 76% of prisoners tested positive for an illicit substance on their admission to prison. The drugs that these prisoners most frequently tested positive for were:

	Percentage of Positive Tests Containing This Substance
Cannabis	47%
Benzodiazepines	41%
Opioids	33%
Cocaine	20%

Of those who tested positive for drugs, 30%–40% of prisoners reported feeling that their drug use was problematic prior to coming to prison and it was noted that women are more likely to report difficulties with illicit substance misuse than men (41% vs. 27%).[17] In Scotland in 2016–2017, the rate of disciplinary action against inmates for use of illicit substances was 154 per 1000 prisoners, roughly one disciplinary action for every 6 prisoners.

Use of illicit substances in prison is associated with an increase in violence and agitation toward both staff and other inmates[18] and is also linked with increased rates of self-harm and suicide.[17] As illicit drug use has increased in prisons, so have reports of violence and aggression. A report from the United Kingdom discusses the negative effects that illicit drug use in prison can have on an individual, including: poorer physical and mental health, drug toxicity, bullying and debts related to drugs, and negative behavioral changes. Of particular importance is the increased risk of psychosis and the heightened chance of contracting a blood-borne virus while using illicit substances in prison. Use of opioids is particularly dangerous around the time of release from prison. Men are 29 times more likely to die in the first 2 weeks after release, and women are 69% more likely to do so when compared to the general population. Whilst take-home naloxone has been considered as a harm-reduction measure, it is not yet standard practice.[17]

A more recent phenomenon surrounding illicit drug use in prison is that of novel psychoactive substances (previously also called "legal highs"). These novel psychoactive substances are mostly synthetic cannabinoids, synthetic opioids, synthetic cathinones, and new benzodiazepines. As these are more recent, the evidence base is still evolving, but current numbers suggest that the use of novel psychoactive substances in prisons in Europe varies from 2% of drug use to 30%.[19]

The rates of substance misuse and dependence are particularly high in the United States, where a study in 2010 showed that 85% of inmates were using an illicit substance and roughly two-thirds of the prison population met criteria for a diagnosis of either illicit substance/alcohol misuse or dependence. This same study also showed that drugs or alcohol were involved in 78% of violent crimes, 83% of property crimes, and 77% of weapons offenses or parole violations leading to incarceration in the first place. In the United States in 2005, $74 billion was spent on incarceration and the associated legal processes for those with a substance misuse problem. Only $632 million (less than 1% of the previous figure) was spent on prevention and treatment of offenders' difficulties. Just 11% of those with a substance misuse disorder receive any form of treatment, with only 16.6% of facilities offering specialized treatment.[20]

Drug and alcohol misuse increases the chances that a person will be involved with a crime carrying a prison sentence, and it can be argued that if all of those with addiction problems in the prison system were offered evidence-based treatment, the investment would pay for itself quickly by the reduced rate of incarceration and the associated benefits of improved health, increased employment, and reduced reoffending.[20] The paper that showed this concluded that every $1 spent on addiction services saved $12 elsewhere within the system. It showed the longer-term impact that using substances in prison has on somebody after release, with reduced rates of employment (27% vs. 32%) and increased likelihood of income from criminal activity (25% vs. 6%). The authors went on to report that those who used drugs in prison had more challenging experiences when growing up:

	Prisoners Who Use Drugs	Prisoners Who Do Not Use Drugs
Family history of criminality	43%	30%
Parental abuse of alcohol or substances	35%	18%
Spent time in foster care	12%	7%
Finished high school	30%	39%

The data from this study suggest that a person's early experiences and their environment as a child have a significant impact on their use of illicit substances and their likelihood of incarceration. This would suggest that resources would be better allocated to supporting younger people who face adversity, rather than punishing those who commit crimes with longer prison sentences (particularly bearing in mind that the US already has the highest incarceration rate globally).

For some, simply going to prison reduces their use of alcohol and/or other illicit substances because of difficulties acquiring them. However, prisons are facing an increasingly complex task to keep alcohol and drugs out. Visitors and staff have been known to bring these in, often under intense pressure or blackmail. This has led to the introduction of searches and in some places scanning of visitors and staff before they enter the prison. In response to this increased surveillance, more advanced methods of supplying drugs have quickly developed. One of the most frequent methods of bringing drugs into a prison is now via drones whereby drugs are flown over the walls of a prison and dropped either onto the grounds or into specific rooms. Another more recent development is using cards or notes which are saturated with a drug dissolved in a liquid. The liquid then evaporates from the card, leaving the substance combined with the card, which can then be posted to inmates who can smoke the paper to utilize the substance. One impact of these increasingly complex methods of delivery is the need for closer monitoring. Such measures can make it more difficult and stressful for family and friends to visit prisoners and potentially reduce these outside contacts, which we know are so important.

Smoking tobacco is another source of significant ill health in the global population. While rates of smoking overall are declining, a significant proportion of the population still do so, and the figure for prisoners is up to 90%. The negative effects of smoking tobacco on health are well-known and the use of tobacco alongside alcohol and other substances only compounds the negative effects already highlighted.

With regard to treatment and rehabilitation of prisoners with addiction problems, the Forward Trust in the United Kingdom has been utilizing the "Rapt" 12-step treatment program, which has been shown to reduce the rate of reoffending after release from prison. This trust is currently working in 7 different prisons in the United Kingdom, and this may be a model which can reduce reoffending rates, reduce substance and alcohol misuse, and reduce overall costs. It focuses on four main areas of change: promoting health and well-being, tackling drug and alcohol misuse, developing positive connections with others, and encouraging and supporting employment. Tackling substance misuse in prisons undoubtedly requires such a broad approach that encompasses biological, psychological, and social factors into any treatment plan.[21]

Special Populations
Prisoners on Remand

Concerningly, the paper on mental illness in Africa mentioned above[14] also reported that in 36% of studies, most prisoners had not been convicted of a crime. This could be attributed to factors such as political changes, but probably also reflects very poor community access to mental healthcare and prisons being used to manage mental health problems by default. In many LMICs, less than 1% of the health budget is spent on mental healthcare, and it is likely that the prison system picks up the slack where appropriate mental healthcare is not available, leading to the increased detention of those who are displaying signs of mental illness, like distressed or agitated behavior, but who have committed no crime.

Women

Women make up approximately 7% of the global prison population.[2] While this may seem low overall, the number of women detained since 2000 has increased by around 50%, compared to a 20% increase for men. In 2014, the United Nations published the *Handbook for Women and Prisons*, also known as *The Bangkok Rules*.[22] These set out basic principles with regard to women in prisons. Female prisoners are more likely to have committed nonviolent offenses compared to male prisoners. Up to 85% of female prisoners report having experienced at least one incident of physical or sexual abuse during their life; 50% report that they are currently a regular user of drugs and 25% report being under the influence at the time of the offense. Research has also shown that female prisoners are more likely than male prisoners to experience mental health problems, with up to 80% suffering with a mental illness[22] and 44% of female prisoners in the United Kingdom reporting that they have attempted suicide at least once.[12]

In a number of countries, the main "crimes" leading to imprisonment for women are related to pregnancy. Infanticide, illegal abortions, and even miscarriages and/or stillbirths may lead to a conviction and time spent in prison. Occasionally they even lead to the death penalty. The pre-trial period for pregnant or recently pregnant women is particularly stressful and inherently risky, and the risk of prosecution may also mean that pregnant women or those having difficulty during childbirth are less likely to seek assistance. This can in turn have a significant effect on both their physical and mental health and increase risks to the unborn child.

High rates of violence and abuse toward women are a global phenomenon, and their link with mental disorder is well established. Verbal, physical, and sexual forms of abuse are also common in female prisons, particularly when male staff are supervising. *The Bangkok Rules* state that male prison guards should not be used in female prisons because of this risk, but their presence is still routine. Women are often the primary or sole caregiver within their family, and being sentenced to time in prison represents a significant change whereby they can no longer take on this role and will often lose the close contact that they had with their family. This change of role and increased feelings of isolation are both risk factors for developing mental health problems. Women also experience the same issues as men in terms of the negative effects of prison overcrowding. Given the rapid increases in the female prison population, resources and space available for female prisoners do not always keep up and this may contribute to lower levels of well-being.

Because of the smaller population, there are fewer female prisons and they are more widely spaced. This can make it logistically and financially difficult for family to visit female prisoners. Some prisons even demand payment just to facilitate a visit,[22] leaving female prisoners more likely to be socially isolated than male prisoners. Families of female prisoners are more likely to become fragmented, and there is an increased chance that children of female prisoners will have to go to alternative care arrangements.[22]

Support around the time of release from prison is also noted to be poor, with little attention paid to female prisoners' needs. As female prisoners are more likely to suffer from mental health problems, mental health follow-up is crucially important but rarely provided, leaving a potentially lasting impact on that person. Women who have been abused or in violent relationships will often have to return to such situations and experience further abuse and humiliation upon release.[22] This undoubtedly places a significant stress on these individuals and will only perpetuate the difficulties that led to them going to prison.

With women experiencing worse conditions in prison, being more likely to experience mental illness and addiction, and being more likely to be a victim of abuse, it is worth considering why prison is an increasingly common choice internationally. The different needs of women probably require an alternative approach to the standard one of incarceration or rates will just continue to rise, further worsening conditions and aggravating the significant mental health problems in this population.

Younger People

There is no clear data with regard to how many people under the age of 18 are prisoners, but it is estimated to be roughly one million globally—approximately 9% of the overall prison population.[2] Rates of youth imprisonment vary greatly between different countries, partly as a result of variations in the age of criminal responsibility from 7 to 16. Despite being illegal under international law, some countries also continue to use the death penalty for crimes committed before the age of 18. In the United Kingdom, young people from a Black, Asian, or Minority Ethnic (BAME) background are significantly more likely to be convicted of a crime leading to a custodial sentence than those of a White British background.[23] This suggests systemic problems in the way that crimes are dealt with and is important because of the longer-term effects as well as the immediate unfairness.

Prison not only restricts a young person's liberty, it limits access to their usual caregivers and has a significant impact on their education. Upon release, younger people may also experience the effects of stigmatization more intensely than the general population.

The first symptoms of mental illness most commonly occur during adolescence and the teenage years,[24] though most individuals do not access treatment until many years later, if at all.[25] Rates of self-harm in young people in custody have been increasing for some time in the United Kingdom. A recent study showed that people who spend time in prison while under 18 have worse outcomes in terms of both their physical and mental health in the long term.[26] Between 50% and 75% of young offenders meet criteria for a diagnosis of mental disorder.[27] The breadth of mental health problems among the young prison population is very similar as in the general population but with higher rates. It is recorded that around 25% of young offenders have an IQ of less than 80, meaning they meet diagnostic criteria for an intellectual disability.[28] One must ask why this is the case and why we choose to incarcerate them rather than offer care.

Another common problem is gang behavior, with up to 16% of male young offenders in the United Kingdom reporting gang-related problems when first imprisoned. One prison recorded members of 48 different gangs at one time![29] The Metropolitan Police report that there are over 250 active gangs in London alone. Even if someone is not involved with gangs before imprisonment, the likelihood of them becoming involved with gangs increases because of these high rates of gang membership and activity in prison. While gangs may provide some sense of identity for younger people who would otherwise lack this, the association with criminal activity proves detrimental for most, and the effects of being in a gang (increased likelihood of criminality, increased chance of being assaulted) provide further stress and anxiety, making mental health problems more likely.

There have been some successful changes made to the way that the prison system deals with young offenders who have mental health problems. In several countries, teams have been set up that will work with young offenders on a biopsychosocial model which often includes psychological therapy as part of this. The principle of restorative justice has also been shown to reduce reoffending rates.[30] Restorative justice involves bringing the victim and the perpetrator of a crime together in communication. This can be done in a number of formats, including by email, letter, or a facilitated face-to-face meeting. It could be suggested that such practices help young offenders to be more mindful of the impact of their actions on others and may also help victims to receive closure.

Older People

As with the general population, the average age in prisons is rising, and those over 50 are the fastest-growing population in prisons. Between 10% and 15% of the UK prison population are over 50.[31] Older people are more likely to experience ill health and, given the known difficulties around accessing the same level of healthcare in prison, this can often have a particularly negative impact on them.[32] Older people are also just as likely as other age groups to experience mental illness. Dementia in particular poses a significant problem for older prisoners, and people with dementia often require more adjustment than others and certainly have greater needs than those of other ages.[33] It has also been suggested that those who spend time in prison will experience the effects of aging sooner than those that do not.

Prisons have very limited access to social work and occupational therapy services, with less than 10% of prisons having access to either. It is important to note that social work and occupational therapy are important not only on release from prison, but also during the period of imprisonment. The majority of prisons were designed for young, able-bodied individuals, and so if a prisoner has difficulties in managing their personal care or mobility, it is often very difficult to manage this appropriately in a prison setting. This can be for a number of reasons, including lack of staff training, inadequate prison facilities, and stigma. In addition to this, most activities in prison are also created with the aim of rehabilitating young people, with classes on literacy and intense physical exercise being less likely to be utilized by the older population.[34] This lack of resource can have a serious impact on individuals, by making their experience of prison life worse, creating and perpetuating difficulties relating to both physical and mental health. The increased risk of mental health problems in those with a chronic physical disorder is well-known, and mismanagement of these symptoms will increase the risk of mental health problems.

Dementia is an increasingly common problem in the aging general population, an issue mirrored in prison. Under-diagnosis due to lack of knowledge and possible lengthening of sentences due to disruptive behavior are both sadly likely. The ethics around detaining people with dementia are complex. People with a diagnosis of dementia may not recall the crime committed. The potential for rehabilitation in prison for those with dementia is reduced and the risk of further offending is probably lower. However, society may consider that people who have committed crimes should receive the same punishment, despite a diagnosis of dementia. It should also be considered, though, that prison may not be an effective way of managing those whose risk of further offending is now significantly reduced and for whom community-based sentences may be more appropriate.

High numbers of older people in the community experience loneliness and isolation. Within prison, older people are more likely to experience bullying and victimization and older prisoners are also often assumed to have committed a sexual offense, leading to further discrimination by other prisoners. Older people may have to move property to an unfamiliar area after imprisonment and build new links for healthcare and social contact. It is important to consider how society may have changed during a prisoner's time in jail, with today's rapid advancements in technology often proving particularly tricky. Inventions such as bank cards, mobile phones, online banking, and email can all pose significant challenges to people who are not familiar with these, and mastery of online processes is increasingly important to get basic benefits and other crucial necessities arranged in many countries.

In the United Kingdom, the Equality Act 2010 states that people should have access to the same facilities regardless of their age. Legislation such as this is key when considering how to improve access to the correct facilities for older people in prison. Not only is access to the correct facilities in prison important, it is also worth considering that older people are more likely to have family and friends who are older and who may find it more difficult to visit prisoners. This, in turn, can further increase isolation when compared to those in other age categories.

Another important aspect of care relating to health in prisoners is the provision of end-of-life care. There is the possibility of release near the end of life, but this rarely happens, and the facilities available for end-of-life care for prisoners remains poor globally.

An interesting (and troubling) phenomenon has been found in Japan, whereby older people who struggle for a variety of reasons in the community (often financial or related to lack of family engagement) will commit crimes with the aim of being imprisoned, whereby their financial and care problems are then less of a concern as they are in a facility which provides shelter, nutrition, and activities.[35] While not mirrored across the globe, this demonstrates the need for us to be alert to the many reasons for imprisonment and their likely variation as people age.

Gender and Sexuality in Prison

Though the global data on the rates of LGBT+ (lesbian, gay, bisexual, or transgender) people in prison is not yet adequate, studies have suggested that there is a higher incarceration rate for those in the LGBT+ population.[2] This population is more likely to experience assault in prison, which in turn means that they may be more likely to experience mental health problems (for example, PTSD) related to this. For some people, their LGBT+ status may be the reason that they are in prison, given that same-sex relationships remain illegal in 74 countries and punishable by death in 13 countries.[36] There may also be difficulties when considering the correct setting in which people from the LGBT+ population should be incarcerated. As we know, the rates of assault when transgender people are imprisoned in their birth gender prison are increased, and this is likely also the case when they are in prisons of the gender with which they identify. One solution that has been proposed by some is to have dedicated prisons for the LGBT+ community. This may, however, create other difficulties and inequalities, such as people being imprisoned far away from their home and having reduced contact with friends, family, and healthcare professionals. There is no doubt, though, that things need to change to mirror the changes in most societies around the world.

Conclusions

This chapter is an attempt to give a broad overview of the complex issues surrounding mental health and prison systems internationally. While there has been some work to analyze and understand global prison populations and their mental health needs, most of this work has been focused on Western countries, meaning that there is less focus on mentally ill prisoners in other areas of the world. This imbalance requires addressing and there should be a focus on research among all groups of prisoners worldwide and not just certain populations.

What is clear is that there is a strong correlation between prison and mental health problems, with one making it more likely that an individual will also experience the other (in both directions). It is also clear that prisoners with mental illness experience significantly negative effects on almost all aspects of their life, with their health, well-being, family life, social life, and occupational life proving more difficult compared to other prisoners.

Evidence is emerging about interventions that can be helpful in reducing reoffending rates, encouraging appropriate engagement with the non-prison community, reducing costs to the state overall, and improving the health of prisoners. There is no consistency of approach within or between individual countries, however. Overall, prison continues to be used primarily as punishment, with rehabilitation playing a smaller part or being absent altogether. This can be through ideology, economy, or both. A global approach to gathering data regarding rehabilitation practices that work is likely to be most productive in the longer term to produce better outcomes for prisoners, the state, and society as a whole.

Care of someone with any form of mental health problem in prison is difficult, and services are almost universally less developed and supported than their "non-prison" comparators. The United Nations states that prisoners should have the same access to healthcare as if they were in the general community, but the evidence suggests that this standard is nowhere near being met globally. Challenges range from the support and education of children with developmental disorders to the humane management of older prisoners with dementia. Investment of time, money, and further research is the only way to improve the mental health and well-being of prisoners. Without work to correct these imbalances, the gaps between prisoners and non-prisoners will only continue to widen, exacerbating all of the difficulties that prisoners experience both in prison and after release. These then affect all of us.

References

1. Walmsley R. *World Prison Population List.* 12th ed. World Prison Brief, Institute for Criminal Policy Research. London; September 2018.
2. Rope O, Sheehan F. Global prison trends 2018. *Penal Reform International,* May 2018.
3. Genocide in Rwanda: detention and prison involvement, Luyt W, Acta Criminologica: Southern African Journal of Criminology, Volume 16, Number 4, 1 January 2003, pp. 96–111(16)
4. Highest to Lowest Occupancy Level, World Prison Brief, Institute for Criminal Policy Research. https://www.prisonstudies.org/highest-to-lowest/occupancy-level?field_region_taxonomy_tid=All. Accessed October 31, 2019.
5. Solitary Confinement, Penal Reform International. https://www.penalreform.org/priorities/prison-conditions/key-facts/solitary-confinement/. Accessed October 31, 2019.
6. Myers B. *"Drapetomania": Rebellion, Defiance and Free Black Insanity in the Antebellum United States.* University of California, Los Angeles; 2014. Retrieved from https://escholarship.org/uc/item/9dc055h5.
7. Wilkinson G. Political dissent and "sluggish" schizophrenia in the Soviet Union. *Br Med J.* 1986 Sept;293(6548):641–642.
8. *United Nations Standard Minimum Rules for the Treatment of Prisoners (the Nelson Mandela Rules).* United Nations General Assembly, Seventieth Session, Agenda Item 106, January 8, 2016.
9. Walker J, Illingworth C, Canning A, et al. Changes in mental state associated with prison environments: a systematic review. *Acta Psychiatr Scand.* 2014;129:427–436.
10. Ramsay M. *Prisoners' Drug Use and Treatment: Seven Research Studies.* Home Office Research, Development and Statistics Directorate. London, UK; July 2003.
11. Fazel S, Hayes AJ, Bartellas K, Clerici M, Trestman R. Mental health of prisoners: prevalence, adverse outcomes, and interventions. *Lancet Psychiatry.* 2016;3:871–881.
12. Singelton N *Psychiatric Morbidity Among Prisoners: A Summary Report.* Office for National Statistics. London, UK; 1997.
13. Baranyi G, Scholl C, Fazel S, Patel V, Priebe S, Mundt A. Severe mental illness and substance use disorders in prisoners in low-income and middle-income countries: a systematic review and meta-analysis of prevalence studies. *Lancet Global Health.* 2019;7:e461–471.
14. Lovett A, Kwon HR, Kidia K, Machando D, Crooks M, Fricchione G, Thornicroft G, Jack HE. Mental health of people detained within the justice system in Africa: systematic review and meta-analysis. *Int J Mental Health Systems.* 2019;13:1–41.
15. World Health Organization. *Preventing Suicides in Jails and Prisons.* Geneva, Switzerland: World Health Organization; 2007.
16. Our World in Data. https://ourworldindata.org/. Accessed October 31, 2019.
17. Crawford C, UK Focal Point on Drugs. *United Kingdom Drug Situation 2017.* Public Health England; 2018.
18. McGuire J. *Understanding Prison Violence: A Rapid Evidence Assessment. Analytical Summary.* 2018.
19. Vandam L, et al. *New Psychoactive Substances in Prison: Results from a EMCDDA Trendspotter Study.* European Monitoring Centre for Drugs and Drug Addiction; July 2018.

20. *Behind Bars II: Substance Abuse and America's Prison Population.* New York: The National Centre on Addiction and Substance Abuse at Columbia University; February 2010.

21. Martin C, Player E, Liriano S. *Results of Evaluation of the RAPt Drug Treatment Programme: Prisoners' Drug Use and Treatment: Seven Research Studies.* Home Office Research, Development and Statistics Directorate: London, UK; July 2003.

22. Atabay T. *Handbook on Women and Imprisonment.* 2nd ed. [The Bangkok Rules]. United Nations: New York, USA; 2014.

23. *The Lammy Review: An Independent Review into the Yreatment of, and Outcomes for, Black, Asian and Minority Ethnic Individuals in the Criminal Justice System.* https://www.gov.uk/government/publicati ons/lammy-review-final-report#history. Accessed November 21, 2019.

24. Kessler RC, Amminger GP, Aguilar-Gaxiola S, Alonso J, Lee S, Ustun TB. Age of onset of mental disorders: a review of recent literature. *Curr Opin Psychiatry.* 2007 Jul;20(4):359–364.

25. Wang PS, Angermeyer M, Borges G, et al. Delay and failure in treatment seeking after first onset of mental disorders in the World Health Organization's World Mental Health Survey Initiative. *World Psychiatry.* 2007 Oct;6(3):177–185.

26. Barnert ES, Dudovitz R, Nelson BB, Coker TR, Biely C, Li N, Chung PJ. How does incarcerating young people affect their adult health outcomes? *Pediatrics.* 2017 Feb; 139(2):2016–2624.

27. Underwood L, Washington A. Mental illness and juvenile offenders. *Int J Environ Res Public Health.* 2016 Feb;13(2):228.

28. Talbot J. *Seen and Heard, supporting vulnerable children in the youth justice system.* London: Prison Reform Trust; 2010.

29. Factor F, Pitts J, Bateman R. Gang involved young people, custody and beyond, *Beyond Youth Custody.* 2015.

30. Latimer J, Dowden C, Muise D. The effectiveness of restorative justice practices: a meta-analysis. *Prison J.* 2005 Jun 1;85(2):127–144.

31. Fazel S, McMillan J, O'Donnell I. Dementia in prison: ethical and legal implications. *J Med Ethics.* 2002;28:156–159.

32. Ginn S. Elderly prisoners. *BMJ.* 2012;345:e5921.

33. Le Mesurier N. Supporting older people in prison: ideas for practice. *Age UK.* June 2011:4–33.

34. Baidawi S, Turner S, Trotter C, Browning C, Collier P, O'Connor D, Sheehan R. Older Prisoners: A Challenge for Australian Corrections. *Trends & Issues in Crime and Criminal Justice.* 2011;426:1–8.

35. Sugie N. When the elderly turn to petty crime: increasing elderly arrest rates in an aging population. *Int Criminal Justice Rev.* 2017;27(1):19–39.

36. LGBT relationships are illegal in 74 countries, research finds. https://www.independent.co.uk/news/ world/gay-lesbian-bisexual-relationships-illegal-in-74-countries-a7033666.html. Accessed November 21, 2019.

Special Topics

In this section we address various topical issues where social pshychiatry is making significant contributions. These range from ongoing social challenges to mental health such as stigma and violence, the impact of technology on mental health and treatment interventions, the impact of the recent COVID pandemic, and the development of social psychiatry in two Eastern European nations.

34

Stigma

Mariam Rahmani, Gabriel Ivbijaro, and
Andres J. Pumariega

Definition of Stigma

The word "stigma" is derived from the Greek word *stizein*, which means marking, puncturing, or tattooing. In ancient Greece, *stizien* was used to describe an identification mark placed on slaves.[1] The modern derivative, stigma, is used to identify someone as being of lesser value or belonging to a lower position in the social structure. Ervin Goffman, an influential sociologist, defined stigma as "an attribute that is deeply discrediting" and reduces the bearer "from a whole and usual person to a tainted, discounted one."[2(p3)]

Stigma is a powerful social process that uses stereotyping, prejudice, and discrimination. It has many forms and it is dynamic. It disqualifies individuals from full social citizenship. It oppresses people based on their membership in a group and hinders their full acceptance by others.

This chapter will review the neurobiology of stigma, different types of stigma, the consequences of stigma against psychiatric illness, and how to counteract their negative impact.

Neurobiology of Stigma

The development and persistence of stigma against psychiatric illnesses can be explained by evolutionary neurobiology.

One explanation is that the survival of early human beings depended on belonging to a tribe whose members would support and defend one another. Tribe members had to quickly identify and protect themselves from outsiders, and anyone who appeared different was viewed as a threat. This "threat theory" is supported by neuroimaging research. For example, activation of the superior colliculus when presented with a threat has been noted in many primates including humans. Functional magnetic resonance imaging (fMRI) studies have shown that activation of the amygdala, the fear center of the brain, is greater when participants view faces from a different race than their own race, particularly if the presentation is very brief.[3,4,5] Another fMRI study showed that people have greater activation of the prefrontal cortex (PFC) in the first two seconds of being shown negative images of stigmatized people (e.g., a homeless or an alcoholic person) versus negative images of non-stigmatized people (e.g., a man holding a gun).[6]

Ethological research has also established the well-known phenomenon of social stratification practiced not only by humans but also by lower species, often termed a "pecking order." The formation of such dominance hierarchies is known to have genetic bases, and to have evolutionary adaptive value for lower species in the distribution of physical resources to "fitter" animals. Stigmatized individuals (often based on appearance or behavior) fall lower within such dominance hierarchies.[7]

Perceived stigma or anticipation of stigma is associated with neurochemical changes in the human body. For example, perception of racial discrimination is associated with elevations of cortisol, dehydroepiandrosterone sulfate (DHEA) and C-reactive protein (CRP), indicating activation of the stress response.[8] Historic stigma and generational trauma have also been associated with different physiological responses. For example, African Americans under stereotype threat exhibited larger increases in mean arterial blood pressure during an academic test than European Americans and African Americans who were not under stereotype threat.[9]

Research has confirmed that the perception of a threat is often subjective and not objectively accurate.[10] Although the biological mechanisms for threat recognition and population survival were adaptive at some point in the human history, they are maladaptive in a complex society where genotypic and phenotypic diversity and associated strengths enhance humanity's ability to address diverse challenges.

Why Stigma Against Mental Illness Exists

Stigma exists in mental illness because of a number of factors. As discussed previously, stigma has a neurobiological basis, and perceiving anything that was different as a threat was once essential for survival, giving rise to the "threat theory."

Another model that may explain the stigma in mental illness is the "attribution theory." People who attribute the cause of mental illness to controllable traits exhibit prejudice, and blame people with mental illness for their own fate.[11]

Other trends that have contributed to stigma are religious beliefs that associate mental illness with immorality and sinfulness;[12] the hierarchical strictures of society where people with power strengthen their power by stigmatizing those with less power;[13] the dehumanizing impact of seclusion and restraints;[14] disempowerment of people with mental illness when they are hospitalized against their will;[15] fear when a psychiatric hospitalization is facilitated by law enforcement; and conditioning by the media through stigmatized portrayals of psychiatrists and psychiatric illnesses.

Types of Stigma

Stigma can be divided into the following categories.

- *Public stigma* is a set of negative attitudes and beliefs that motivate individuals to fear, reject, avoid, and discriminate against people with mental illness.[16] It includes stereotyping (e.g., believing that mental illness leads to violence), prejudice (e.g., fearing people with mental illness), and discrimination (e.g., excluding mentally ill persons from employment or housing opportunities). Stigma against mental health is common and is experienced even by children. For example, parents and teachers perceive children with attention deficit hyperactivity disorder (ADHD) to have lower math and reading abilities than those without ADHD.[17]
- *Self-stigma* develops when an individual internalizes public stigma. Like public stigma, it includes stereotyping or negative belief about the self (e.g., character weakness, incompetence), prejudice or agreement with the negative belief leading to negative emotional reaction (e.g., low self-esteem, low self-efficacy), and discrimination or behavioral response to prejudice (e.g., fails to pursue work and housing opportunities).[18]
- *Courtesy stigma* is transferred from an already stigmatized person to individuals connected through familial or professional relationships. Examples include blaming the "refrigerator mother" for causing autism in a child and perceiving psychiatry as a less prestigious medical specialty.[19] Courtesy stigma against psychiatry is found in both psychiatric and non-psychiatric health professionals.[20]
- *Affiliate stigma*, which can be conceptualized as the self-stigma experienced by the family members of a stigmatized person, relates to the internalization of courtesy stigma.[21] It has been found that low education level, low social support, and high courtesy stigma are associated with the development of affiliate stigma.[21]
- *Health system stigma*, or *institutional stigma*, takes place when public stigma affects healthcare systems, e.g., a healthcare plan that covers physical illnesses but not mental illnesses. Practices in psychiatric hospitals that contribute to courtesy stigma are involuntary hospitalization of a psychiatric patient, which is often accompanied by restricting visitors, even the patient's family members. While these practices contribute to safety, they also contribute to overriding a patient's civil liberties, isolating the patient, and subliminal messaging that the psychiatric patient needs to be separated from the family.

Sometimes different types of stigma are experienced together, giving rise to more complex forms such as cultural or societal stigma (combination of courtesy and institutional stigma), or double stigma with minority populations (racial/ethnic discrimination works at same levels). For example, African Americans with bipolar disorder are more likely to be misdiagnosed with schizophrenia. African Americans who are accurately diagnosed with bipolar disorder receive less adequate treatment compared to bipolar patients from other races.[22] As another example, low-income and racial/ethnic minority youth on the autism spectrum are less likely to participate in transition planning meetings, enroll in postsecondary education, find competitive employment after high school, live independently, participate in social activities, and receive healthcare transition services than their White and higher income peers on the autism spectrum.[23]

Consequences of Stigma Against Mental Health

Stigma against mental health leads to many negative outcomes, including shame, health disparities, decreased social support, and delay in diagnosis and treatment.

Shame and Secrecy

Many people hide their mental illness because of stigma. For example, a majority of the medical students surveyed in the Midwest United States indicated that, if depressed, they would feel embarrassed if classmates knew. Many believed that revealing depression could negatively affect professional advancement.[24] Less than half of U.S. military servicepersons who screened positive for depression, anxiety, and post-traumatic stress disorder (PTSD) sought care for mental health problems because they were afraid they would be branded as weak or would lose the respect and trust of their peers and leaders.[25] Other populations have identified "preserving dignity," "saving face," "loss of friends", and "harm to career" as reasons to keep their mental illness a secret from family and friends.[26,27]

Decreased Social Support

As a result of secrecy and shame around mental illness, people with psychiatric illness do not receive the social support they need. Low levels of family and peer support are related to higher severity of mental illness.[28] Among LGBTQ adolescents, lack of social support is associated with higher levels of depression, anxiety, alcohol and drug misuse, low self-esteem, and risky sexual behaviors.[29] Even clinicians are even known to "emotionally withdraw" or distance themselves from patients with severe psychiatric illnesses, especially personality disorders.[30] Decrease in perceived social support is also associated with depression for the caregivers of patients with mental illness.[31]

Health Disparities

Stigma results in disparities in psychiatric diagnoses and treatment. For example, U.S. minorities are less likely than White majorities to be diagnosed with depression, due to a variety of factors including stigma, socioeconomic status, and cultural beliefs about depression.[32] Students from racial minorities are less likely to use in-school and out-of-school mental health services than their White peers.[33]

Shortage of Mental Health Workforce

Stigma has contributed to fewer physicians specializing in psychiatry, although this trend is recently reversing in the United States. According to a World Health Organization (WHO) report, stigma against mental illness is a barrier in recruitment, retention, and professional development of psychiatric nurses.[34]

Delay in Diagnosis and Treatment

Stigma is associated with reluctance to seek treatment for psychiatric disorders in different age groups across different cultures.[35,36] Adolescent-perceived stigma about ADHD is an influential factor in whether the adolescent receives treatment for ADHD.[37] Self-stigma influences whether people seek professional help for mental health problems and adhere to psychiatric treatment.38,39

Misdiagnosis of Mental Illness

Stigma, implicit biases, and a shortage of psychiatric experts leads to misdiagnosis of mental illness. As mentioned previously, African Americans with bipolar disorder are more likely to be misdiagnosed with schizophrenia. Recent studies speculate that implicit bias may have contributed to a higher prevalence of certain psychiatric disorders, e.g., autism and ADHD, being more commonly diagnosed in boys than girls.

Withholding Accurate Diagnosis and Treatment

Several studies have shown that clinicians are reluctant to diagnose borderline personality disorder (BPD) and offer appropriate treatment for it to adolescents because of stigma about the diagnosis.[40,41] A survey of U.S. mental health practitioners and patients showed that the majority of clinicians sampled did not actively share the BPD diagnosis with their patients, even when they felt it was the most appropriate diagnosis, and patients who later discovered that their diagnosis had been withheld consistently left treatment.[42]

Other notable harmful effects of stigma can include a lack of understanding by family, friends, and co-workers; fewer opportunities for work, school, housing, and social activities or trouble finding housing; and experiencing bullying, physical violence or harassment, all of which further compound the effects of having a mental illness.

Approaches to Address Stigma

Several approaches have been taken to address stigma against mental illness. Some of these efforts are described below.

Advocacy for Mental Health Parity

Advocacy for mental health parity can take several forms, such as educating patients and families about the importance of mental health treatment, partnering with professional organizations, urging insurance companies to provide coverage for psychiatric illnesses, and advocating for medical licensing boards to ask for only relevant mental health information because it may make physicians reluctant to seek needed psychiatric treatment.

Neurobiological Approach to Mental Illness

It had been thought that a neurobiological approach would reduce blaming a person for their mental illness; however, the results of this approach are not as positive as once expected. One study showed the educating people about depression through neurobiological models reduced their social distance from depressed individuals.[43] Another study found that neurobiological models were associated with less attribution and blame, but more social distance from people with mental illness among the general public.[44] On the other hand, a meta-analysis found that neurobiological explanations of mental illnesses did not reduce stigma and were associated with greater desire for social distance, greater perceived dangerousness, and greater prognostic pessimism.[45] One study even found that biological explanations evoked significantly less empathy in clinicians.[46]

Destigmatizing Language

An important way of destigmatizing mental illness is using respectful language. For example, in 2008, Rosa's Law was passed in the United States, which replaced the terms "mental retardation" and "mentally retarded" with "intellectual disability" and "person with intellectual disability" in all federal policies. Hospital staff can be respectful by using the term "support-seeking" or "comfort-seeking" behaviors instead of "attention-seeking"; saying that "a person with a substance use disorder is abstinent" instead of saying that "an addict is clean."

Approaches by Psychiatrists

Psychiatrists can help reduce stigma by having open discussions about diagnosis and prognosis with patients and families, including openness to questions, transparency about the pros and cons of treatment, acknowledging the limitation of their knowledge, and providing support and psychoeducation for families and youth dealing with family member and peers who stigmatize; empowering patients to distinguish who they self-disclose to; and volunteering for public presentations and media interviews that increase awareness and empathy toward people with mental illness.

Systems-Based Approaches

Reducing stigma toward mental health requires efforts from all sectors of society. For example, in Australia, all state and territory governments share the responsibility to provide education and treatment for mental illness.[47] Other approaches include integration of mental health education into school curricula and requiring all healthcare professionals, regardless of specialty, to have some experience in psychiatry. Additionally, advocacy organizations such as the National Alliance for the Mentally Ill in the United States serve an important role in educating the public against stigmatizing perceptions of mental illness, as well as serving as an agentistic venue for self-advocacy by individuals with mental illnesses and their family members, thus countering against self-stigma.

Positive Role Models with Mental Illness

Acknowledging that many historical figures made major contributions in the context of their illness can serve as an antidote to stigma. For example, it has been speculated that Abraham Lincoln's depression deepened his sensitivity to losses in the Civil War. Sir William

Churchill, who referred to his depression as "the black dog," provided purposeful leadership to Britain during the Second World War.

Public figures can help reduce stigma by being transparent about their own experiences with mental health. Some notable examples are below.

- American politician Patrick Kennedy publicly disclosed his struggle with bipolar disorder and cocaine use; his treatment for opioid use disorder and alcoholism; and helped the U.S. government battle the opioid crisis.
- Pope Francis revealed that he sought the help of a psychoanalyst for 6 months when he was 42 and the leader of the Jesuit order in Argentina during the country's military dictatorship.
- Marsha Linehan, PhD, developer of dialectical behavior therapy (DBT), came out about her own struggle with borderline personality disorder (which informed her treatment approach) and even visited her former seclusion room at the Institute of Living residential program in an attempt to reduce stigma.
- Elyn Saks, JD, professor of law at the University of Southern California, has been open about her diagnosis and treatment for schizophrenia.
- Hollywood actor Dwayne Johnson (the Rock) has publicly vocalized his personal experience with depression.
- Earl Campbell, running back for the Houston Oilers, has been open about his anxiety disorder.

Summary

Stigma toward mental illness is rooted in history, neurobiology, and social hierarchy. It is prevalent in all cultures. Stigma extends beyond the person who has a mental illness, to people associated with that person, resulting in dire consequences including developing shame, social isolation, no treatment or under-treatment of treatable psychiatric illnesses, health disparities, and discrimination. Addressing stigma is an important step toward improving public mental health. It requires efforts from all stakeholders. Notable approaches include educating the public and lawmakers, disclosing personal experiences of mental illness, and sharing the responsibility of reducing stigma.

References

1. Arboleda-Flórez J. What causes stigma? *World Psychiatry.* 2002;1(1):25–26.
2. Goffman E. Stigma and social identity. In: Goffman, *Stigma: Notes on the Management of Spoiled Identity.* New York and London: Simon and Schuster, 1963, Chapter 1, page 3.
3. Amodio DM. The neuroscience of prejudice and stereotyping. *Nat Rev Neurosci.* 2014;15:670–682.
4. Chekroud AM, Everett JA, Bridge H, et al. A review of neuroimaging studies of race-related prejudice: does amygdala response reflect threat? *Front Hum Neurosci.* 2014;8:179.
5. Cikara M, Van Bavel JJ. The neuroscience of intergroup relations: an integrative review. *Perspect. Psychol Sci.* 2014;9:245–274.

6. Krendl AC, Kensinger EA, Ambady N. How does the brain regulate negative bias to stigma?. *Soc Cogn. Affect Neurosci.* 2012;7(6):715–726. doi: 10.1093/scan/nsr046.

7. Sapolsky R. *Behavioral Genetics I (Human Behavioral Biology)*. Stanford University; 2010. https://www.youtube.com/watch?v=e0WZx7lUOrY.

8. Lucas T, Wegner R, Pierce J, Lumley MA, Laurent HK, Granger DA. Perceived discrimination, racial identity, and multisystem stress response to social evaluative threat among African American men and women. *Psychosom Med.* 2017;79(3):293–305. doi: 10.1097/PSY.0000000000000406.

10. Major B, Quinton WJ, McCoy SK. Antecedents and consequences of attributions to discrimination: theoretical and empirical advances. *Adv Exp Soc Psychol.* 2002;34:251–330.

11. Hegarty P, Golden AM. Attributional beliefs about the controllability of stigmatized traits: antecedents or justifications of prejudice? *J Appl Soc Psychology.* 2008;38:1023–1044. doi: 10.1111/j.1559-1816.2008.00337.x.

12. Wesselmann ED, Day M, Graziano WG, Doherty EF. Religious beliefs about mental illness influence social support preferences. *J Prev Interv Community.* 2015;43(3):165–174. doi: 10.1080/10852352.2014.973275. PMID: 26151166.

13. Gwinn JD, Judd CM, Park B. Less power = less human? Effects of power differentials on dehumanization. *J Exper Soc Psychology.* 2013;49:464–470.

14. Wilson C, Rouse L, Rae S, Kar Ray M. Is restraint a "necessary evil" in mental health care? Mental health inpatients' and staff members' experience of physical restraint. *Int J Mental Health Nurs.* 2017;26:500–512. doi: 10.1111/inm.12382.

15. Seed T, Fox J, Berry K. The experience of involuntary detention in acute psychiatric care. A review and synthesis of qualitative studies. *Int J Nurs Studies.* 2016;61:82–94.

16. Corrigan PW, Penn DL. Lessons from social psychology on discrediting psychiatric stigma. *Am Psychologist.* 1999;54(9):765–776.

17. Eisenberg D, Schneider H. Perceptions of academic skills of children diagnosed with ADHD. *J Attention Disorders.* 2007;10(4):390–397. https://doi.org/10.1177/1087054706292105.

18. Corrigan PW, Watson AC. Understanding the impact of stigma on people with mental illness. *World Psychiatry.* 2002;1(1):16–20.

19. Feifel D, Moutier CY, Swerdlow NR. Attitudes toward psychiatry as a prospective career among medical students entering medical school. *Am J Psych.* 1999;156:1397–1314.

20. Natan MB, Drori T, Hochman O. Associative stigma related to psychiatric nursing within the nursing profession. *Arch Psychiatr Nursing.* 2015;29(6):388–392.

21. Werner P, AboJabel H. Who internalizes courtesy stigma and how? A study among Israeli Arab family caregivers of persons with dementia. *Aging Ment Health.* 2020 Jul;24(7):1153–1160. doi: 10.1080/13607863.2019.1584790. Epub 2019 Mar 5. PMID: 30836018.

22. Johnson KR, Johnson S. Inadequate treatment of Black Americans with bipolar disorder. *Psychiatr Services.* 2014;65(2):255–258.

23. Eilenberg JS, Paff M, Harrison AJ, et al. *Curr Psychiatry Rep.* 2019;21:32. https://doi.org/10.1007/s11920-019-1016-1.

24. Wimsatt L, Schwenk T, Ananda S. Predictors of depression stigma in medical students: potential targets for prevention and education. *Am J Prevent Med.* 2015;49(5):703–714. https://doi.org/10.1016/j.amepre.2015.03.021.

25. Hoge CW, Castro C, Messer S, McGurk D, Cotting D, Koffman R. Combat duty in Iraq and Afghanistan, mental health problems, and barriers to care. *N Engl J Med.* 2004;351:13–22. doi: 10.1056/NEJMoa040603.

26. Chen, F-P, Lai GY-C, Yang L. Mental illness disclosure in Chinese immigrant communities. *J Counsel Psychology.* 2013;60(3):379–391. https://doi.org/10.1037/a0032620.

27. Mulfinger N, Rüsch N, Bayha P, et al. Secrecy versus disclosure of mental illness among adolescents: I. The perspective of adolescents with mental illness. *J Mental Health.* 2019;28(3):296–303. doi: 10.1080/09638237.2018.1487535.

28. Jibeen, T. Perceived social support and mental health problems among Pakistani university students. *Community Ment Health J.* 2016;52:1004. https://doi.org/10.1007/s10597-015-9943-8.

29. McDonald K. Social support and mental health in LGBTQ adolescents: a review of the literature. *Issues Ment Health Nursing*. 2018;39(1):16–29. doi: 10.1080/01612840.2017.1398283

30. Hinshelwood R. The difficult patient: The role of "scientific psychiatry" in understanding patients with chronic schizophrenia or severe personality disorder. *Br J Psychiatry*. 1999;174(3):187–190. doi:m10.1192/bjp.174.3.187.

31. Chai YC, Mahadevan R, Ng CG, Chan LF, Md Dai F. Caregiver depression: the contributing role of depression in patients, stigma, social support and religiosity. *Int J Soc Psychiatry*. 2018;64(6):578–588. doi:m10.1177/0020764018792585.

32. Shao Z, Richie WD, Bailey RKJ. Racial and ethnic disparity in major depressive disorder. *Racial Ethnic Health Dispar*. 2016;3:692. https://doi-org.lp.hscl.ufl.edu/10.1007/s40615-015-0188-6.

33. Locke J, Kang-Yi CD, Pellecchia M, Marcus S, Hadley T, Mandell S. Ethnic Disparities in school-based behavioral health service use for children with psychiatric disorders. *J School Health*. 2017;87:47–54. doi: 10.1111/josh.12469.

34. World Health Organization. *Atlas: Nurses in Mental Health*. Geneva: World Health Organization; 2007.

35. Wang X, Li H, Peng Y, Peng S. How depression stigma affects attitude toward help seeking: the mediating effect of depression somatization. *Soc Behav Personality*. 2015;43(6):945–953.

36. Vogel DL, Wade NG. Hackler AH. Perceived public stigma and the willingness to seek counseling: the mediating roles of self-stigma and attitudes toward counseling. *J Counsel Psychol*. 2007;54(1):40–50. doi: 10.1037/0022-0167.54.1.40.

37. Bussing R, Zima B, Mason D, Porter P, Garvan C. Receiving treatment for attention-deficit hyperactivity disorder: do the perspectives of adolescents matter? *Adolesc Health*. 2011;49(1):7–14. doi: 10.1016/j.jadohealth.2010.08.014.

38. Jennings KS, Cheung JH, Britt TW, et al. How are perceived stigma, self-stigma, and self-reliance related to treatment-seeking? A three-path model. *Psychiatr Rehabil J*. 2015;38(2):109–116. https://doi.org/10.1037/prj0000138.

39. Yilmaz E, Okanlı A. The effect of internalized stigma on the adherence to treatment in patients with schizophrenia. *Arch Psychiatr Nursing*. 2015;29(5):297–301. https://doi.org/10.1016/j.apnu.2015.05.006.

40. Miller A, Muehlenkamp J, Jacobson C. Fact or fiction: diagnosing borderline personality disorder in adolescents. *Clin Psychol Rev*. 2008;28(6):969–981. doi: 10.1016/j.cpr.2008.02.004.

41. Laurenssen EM, Hutsebaut J, Feenstra DJ, Van Busschbach JJ, Luyten P. Diagnosis of personality disorders in adolescents: a study among psychologists. *Child Adolesc Psychiatry Ment Health*. 2013;7(1):3. doi: 10.1186/1753-2000-7-3.

42. Sulzer SH, Muenchow E, Potvin A, Harris J, Gigot G. Improving patient-centered communication of the borderline personality disorder diagnosis. *J Ment Health*. 2016;25(1):5–9. doi: 10.3109/09638237.2015.1022253.

43. Han D-Y Chen S-H. Reducing the stigma of depression. *Psychiatry Clin Neurosci*. 2014;68: 666–673. doi:10.1111/pcn.12174

44. Rüsch N, Todd AR, Bodenhausen GV, Corrigan PW. Biogenetic models of psychopathology, implicit guilt, and mental illness stigma. *Psychiatry Res*. 2010;179(3):328–332. doi: 10.1016/j.psychres.2009.09.010.

45. Loughman A, Haslam N. Neuroscientific explanations and the stigma of mental disorder: a meta-analytic study. *Cogn Res Princ Implic*. 2018;3(1):43. doi:10.1186/s41235-018-0136-1.

46. Lebowitz MS, Woo-kyoung A. *Proc Natl Acad Sciences*. 2014;111(50):17786–17790. doi: 10.1073/pnas.1414058111.

47. Australian Institute of Health and Welfare. Mental health services in Australia: Mental health services. Last updated 7 July 2022. https://www.aihw.gov.au/reports/mental-health-services/mental-health-services. Accessed December 3, 2022.

35

Terrorism and Other Forms of Violent Extremism

The Role of Social Psychiatry

Debasish Basu

Introduction

At its 75th anniversary in 2020, the special webpage of the United Nations shows as its heading: *A new era of conflict and violence.*[1] Interestingly, its masthead reads: "shaping our future together." This is not surprising. A secure future cannot be achieved if conflicts and violence cannot be maintained at a manageable level.

Although the number of deaths due to wars between states has come down, the number of people dying of various kinds of violent conflicts has increased. Organized crime, gang wars, domestic violence, politically motivated violence, protest-based violence, gender-based violence, violence against children, use of progressively sophisticated and deadly weapons, and use/misuse of the combination of internet and technology in various forms to achieve an unprecedented reach globally are some of the worrisome trends. Violent extremism (VE), including acts of terrorism, has become more globally spread. As the UN webpage notes, "The nature of conflict and violence has transformed substantially since the UN was founded 75 years ago."[1]

Of the various kinds of violence and conflicts, terrorism and other forms VE occupy a special place. Although the number of deaths due to terrorist incidents has come down since 2014, the number of countries where terrorist activities have been reported has actually gone up.[2] There is tremendous economic, social, and psychological fallout of terrorism. The drivers of, and pathways to, terrorism and other forms of VE are diverse, complex, and multilayered. However, "social" and "psychological" are two recurrent and persistent themes in this literature for the past decades. Hence it is important to understand the role of social psychiatry, and socially minded mental health professionals, in this area.

Definitions and Concepts

Before moving further, it is important to clarify some relevant terms. It is important to note that there are many different definitions and conceptualizations of some of the key terms, some of them conflicting or confusing.

Although the term "extremism" literally means "advocacy of extreme measures or views" about anything (food, sports, hobbies, scientific theories), in the current context it usually refers to political, religious, or other ideological spheres. As such, there is nothing wrong in holding and advocating non-hateful and nonviolent extremist views. Trouble starts when extremism becomes "hateful" (typically against an identified "enemy" or "out-group") and then "violent" (with overt support or use of violence to achieve a particular political, religious, or other ideological goal and in the process intending to or actually harming the object of hatred and violence). Terrorism, however defined in myriad ways, is essentially a special case of VE where the intent of the VE act is to achieve the goals by intentionally *inducing terror* in the minds of these targets of hatred and violence, beyond the direct victims of the violent act. Other VE acts can follow ideologies that are far-right (e.g., various supremacist theories like white supremacy or neo-nazism), far-left (e.g., anti-capitalist), or single-issue (e.g., anti-gay rights). Note that all these instances of VE can also lead to terrorist acts as long as these acts are carried out with the motive of achieving their respective goals with the *coercive strategy of instilling fear, terror, or panic among those beyond the direct victims of the violent act.* Thus, there is some degree of overlap between terrorism and other forms of VE, though conventionally terrorism focuses on achieving political, religious, or economic goals. Radicalization (again, a somewhat controversial but now widely accepted term) refers to the process of a positional shift of an individual from a "moderate" or "mainstream" position to progressively extremist positions, usually reaching up to the state of cognitively endorsing violence (cognitive radicalization) or actually using violent means (behavioral radicalization). Finally, on the reverse path, preventing or countering VE (P/CVE) policies or strategies aim to de-radicalize and/or disengage the individual from VE. Whereas disengagement is primarily a process of behavioral change, de-radicalization refers to cognitive adaptations.[3]

Magnitude and Consequences

The Global Terrorism Index (GTI)[2] provides the updated figures on terrorist incidents and their impact, using data from the Global Terrorism Database (GTD) and other sources. Data for the GTD are collected and collated by the National Consortium for the Study of Terrorism and Responses to Terrorism (START)[4] at the University of Maryland. The GTD contains nearly 200,000 terrorist incidents from 1970 onwards.

According to GTI 2019, which shows the terrorist incident data until 2018, deaths from terrorism fell for the fourth consecutive year, after peaking in 2014, the downward trend being ascribed to the fall of the terrorist organization Islamic State of Iraq and the Levant (ISIL), though many other large-scale terrorist organizations are still active. Presently, South Asia remains the region most impacted by terrorism. In fact, 2018 was the first year since 2012 that South Asia recorded more deaths than any other region, largely ascribed to terrorist activities in Afghanistan and neighboring states. Sub-Saharan Africa recorded the second-highest number of deaths from terrorism, overtaking the Middle East and North Africa (MENA), which is now ranked third. Bombings and armed assaults have been the most common type of terrorist attack over the past two decades. Between 2002 and 2018, South Asia, MENA, and Sub-Saharan Africa accounted for 93% of all deaths from terrorism. The largest number was recorded in MENA, with more than 93,700 fatalities.

After recording the overall hopeful longitudinal trend, however, GTI 2019 notes with concern:

> Although the intensity of terrorism has diminished its breadth has not, with 103 countries recording at least one terrorist incident in 2018, and 71 countries suffering at least one fatality in the same year. This is the second worst year on record for the number of countries suffering at least one death, and highlights the need for continued assertive international action to combat terrorism. . . . Conflict remains the primary driver of terrorism, with over 95 percent of deaths from terrorism occurring in countries already in conflict. The ten countries most impacted by terrorism according to GTI 2019, in order of descending order, were; Afghanistan, Iraq, Nigeria, Syria, Pakistan, Somalia, India, Yemen, Philippines and the Democratic Republic of Congo.[2(p2)]

Although GTI 2019 mentions Europe as one of the stable regions with low impact of terrorist activities, recent events in France, Germany, Austria, Turkey, and elsewhere in 2019 and 2020 would force us to revise this notion. The terrorist incidents in these countries would further add to the increasing breadth of the global spread of terrorism.

One of the more worrying trends is the surge in far-right political terrorism over the past 5 years, although the absolute number of far-right attacks remains low when compared to other forms of terrorism. In North America, Western Europe, and Oceania, far-right attacks increased by 320% over the past 5 years, motivated by such issues as white supremacy, xenophobia, and anti-immigrant beliefs. These attacks took place in 23 different countries between 2015 and 2019. In 2019 there was a sharp increase in the lethality of terrorist attacks that were racially or ethnically motivated. This increase was largely a result of exceptionally deadly attacks targeting Hispanic Americans in the United States and Muslims in New Zealand.[5]

Finally, there has been a growing trend of increased female participation in terrorism, although still a small percentage of all attacks. Between 1985 and 2018 there were 300 suicide attacks involving at least one female. These attacks killed over 3,000 people. The trend has intensified over the past 5 years, with the number of female suicide attacks increasing 450% between 2013 and 2018.

The 2022 update of the GTD,[5] largely reflects the same pattern as GTI 2019. However, an interesting pattern noticed recently is that

> Politically motivated terrorism has now overtaken religiously motivated terrorism, with the latter declining by 82 per cent in 2021. In the last five years, there have been five times more politically motivated terrorist attacks than religiously motivated attacks.[5(p2)]

Further, and of our relevance, is the observation that:

> The decline is terrorism in the West coincided with the COVID-19 pandemic. Restrictions on freedom of movement, public gatherings, travel and an immediate threat to personal health may help to explain some of this fall. Once the emergency measures are removed and societies begin to live with COVID-19, there is the possibility of an uptake in terrorism activity. This would require addressing the underlying issues of alienation.[3(p3)]

A complementary document, Global Peace Index 2020,[6] looks at the issue from the obverse lens. The GPI covers 99.7% of the world's population, using 23 qualitative and quantitative indicators from highly respected sources, and measures the state of peace across three domains: the level of *Societal Safety and Security*; the extent of *Ongoing Domestic and International Conflict*; and the degree of *Militarization*.[6] The overall results show that the level of global peacefulness has deteriorated. Afghanistan is the least peaceful country in the world for the second year in a row, followed by Syria, Iraq, South Sudan, and Yemen. Terrorism and internal conflict have been the biggest contributors to the global deterioration in peacefulness. Ninety-seven countries recorded increased terrorist activity, while only 43 had lower levels of terrorism.

The latest Global Burden of Disease publication[7] compared the disability-adjusted life years (DALYs) and other metrics of burden of disease due to 369 diseases and injuries, for two sexes, and for 204 countries and territories, between 1990 and 2019. It found that over these 20 years, ranking of "conflict and terrorism" as a contributor to DALYs came down from 16 in 1990 to 46 in 2019 in the young age group (10–24 years). While this is good news, the fact that it still featured among the top 50 causes is a matter or worry, especially because the young are affected disproportionately more.

Impact and Consequences of Terrorism

Although the total number of deaths from terrorism has fallen, the impact of terrorism remains widespread. A recent publication used different metrics for combining the effects of death and injuries specifically due to terrorism, placed terrorism in the context of global burden of diseases 2010, and found that terrorism lies in the bottom 9% of the global burden of disease.[8] Year after year, road traffic accidents, cardiovascular and cerebrovascular disease, neonatal disorders, infections, cancers, and diabetic complications kill far more people and cause far more burden of disease than terrorism.[7] However, the impact and consequences of terrorism and other violent extremism go far beyond death and trauma.[9] The very purpose of terrorist acts is to create "terror," not only in the minds of those directly affected by such acts, but more importantly, in the larger society as an overt threat. Thus, the social impact of terrorism and extremism goes beyond individual psyche (where it can cause several psychiatric disorders and/or psychological sequelae), to the collective psyche or the social mindset. These acts set in motion a series of counter-terrorist measures and generate a sense of paranoia in the society, which, paradoxically, may further fuel the cycle of terrorism in the long run.[10]

The economic impact of violence on the global economy in 2019 was $14.5 trillion in purchasing power parity (PPP) terms. This figure is equivalent to 10.6% of the world's economic activity (gross world product) or $1,909 per person.[2]

At the individual level, terrorism instills fear and unpredictability, hence apprehension, in the minds of those directly afflicted by an attack, those who witnessed or were close associates of the victims, and the society at large. The psychiatric disorders can range from acute stress reaction, which may or may not escalate or persist as prolonged adjustment disorders, anxiety disorders, depressive disorders, substance misuse, or post-traumatic stress disorder (PTSD). Of these, PTSD has received a great deal of attention, though a recent review argues that the prevalence and impact of PTSD may have been overemphasized, and the reliance from such conditions underemphasized.[11] In any case, terrorist attacks usually instill deep and lasting fear in a society which is targeted. They serve a dual purpose by drawing the attention of the media worldwide and disrupting the social functions and the infrastructure of the targeted societies. It might be apt to draw the conclusion that terrorism is psychological warfare and that terrorists design attacks to have a maximum impact on target population. All this has an impact on the health-related behaviors of the population.[12]

The social impact of terrorism and other forms of violent extremism can be far more devastating, multilayered, complex, and lasting. These include, but are not limited to, the effects on migration and displacement, social trust, job stability, living security, cultural changes, participation in social-cultural-religious events, and on tourism and migration.[10]

Progression of VE/Pathways to VE

The usual understanding is that the progression of an apparently average, ordinary, "normal" individual to a bomb-exploding, vehicle-ramming, or suicide-pledging hard-core terrorist is not a simple, linear, logical, and predictable progression. Instead, the progression of a career in violent extremism can be tortuous, multi-phasic, and unpredictable.

The major focus in understanding the progression of events has been two facts:

(a) There are different spheres of beliefs and activities in the context of what is socially acceptable: "mainstream" (reflecting the majoritarian dominant mode or norm of beliefs, attitudes, and behaviors in a particular society at a particular epoch), deviation and dissent from mainstream, extremism, and violent extremism including terrorism. "Radicalization" is the term given for this process of shifting attitudes and actions. Violent radicalization (or the more commonly used phrase, "radicalization into violent extremism") is often seen as this process.

(b) However, not all those who shift from the mainstream to the extremes endorse violence. Further, not all those who endorse or justify violence at an ideological level actually indulge in an act of violence. On the contrary, not all who commit terrorist acts are necessarily indoctrinated into violent extremist ideology first. This fact argues against the smooth and continuous transitional nature of radicalization.

The earlier theories did not take into account this nonlinearity of progression or pathways to VE, but rather posited linear incremental models.[13,14] An early one proposed a four-stage model for "understanding the terrorist mindset."[15] "Fundamentally, the four-stage process begins by framing some unsatisfying event, condition, or grievance (*It's not right*) as being unjust (*It's not fair*). The injustice is blamed on a target policy, person, or nation (*It's your fault*). The responsible party is then vilified—often demonized—(*You're Evil*), which facilitates justification or impetus for aggression. The model was developed originally as a training heuristic for law enforcement, not as a formal social science theory."[13(p39)]

In the second model, called the "staircase to terrorism," six floors are conceptualized, with fewer and fewer people progressing to the top floor. It starts from the psychological interpretation of material conditions, progressing to perception of unfair treatment, displacement of aggression, moral engagement with extremist ideology, solidification of categorical thinking and legitimacy of the terrorist organization, and finally overcoming inhibitions to the commitment of terrorist acts.[16]

Both of these, and similar "stage" or "staircase" models, assume linear progressive causality and are heavily psychologically oriented. Further, empirical research has been lacking.

In order to accommodate these two apparently conflicting facts stated above, and to explain the crucial disconnect between cognitive vs. behavioral radicalization, different conceptualizations of the "pathways" to VE (the "how" of it) have been formulated. One such influential conceptualization is the "Two Pyramids Model."[17] This model separates out the "pyramid" of opinion from the pyramid of action related to radicalization to VE. While both are pyramid-shaped, with fewer and fewer people on the narrowing tip of the pyramids, the opinion pyramid consists of people from bottom to top comprising rungs of "neutrals," "sympathizers," "justifiers," and finally "those who feel a personal moral obligation to take up violence in defense of the cause." From the bottom to the top of the "action pyramid" are those who are "inert," followed by "activists," "radicals," and finally "terrorists." A person does not have to necessarily reach each of the levels successively to reach a higher level. This model explicitly separates the process of cognitive radicalization from that of behavioral radicalization. This is currently an influential model with some research support.

A most recent model called the Attitudes-Behaviors Corrective (ABC) model has conceptualized this cognitive-behavioral distinction in a two-dimensional graph.[14] The x-axis refers to attitude toward in terms of sympathy for (toward the right of the y-axis) or opposition to (toward the left of the y-axis) ideologically justified violence. The y-axis refers to the extent of involvement in ideologically justified violence. An individual's location at a given time can be located on this x-y matrix. For example, a person may be highly sympathetic to ideology-driven violence (i.e., highly cognitively radicalized) but may (still) be quite low in his/her intent to engage in an actual act of violence (i.e., not behaviorally radicalized). Another person may be high on action-oriented radicalization but due to reasons other than ideological justification (e.g., for monetary gain, power and position, reward in afterlife, or simply coercion into VE). In addition, a person's location can change on this two-dimensional map later, thus emphasizing the dynamic nature of the process over time and circumstances. This model also mentions a three-point system of the "drivers of VE" (see below), which can explain a person's location on this map at a given time and circumstances. Finally, this model can map a person's reverse journey into de-radicalization from the cognitive component of VE and/or disengagement from violent action. Thus this is a very promising and intuitively appealing model which needs empirical research validation.

Yet another recent way of looking at the pathway to VE issue is the life-course analysis. This focuses on the fact that most radicalizations take place when the person is young, often late adolescence to the early twenties. In this analysis, "it is suggested that the process of engagement consists of three steps: (1) a weakening of informal social controls, followed by (2) an interaction with individuals in proximity to the group and (3) a stage of meaning-making in relation to the group and one's identity, resulting in an individual's willingness and capacity to engaging in the group's activities, including violence."[18(p82)] Though it appears like one of the linear models mentioned above, it focuses on the crucial importance of age, and three things that are important at this stage: informal social control (as from the family, school, and neighborhood), an active seeking out and the formation of a new social identity based on peer groups. It thus emphasizes "the intricate intersections of biography, social context and life-course contingent dynamics" in understanding the pathways to VE.[18(p85)] We will return to this later, to highlight the crucial importance of the concept of social identity, social context, and socially facilitated meaning-making in the pathway to VE.

Drivers of VE

If the previous section on progression and pathways to VE asked the question "how," this section focuses on the all-important question of "why"? Why does an apparently normal individual living in the mainstream society become a sympathizer for VE, and why do some indulge in terrorist or other VE acts?

The earlier quest was for the "root causes" of VE and terrorism. There were two main schools of thoughts—the ones focusing on the structural/sociological root causes, and the other on the individual/psychological factors. However, as later research showed, just as there is no single pathway to VE, similarly, there is no single group of "root causes" of VE. Thus, the narrative changed to finding the "conditions conducive to VE." The current focus simply is on the various levels of "drivers of VE." This is achieved by the appreciation of the principles of "equifinality" and "multifinality," both derivatives of the general systems theory. "Equifinality refers to the observation that in any open system a diversity of pathways may lead to the same outcome. Multifinality suggests that any one component may function differently depending on the organization of the system in which it operates."[19(p597)] Thus, the emphasis shifts from a single factor or factors to the system within which such factors operate. Translated in the context of VE, it means that very different sets of factors, in several permutation-combinations, may give rise to either cognitive or behavioral radicalization to VE (equifinality). It also means that, the same "conducive" factors may give rise to very different outcomes in terms of the different levels espoused in the two-pyramid model. System characteristics (including the most important role of social context) are important in defining the final outcome. Thus, there are no "root causes" that are both necessary *and* sufficient to explain VE, but all are important to varying degrees depending upon circumstances.

An influential way of combining this multitude of factors is by categorizing them into "push" and "pull" factors.[20,21] Push factors refer to the antecedent distal predisposing factors of structural nature, which may "push" an individual toward extremist ideology and action. Usually these factors operate at a macro level (societal, cultural, political, and economic inequities). However, while many (not all) violent extremists came from socio-economically disadvantaged and inequitable backgrounds, most from these backgrounds do *not* turn to VE. On the other hand, pull factors refer to individual characteristics that may attract ("pull") him/her toward the VE outcome. Thus these factors are relevant at a micro level (individual needs, ambitions, frustrations, psychological characteristics, perhaps psychopathology—but see later). Again, while many (not all) violent extremists display these characteristics, most with these characteristics do *not* turn to VE.

An indicative, though incomplete, list of these putative push and pull drivers of VE is mentioned below.

Along with the push and pull factors, Vergani et al.[22] made an important third category of drivers of VE: *personal factors* (they titled their categorization "the Three Ps of radicalization"). The personal factors include: "individual psychological vulnerabilities independent of push and pull factors (e.g., mental health conditions, depression, trauma), personality traits (such as narcissism and impulsivity), biographic factors (substance abuse, prior involvement in crimes) and individually specific demographic characteristics (e.g., age, gender, country of birth) that constitute subjective states that make the individual more vulnerable to extremism."[22(p4)]

Finally, Khalil et al.[14] in their ABC model categorized the drivers into three groups:

- "*Structural motivators*: Contextual factors that may be of relevance in specific locations include, for instance, state repression, political exclusion, corruption, poverty, deprivation, injustice, inequality and discrimination. Depending on the ideology and objectives of the violent extremists in question, they may also include factors as varied as an absence of self-rule, state interventions into the affairs of other nations, the lack of Sharia law, and the presence of migrant communities deemed harmful to existing cultures.
- *Individual incentives*: This second category is comprised of economic, security based, and psychosocial benefits that are contingent on the individuals in question acting in a manner that contributes to violence. These include, for instance, material incentives

(salaries and so on), protection, status, a sense of adventure, belonging, vengeance, expected rewards in the afterlife, and a sense of purpose gained through acting in accordance with perceived ideological tenets."[14](p9) Note that some of these individual factors are categorized as "pull" factors in the scheme of Vergani et al.[22]

- "*Enabling factors*: This third category is distinguished from the previous two through being comprised of factors that enable, facilitate or channel movements within their two-dimension attitude-behavior map, rather than motivate them per se (thus, corresponding more to the 'how' questions). These include 'radical' mentors, recruiters, wider social networks, and online communities, other forms of traditional and modern media, access to weaponry and other technology, territorial control maintained by violent extremist groups, and so on."[14](p9) Again, these are categorized as "pull" factors in the scheme of Vergani et al.[22]

Thus, there is some degree of overlap and confusion between different categorizations of the drivers of VE. Despite these differences, the agreed-upon notion is that there are multiple factors acting at various levels and proximity to result in VE as a final outcome, and that there are three units of analysis: individual, group, and mass.

At the individual level of analysis, along with demography (age, sex, original location, migratory location) and biography (prior involvement in crimes and drug use), an important if controversial issue of direct interest to mental health professionals is the role of personality and especially psychopathology.

Personality, Mental Illness, and VE

Vergani et al.'s[22] scoping review identified a number of personality and psychological issues reported in the literature. These ranged from "depression, low self-esteem, personal alienation, isolation, friendless, loneliness, and misfit, and personality traits such as narcissistic personality, low tolerance of ambiguity, high personal uncertainty, black-and-white type of thinking, and impulsiveness."[22](p11)

However, it is widely agreed that there is no consistent "terrorist personality," nor is there any cognitive-psychological constellation that can confidently associate with VE, let alone predict it.

Further controversy has raged around psychopathology, mental illness, and their association with VE. At one time, almost all terrorists were thought to be psychopathic, harboring serious mental illnesses, or in some way not "normal." We have come a long way from that position. It is generally established now, barring an interesting category called "lone-actor" or "lone-wolf" or "fringe" terrorists, that there is not an increase in rates of serious mental disorders in those committing terrorist or other VE acts.

Although not a large literature, there are now a reasonable number of studies in this area, though there are methodological issues. An earlier systematic review found that "the only one common characteristic determined that terrorists are generally well-integrated, 'normal' individuals."[23](p45) Misiak et al.[24] performed a systematic review of 12 studies addressing the relationship between mental health characteristics, radicalization and mass violence acts. The authors concluded: "Results of this systematic review indicate that a unique profile of psychopathology or personality traits that makes individuals more prone to radicalization cannot be proposed based on available evidence."[24(p56)] In an earlier editorial, Bhui et al.[25] cautioned against the tendency to oversimplify matters with lack of evidence to further stigmatize those with mental illness.[25]

In contrast, a very recent study[26] systematically reviewed 25 studies on 28 samples and found an overall prevalence of mental illness to be 14% in the 19 studies with confirmed diagnoses. The authors wrote, "these results largely dispel the myth there is no mental disorder presence within terrorist samples. What we see is that mental health problems are relatively common within such studies, and are more easily identifiable when research teams are in proximity to the subjects, using standardized measures and/or have access to privileged closed-sources."[26(p8)] There is no "typical" or "common" mental disorder, diagnoses ranging from mood and anxiety disorders, psychotic disorders, personality disorders to autism spectrum disorders. The relevance of these disorders in the genesis or maintenance of VE was difficult to delineate. More importantly, these disorders and other psychological conditions, when present, were relevant only in the context of other complex needs—those of personal lives and relationships, work and (un)employment, discrimination, life changes, traumatic experiences, and substance use and addiction. Thus, mental illnesses and issues, when present, were best seen in the context of various other factors influencing the pathways to VE.

It is quite well established that mental disorders are more common in the "lone-actor" or "lone-wolf" or "fringe" terrorists, as opposed to those who operate in groups (group-actor terrorists), with some estimates reporting that 43% of the lone actors assessed had a history of mental illness and that a lone-actor terrorist was 13.5 times more likely to have a mental illness than a group actor.[27]

This area is fraught with methodological hurdles, from definitions of "terrorist" and "mental illness," sample selection, control group, assessment issues, analysis, and inference.[28,29] Very importantly, such research does not tell us which led to what, because both the "outcomes" (mental illness and terrorist or other VE act) have already occurred. Another strand of research has been done with those who express "sympathy for violent radicalization or actions" drawn from the general population but not categorized as VE or terrorists. This strategy can potentially identify those with a future risk of behavioral radicalization, though presently this has more to do with cognitive radicalization. The role of depression in this case has been demonstrated in a series of studies conducted in the United Kingdom.[30,31] The causal pathways remain to be determined. The complexity of the situation is captured in a recent study where depression, religiosity, and social support moderated the association between social adversity and sympathy for violent radicalization.[32] Thus, there is clear implication for the mental health professional.

Perhaps Al-Attar,[33] in his recent formulation, captures the situation aptly:

> There is consensus that mental illness is not a direct risk factor and that a more nuanced understanding of the links between mental illness and terrorism is warranted in order to inform sound practice. . . . Where such mental illnesses

contribute to push and pull factors for terrorism in an individual, they often do so in complex and often indirect ways and through specific symptoms and their experience by the individual. Such symptoms typically interact with other factors such as social, attitudinal, ideological and environmental factors, to shape vulnerability (to terrorism).[33(p17)]

Comprehensive Theories

Keeping in view the diverse range of drivers and pathways of radicalization to VE, and the principles of equifinality and multifinality, it is very difficult to arrive at any one comprehensive theory to explain both the why and how of radicalization to VE including terrorism. Individual theories have tried to capture parts of the complex phenomenon. For example, there have been attempts to find biological correlates of VE behavior by neuroimaging and social neuroscience.[34,35] Many sociological theories have been invoked. These include: functionalism, social movement theory, social control theory, relative deprivation theory, and so on.[36] Social psychology theories have focused on social forces influencing individual actions.[36] Individual psychology theories include rational choice theory and conflict theory, among others.

However, none of these in isolation can explain the complexity of the VE phenomenon. Hence combined theories have been developed. Two recent and promising theories are briefly presented here.

Needs, Narrative, Network ("3N") Theory

This theory, developed by Arie Kruglanski, David Webber, and their associates from the United States, is an elaboration of their primary theory of quest for significance. In essence, it posits that radicalization to VE occurs by the combination of three essential elements or ingredients—the universal *need* of every human being to achieve "significance" in some form (esteem, achievement, status, power, control, meaning) and the frustration/grievance from loss of such significance by whatever means (deprivation, humiliation, loss, threat, etc.); a *narrative* that makes sense of the world in a particular way for a particular audience—in this case, an ideology justifying violence; and a social *network* of persons (which may be physical or virtual) which makes this narrative accessible to the person and validates the reality of the violence-justifying narrative by sharing and reinforcement and thus makes it morally acceptable. It is the combination of these elements that goes into the "making of violent extremists."[37,38] This theory, other than making good intuitive and logical sense, has been gaining some empirical research ground recently and has provided heuristic impetus for new research in this area.[37,39,40]

Person-Situation Theory

The other very recent theory, again by Arie Kruglanski along with Preben Bertelsen from Denmark, is actually a hybrid model that integrates the 3N model with Bertelsen's Life Psychology Model.[41] The latter provides the theoretical framework for the influential mentoring program for counter-terrorism initiatives in Denmark, also known as the Aarhus/ Denmark model.[42,43] According to this framework, "the root factor underlying extremism is an insecure or disordered life attachment and the primary risk factor in extremism is a deficiently formed set of general human life skills. For the state of non-flow to lead to violent extremism, reinforcing personal, external and structural factors may be at work. These reinforcing risk factors are classifiable into the categories of social and societal factors on the one hand and psychological and/or cognitive factors on the other."[42(p162)] There is cross-national (U.S. and Denmark) support for this model as well.[43] While this model, like the 3N model, is individually focused, the life psychology model places more explicit emphasis beyond individual psychology, on the socioeconomic as well as sociocultural factors in the meso- and macro-domains as objective risk factors.

The Person-Situation (P-S) model captures this social-situational dimension and places it in perspective to explain radicalization to VE. In this integrated hybrid model, it is the *position* of a person in social, cultural, and societal networks, rather than only his needs as envisaged in the 3N model, that influences the vulnerability to radicalization. Once the adverse position in social, cultural, and societal networks makes the person vulnerable, this, in conjunction with the narrative and network ingredients, influences a full-blown shift to radicalization into VE. The position is a fluid state and is more than the person's quest for significance; it also means the person's quest for life attachment. The position is determined by two categories of factors: person and situation. The *person* factor comprises the needs as in the 3N model, plus the deficit in life skills in various domains. The second, and important, factor that determines a person's position is called *situation*. "The situation category refers to the socio-political, social, cultural and societal environment in which the persons exist. It includes the nature of the political system, and its affordance of legal recourses for addressing grievances and felt injustices. It also includes the degree of state control over population's actions, and its ability to enforce the laws of the land."[41(p17)] Thus the situation factor is the crucial addition in the P-S model. It implies that not only subjective, internal, and evaluative cognitive factors, but also objective, external sociopolitical factors, are important in determining a person's position with respect to the society as the drivers of radicalization. The P-S model emphasizes the social, cultural, and sociopolitical task of facilitating human life conditions and positioning, marked by personal significance and secure life attachment. Hence it has obvious implications for de-radicalization policies as well—that, "countering radicalisation cannot be fully accomplished by interventions (e.g. of a psychological nature) aimed exclusively at the individual. Instead, a whole society approach is required."[41(p18)] Although very promising in its intuitive appeal, it is at a rather abstract level at this stage, and would require empirical research and validation.

Role of "Social" and "Psychiatry" in Terrorism and Other Forms of VE

It has become progressively clearer over the years that terrorism and other forms of VE cannot be understood, let alone prevented or countered (the P/CVE initiatives), by looking

TABLE 35.1 Various Levels of Explanatory Analytic Factors and Models

Levels of Analysis	Macro	Meso	Micro
Units of analysis	Structural	Group	Individual
Drivers of VE	Push	Pull	Personal
Social science discipline	Sociology, politics, economics, history, religion	Social psychology	Individual psychology
3N Model	Narrative	Network	Needs
P-S Model	Situation	Position	Person

through simplistic, linear, one-cause and one-path theories and measures. No single perspective or explanatory perspective—strictly psychological-psychopathological, strictly sociological, or strictly structural (political-economic-institutional)—is sufficient to explain, predict, and counter the processes and drivers of radicalization to, and de-radicalization from, VE. It is a complex mixture—in various permutation-combinations—of all or most of the factors reviewed above.

However, in all these things, two essential facts are inescapable: first, the role of the "social" factors at all levels of analysis, across all theories, models, and hypotheses; and second, the ultimate focus on the individual. The P-S model captures this dual element quite well at a conceptual level.

Table 35.1 provides a summary of various models and conceptualizations.

Central Importance of the "Meso" Level

Of these levels, it is the "meso" level that is the most essential. It connects the macro and the micro levels. For example, in a recent conceptualization of religious radicalization, it has been argued that "meso-level approaches best explain religious radicalization. These meso-level approaches explain how members of extreme religious groups appraise societal conditions and find redemption in radical beliefs.[44] Similarly, Rousseau and Hassan,[45] talking about the challenges in addressing youth mental health in the context of violent radicalization (VR), have emphasized that "(a) social changes explain some, but not all, of VR; (b) the internet explains some, but not all, of VR; and (c) psychopathology explains some, but not all, of VR."[45(p747)] Another study by the same group found that depression, religiosity, and social support mediated or moderated the link between social adversity (as experienced discrimination or violence) and sympathy toward VR in a large college student sample in Quebec, Canada.[46]

Such studies underscore the need to understand this complex issue through the lens of social psychology and social psychiatry. The authors make the important conclusion that "such results support the importance of adopting an ecological and public health approach to the study of violent radicalization phenomena, able to take into account the interplay of individual, contextual and social variables in determining the risks associated with SVR, while focusing on prevention."[46]

Social Identity, Collective Identity, Identity Fusion

Indeed, social psychology and social psychiatry are disciplines best suited to study the interaction of a person within the matrix of social network to lead to outcomes that cannot be explained in isolation of each other. A decade ago, Jerrold Post put it candidly and emphatically, worth citing in full:

> It is not individual psychology, but group, organizational, and social psychology, with a particular emphasis on "collective identity," that provides the most powerful lens to understand terrorist psychology and behavior. . . . The importance of collective identity and the processes of forming and transforming collective identities cannot be overemphasized. This in turn emphasizes the sociocultural context, which determines the balance between collective identity and individual identity. A clear consensus exists that it is not understanding individual psychopathology but group, organizational, and social psychology, which provides the greatest analytic power in understanding this complex phenomenon, a phenomenon where collective identity is paramount. Terrorists have subordinated their individual identity to the collective identity, so that what serves the group, organization, or network is of primary importance.[47(pp15-16)]

Even for the individual psychology–oriented 3N model, there are several clear "social" elements. The authors themselves commented on the "social psychological makings of the terrorist" while explaining their model.[38] Social network is the obvious enabler and validator of the "shared reality" of the violence-justifying narratives to the person on the quest for significance in life position. As the authors say, "individuals who both experience a quest for significance and are embedded in a social network that subscribes to a violence justifying narrative will be more likely to engage in violent extremism than individuals who experience only one, or neither, of those."[37(p116)] However, both the personal needs as well as the narratives are also influenced and co-produced by social factors. For example, "individuals gain personal significance from belonging to important social groups. When these groups are socially, economically, or politically discriminated against, these conditions can be a potent source of significance loss. In such cases, the group members experience a threat to their social identity that may prompt aggression against the groups' perceived detractors."[37(p117)]

In this regard, it is noteworthy that the study which found empirical validation of the 3N model explicitly used social alienation as the variable for measuring "need."[39] A recent study found significant interactions between social context and quest for significance on violent extremism; in particular, across 4 studies set in Sri Lanka, Morocco, and Indonesia, the authors "found evidence that radical social contexts strengthen the link between quest for significance—particularly collective significance—and support for political violence."[48(p1182)]

One of the important constructs that can help to understand the phenomenon of VE at a social-psychological level is that of social identity.[49] As originally proposed by Tajfel et al.,[50] social identity is a person's sense of who they are based on their group membership(s). While this is a normal cognitive process of categorizing those around us and to identify where we "belong," and hence define "in-groups" and "out-groups," it can become extreme and lead to stereotypy, xenophobia, and even violence against the perceived "out-groups." One of the most vicious instances can arise "when people become fused with a group, their personal and social identities become functionally equivalent" giving rise to "identity fusion."[51(p1008)] Extreme forms of behavior, including terrorism and other VE, can result from this identity fusion with a violence-justifying and violence-promoting in-group (religious, supremacists, or other group characteristics) perpetrated against socially categorized out-groups.

This fused "collective identity" has recently been studied in the same large Canadian student sample mentioned above, in relation with social adversity (discrimination and exposure to violence), and sympathy for violent radicalization.[32] The results, although complex and multifaceted, confirmed that "group belonging, collective identity perception, and its negotiation in the public space may be a source of hurt and threat for college students in the present context, confirming the triad of injustice, identity, and belonging, identified as key in the radicalization."[32(p10)]

A very recent and comprehensive meta-analysis of putative risk and protective factors for various radicalization outcomes (attitudes, intention, action) was conducted on 57 studies on 62 individual factors.[52] As a surprising finding, the authors found very little support for the role of traditional sociodemographic factors and higher role of criminogenic (past history or involvement with crime) and criminotrophic factors (low self-control, thrill seeking). However, even these authors, studying from a criminological perspective, conceded that "factors associated with social controls and bonds, such as parental involvement, school bonding, types of peers (e.g. deviant, similar, out-group), integration, attitudinal factors relating to the law and institutions, moral neutralizations, and radical attitudes themselves, had the largest estimates."[52(p437)] Again, the focus was on social controls and bonds.

Box 35.1 summarizes the various terms involving "social" in context of VE, at the "meso" analytic level.

The Paradox of the "Lone-Actor" Terrorist

Most of the discussion above has revolved around terrorists or other violent extremists who act in a group. This "in-group" to which they belong provides them with the rationale and moral justification for violence, provides them direction and support of various kinds, and help them maintain their identity (though it may be a "fused" collective identity) and goals. As mentioned above, most of these people do not appear to have overt psychopathology or serious mental illnesses. Most importantly, they operate within the rules, norms, and directives of the defined group to which they belong.

The "lone-actor" terrorists (variously also known as "lone wolf" or "fringe" terrorists), on the other hand, appear to be of a different kind. As the name suggests, they do not align themselves to a specified terrorist or other VE group membership. They tend to be reclusive, and operate alone. Most importantly, in contrast to the group-actor terrorists, they have a much higher prevalence of documented psychiatric disorders (most notably

---

BOX 35.1. Various Terms Involving "Social" in the Context of VE, at the "Meso" Analytic Level

(Loosening of) social controls and social cohesion

De-socialization from the mainstream

Re-socialization into radicalized groups

Social context

Social (group) dynamics

Social cognition

Social appraisal

Social identity/collective identity

In-group/out-group phenomenon ("us vs. them")

Social networks

Social narratives

Socially mediated quest for significance

Social narratives—discourses of threat, injustice, salvation, and significance

---

schizophrenia and other psychotic disorders), 13.5 times higher in one oft-cited series.[27] They appear to challenge the social-based discourse narrated above, and appear to correspond more closely with the stereotype of "crazed fanatics" referred to by Post.[47] Social theories and relevance to social psychology and psychiatry do not appear applicable to them, thus posing an apparent paradox.

However, a number of studiers and publications in the recent years have challenged this concept.[53-56] It now appears that, with the right kind of painstaking analysis with social network modeling and other in-depth analysis, the lone actors are not so "alone" after all. "Put simply, the current empirical scholarship on lone-actor terrorism argues that their motivations, methods, and ideologies are influenced by their larger socio-political environments and by their interactions and relationships with other people."[53(p15)] In Schuurman et al.'s in-depth study of 55 lone-actor terrorists, it was found that 62% turned out to have contacts with clearly radical, extremist, or terrorist individuals. Moreover, 33% socialized with individuals who could be designated as leaders or authority figures within radical, extremist, or terrorist groups. Finally, 31% were recognized members or participants in radical, extremist, or terrorist groups at some point in their lives. Further, 78% of the sample were exposed to external sources of encouragement or justification for the use of violence, i.e., they were immersed in a "radical milieu." "In short, our findings suggest that social settings supportive of radicalism, extremism, or terrorism play an important role part in the commission of extremist events, even for those thought of as "lone" actors."[55] Based on this and other facts and considerations, these same authors have actually questioned the categorization of lone actor terrorism itself.[3] The study by Bright et al.[54] also echoes similar findings and conclusions. Thus, it appears that the "social" concept is very much relevant for the so-called lone actor terrorists too.

Role of Social Psychiatry and Socially Oriented Mental Health Professionals

The essential nature of the "social" component of terrorism and other VE in all its shapes and sizes, along with the fact that eventually one is dealing with cognitively or behaviorally radicalized individuals who intend to enact, or actually engage in, "extremes" of behaviors with the potential to cause harm, makes a strong case for the involvement of social psychiatry.

A few caveats are important. First, conflicts and extremism, however violent, are not medical conditions themselves, though they may lead to many. By the same token, terrorism and other VE are not mental illnesses per se, though these are aberrant behaviors. Second, the role of a psychiatrist or other mental health professionals should not include "screening for VE" or "terrorist profiling" as part of the government's counter-terrorism or P/CVE strategies, due to lack of evidence of such an approach, and serious ethical issues including obvious role conflict, loss of therapist-patient relationship, loss of trust, and impaired privacy and confidentiality. Finally, forensic psychiatry's role in assessing and treating severe mental illnesses in the conspicuous minority of those engaged in terrorist or other VE acts is much focused and very different from the broader role of social psychiatry and socially oriented mental health professionals.

With these caveats, let us see in which ways can social psychiatry and socially oriented mental health professionals contribute to the area of VE (Box 35.2).
A brief description of each follows.

Catering to the Needs of Those Affected by Terrorism and other VE

This is intuitively obvious, keeping in view the mental health impact of such events on not only the directly affected person but also the family, other witnesses, and larger society

---

BOX 35.2. Role of Social Psychiatry and Socially Oriented Mental Health Professionals*

Catering to the needs of those affected by terrorism and other VE

Countering stigma

Theoretical understanding and research

Clinical, risk, and psychosocial assessment

Prevention/countering of VE (P/CVE)

Advocacy

Multi-sector coordination

Community-based working

Public health perspective

*Adapted and enlarged from Dom et al. (2018), Ho et al. (2018), and Weine et al., (2017).[28,57,58]

members. This process can be tortuous, long, and complicated. "Social-mindedness" is highly desirable to assess, empathize, and manage the multilayered trauma, rather than only prescribing medications. As the *Lancet Psychiatry* editorial put it quite succinctly:

> First, individuals with ongoing traumatic stress disorders, mood disorders, and other mental health problems require treatment for many years after the violence stops. Second, there is the broader issue of the economic damage wrought by conflict, which can increase the ongoing population risk for mental disorders and suicide. Finally, there are the less tangible, but no less important, problems faced by a society that shares a history viewed from radically different perspectives. For societies to recover after years—sometimes decades—of conflict, mental health professionals must be prepared to help people individually and collectively to reconcile themselves with the past, and to construct a stable and equitable future.[9]

Countering Stigma

Social psychiatry has an important role in preventing and countering stigma. Stigma may be associated with victims of VE, or with the stereotyped perpetrators of such attacks, either at the governmental level (e.g., as a fallout of strict counter-terrorism measures) or at the societal level (e.g., Islamophobia—a paranoid attitude toward, and phobic avoidance of, all Muslims because of their purported association with religious-based terrorism). Stigma is of course directed against many of the far-right VE targets (e.g., LGBTQ community, people of color or particular communities etc.).

Theoretical Understanding and Research

As demonstrated above, social psychology and psychiatry are best equipped to capture the confluence of structural macro level and the intrapersonal micro level—i.e., the meso level, where society and the person meet, shape, and influence each other. Thus, research in the understanding of various aspects of the genesis, maintenance, and exit from VE can benefit greatly by contributions from these disciplines.

Clinical, Risk, and Psychosocial Assessment

At the individual level, an enhanced understanding of the social principles of mental health can inform the assessment of individuals involved in VE and their family and/or network members. Assessment can also be important for the so-called lone-actor VE because of their unusual characteristics.

Prevention/Countering of VE (P/CVE)

This is an area of intense attention at the national and international arenas for a number of years now, especially since the last decade or so. The original focus was on counter-terrorism, which concerned itself with detecting, disrupting, and dealing with terrorist groups, preventing terrorist attacks, and managing the aftermath of terrorist acts using security force and criminal justice systems. While this of course has to continue, gradually the focus also has highlighted VE and how to counter it. Language changed later to the prevention of VE, with similar content, though with some controversy. The two terms are used more or less synonymously in the context of VE. Essentially, the P/CVE approach emphasizes addressing the conditions conducive to the genesis, spread, and maintenance of terrorism; in other words, the drivers of radicalization to VE. While most of these are at the macro level (international, national, regional), addressing the structural "push" factors (repression, inequities, corruption, deprivation, etc.), quite a few address the "pull" and "personal" factors operating at the meso and micro levels, respectively, for example, by empowering youth, families, women, religious, cultural, and education leaders, and all other concerned groups of civil society, and promoting social inclusion and cohesion. At the micro levels, attention to adverse childhood traumatic experiences, psychological and personality factors, and early detection and treatment of any psychiatric disorder could be of help. Mental health professionals can take part in these.

Advocacy

It is imperative upon social psychiatry to advocate the structural and social determinants of health, including mental health, to liaise with the government, to contact the electronic, print, and social media, and to talk about increasing social inclusivity, respect for diversity, and enhancing equity. Social psychiatry can help to develop counter-narratives and build counter-networks by their presence and advocacy.

Multi-Sector Coordination

Sestoft et al.[59] described a system operating in Denmark since 2009. Called the PSP model, it is a system of coordination among the police, social system, and psychiatrists, which provide a joint platform for detecting, managing, and monitoring risk in the community. The PSP cooperation already facilitates the identification of citizens at many kinds of risk (e.g., suicide, substance abuse, social decline, mental illness), and coordinates relevant intervention and treatment. The existing PSP cooperation is, therefore, an obvious forum for identifying and handling concerns of radicalization and extremism.[59] The Aarhus Model is another mentoring program in Denmark utilizing the life psychology model mentioned above[42] for guiding deradicalization efforts. Socially oriented mental health professionals can play a significant contributory part in such coordinated efforts.[45]

Community-Based Working

Weine et al.[58] have provided an excellent overview of the many ways mental health professionals can become involved with community-based targeted violence prevention. They describe a model of such a community-based program. As the authors write: "This model consists of a multidisciplinary team that assesses at-risk individuals with comprehensive threat and behavioral evaluations, arranges for ongoing support and treatment, conducts follow-up evaluations, and offers outreach, education, and resources for communities. This model would enable mental health professionals in local communities to play key roles in preventing violent extremism through their practice and leadership."[58(p56)] In fact, they have provided a useful summary of the practical ways a mental health professional can contribute:

- "*Attend*: Provide a safe space for a client to express their views on identity, grievances, discrimination, profiling, politics, foreign policy, or violence.
- *Ask*: Consult with religious leaders or cultural experts to better understand the context of their client's experience.
- *Build trust*: Help community members to understand how community-based violence prevention works and why they [*sic*] are needed.
- *Mobilize*: Enlist a professional peer group, including other disciplines/cultures, to discuss violent extremism.
- *Partner*: Get to know your local law enforcement agencies and give them a directory of local providers.
- *Remember*: Consider ideologically inspired violence when assessing for violence.
- *Self-educate*: Get trained in threat assessment.
- *Educate*: Teach students and trainees about the causes and responses to violent extremism."[58(p56)]

Public Health Perspective

Last but not the least, mental health professionals can play an important role when VE is viewed "through a public health prevention lens"[60(p341)] and dealt with on par with prevention efforts for interpersonal violence and gang violence in the community. In fact, the social-ecological model for potential risks factors for ideologically motivated violence[61] fits in quite well with the current push-pull-personal model for radicalization into VE.[22] Thus, the WHO model for preventing violence by public health approach should also be at least partly applicable to P/CVE. The advantage would be to connect the programs together in the local and national contexts. The recent document from the United Kingdom also highlights several possible integration pathways for P/CVE with public health initiatives.[62]

Conclusion

In this chapter, I have argued that social psychiatry has a central role to play in understanding the origin, spread, consequences, and possible mitigation of VE including terrorism. Such phenomena essentially build upon the interaction of an individual with his/her sociocultural-economic-political milieu. This applies even to the "lone-actor" terrorist. A currently influential psychological theory of VE—the 3N model (needs, narrative, and network)[37]—is actually psychosocial. A socially oriented psychiatrist or related mental health professional is hence particularly enabled to appreciate the psychological/psychiatric aspects of the individual involved/inducted in VE and the socio-environmental factors that generate and mediate the needs, narrative, and network which goes into the making, maintenance, and possible exit from VE.

References

1. United Nations. *A New Era of Conflict and Violence.* 2020. Available at: https://www.un.org/en/un75/new-era-conflict-and-violence. Accessed November 6, 2020.

2. Institute for Economics & Peace. *Global Terrorism Index 2019: Measuring the Impact of Terrorism.* Sydney: IEP; November 2019. http://visionofhumanity.org/reports. Accessed November 6, 2020.

3. Schuurman B, Bakker E. Reintegrating Jihadist extremists: evaluating a Dutch initiative, 2013–2014. *Behav Sci Terror Political Aggress.* 2015;8(1):66–85.

4. National Consortium for the Study of Terrorism and Responses to Terrorism (START). Global Terrorism Database (GTD). 2020. https://www.start.umd.edu/research-projects/global-terrorism-database-gtd. Accessed November 8, 2020.

5. Institute for Economics & Peace. Global Terrorism Index 2022: Measuring the Impact of Terrorism, Sydney, March 2022. Available from: http://visionofhumanity.org/resources. Accessed November 22, 2022.

6. Institute for Economics & Peace. *Global Peace Index 2020: Measuring Peace in a Complex World.* Sydney: IEP; June 2020. http://visionofhumanity.org/reports. Accessed November 6, 2020.

7. GBD 2019 Diseases and Injuries Collaborators. Global burden of 369 diseases and injuries in 204 countries and territories, 1990–2019: a systematic analysis for the Global Burden of Disease Study 2019. *Lancet.* 2020;396(10258):1204–1222.

8. Arce DG. On the human consequences of terrorism. *Public Choice.* 2019;178:371–396.

9. *The Lancet Psychiatry.* Terrorism and conflict: effects beyond trauma. *Lancet Psychiatry.* 2019;6(1):1.

10. Basu D, Hans G. Social impact of terrorism and extremism. In: Chadda R, Kumar V, Sarkar, S, eds. *Social Psychiatry: Principles and Clinical Perspectives.* New Delhi: Jaypee; 2018:458–468.

11. Durodié B, Wainwright D. Terrorism and post-traumatic stress disorder: a historical review. *Lancet Psychiatry.* 2019;6(1):61–71.

12. Grieger TA. *Psychiatric and Societal Impacts of Terrorism.* June 1, 2006. http://www.psychiatrictimes.com/disaster psychiatry/psychiatric and societal impact of terrorism. Accessed November 8, 2020.

13. Borum R. Radicalization into violent extremism II: a review of conceptual models and empirical research. *J Strateg Secur.* 2011;4(4):37–62.

14. Khalil J, Horgan J, Zeuthen M. The Attitudes-Behaviors Corrective (ABC) model of violent extremism. *Terror Political Violence.* 2019:1–26. doi: 10.1080/09546553.2019.1699793.

15. Borum R. Understanding the terrorist mindset. *FBI Law Enforce Bull.* 2003;72(7):7–10.

16. Moghaddam FM. The staircase to terrorism: a psychological exploration. *Am Psychol.* 2005;60:161–169.

17. McCauley C, Moskalenko S. Understanding political radicalization: the two-pyramids model. *Am Psychol.* 2017;72(3):205–216.

18. Carlsson C, Rostami A, Mondani H, et al. A life-course analysis of engagement in violent extremist groups. *Br J Criminol.* 2020;60:74–92.

19. Cicchetti D, Rogosc, FA. Equifinality and multifinality in developmental psychopathology. *Devel Psychopathol.* 1996;8(4):597–600.

20. United Nations Development Programme (UNDP). *Preventing Violent Extremism Through Promoting Inclusive Development, Tolerance and Respect for Diversity.* Vienna: UNDP; 2016.

21. UNODC. *Drivers of Violent Extremism.* 2018. https://www.unodc.org/e4j/en/terrorism/module-2/key-issues/drivers-of-violent-extremism.html. Accessed November 10, 2020.

22. Vergani M, Iqbal M, Ilbahar E, Barton G. The three Ps of radicalization: Push, Pull and Personal: a systematic scoping review of the scientific evidence about radicalization into violent extremism. *Studies Conflict Terror.* 2018:1–32. doi: 10.1080/1057610X.2018.1505686.

23. McGilloway A, Ghosh P. Bhui, K. A systematic review of pathways to and processes associated with radicalization and extremism amongst Muslims in Western societies. *Int Rev Psychiatry (Abingdon, England).* 2015;27(1):39–50.

24. Misiak B, Samochowiec J, Bhui K, et al. A systematic review on the relationship between mental health, radicalization and mass violence. *Eur Psychiatry.* 2019 Feb;56:51–59.

25. Bhui K, James A, Wessely S. Mental illness and terrorism. *BMJ (Clinical Research Ed.).* 2016;354:i4869.

26. Gill P, Clemmow C, Hetzel F, et al. Systematic review of mental health problems and violent extremism. *J Forens Psychiatry Psychol.* 2020:1–28. doi: 10.1080/14789949.2020.1820067

27. Corner E, Gill P. A false dichotomy? Mental illness and lone-actor terrorism. *Law Human Behav.* 2015;39:23–34.

28. Ho CSH, Quek TC, Ho RCM, Choo CC. Towards an integrated pragmatic approach in terrorism and mental illness. *B J Psych Advances.* 2019;25:101–109.

29. Gill P, Corner E. There and back again: the study of mental disorder and terrorist involvement. *Am Psychol.* 2017;72:231–241.

30. Bhui K, Silva MJ, Topciu RA, Jones E. Pathways to sympathies for violent protest and terrorism. *Br J Psychiatry.* 2016;209:483–490.

31. Bhui K, Otis M, Silva MJ, Halvorsrud K, Freestone M, Jones E. Extremism and common mental illness: cross-sectional community survey of White British and Pakistani men and women living in England. *Br J Psychiatry.* 2020;217(4):547–554.

32. Rousseau C, Hassan G, Miconi D, et al. From social adversity to sympathy for violent radicalization: the role of depression, religiosity and social support. *Arch Public Health.* 2019;77:45. https://doi.org/10.1186/s13690-019-0372-y.

33. Al-Attar Z. Severe mental disorder and terrorism: when psychosis, PTSD and addictions become a vulnerability. *J Forens Psychiatry Psychol.* 2020:1–22. https://doi.org/10.1080/14789949.2020.1812696. Accessed November 10, 2020.

34. Bogerts B, Schone M, Breitschuh S. Brain alterations potentially associated with aggression and terrorism. *CNS Spectrums.* 2018;23:129–140.

35. Decety J, Pape R, Workman CI. A multilevel social neuroscience perspective on radicalization and terrorism. *Social Neurosci.* 2018;13(5):511–529.

36. Borum R. Radicalization into violent extremism I: a review of social science theories. *J Strateg Secur.* 2011;4(4):7–36.

37. Kruglanski A, Jasko K, Webber D, Chernikova M, Molinario E. The making of violent extremists. *Rev Gen Psychol.* 2018;22(1):107–120.

38. Webber D, Kruglanski AW. The social psychological makings of a terrorist. *Curr Opin Psychol.* 2018;19:131–134.

39. Bélanger JJ, Moyano M, Muhammad H, et al. Radicalization leading to violence: a test of the 3N model. *Front Psychiatry.* 2019;10:42. https://doi.org/10.3389/fpsyt.2019.00042.

40. Lobato RM, Moyano M, Bélanger JJ, Trujillo HM. The role of vulnerable environments in support for homegrown terrorism: fieldwork using the 3N model. *Aggress Behav.* 2020;10.1002/ab.2193. https://doi.org/10.1002/ab.21933.

41. Kruglanski AW, Bertelsen P. Life psychology and significance quest: a complementary approach to violent extremism and counter-radicalisation. *J Polic Intel Counter Terror.* 2020;15(1):1–22. doi: 10.1080/18335330.2020.1725098.

42. Bertelsen, P. The fight against violent extremism: the Aarhus model. In: J. Kärgel, ed. *"They Have No Plan B.": Radicalization, Departure, Return—Between Prevention and Intervention.* Bonn: Bundeszentrale für politische Bildung; 2018:154–170.

43. Ozer S, Bertelsen P. Countering radicalization: an empirical examination from a life psychological perspective. *Peace Conflict.* 2019;25(3):211–225.

44. de Graaf BA, van den Bos K. Religious radicalization: social appraisals and finding radical redemption in extreme beliefs. *Curr Opin Psychol.* 2021;40:56–60.

45. Rousseau C, Hassan G. Current challenges in addressing youth mental health in the context of violent radicalization. *J Ame Acad Child Adolesc Psychiatry.* 2019;58:747–750.

46. Rousseau C, Oulhote Y, Lecompte V, Mekki-Berrada A, Hassan G, El Hage H. Collective identity, social adversity and college student sympathy for violent radicalization. *Transcult Psychiatry.* 2019:1363461519853653.

47. Post JM. "When hatred is bred in the bone": the social psychology of terrorism. *Ann NY Acad Sci.* 2010;1208:15–23.

48. Jasko K, Webber D, Kruglanski AW, et al. Social context moderates the effects of quest for significance on violent extremism. *J Pers Soc Psychol.* 2020;118(6):1165–1187.

49. McLeod SA. *Social Identity Theory*. Simply Psychology. 2019, October 24. https://www.simplypsychology.org/social-identity-theory.html. Accessed November 12, 2020.

50. Tajfel H, Turner JC, Austin WG, Worchel S. An integrative theory of intergroup conflict. *Organizational Identity: A Reader*; 1979:56–65.

51. Swann WB Jr, Gómez Á, Seyle DC, Morales JF, Huici C. Identity fusion: the interplay of personal and social identities in extreme group behavior. *J Pers Soc Psychol*. 2009;96(5):995–1011.

52. Wolfowicz M, Litmanovitz Y, Weisburd D, et al. A field-wide systematic review and meta-analysis of putative risk and protective factors for radicalization outcomes. *J Quant Criminol*. 2020;36:407–447.

53. Hofmann DC. How "alone" are lone-actors? Exploring the ideological, signaling, and support networks of lone-actor terrorists. *Studies Conflict Terror*. 2018:1–22. doi: 10.1080/1057610X.2018.1493833.

54. Bright D, Whelan C, Harris-Hogan S. Exploring the hidden social networks of "lone actor" terrorists. *Crime Law Soc Change*. 2020;74:491–508.

55. Schuurman B, Bakker E, Gill P, Bouhana N. Lone actor terrorist attack planning and preparation: a data-driven analysis. *J Forens Sci*. 2018;63(4):1191–1200.

56. Schuurman B, Lindekilde L, Malthaner S, et al. End of the lone wolf: the typology that should not have been. *Studies Conflict Terror*. 2019;42(8):771–778.

57. Dom G, Schouler-Ocak M, Bhui K, et al. Mass violence, radicalization and terrorism: a role for psychiatric profession? *Eur Psychiatry*. 2018;49:78–80.

58. Weine SM, Stone A, Saeed A, et al. Violent extremism, community-based violence prevention, and mental health professionals. *J Nerv Mental Dis*. 2017;205(1):54–57.

59. Sestoft D, Hansen SM, Christensen AB. The police, social services, and psychiatry (PSP) cooperation as a platform for dealing with concerns of radicalization. *Int Rev Psychiatry*. 2017;29(4):350–354.

60. Eisenman DP, Flavahan L. Canaries in the coal mine: interpersonal violence, gang violence, and violent extremism through a public health prevention lens. *Int Rev Psychiatry*. 2017;29(4):341–349.

61. Butchart A, Phinney A, Check P, Villaveces A. *Preventing Violence: A Guide to Implementing the Recommendations of the World Report on Violence and Health*. Geneva: World Health Organization (WHO); 2004:1–92.

62. Bellis MA, Hardcastle K. *Preventing Violent Extremism in the UK: Public Health Solutions*. Cardiff; Public Health Wales; 2019.

36

Youth Violence

A Social Psychiatry Perspective

Eugenio M. Rothe, Yoshiro Ono, and
Andres J. Pumariega

Introduction

The World Health Organization (WHO)[1(p5)] defines violence as "the intentional use of physical force or power, threatened or actual, against oneself, another person, or against a group or community, which either results in or has a high likelihood of resulting in injury, death, psychological harm, maldevelopment or deprivation." The WHO divides violence into three broad categories according to the characteristics of those committing the violent act: (1) self-directed violence, (2) interpersonal violence, and (3) collective violence. Self-directed violence typically includes suicidal behaviors, attempted suicides, completed suicides, and self-abusive acts such as self-mutilation. Interpersonal violence has two major domains; family–intimate partner violence and community violence. Collective violence refers to violence committed by larger groups of individuals, and can be subdivided into social, political, and economic violence. Violent acts are classified into four types by their nature: (1) physical, sexual; (2) psychological; and (3) deprivation or neglect.[2] From a clinical perspective, violence is considered to be interpersonal aggressive behavior, including aggressive behaviors toward the self, objects, or authorities. In the social context, violence is considered to be illegal or deviant behavior differing from the norm of the community one belongs to. Although violence has existed in all of human history, it has only recently been recognized as a public health issue because of its major impact on the physical and mental health of both victims and perpetrators.[3] Societal reactions toward violence vary and depend on the geographic region, the current historical events, and the social context in which it occurs. People who injure or kill, destroy property, or violate laws are typically held accountable in a manner appropriate for their developmental level, and children are often the victims of violence in the midst of wars, terrorism, or riots. They sometimes also commit violent acts during wars or significant violent criminal offenses in the community. In addition to the visible violence that is perpetrated by and toward children and adolescents, there are also hidden forms of violence, such as child abuse and neglect and school bullying, that can have devastating and long-lasting impact on the minds of young people.[3]

Epidemiology of Youth Violence Worldwide

Only a small proportion of acts of violence against children are reported and investigated, and few perpetrators are held to account. In terms of youth perpetrators, the scant data that exist point to regional differences. According to the WHO data on homicide rates per 100,000 population age 10–29 years in 2000, the rates are highest in Latin America, the Caribbean, the Russian Federation, and some countries of southeastern Europe. On the other hand, countries in western Europe (such as France, Germany, and the United Kingdom), or in Asia (such as Japan) have the lowest rates, at below 1.0 per 100,000. The homicide rate in the United States was 11.0 in the year 2000, which was rather high among the industrialized countries, and most homicide deaths in the United States are characterized by firearm assault, as compared to other high-income countries where violent death by firearm assault is quite rare. Thus, there is a substantial difference not only in rate but also in means of homicide between countries or regions, suggesting sociocultural influences on the epidemiology of violent behaviors in children and adolescents. A cross-national study of non-fatal violence-related behaviors, such as physical fighting, bullying, carrying weapons, and injuries from fighting in adolescents among five countries (Ireland, Israel, Portugal, Sweden, and the United States), revealed that the most frequent behavior was physical fighting (40.3%), followed by bullying (33.7%) and injuries from fighting (15.8%), with carrying weapons being the least frequent response (10.7%). Those frequencies of violence-related behaviors were similar in all five countries, except for bullying perpetrated by adolescents, with the prevalence rates ranging from 14.8% in Sweden to 42.9% in Israel.[4]

Violence against children and adolescents has been increasingly acknowledged to have an immediate and long-term impact on the victim's health. Young children are particularly vulnerable to any form of violence, including child abuse, and are likely to experience devastating consequences for their physical and emotional development and mental health. Older children and adolescents are also likely to be victimized, but at the same time are likely to also be perpetrators, and there is a direct relationship with having been a victim of violence in childhood and later becoming a perpetrator.[3] In addition, exposure to violence in early life is particularly critical because it can have an impact on early brain development. Infants and toddlers who witness violence either in their homes or in their communities show excessive irritability, immature behavior, sleep disturbances, emotional distress, fears of being alone, and regression in toileting and language. In older children and adolescents, associations have been established between exposure to community violence and post-traumatic stress disorder, depression, antisocial behaviors, substance abuse, decline in academic performance, problematic relations, and greater involvement with the criminal justice system.[5] Social cognition in youth exposed to violence changes their interpretation of their surrounding reality through several mediating factors, such as the creation of new normative beliefs about violence and aggression, an increase in aggressive fantasies, and feelings of subjective alienation in a dangerous world. Exposure to violence may also lead to gang involvement and therefore gang-related aggressive behavior, as exposed individuals search for means for protection in a violent neighborhood. It also affects the parent's capacity to parent and may indirectly increases conflicts at home.[6]

Kirk and Hardy[7] examined the enduring psychological effects on youth who were exposed to violence in the form of aggravated assault via a knife, bat, or gunshot, and found that these youth displayed heightened levels of aggression over 2.5 years later. In addition, a large body of research has demonstrated that being raised in disorderly, violent neighborhoods is highly predictive of psychological distress because the environment is subjectively alienating, and that this may also lead to violent behaviors in youth because neighborhood controls have broken down. These effects endure even after the person has relocated, with no improvement in psychological distress, and these youth continue to engage in risky behaviors.[8] Sharkey and Elwert[9] found evidence that the characteristics of the neighborhood environment in which a parent was raised as a child affect the children's cognitive ability a generation later (through their impact on the parent's educational attainment, occupation, income, marriage, and mental health). Thus, there is evidence that neighborhood effects of various forms endure, even for generations. In contrast, not all adolescents who are exposed to violence or live in a violent neighborhood ultimately become aggressive, and they can be sheltered from these effects by the buffering effect of supportive parents and the role of genetic characteristics.[10]

The Neurobiology of Adolescence

Adolescence is a time of dramatic changes, including rapid physical growth, the onset of sexual maturation, the activation of new drives and motivations, and a wide array of social and affective changes and challenges. Two of these motivational changes are: (1) increases in sensation-seeking (motivational tendency to want to experience high-intensity, exciting experiences); and (2) stronger natural interest in, and pursuit of, contact with peers and potential romantic partners. These motivational changes promote exploration of social experiences, development of skills and knowledge relevant to taking on adult social roles, individuation from family, and establishment of an individual identity, all of which represent core developmental tasks during this period in the life span. Another feature that explains behavior in adolescence is related to the notion that immature neuronal processing in the prefrontal cortex and other cortical and subcortical regions, along with their interaction, leads to behavior that is biased toward risk, reward, and emotional reactivity. During adolescence the dopamine-modulated neurobehavioral system that underlies incentive-driven behavior undergoes important changes; studies showing differences in the hedonic value of sucrose solutions in the brains of adults versus adolescents reveal marked differences in brain functioning during these periods of life. Some studies show that adolescents, compared to adults, experience more negative affect and depressed mood, and may feel less pleasure from stimuli of low or moderate incentive value; therefore they seek stimuli of greater hedonic intensity to satisfy a deficiency in their experience of reward. Adolescents and adults may also differ in the way they integrate emotional information in decisions: adolescents may be less adept at interpreting or integrating relevant emotional content, or less effective at forming such associations. All of these changes, which may translate into propensity toward impulsive behaviors, may also confer positive evolutionary advantages as the adolescent moves to explore new social environments, acquiring relevant knowledge and skills and moving toward increasing independence.[11,12] The ability known as mentalizing, or theory of mind, enables us to understand other people's behavior and actions in terms of underlying mental states such as intentions, desires, and beliefs. Functional magnetic resonance imaging (fMRI) studies have demonstrated how in early adolescence the areas of the brain involved in self-awareness and mentalizing become progressively more activated, and youth at this age become increasingly self-conscious and more aware of, and concerned with, others' opinions and social brain functions. Also, the pubertal rise in reproductive hormones activates increasing motivations to attract friends, to attain social status, and more generally, in their natural tendencies to pay more attention and to care about and react to peer, romantic, and sexual contexts; thus adolescence is a time during which peers, rather than parents, become influential in shaping social behavior.[13]

As peer relationships become more important in adolescence, the potential negative consequences of rejection or victimization by peers increase, and hypersensitivity to social rejection during adolescence can be explained by the neurobiological changes that take place at this stage of development. Relational aggression in adolescence can occur in various forms, such as socially excluding the victim using the "silent treatment," or by spreading rumors about the victim. Victims of relational aggression often have social-psychological adjustment problems, including low self-esteem, depression, and rage.[14]

Bullying

Bullying is defined as the systematic abuse of power utilizing aggressive behavior or intentional harm, perpetrated by peers, that is carried out repeatedly and involves an imbalance of power, either actual or perceived, between the victim and the bully. In the United Kingdom, for instance, being bullied by peers is the most frequent form of abuse encountered by children, much higher than abuse by parents or other adult perpetrators.[15] Bullying can take the form of direct bullying, which includes physical and verbal acts of aggression such as hitting, stealing, or name calling, or indirect bullying, which is characterized by social exclusion and rumor spreading. Children can be involved in bullying as victims or bullies, and also as bully-victims, a subgroup of victims who also display bullying behavior.[16] Children bullying others, those being bullied, and those who were both bullying others and being bullied had significant common health problems, including psychosomatic symptoms, and psychiatric problems including depression, suicide attempts, anxiety, externalizing behaviors, hyperactivity, substance abuse, and eating disorders. Bullying is associated with various psychopathological behaviors, including social problems, aggression, and externalizing behavioral problems. Bullying is found in all societies, including modern hunter-gatherer societies and ancient civilizations. It is considered an evolutionary adaptation, the purpose of which is to gain high status and dominance, get access to resources, secure survival, reduce stress, and allow for more mating opportunities. Bullies are often bi-strategic, employing both bullying and also acts of aggressive "prosocial" behavior to enhance their own position by acting in public and making the recipient dependent as they cannot reciprocate. Thus, pure bullies (but not bully-victims or victims) have been found to be strong, highly popular, and to have good social and emotional understanding. Hence, bullies most likely do not have a conduct disorder. Moreover, unlike conduct disorder, bullies are found in all socioeconomic and ethnic groups. In contrast, victims have been described as withdrawn, unassertive, easily emotionally upset, and as having poor emotional or social understanding, while bully-victims tend to be aggressive, easily angered, low on popularity, frequently bullied by their siblings, and come from families with lower socioeconomic status (SES), similar to children with conduct disorder.[16] Often bullying occurs in settings where individuals do not have a say concerning the group they want to be in. For these children, being in school classrooms or in the home with siblings has been compared to being "caged" with others. In an effort to establish a social network or hierarchy, bullies will try to exert their power with all children. Those who have an emotional reaction and have nobody or few to stand up for them are the repeated targets of bullies. Bullies may get others to join in as bystanders or even as henchmen (these then become bully-victims). It has been shown that conditions that foster higher density and greater hierarchies in classrooms, homes, or even in nations tend increase the frequency in which bullying occurs. Childhood bullying has serious effects on health, resulting in substantial costs for individuals, their families, and society at large. Many bullied children suffer in silence and are reluctant to tell their parents or teachers about their experiences, for fear of reprisals or because of shame. Health professionals should always ask children about their peer relationships, and it is important to remember that many children abstain from school due to bullying and related health problems, and that being bullied throws a long shadow over their lives.[16,17]

Violence and Social Media

Cyberbullying has become an international public health concern among adolescents, and as such, it deserves further study. It can be broadly defined as any bullying which is performed via electronic means, such as mobile phones or the internet. In general, cyberbullying involves hurting someone else using information and communication technologies. This may include sending harassing messages (via text or internet), posting disparaging comments on a social networking site, posting humiliating pictures, or threatening/intimidating someone electronically. Adolescents who are targeted via cyberbullying report increased depressive affect, anxiety, loneliness, suicidal behavior, and somatic symptoms. Perpetrators of cyberbullying are more likely to report increased substance use, aggression, and delinquent behaviors. Compared to traditional bullying, cyberbullying is unique in that it reaches an unlimited audience with increased exposure across time and space, preserves words and images in a more permanent state, and lacks supervision. The perpetrators of cyberbullying do not see the faces of their targets, and subsequently may not understand the full consequences of their actions, thereby decreasing important feelings of personal accountability. This has often been referred to in the literature as the "disinhibition effect."[18] A study of American middle school students examined the relationship between involvement in cyberbullying (either as a victim or perpetrator) and suicidality. The results revealed that both targets and perpetrators of cyberbullying were more likely to think about suicide, as well as attempt suicide, when compared to their peers who were not involved with cyberbullying. This relationship between cyberbullying and suicidality was stronger for targets, as compared to perpetrators of cyberbullying. Specifically, targets of cyberbullying were almost twice as likely to have attempted suicide (1.9 times), whereas perpetrators were 1.5 times more likely compared to their uninvolved peers, and that cyber-victims and cyberbully-victims were more likely to experience somatic problems, including difficulty sleeping, headaches, and stomachaches, as compared to their unaffected peers.[19] A study of adolescents who were harassed online found that they were more likely to use alcohol, drugs, and carry a weapon at school. In fact, victimized youth were 8 times more likely than their peers to carry a weapon to school in the past 30 days.[20] Perpetrators of cyberbullying have been positively associated with hyperactivity, relational aggression, conduct problems, smoking, and drunkenness and with decreased levels of self-esteem, self-efficacy, prosocial behavior, perceived sense of belonging, and safety at school. Cyberbullying perpetration has also been associated with adolescents' negative emotions such as anger, sadness, frustration, fear, and embarrassment. Disruptions in relationships have also been associated with cyberbullying perpetration among youth, including lower levels of empathy, increased levels of depression, weaker emotional bonds with caregivers, lower parental monitoring, and increased use of punitive discipline. Finally, perpetrators of cyberbullying were more likely to rationalize their destructive behaviors by minimizing the impact they had on others. In contrast, adolescents who have been both victims and then perpetrators of bullying experienced the most adverse health outcomes, including decreased psychological and physical health, increased levels of depression, substance use, and conduct problems compared to their peers who were either only targets or perpetrators. Adolescents who were both targets and perpetrators of cyberbullying also reported poorer relationships with their caregivers, and higher levels of victimization and perpetration offline, compared to their peers. These results suggest that this group of adolescents may require extra support from healthcare professionals, educators, and caring adults.[18] Adolescents involved in cyberbullying may be less inclined to experience empathy for targets online, in part because they are not privy to the targets' facial expressions. Future prevention and intervention efforts should be targeted toward increasing adolescents' affective and cognitive empathy in an effort to reduce participation in cyberbullying. Efforts should also address adolescents' self-esteem, as well as specific problem behaviors, and healthcare professionals and educators should work toward helping adolescents and their parents establish warm, nurturing relationships that include close adult monitoring and to encourage parents to participate in open discussions with children and adolescents about their online behavior, as well as to implement the necessary safeguards to protect youth from engaging in cyberbullying behaviors.[21,22]

School Shootings

Situations involving active firearms shooters in schools have increased in recent years, with each of the past several decades having one significant school shooting resulting in death and psychological traumatization, not just to the involved school and community, but also across the United States and other countries. Targeted violence at a school is defined as any premeditated incident where a known or knowable attacker deliberately chooses the school as the location for the attack, and an "active shooter incident" as an occurrence where one or more individuals participate in an ongoing, random, or systematic firearms shooting spree with the objective of multiple or mass murders.[23] In an examination of 37 incidents of targeted school violence in the United States, Vossekuil et al.[24] found that the great majority of the attackers were males, and 95% of them were current students, with 5% being former students. Attackers worked alone in 81% of the incidents. Assistance from at least one other peer in the planning of the attack occurred in 11% of the incidents, but the attackers in those incidents ultimately carried out the attack alone. Two or more attackers committed the assault together in 8% of the incidents. In terms of weapons, 76% of the attackers used only one weapon, whereas 46% of the attackers had more than one weapon with them at the time of the attack. Handguns were used by 61% of the attackers, and 49% of the attackers used rifles or shotguns. In 73% of the incidents, the attacker killed one or more individuals at the school, and in the remaining incidents, at least one person was injured by a weapon. Fifty-nine percent of the incidents occurred during the school day, indicating that fewer were carried out before school (22%) or after school (16%). Targets were not necessarily random, although persons in addition to targets were also harmed. Attackers had selected at least one administrator, faculty member, or staff member as a target in 54% of the incidents. Students were chosen as targets in 41% of the cases, and attackers selected more than one target prior to the attack in 44% of the incidents. Persons who were targeted before the attack were actually harmed in the attack in 46% of the cases. Individuals not identified as original targets of the attack were also injured or killed, and of these individuals, 57% were students and 39% were administrators, faculty, or staff. According to Vossekuil et al.,[24(p11)] there is no "profile," or "set of demographic and other traits that a set of perpetrators of a crime have in common" for student attackers. Attackers came from a variety of family situations, and they differed considerably in social relationships. At the same time, 71% of the attackers felt bullied, threatened, or injured by others before committing the attack, a significant finding to note if one were to attempt to categorize traits of active shooters. In addition, most attackers had some history of suicidal ideation or attempts, or a history of extreme depression. Most attackers were known to have had difficulties coping with "significant losses or personal failures."[24(p35)] Academic achievement ranged from failing to excellent grades. Some attackers had no behavioral problems, whereas others had histories of disciplinary problems. Although most attackers had no history of violent or criminal behavior before the attack, 59% demonstrated some interest in violence, whether it was through video games, movies, books, or other media. Most attackers did not display any significant change in academic performance, friendship patterns, interest in school, or disciplinary problems before the attack. At the same time, the study noted that 93% of the attackers engaged in some behavior before the attack that made others, such as parents, school officials, teachers, or fellow students concerned about their behavior. Targets did not seem to know about the attack beforehand, as most attackers did not threaten their targets directly before the attack. The targeted violence at school was often planned ahead of time, with some attackers devising the idea as few as 1 or 2 days before the attack and others holding the idea of the attack for as long as a year before its execution. Motives for attacks varied, and 54% of the attackers held multiple motives or reasons. For 61% of the attackers studied, revenge was a reason for the attack, 81% of the attackers had some type of grievance at the time of their attack, and 66% of the attackers had told other people about the grievance before the attack. Additional but less common motives of attackers were trying to solve a problem (34%), suicide or desperation (27%), and attempts for attention or recognition (24%). In terms of advancing the attack, many attackers had experience using weapons and had access to weapons. Fifty-nine percent of the attackers had some experience with a gun, and 68% used firearms that they obtained from their own home or that of a relative. Most school shootings were not stopped by law enforcement despite prompt response times. Instead, the shooter surrendered to or was apprehended by school staff (27% of the incidents) or by students (5% of the incidents). The attacker stopped on his or her own or left the school in 22% of the attacks, and in 13% of the attacks, the shooter killed himself. Law enforcement stopped only 27% of the shootings and only discharged weapons in three of the incidents examined. Most school shootings were not stopped by law enforcement, in part, because of their short duration. School shootings have occurred with increasing frequency in the past 20 years, and research is needed on prevention, particularly in the areas of security of the physical plant, school climate, and promoting prosocial behavior among students, faculty, and staff. Professional development activities that consist of pertinent information regarding known characteristics of school shooters should be a regular part of all school personnel's continuing education. School districts need to form partnerships with law enforcement personnel who are specialists in threat assessment, with the goal of policy and program development as prevention measures.[23]

Psychopathology, Aggression, and Violence among Youth

A wide range of psychopathology has been associated with aggression and violence in children and youth. These disorders include the disruptive behavior disorders (such as conduct disorder, oppositional defiant disorder and attention deficit/hyperactivity disorder [ADHD]), post-traumatic stress disorder (particularly in youth who have been traumatized through violence and re-enact the violence as part of their symptomatology), mood disorders (primarily bipolar disorder in the manic phase, but sometimes major depressive disorder as a result of anger and irritability), substance abuse disorders, and delirium/organic mood disorders (contributing to disinhibition and impulsivity), psychosis of various

types (schizophrenic, substance-induced, organic, and brief reactive), and various personality disorders, such as borderline and antisocial.[25-27]

The diagnostic entity of intermittent explosive disorder in itself characterizes violent
behavior as part of the diagnostic criteria, although this diagnosis has been often called
into question. Even the diagnosis of conduct disorder has some questionable validity, particularly since it has been found to be highly comorbid in children and youth (usually associated with another Axis I disorder that typically precedes it). Conduct disorder is also
disproportionately diagnosed in minority youth, either in significantly higher rates than
Caucasian youth or with underlying comorbid conditions missed, such as post-traumatic
stress disorder and ADHD.[26,28,29] Additionally, researchers have pointed out that only a
small percentage (no more than 10%) of youth with conduct disorders go on to be diagnosed with antisocial personality disorder.[30] Two national organizations in the United States
(the American Society of Adolescent Psychiatry and the American Community Psychiatry
Association) called for the removal of the diagnosis of conduct disorder from the DSM-5
but were unsuccessful.

Aggression can be a consequence of the challenges associated with autism spectrum
disorder (ASD). A number of sensory, processing, and emotional-regulation problems can
result in aggression and violence by youth with ASD, or toward youth with ASD by other
youth. These include: the need for sameness and sensitivity to environmental disruption,
sensory sensitivity to various stimuli (such as loud sounds), interpersonal discomfort and
social skills challenges, difficulty with theory of mind and assessment of the intention-
ality of others, and difficulty with determining the context of interpersonal boundaries.
These challenges when triggered can result in irritability and even aggressive and violent
behavior. Comorbid ADHD (which occurs with some frequency in youth on the autism
spectrum) can heighten impulsivity and aggravate aggressive behavior.[25,31] Some clinicians
and researchers have observed that the onset of puberty and hormonal dysregulation have
been associated with increased aggressive behavior in youth on the autism spectrum, particularly males.[31] However, youth on the autism spectrum are also often the victims of
violence and traumatization through bullying by neurotypical youth.[32] Aggression is a frequent reason why youth with ASD fall out of mainstream education, especially given the
shortages of behavioral therapy and social skills training in schools. Aggressive behavior
by youth with ASD often results in disciplinary action and even juvenile justice involvement in spite of fact that aggression is reactive/non-predatory and resulting from their
disabilities.

An important distinction can be made between predatory aggression versus reactive
aggression. Predatory aggression is more typically associated with youth who have antecedents of antisocial personality disorder, particularly in youth who have been subjected
to severe emotional neglect or abuse that has contributed to failures in empathy. Reactive
aggression occurs in the moment as a result of the interaction between mood or anxiety
disturbance, impulsivity, and significant triggering events in the youth's environment.
Reactive aggression and violence are much more frequent than predatory aggression, yet
most funding and law enforcement efforts are directed at predatory aggression.[25,26,33]

Youth Violence, Prejudice, Marginalization, and Hate Crimes

Increases in racial/ethnic/sexual hate rhetoric, seen in many societies worldwide, have had a significant adverse impact on youth, promoting aggressive and violent behavior to serve the cause of various ideologies. Such violence is often associated with racist, xenophobic, and fundamentalist/ultra-religious beliefs. It can also be a reaction to the increasing globalization of cultures and economies, increasing technological and educational demands, and resulting threats perceived by traditionalist groups and cultures. Youth who engage in such violence are typically marginalized from their own mainstream cultural/ethnic groups, or are children of immigrants marginalized from the mainstream cultures within which they reside. Their sense of alienation and idealism make them easy recruits to organized hate groups or terrorist organizations. The majority of hate crimes appear to be perpetrated by youth, though the majority of hate crimes perpetrated by youth are not associated with organized groups.[34,35]

On the other hand, youth who have been victimized by xenophobia or racial discrimination can also resort to violence out of frustration and desperation, which can start out as part of a protest but can become violent. Their deep sense of frustration with injustice and socioeconomic disparities often has its roots in historical trauma perpetrated against their racial/ethnic groups across generations.

Treatment and Preventive Interventions

A number of treatment interventions used to treat youth with emotional/behavioral and psychiatric disorders have developed evidence for the management of aggressive behavior, both as a target symptom and as part of overall treatment for a primary disorder. Cognitive behavioral therapy and mindfulness approaches directed at emotional regulation and anger management have demonstrated effectiveness.[36] Parent behavioral management has demonstrated evidence in managing aggressive behavioral in children with ADHD and conduct disturbances.[37] Other more comprehensive interventions using principles of parent behavioral management along with community services and supports, functional family therapy (FFT) and multisystemic therapy (MST), both have evidence in diverting youth from juvenile justice and even psychiatric admissions.[38,39] For youth on the autism spectrum, applied behavioral analysis and social skills training have well established evidence for reducing aggressive behaviors triggered by change disruption and social and academic demands.[31] Pharmacotherapy, including stimulants, alpha agonists, atypical antipsychotics, anticonvulsants, and lithium carbonate, has been used for the management of aggression with youth with a wide variety of disorders with demonstrated efficacy, though larger-scale placebo controlled trials have primarily focused on use with youth with ADHD and ASD.[31,40]

The community-based system of care model, which was originally proposed by Stroul and Friedman,[41] has been increasingly implemented in the United States to guide services for seriously emotionally disturbed children in the least restrictive setting within the communities where they live. This model has also been found to be effective in addressing populations of youth at risk for youth violence. The community-based system of care model proposes access to a comprehensive array of services, addressing individual needs and strengths in the least restrictive environment, with the family as full participants, as well as inter-agency efforts that are closely coordinated. These programs rely heavily on case management and coordination, smooth transitions among levels of care and services, and the use of evidence-based interventions, and they particularly focus on services that are culturally competent and meet the needs of special populations.[42] Over 100 systems of care demonstration programs, particularly those funded by the U.S. federal government, are being infused with evidence-based interventions and are targeting many populations of youth at risk for youth violence, with significant positive outcomes.[43]

One of the original systems of care programs funded by the Center for Child Mental Health Services, called the Village Project, serves as a good example. This program, located in Charleston, South Carolina, served a population that was 62% male, 70% African American, with a mean age of 11.4 years and a high prevalence of contacts with law enforcement and courts. This program reduced the rate of incarceration within that community by over 80%, with a low rate of recidivism. It similarly reduced in-patient service utilization by similar levels, and state hospital utilization to near zero. The Village Project accomplished these impressive outcomes through a network of services that included school-based mental health services in most county schools; community mentoring and vocational programs; case management; wrap-around and home-based services, and even community-based sex offender programs. It also included psychopharmacological services that were supported by parent advocates to facilitate the interactions between families and child psychiatrists. They also promoted a major cultural competence initiative across the various participating agencies to enhance their effectiveness in serving the area's diverse population. The program held weekly inter-agency child and family consultations, focusing on youth with particularly difficult problems and multi-level intervention needs. They also worked closely with the juvenile court around youth drug arrests, with the juvenile drug court, with assigned staff, and worked very closely with the juvenile judge. There was an extensive program of parent volunteers and advocates closely linked to the predominately African American community. All these services were headquartered and co-located in a one-stop shopping center, including mental health, juvenile justice, and child welfare services. The community-based system of care model shows significant promise in maximizing the resources of the various agencies that serve children and youth involved in juvenile justice with violent or aggressive potential, and it impacts youth violence and aggression at multiple levels (clinical, psychosocial, socioeconomic, and cultural).[44]

Another model being promulgated within the United States, the National Child Traumatic Stress Network, is a program to address traumatic stress suffered by children, youth, and families exposed to family or community violence, terrorism, and other natural or man-made disasters. It has created various training and service programs throughout the nation, supported by two technical assistance centers. These programs have been charged with improving the standard of care for traumatized children and increasing access to care. They are involved in developing and/or disseminating evidence-based community interventions, trauma-informed services, and public and professional education.[45,46] An intervention developed within one of these programs, Cognitive Behavioral Intervention for Trauma in Schools (CBITS), has been designated as an evidence-based intervention for traumatic stress for children and youth. It involves structured group sessions for children, individual sessions, and parent sessions that teach children and youth (from the elementary to the high school level) to manage anxiety and mood problems resulting from exposure to violence and to improve interpersonal skills. This intervention has demonstrated significant outcomes in reduced symptoms of post-traumatic stress, improved academic performance, and improved behavioral function in its participants.[47]

Prevention science has already demonstrated that addressing developmental, educational, socioeconomic, and financial disparities are effective in promoting healthy socioemotional development and preventing social margination and reactive aggression, and as a consequence preventing youth violence.[48,49] In a more focused manner, various models have been developed to address offending and violent behaviors in a constructive and prosocial manner. These range from restorative justice approaches with youth offenders to peace and reconciliation councils in response to community and national conflicts.[46] Trauma-informed approaches have been developed to address ideological indoctrination and trauma with child combatants in war zones and with youth recruited into gangs and terrorist organizations.[50,51] Some researchers have demonstrated that programs and movements that promote youth agency, which can give voice to youth grievances and concerns, contribute to the reduction of violence and promotion of public health prevention.[52]

Conclusions

There is a global consensus that "no violence against children is justifiable; all violence against children is preventable."[53] To prevent all violence against children and by children and youth, violence should be a matter of public health, not merely a matter of juvenile justice or child welfare. In this context, child and adolescent mental health has an important role to prevent violence against children.

Although further research is needed to understand violent behaviors in children and youth, cross-cultural and interdisciplinary collaboration is particularly important because of its multifaceted and multifactorial nature. Since the occurrence of youth violence varies by location and setting, preventive efforts should be tailored to be most effective and appropriate for each context. The need for sufficient mental health services for both victims and perpetrators of violent behaviors is universal, regardless of the national or regional situation. Such mental health services should be community-based and easily accessible for every child and adolescent and their family in the community. Programs based on community-based systems of care philosophy and on preventive science are good examples of the potential contribution of child and adolescent mental health to reduce youth violence within communities.

References

1. World Health Organization. *World Report on Violence and Health*. Geneva: World Health Organization; 2002.
2. Dahlberg LL, Krug EG. A global public health problem. In: World Health Organization, ed. *World Report on Violence and Health*. Geneva: World Health Organization; 2002:1–22.
3. Ono Y, Pumariega AJ. Violence in youth. *Int Rev Psychiatry*. 2008;20(3):305–316.
4. Smith-Khuri E, Iachan R, Scheidt PC, et al. A cross-national study of violence-related behaviors in adolescents. *Arch Pediatr Adolesc Med*. 2004;158:592–594.
5. Osofsky JD. The impact of violence on children. *Future Children*. 1999;9:33–49.
6. Osofsky JD. The effects of exposure to violence of young children. *Am Psychol*. 1995;50:782–788.
7. Kirk DS, Hardy M. The acute and enduring consequences of exposure to violence on youth mental health and aggression. *Justice Q*. 2014;31:3, 539–567. doi: 10.1080/07418825.2012.737471.
8. Sanbonmatsu L, Ludwig J, Katz LF, et al. *Moving to Opportunity for Fair Housing Demonstration Program: Final Impacts Evaluation*. Washington, DC: US Department of Housing and Urban Development, Office of Policy Development and Research; 2011.
9. Sharkey P, Elwert F. The legacy of disadvantage: multigenerational neighborhood effects on cognitive ability. *Am J Sociol*. 2011;116:1934–1981.
10. Caspi A, McClay J, Moffitt TE, Mill J, Marti J, Craig IA. Role of genotype in cycle of violence in maltreated children. *Science*. 2002;297:851–854.
11. Blakemore SJ. The social brain in adolescence. *Nature Rev Neurosci*. 2008 April;9:267–276.
12. Wahlstrom D, Collins P, White T, Luciana M. Developmental changes in dopamine neurotransmission in adolescence: behavioral implications and issues in assessment. *Brain Cogn*. 2010;72:146–159.
13. Forbes EE, Dahl RE. Pubertal development and behavior: hormonal activation of social and motivational tendencies. *Brain Cogn*. 2010;72:66–72.
14. Sebastian C, Viding E, Williams KD, Blakemore SJ. Social brain development and the affective consequences of ostracism in adolescence. *Brain Cogn*. 2010 Feb;72(1):134–145. doi: 10.1016/j.bandc.2009.06.008. Epub 2009 Jul 22.
15. Radford L, Corral S, Bradley C, Fisher HL. The prevalence and impact of child maltreatment and other types of victimization in the UK: findings from a population survey of caregivers, children and young people and young adults. *Child Abuse Negl*. 2013;37:801–813.
16. Wolke D, Lereya ST. Long-term effects of bullying. *Arch Dis Child*. 2015;100:879–885. doi: 10.1136/archdischild-2014-306667.
17. Dale J, Russell R, Wolke D. Intervening in primary care against childhood bullying: an increasingly pressing public health need. *J Royal Soc Med*. 2014 Jun;107(6):219–223. doi: 10.1177/0141076814525071.
18. Nixon CL. Current perspectives: the impact of cyberbullying on adolescent health. *Adolesc Health Med Ther*. 2014;5:143–158.
19. Hinduja S, Patchin JW. Bullying, cyberbullying, and suicide. *Arch Suicide Res*. 2010;14(3):206–221.
20. Ybarra ML, Diener-West M, Leaf PJ. Examining the overlap in internet harassment and school bullying: implications for school intervention. *J Adolesc Health*. 2007;41(6 Suppl 1):S42–S50.
21. Davis S, Nixon C. Empowering bystanders. In: Patchin J, Hinduja S, eds. *Cyberbullying Prevention and Response: Expert Perspectives*. New York: Routledge; 2012:93–113.
22. Schurgin O'Keeffe G, Clarke-Pearson K. Council on Communications and Media. Clinical report: the impact of social media on children, adolescents, and families. *Pediatrics*. 2011;127:800–804.
23. Bonanno CM, Levenson RL. School shooters: history, current theoretical and empirical findings, and strategies for prevention. *SAGE Open*. 2014 Jan–Mar;4(1):1–11. doi: 10.1177/2158244014525425.
24. Vossekuil B, Fein RA, Reddy M, Borum R, Modzeleski W. *The Final Report and Findings of the Safe School Initiative: Implications for the Prevention of School Attacks in the United States*. Washington, DC: U.S. Secret Service and U.S. Department of Education; 2002.
25. Jensen P, Youngstrom E, Steiner H, et al. Consensus report on impulsive aggression as a symptom across diagnostic categories in child psychiatry: implications for medication studies. *J Am Acad Child Adolesc Psychiatry*. 2007;46(3):309–322.

26. Steiner H, Silverman M, Karnik N, et al. Psychopathology, trauma and delinquency: subtypes of aggression and their relevance for understanding young offenders. *Child Adolesc Psychiatry Mental Health.* 2011;5:21:1–11.

27. American Psychiatric Association. *Diagnostic and Statistical Manual of Mental Disorders.* 5th ed. Arlington, VA: American Psychiatric Publishing; 2013.

28. Fabrega H, Ulrich R, Mezzich JE. Do Caucasian and Black adolescents differ at psychiatric intake? *J Am Acad Child Adolesc Psychiatry.* 1993;32(2):407–413. https://doi.org/10.1097/00004583-199303 000-00023

29. Kilgus MD, Pumariega AJ, Cuffe SP. Influence of race on diagnosis in adolescent psychiatric inpatients. *J Am Acad Child Adolesc Psychiatry.* 1995;34(1):67–72. https://doi.org/10.1097/00004583-199501 000-00016

30. Rappaport N, Thomas C. Recent research findings on aggressive and violent behavior in youth: implications for clinical assessment and intervention. *J Adolesc Health.* 2004;35(4):260–277. https://doi.org/ 10.1016/j.jadohealth.2003.10.009

31. Fitzpatrick S, Srivorakiat L, Wink L, Pedapati E, Erickson C. Aggression in autism spectrum disorder: presentation and treatment options. *Neuropsychiatr Dis Treat.* 2016;12:1525–1538.

32. van Roekel R, Scholte R, Didden R. Bullying among adolescents with autism spectrum disorders: prevalence and perception. *J Autism Dev Disord.* 2010;40:63–73.

33. Connor D, Steingard R, Cunningham J, Anderson J, Melloni R. Proactive and Reactive Aggression in Referred Children and Adolescents. *Am J Orthopsychiatry.* 2004;74(2):129–136.

34. Steinberg A, Brooks J, Remtulla T. Youth hate crimes: identification, prevention, and intervention. *Am J Psychiatry.* 2003;160:979–989.

35. Michener W. The individual psychology of group hate. *J Hate Studies.* 2012;10(1):15–48.

36. Sukhodolsky D, Scahill L. *Cognitive-Behavioral Therapy for Anger and Aggression in Children.* New York: Guilford Press; 2012.

37. Forgatch MS, Patterson GR. Behavioral family therapy. In: Dattilo FM, ed. *Case Studies in Couple and Family Therapy: Systematic and Cognitive Perspectives.* New York: Guilford Press; 1998:85–107.

38. Catalano RF, Loeber R, McKinney KC. School and community interventions to prevent serious and violent offending. *Juvenile Justice Bull.* 1999:1–12. https://ojjdp.ojp.gov/library/publications/school-and-community-interventions-prevent-serious-and-violent-offending

39. Henngeler S, Sheidow A. Empirically supported family-based treatments for conduct disorder and delinquency in adolescents. *Marital Fam Ther.* 2012;38(1):30–58.

40. Pappadopulos E, Woolston S, Chait A, Perkins M, Connor D, Jensen P. Pharmacotherapy of aggression in children and adolescents: efficacy and effect size. *J Canadian Acad Child Adolesc Psychiatry.* 2006;15(1):27–39.

41. Stroul B, Friedman R. *A System of Care for Severely Emotionally Disturbed Children and Youth.* Washington, DC: Georgetown University Child Development Center, CASSP Technical Assistance Center; 1986.

42. Pumariega AJ, Winters NC, Huffine C. The evolution of systems of care for children's mental health: forty years of community child and adolescent psychiatry. *Commun Mental Health J.* 2003;39:399–425.

43. Stephens RL, Connor T, Nguyen H, Holden EW, Greenbaum P, Foster EM. The longitudinal comparison study of the national evaluation of the Comprehensive Community Mental Health Services for Children and Their Families Program. In: Epstein MH, Kutash K, Duchnowski AJ, eds. *Outcomes for Children and Youth with Emotional and Behavioral Disorders and Their Families: Programs and Evaluation Best Practices.* Austin, TX: Pro-Ed, 2005:525–550.

44. Heffron W, Pumariega A, Fallon T, Carter D. Youth in the juvenile justice system. In: Pumariega A, Winters N, eds. *Handbook of Community-Based Systems of Care: The New Child and Adolescent Psychiatry.* San Francisco: Jossey Bass; 2003:224–249.

45. Gurwitch RH, Pfefferbaum B, Montgomery JM, Klomp RW, Reissman DB. *Building Community Resilience for Children and Families.* Oklahoma City: Terrorism and Disaster Center at the University of Oklahoma Health Science Center; 2007.

46. U.S. Department of Health and Human Services: *Youth Violence: A Report of the Surgeon General.* Washington, DC: Center for Mental Health Services, Substance Abuse and Mental Health Services Administration, U.S. Department of Health and Human Services; 2001.

47. Stein BD, Jaycox LH, Kataoka SH, Wong M, Tu W, Elliott MN, et al. A mental health intervention for school children exposed to violence: a randomized controlled trial. *JAMA.* 2003;290:603–611.

48. Olds DL, Pettitt LM, Robinson J, et al. Reducing the risks for antisocial behavior with a program of prenatal and early childhood home visitation. *J Community Psychol.* 1998;26:65–83.

49. Shonkoff J, Phillips D. *From Neurons to Neighborhoods: The Science of Early Childhood Development. Committee on Integrating the Science of Early Childhood Development, Board on Children, Youth, and Families, Commission on Behavioral and Social Sciences and Education, National Research Council and Institute of Medicine.* Washington, DC: National Academy Press; 2000.

50. Peltonen K, Punamaki RL. Preventive interventions among children exposed to trauma of armed conflict: a literature review. *Aggress Behav.* 2010 Mar–Apr;36(2):95–116. doi: 10.1002/ab.20334.

51. Higginson A, Bernier K, Shenderovich Y, Bedford L. Preventive interventions to reduce youth involvement in gangs and gang crime in low- and middle-income countries: a systematic review. *Campbell Syst Rev.* November 2015;11(1):1–176. doi: 10.4073/csr.2015.18.

52. Earls, F. *The Child as Citizen.* New York: SAGE Publications; 2011.

53. Harrington ER. The Social Psychology of Hatred. *J Hate Stud.* 2004;3:49–82.

37

The COVID-19 Pandemic

Social Psychiatric Perspectives

Andres J. Pumariega, Marianne Kastrup, and
R. Srinivasa Murthy

Introduction

It was December 2019 when COVID was identified in China and its potential to become a global pandemic was recognized. Since then, nations across the globe have raced to both immediately protect its citizens and come to terms with its immediate and longer-term health, educational, and societal implications. This process has been very distinctly national and regional, though it often involved international actions such as the sudden closure of borders, cessation of travel, and diplomatic exchanges and tensions around public health, economic, and political responses.

There have been clear implications of sociocultural and mental health factors within the vulnerability and responses to the pandemic. This chapter examines these factors through an analysis of the impact and response of the pandemic in three national examples: the United States, the nations of the Scandinavian region, and the world's most populous nation, India. These analyses have focused on their unique sociocultural factors and embedded lessons, as well as the mental health implications of this public health crisis.

COVID-19: The American Pandemic

With some exceptions, governments have made great efforts to put the well-being of their people first, acting decisively to protect health and to save lives. The exceptions have been some governments that shrugged off the painful evidence of mounting deaths, with inevitable, grievous consequences. But most governments acted responsibly, imposing strict measures to contain the outbreak.

Yet some groups protested, refusing to keep their distance, marching against travel restrictions—as if measures that governments must impose for the good of their people constitute some kind of political assault on autonomy or personal freedom! Looking to the common good is much more than the sum of what is good for individuals. It means having a regard for all citizens and seeking to respond effectively to the needs of the least fortunate.
It is all too easy for some to take an idea—in this case, for example, personal freedom—and turn it into an ideology, creating a prism through which they judge everything.

> —Pope Francis,[1] in an editorial in the *New York Times*, written and published immediately after the U.S. Supreme Court ruled against the State of New York for enforcing attendance limits on religious services

Statistics and Epidemiological Course of the COVID Pandemic

As of June 2021, there were 33.4 million total cases and almost 600,000 deaths in the United States alone since the beginning of the pandemic (out of 176 million cases and 3.8 million fatalities worldwide), making it the leading nation both in number of infections and deaths. The current daily rate of new infections has dropped to approximately 15,000, after a period of time where this rate had risen to 250,000 new infections daily, also highest in the world. The number of deaths exceeded those associated with World War II and were only exceeded by the U.S. Civil War (estimated at total of 2 million and 650,000 combat deaths) and the 1918 influenza pandemic (650,000). Forty-eight out of 50 states are at positivity rates of over 5%, many in the twin digits.[2]

The hope of overcoming the pandemic in the United States has been placed primarily around the mass vaccination of the American population. Scientific advances stimulated by federal government funding and international competition and cooperation led to the rapid development of multiple vaccines, with two (by Pfizer/BioNtec and Moderna Pharmaceuticals) receiving emergency authorization by the U.S. Food and Drug Administration in December 2020. This set the stage for what has become a rapid mass vaccination campaign, nearly matching the speed of vaccine development, but with uneven implementation within and across nations. However, the poor planning by the administration of former President Trump led to multiple missteps in distribution (see contributing factors below). Where there was a promise of vaccinating 100 million citizens (about 30%) by the spring of 2021, only 27 million doses had been administered, most of dose being first shots.[3] The new Biden administration has been progressively ramping up vaccine distribution and vaccination rates, with a goal of 70% of the U.S. population receiving at least one shot by July 4, at times reaching 3 million daily vaccinations (note that the main vaccines require two vaccinations and the total U.S. population totals almost 350 million) but recently slowing down due to vaccine hesitancy and sociocultural obstacles aggravated by the politization of the pandemic. Additionally, they have worked to re-establish a more centralized and coordinated approach to public health measures, reopening schools and maintaining essential services, and addressing economic impact and disparities. They have also become more involved in the global fight against the pandemic, recently promising 500 million vaccine doses by early 2022.

The emphasis on vaccination, however, has been in part the result of the rejection of public health population mitigation measures by many in the U.S. population (especially those from conservative orientations). Mask wearing only recently increased to approximately 70% of adults from 50% after much resistance, hypothesized to result in the aforementioned recent reduction in the daily rates of infection. Only 26 states had some form of travel restrictions and about the same numbers had restrictions around school attendance (shifted to virtually), shopping, eating out, gatherings, etc.—mostly those with more liberal political leanings which are willing to enforce such mitigating restrictions. Many of these mitigating measures and restrictions are in the process of being lifted under both political pressure as well as due to declining rates resulting from the success of the U.S. vaccination campaign.[4]

As presented below, multiple sociocultural and political factors have hindered the American response to the COVID pandemic, many of which have been endemic in U.S. culture and values. Some of these factors have in themselves been exacerbated to the level of becoming pandemics themselves, threatening the economic and social progress made in the U.S. over the past 70 years since World War II.

Brief History of the American Pandemic

Recent historians point to U.S. intelligence agencies having information about the severity of the pandemic in Wuhan by December 2019 and warning the U.S. government, with mixed concern. Latter revelations showed that U.S. President Trump knew as far back as January/February 2020 of the seriousness of the COVID-19 threat but minimized its severity of the virus, purportedly so as not to alarm/demoralize the U.S. population, but most likely in an attempt to avoid derailing the economic expansion he was presiding over (often stating the "virus will just go away . . .").[5]

Though the initial cases and clusters occurred in the Northwest and Western U.S. (possibly tied to spread from China), the initial major wave and lockdowns occurred in the Northeast (spread coming from Europe) from March through June 2020. An exponentially rapid rise in cases and number of deaths occurred that overwhelmed cities in the Northeast (over 20,000 deaths in 3 months in New York City alone). The governors and mayors in this region called for swift national response to the growing pandemic with broad restrictions in movement and travel, but these were rebuffed by the federal government.

It is important to note that the elements of the Republican Party in power had been elected on an anti-government platform, which has been highly popular in many segments of the United States for over 40 years. Therefore, a nationalized public health response ran totally counter to the core beliefs held by the government and its most ardent supporters. The Northeast is often viewed as a liberal and elitist enclave due to its higher education and much greater wealth, so reports about the virus's spread were mistrusted in more conservative regions of the country, viewing the problem as primarily an urban problem and their requests an infringement on their "freedoms."

The growth of the pandemic did eventually lead to a national lockdown in April 2020, though it was relatively short-lived, and ended suddenly due to the severe economic impact that resulted (rapid rise in unemployment, rental evictions, and homelessness), with demands for economic stimulus and support by the government. Some stimulus support was passed legislatively, but the federal government continued to struggle with pushing for supplies of personal protective equipment (PPE), disinfectants, and ventilators, shifting responsibilities for acquiring these to state governments. A backlash by conservative governors, the party in power, and the president called for opening up states and reversing restrictions to revive the economy. Right-wing protests against masking and social distancing, pushing for bars and restaurants and resorts to open, were stoked by extremist groups which rose to gain great power and support. Some went as far as making death threats to public health officials and even plotting the kidnapping and murder of the governor of Michigan, who had enforced public health protections.

Widespread disregard for public health measures likely led to a summer wave of the pandemic in the more conservative Southern and Midwestern states, and eventually a third massive wave in the fall and winter of 2020–2021. These were associated with lack of restraint around family gatherings, parties, clandestine group entertainment, and even mass travel and gatherings for the national Thanksgiving holiday and Christmas/New Year's holidays, in spite of public health warnings.

The psychosocial and political impact of the pandemic became evident in other ways by the summer of 2020. Racial/ethnic economic disparities associated with the pandemic became recognized publicly, with much higher rates of mortality and morbidity suffered by underserved minority populations. The rates of morbidity and mortality for Latinos and African Americans in the United States range from 3 to 4 times that of their White counterparts. This is a result of such risk factors as high percentages of front-line workers with high exposure and little possibility of remote work or sheltering at home, few savings to fall back on, high rates of physical health disparities/comorbidities (such as diabetes and obesity), working in high-risk workplaces (meatpacking, agribusiness, manufacturing, delivery services) with little PPE or mitigating procedures or government regulation, low rates of health literacy, living in multigenerational families, and lack of childcare, and thus dependent on children attending school. Outrage around these disparities added to the mounting outrage around police killings and the rise of racist White supremacist groups (allied with anti-government groups). These resulted in multiple demonstrations during the summer of 2020 that were associated with civic unrest, and frequent and at times violent confrontations between minority and leftist groups versus white supremacist groups. These mass gatherings likely further fueled the virus's spread.[6,7]

The election of 2020 placed some of the issues around the pandemic squarely in the public domain, both through behavior and policy. The president's party held campaign rallies and events where masks were discouraged and were not socially distant. This led to many cases of COVID, including the president himself. However, he continued to deny the pandemic's impact on the country and boasted of his economic accomplishments. The opposition Democratic Party challenged his denial and lack of leadership around the pandemic, putting forth many policy proposals on how to respond to the pandemic's public health and economic impact, while they held rallies that were socially distant, used distance technologies, and actively promoted mask wearing and social distancing. By the time of the election and shortly thereafter, just about every region of the United States had high positivity rates and were experiencing crisis levels of hospital occupancy due to severe illness and high numbers of deaths. The presidential election became a referendum on the management of the pandemic. However, in spite of the victory by the Democrats, the more extreme elements of the losing Republicans fought to hang on to power, presenting themselves as the defenders of threatened traditional American values.

Mental Health Impact of the American Pandemic

The pandemic has had definite and significant psychosocial impacts on the U.S. population, both due to the impact of illness and the impact of the mitigation measures. This has included disruption of general routines in personal and family life with increased significant social isolation, disconnection from extended families (out of fear of contagion), postponed or disrupted life plans/activities that involve gatherings or travel (such as graduations, college plans, travel, sports activities, family celebrations, etc.). For children this has included disruption of education with the transition to online learning, the latter being both a technical and interactional challenge for teachers and students. As many as 20% of the adult workforce has been able to work virtually from home to mitigate exposure for themselves and family members, but managing work and the care of children within the confines of their homes has proven to be highly stressful. Quarantine fatigue, setting in over months, led to testing of parental limits and controls, physical abuse, domestic violence, and even substance abuse out of mounting frustration, and breaking of social distancing rules and taking risks that led to exposure. The fear of illness exposure (personal and that of vulnerable family members) also has raised individual and collective anxiety, especially when neighbors and friends may not follow mitigation rules due to their beliefs.[8] Overall, the U.S. adult population has seen a rise in anxiety, depression, suicidality, and substance abuse, with over 40% suffering at least one of these mental health morbidities during a week in June 2020.[9]

There is also significant stress experienced by healthcare workers, both as a result of fears of illness exposure due to inadequate PPE and their facing the high morbidity and mortality of their patients, leading to high levels of anxiety and depression.[10] There has been similar impact on front-line workers, both out of fear for their safety and uncertainty of the safety of their families, while having to perform jobs that provide them their living wage. There has also been significant impact on older adults and their families, as elders both living independently and in nursing or group facilities have had to isolate and forgo visitations from family members. The ultimate tragedy has been many elders who have died alone in hospitals which limit visitations and only being able to say goodbye over televideo through a cell phone.[11]

The impact on children with mental health needs has been closely examined. For example, online school and home confinement have posed a major challenge for many children, especially those with ADHD, autism spectrum disorder (ASD), and learning disorders, with lack of structure and added barriers to learning. For children with ASD, this often results in the ramping up of perseverations and aggression within the pressure-cooker environment of home confinement with high sensory overload.[12,13] Depression and anxiety are greatly aggravated by social isolation, especially for teens, with increases in rates of mental health service need and hospitalizations.[14] Youth with gender dysphoria are also a particularly vulnerable group, at a time when there has been greater openness, but who now face lack of validation by peers and extra-familial adults, while confined with often non-validating family members.[15]

Cultural and Psychosocial Factors Fueling and Aggravating the American Pandemic

The COVID pandemic laid bare many anachronisms and conflicts among elements of American sociocultural values. The conflict between capitalism/materialism versus existentialism/safety/security has been present throughout U.S. history, often with the promotion of material wealth over social well-being and even over family ties and community cohesion.

Fear and mistrust of government is deeply engrained in the American psyche, even seen as the main impetus for the formation of the nation (in rebellion against British governance). This was expressed as a fear of government intrusion on individual rights and freedoms in the face of a public health emergency, which by its widespread nature is best dealt with by coordinated government and communal action and restrictions. The Republican Party is avowedly anti-government, so the federal government did not take over public health planning and regulations and the production of needed supplies and equipment. Above all, there was reticence to guide the population to practice individual public health measures and impose activity restrictions with needed financial compensation.

Even though the United States has been one of the engines of science, technology, and ingenuity in the world, the anti-government movement has come to include an anti-science and anti-expertise element, in which those with higher levels of education are seen as elitists seeking to obtain power over the masses. The segment of the population that engaged in mistrust of government came to also mistrust science and education, which are largely promoted and funded by government, and have even romanticized being uneducated. The messages of denial about the severity pandemic were associated with a mistrust of scientists as also wanting to excessively control people's lives by the promotion of mitigation measures, such as mask wearing. The fear of different perspectives and ideas, especially coming from abroad, is also associated with these beliefs, leading to xenophobia and international isolation. Ultimately, this anti-science and anti-knowledge mentality may serve to undo the power and greatness of the United States as a nation.

Entrenchment of individualistic culture over collectivist values (which has been a thread throughout U.S. history) was another reaction to the pandemic. This was adopted to the point of near rebellion against any government measures (and ultimately the government itself, as witnessed by the January 6th anarchic action against the Congress). It was also seen in the lack of caution or concern for older or vulnerable family members and relatives, with many young adults not refraining from socialization or entertainment and infecting parents and grandparents in congregate households, with unwillingness to practice mitigating practices across households in gatherings. The United States has practiced collectivism and cohesion in response to major existential crises (wars, disasters, etc.) but the minimization of this crisis contributed to this psychosocial defense not being recruited or promoted. The loss of collectivist values has also contributed to the social and economic inequalities seen both through the pandemic and chronically in denial of racial/ethnic disparities and inequalities. The pandemic and its response have also exacerbated discrimination, racism, and xenophobia directed at minority populations beyond the structural disparities it uncovered. For example, the purported origins of the virus in China led to strident xenophobia directed at Asian Americans, including from U.S. president Trump himself. Racism and discrimination have also aggravated the high levels of anomie, loneliness, and hopelessness seen among diverse youth and isolated elders (the latter affected by high death rates in nursing facilities), with reactions ranging from rage to despair.

Technology has been one of the saving graces in the American response to the pandemic. This has included the use of distance web-based telecommunication for students and workers to operate from home (including healthcare services), and the use of the internet to conduct socially distanced commerce and socially distanced education for millions of children, saving millions of infections and thousands of lives by enabling social distancing and reduction in transmission. Telehealth has not only sustained a certain level of general health services not requiring face-to-face interaction, but has promoted a literal revolution in mental healthcare delivery, with many clinics providing as much as 70% of their services by televideo, directly to personal and home devices.[16] American scientific ingenuity led the way to the discovery of effective vaccines, which are rolling out to the population, and to the development and discovery of various medications and procedures which have saved multiple lives of individuals at high risk for COVID complications. However, the American idealization of technological solutions reduces motivation to use low-tech ground-level public health measures to prevent viral spread which have been well proven in the developing world (and often developed by American public health scientists themselves).

History Revisited from the 1918 Spanish Flu Pandemic in the United States

Many of the unique elements of the U.S. response to the current COVID pandemic were already identifiable in the U.S. experience with the 1918–1920 Spanish flu. That pandemic had a total of three waves in the United States from 1918 to early 1920, resulting in 550,000 to 850,000 deaths in a relatively smaller population of 103 million (about 28% infected). The wave affected larger cities but then reverberated to smaller towns and rural regions, with no region being unaffected. The 1918 pandemic struck the United States just as it was undergoing massive mobilization to assist the Allies fighting in Europe in World War I. There was intentional censoring of information by U.S. government and business leaders, who were fearful of demoralizing the U.S. populace as it was entering the war, and causing an economic downturn right after the war. There was clearly a lack of U.S. federal government leadership and coordination in fighting that pandemic, much as in today's pandemic. This was likely a result of distraction by participation in the war and deliberate prioritization by the U.S. president, Woodrow Wilson, of a victory in the war.

Once the pandemic was recognized (in a fragmented awareness due to lack of coverage by the media), there was majority rebellion against mitigating restrictions, be they masks, numbers gathering, or businesses closures. When these measures were undertaken (mask wearing, conducting businesses and even government functions such as courts outdoors, etc.), they were taken at the local and regional level, as the pandemic was never officially acknowledged by the federal U.S. government. There was even the development of rudimentary vaccines at that time that had some effectiveness.

The city of San Francisco had one of first mask mandates in the United States, which was successful in stemming the first wave of the pandemic in that city, When the second wave arrived in 1919, efforts to reimpose mask wearing led to the formation of the Anti-Mask League which fought infringement of the rights of Americans and led to the reversal of the mandate, with a resulting return of a peak in infection. The city of Philadelphia had a disastrous public parade in support of the war and purchase of war bonds, which public health officials had requested be canceled but to no avail. That event led to thousands of deaths in the Northeast United States alone.

The lack of official acknowledgment by the U.S. federal government and populace left a level of mass amnesia about the events of the 1918–1920 pandemic, with people alive in those days having little memory of the events. It was only with renewed journalistic and historical interest and investigation during today's pandemic that the severity and extent of that pandemic is now known, with amazement considering its mortality and devastation vis-à-vis the low level of interest it aroused. There is definitely a stronger memory of that pandemic in Europe and other parts of the world.[17,18]

COVID-19 in the Scandinavian Region

Good mental health should be front and center of every country's response to and recovery from the COVID-19 pandemic.[1] Even though the COVID-19 pandemic is primarily a physical health pandemic, the mental health and well-being of the affected have been severely impacted by this health crisis.

The mental health consequences are extensive and manifest themselves in many ways. In general populations are reporting high levels of distress, increased anxiety, and fear of the virus, either for themselves or their relatives. Insufficient or misleading information has resulted in high level of distress and mistrust in authorities. Quarantine measures—whether voluntary or forced—have for many had an impact on their mental health, and thousands of vulnerable individuals have been left for months without adequate social contacts.

The economic crisis following the outbreak has resulted in huge numbers worldwide losing their employment and source of income. The economic hardship, as well as the increased amount of time spent in confinement, has had another unfortunate consequence in the form of increase in domestic violence. Many also tend toward various types of risky behavior, increased alcohol intake, drugs, binge eating, heavy smoking, or self-harm, to mention only a few.

The above consequences are to a large degree common to all countries, but certain population groups run a higher risk of mental distress and even manifest psychiatric illness.

Particular focus should be directed toward the front-line healthcare workers who report increased distress, insomnia, or even clear depressive symptoms.

Statistics show that a large proportion of those infected by the virus are residents of different kinds of long-term institutions, e.g., old people's residences, and the social isolation they have been subjected to may increase the likelihood of cognitive decline and aggravate dementia symptoms. In fact, increasing age is an overall risk factor, not least due to that with increasing age one may suffer concomitant physical disorders; combined with the loneliness resulting from social isolation, the mortality rate goes up. But also residents of different psychiatric homes, prisoners, refugees living in camps, etc., all constitute high-risk populations, and refugees and others living in conflict zones deserve special attention as their mental condition may deteriorate due to the setting in which they live with inadequate hygiene, lack of access to care, etc.

The Scandinavian Countries

These general aspects are also part of the situation in the Scandinavian region of Europe, but there are particularities that deserve describing.

First, one should be reminded that the Nordic countries have many similarities, including a long common history and common values and have over generations developed a close collaboration. Among their core values could be mentioned the existence of a stable environment with long-term political stability. The societies have a high degree of transparency, and a low level of corruption. There is an efficiency in public decision-making and public institutions.

Furthermore, there is a considerable social trust in government, and labor unions are positive toward new technology and innovation. The general level of education is high and there is a focus on gender equality. Characteristically the countries tend to promote confidence in institutions and rule of law, as well as individual autonomy that is institutionalized in law and policies. The countries have had social democratic governments for long periods, emphasizing social solidarity and a willingness to subordinate individual interests to collective rationality.

As regards health services, all the countries in the region have a public health system with expenses covered for all residents in the countries. Services are generally not based on an insurance system but are financed via the taxes.

History of COVID-19 in Scandinavia

The countries had the first infections almost simultaneously. Despite many similarities regarding their health systems, the countries chose, however, different paths in tackling the pandemic.

In Denmark—that I am most familiar with—the first case was documented on February 27: a Dane returning from holiday in northern Italy. At the same time as WHO declared the pandemic, the prime minister held a press conference on March 11, together with key ministers and directors of the Danish Health Authority and Danish Police. Here the national lockdown was outlined, and subsequently extensive steps were taken to minimize the pandemic. This included simple measures to be followed by all: to keep social distance of minimum 2 m, to carry out scrupulous hand hygiene, to cough or sneeze in your sleeve, to clean all surfaces handles, etc., very frequently, stop shaking hands, hugging, etc.[2] In contrast to many countries, citizens were not in the first phase required to wear masks, even on public transport, and domestic travels were reduced but not restricted. Extensive testing did not take place in the first phases and how those affected were placed in quarantine was a matter of debate.

These recommendations were later followed by a number of restrictions—supported by the entire Parliament—in public transport, closure of schools, educational institutions, closing the borders, closure of restaurants, bars, sports events, etc., and no assembly anywhere of more than 10 persons (later changed to 5). Public institutions were closed, and all staff members worked electronically from home; this was also recommended for private companies if at all possible. From the beginning, authorities stressed that every single citizen must assume responsibility to reduce social contact and maintain social distancing, including among family and friends.

In the following months, restrictions were constantly monitored in the light of the number of new cases, and different adjustments took place as presented at regular press conferences. Already after one month, the Danish Health Authority published its expert plan for the transition and for gradually increasing activities in the national health service by allowing many health professions to reopen. A number of multi-sector partnerships were now be established as fora to further the dialogue between authorities, relevant organizations, and trade unions about how to reopen the society in a responsible manner.

In the subsequent months, a gradual reopening of society took place, schools partly reopened, public employees returned, various institutions returned to normal, and so did most private companies. International traffic has been one of the last areas, and free international travel has returned to normal. Extensive testing continues and the individual hygienic measures have not been canceled. The reopening of society has not led to a new wave of COVID-19 and there are now (July 2020) very few hospitalized due to the virus.

In Sweden, the government issued a number of measures to limit the spread of the COVID-19 virus and emphasized a close dialogue with relevant expert government agencies on effective measures to counter the spread of the coronavirus. The Swedish authorities stated from an early point that the citizens should keep a distance and take personal responsibility, thereby stressing a high trust in the Swedish population to take individual responsibility on how to avoid the pandemic.

Sweden carried out extensive COVID-19 testing per capita, meaning that a large proportion of critical workers would not need to stay home when in fact they are able to work.[3] Public gatherings of more than 50 persons were banned, together with visits to retirement homes. Further travels to Sweden from outside the European Union were banned. But contrary to other Nordic countries, Sweden chose a less restrictive policy, e.g., kept restaurants and bars open and did not close schools down completely. The Swedish Public Health Agency's chief epidemiologist played a decisive role in the overall strategy and was advocating for the development of herd immunity. However, the mortality rate was clearly higher than in the other Nordic countries, and subsequently there have been critical comments regarding this strategy. Sweden's government has been, at all times, prepared to introduce further measures recommended by the expert authority of the Public Health Agency. The Swedish prime minister has later said that Sweden should have done more to halt the outbreak.[4]

As the only EU country not to adopt a strict lockdown, the Swedish "light-touch" coronavirus strategy has created significant international attention. Sweden has chosen to focus on public health in the broadest sense, aiming to keep as much of society open as possible. It has relied on citizen responsibility, voluntary recommendations for social distancing, and homeworking in its effort to flatten the curve enough to allow its healthcare system to keep functioning.

Many Swedes were initially reassured that the crisis had been led by healthcare experts, not politicians, with a belief that the country acted rationally as other countries responded emotionally. But the continuous high death rate has led to sharper domestic criticism. The result is that everything is now up for discussion and the debate about whether Sweden's approach has been right or wrong has started.

In Norway, the Norwegian Directorate of Health introduced a number of measures from March 12, 2020. All educational institutions were closed, and organized sports activities were discontinued. Many events and businesses were closed, and all establishments in the hospitality industry were to close. Healthcare professionals were prohibited from traveling abroad, and the ban applied to both business and private travel. Residents were prohibited from staying in cabins outside their home municipalities, leisure travel was strongly discouraged, and non-residents were banned from entering Norway.[5]

The Directorate discouraged traveling to work unless strictly necessary and encouraged avoiding public transport if possible, as well as avoiding crowded places. People were requested not to visit institutions with vulnerable groups and generally were encouraged to limiting close contact with others. People suspected or confirmed to be infected were to follow strict home isolation rules. The government established fines for people violating home quarantine, home isolation rules, or organizing events.

Statistics

Table 37.1 shows the official number of reported cases, deaths, mortality rate per million, as well as last 14 days cumulative deaths. It should be pointed out that there may be slight differences between countries in what is included in the number of deaths. A higher mortality rate per capita in Sweden than its Nordic neighbors has led these—all of whom were locked down—to open their borders to each other (June 2020) but keep them closed to Swedes, thus a change in the usual Nordic openness toward each other.

General Considerations

As pointed out above, countries that are considered very comparable and usually similar in values nevertheless show large differences in COVID-19 morbidity and mortality patterns, as well as in the restrictions that governments have issued. In that respect it is worth considering what steps were taken when a successful management of the pandemic was achieved.

Let us consider another Nordic country, Iceland, as an example.[6] Here the pandemic was under control in July 2020, and no new cases were seen. From the very start the country

TABLE 37.1 July 1–5, 2020

Country	Cases	Deaths	Deaths/million	14-Day Cum. Deaths
Sweden	54,562	5,333	523.7	2.7
Denmark	12,294	598	104.3	0.1
Norway	8,660	243	47.0	0.0
Finland	7,117	326	59.4	0.0
Island	1,815	10	27.4	0.0

Source: https://www.statista.com/statistics/1104709/coronavirus-deaths-worldwide-per-million-inhabitants/.

focused on three simultaneous steps: testing, contact tracing, and quarantine. Prior to the verification of the first case, a contact tracing group was formed. This group carried out interviews with all those infected, and all identified contacts were placed in quarantine for 2 weeks irrespective of whether they were sick or not. The contact tracing group increased in number as the pandemic increased, but they continued with great professionalism to trace more than 95% of all possible contacts.[6] Further early definition of high-risk areas took place, and quarantine requirements were extended, not only for those in contact with the infected, but also for all returning from abroad.[6]

On the official Icelandic website there is clear day-by-day information of any changes in restrictions, thereby providing transparency to all citizens what goes on. The Icelandic government has focused on evidence-based measures that have a successful track record, such as quarantine at home (self-quarantine), isolation for infected persons, early diagnosis of infection, and effective information disclosure to the public.[6] Kristensen[7] pointed out that Iceland—along with some other countries successful in combating the pandemic—are led by women who are highly supported by the population and in general politically to the left.

Mental Health Consequences

COVID-19 has a number of mental health consequences, in relation to those without previous mental health problems as well as to psychiatric patients. As pointed out in the WPA Position paper on Psychiatry and the COVID-19 Pandemic,[8] individuals with mental disorders may be at higher risk for COVID-19. This may be due to social disadvantages, e.g., stigma, poverty, homelessness, or an inability to follow public health advice. Others may be unable to comply due to depression or psychotic symptoms. The pandemic may also disrupt ongoing treatment, resulting in early discharge from hospitals and shortage of social support. While quarantines decrease the spread of the virus, they also increase the risks of excessive alcohol use, domestic violence, and suicidality.

The Nordic region is no exception, despite the easy availability of mental health services. Here there has been a particular focus on the restrictions toward persons residing in various institutions due to mental illness or physical handicaps and deprived from social contacts. Furthermore, the homeless population and persons with different kinds of severe substance abuse are also considered high-risk populations, and many migrants are also found to belong to high-risk groups. The emphasis on physical health and a lack of focus on the emotional dimension have led to increased loneliness and depressive symptoms, as well as cognitive impairment among the elder population.

Among initiatives to overcome the negative consequences could be mentioned the following: (1) The Norwegian Psychiatric Association published on their website a comprehensive overview[9] on mental health issues related to COVID-19 in relation to both patients and health personnel. (2) The Swedish Psychiatric Association[10] has published an overview "COVID-19 and Psychiatry" with an extensive and useful list of relevant links for patients, relatives, and professionals. (3) In Denmark all regions (health authorities) describe on their websites how persons with mental problems or their relatives should manage when seeking psychiatric help during the pandemic and describe the restrictions issued by authorities.[11] Further detailed information to staff regarding how to increase their competence in dealing with the issue was provided.[12]

And yet, following the pandemic outbreak, Denmark experienced a decline in the contacts with the psychiatric institutions in all parts of the country.[13] All regions reported a significant reduction in the number of psychiatric admissions and acute contacts with mental health services following the outbreak. One reason could be due to a fear of getting infected if in contact with an institution.

Research

We are already seeing several research projects trying to elucidate the mental health aspects of the pandemic.[14] In the Copenhagen region, initiatives have been taken to screen hospital personnel employed in psychiatric services for antibodies against SARS-CoV-2. Another project will map and monitor the extent of COVID-19 infection with a focus on high-risk groups such as persons with substance abuse. Others are investigating the neurological and psychiatric complications of COVID-19 and mechanisms of the disease. The Nordic Psychiatric COVID-19 Consortium—a research group from different Nordic and Baltic countries—is analyzing the pandemic with respect to stress, loneliness, and fear of developing mental disorder. Finally, an ongoing research project Psych-Flame is including testing of psychiatric patients for SARS-CoV-2.

Summarizing

The first wave of the pandemic is almost over in the Nordic countries, and the reopening of society led to a second wave in the winter of 2021–2022 but now the pandemic is no longer a serious health issue. has not led to a second wave. In summary, the importance of a comprehensive public health system should be emphasized. Clear transparent communication by authorities to all citizens is essential, stressing the need for the individual to accept the restrictions for the benefit of those frail and vulnerable in society and emphasizing the importance of mutual trust between the population and government.[7] The welfare model has shown its strength, but from a social psychiatric perspective there are still many pertinent issues. Authorities were focusing on the physical dimension, and in general the psychological aspects and how to cope with, e.g., increased anxiety or social isolation received less attention. Looking ahead we have to develop strategies in order to be better prepared in the future with a focus on the social psychiatric dimensions.

COVID 19 and India: Challenges and Opportunities

Disasters challenge individuals and communities; yet they are both a challenge and an opportunity for growth and development. The Indian experience of the past 6 months (March 2020–October 2022) of the COVID-19 pandemic illustrates the challenges that the pandemic presents to the individuals, families, communities, and governments. On the other side of this period are opportunities for restructuring society and the development of mental health interventions.

Historical Aspects

India, like all other countries, has experienced disasters of a wide variety. Limiting to the last 100 years, India was the country most affected by the Spanish flu (1918) with over 20 million deaths.[1] The other major disasters are the Bengal famine of the 1940s, the Partition with millions displaced in 1947, the Bhopal disaster in 1984, plague in the early 1990s, a supercyclone in 1989, the tsunami in 2004,[2,3,4] in addition to the HIV epidemic from the early 1980s.

In India, there has been growth in the response to disasters at the level of policymaking in the form of the establishment of the National Disaster Management Agency (NDMA) with a strong component of psychosocial care.[5] Professionals have developed innovative ways of addressing the needs at the level of people, volunteers, health personnel, schoolteachers, and vulnerable groups like children and women. A positive impact of these measures in the past, in programs such as those for the control of HIV, has been the inclusion of mental health as an essential part of the disaster response and development of culturally relevant psychosocial interventions.

COVID 19 Pandemic

In spite of over 4 decades of disaster care in general and mental health care specifically, the current epidemic has presented unique and formidable challenges to India. For example, as recently as March 2020, there was only one certified laboratory in Pune to test the COVID-19 viral infection. The blood sample of the first suspected case, in Kerala, was sent to Pune (nearly 500 km away) for testing. In 3 months over 1100 test centers became operational. The health infrastructure was seriously limited to test, trace, isolate, care, and rehabilitate the affected persons. The required protective equipment was not readily available. More importantly, India is a country with massive internal migration of laborers.

When the lockdown was implemented and there was uncertainty of the work situation, millions started returning from their places of work to their home states. This was both a logistical challenge and a health challenge. The elderly population, estimated in the country to be about 7% (nearly 100 million persons), was the most vulnerable and needed to be "cocooned," and most of them had a limited social security net to depend on for their basic needs. The urban centers like Delhi, Mumbai, Chennai, and Bangalore had a large proportion of the population living in crowded settlements (urban slums), potentially becoming centers for the rapid spread of infection.

Impact on Mental Health of the Population

There is growing awareness of the four dimensions of mental health impact of the pandemic. The first is the need to innovatively continue medical care for those with preexisting mental disorders and for the new needs of persons developing episodes of mental disorders like post-traumatic stress disorder (PTSD). The second need is to address behavioral changes like domestic violence, increased health seeking, substance use, and addiction to gadgets, which are common in disasters. The third need is of the larger population experiencing "distress" due to the uncertainties of the situation, fear, stigma, and as a response to the measures like social distancing, loss of earning, and migration. The fourth need is to build community resilience, through addressing social issues of inequities in the community, local-level social supports, welfare measures, strengthening of spirituality, etc. All of these were recognized as important by the Indian mental health professionals. In the Indian situation, one of most specific challenges is the nearly 100 million laborers who were displaced from their places of work, back to their villages. They and their families face the challenge of day-to-day survival. As a recognition of this survival challenge, the government provided essential food support to 800 million of the population for 8 months.

Mental Health Interventions

The striking aspect of the mental health responses to the COVID-19 pandemic in India has been the wide range of responses and the rapidity with which this has occurred during the 4 months from March to July 2020. The *Hindu National* newspaper was one of the early news agencies to recognize the mental health implications of the pandemic. It published an article on March 20, 2020 (3 days before the first lockdown), and an associated podcast.[6]

The following summarizes the activities, with the focus on the initiatives as they relate to social psychiatry.

The Indian Psychiatric Society (IPS) has undertaken a number of activities, including a position statement for the government/public, a guidance for professionals, guidelines for management of opioid dependence, and survey of the general public for emotional responses to the COVID-19 pandemic.[7]

The Ministry of Health and Family Welfare (MOH and FW) included mental health as a part of the health response. It designated the National Institute of Mental Health and Neurosciences (NIMHANS), Bangalore, as the resource center. A number of educational materials in the form of pamphlets, posters, self-care documents, and brief videos are in the MOH and FW website and are accessible to professionals and the general public. The emphasis of the materials has been on "normalising the emotional reactions," reassurance, and measures of self-care. A new guideline for tele-psychiatry has been approved for delivering services.

NIMHANS, Bangalore, set up a cloud-based helpline (080-4611 0007), stretching to over 20 states. This service has been extensively used by the general public. NIMHANS has organized webinars on various aspects of mental healthcare, including a manual of mental healthcare, telepsychiatry, and a guide for online training of psychologists for providing brief and basic telephonic psychological support in the context of COVID-19.[8] Similar efforts have been offered by the other leading mental health centers like the All India Institute of Medical Sciences, New Delhi, IHBAS, Delhi, and PGIMER, Chandigarh.

There have been many professional groups providing tele-counseling in individual cities like Chennai, Kolkata, and across states. The Association of Psychiatric Social Workers has brought out a handbook for parents about childhood emotional issues.[9] There have also been initiatives by voluntary organizations like Kutumbashree in Kerala, training counselors and providing services. Existing online mental health services like the Mind Specialists, located in New Delhi, and Your Dost, located at Bangalore, have recognized the new need and have developed resources for the general population.

Paradoxically, the current pandemic has brought the social realities to the forefront. This is best illustrated by the example of Kerala.

Case Study of Kerala

The importance of the social contract in the community is illustrated by the example of Kerala state.[10,11] Kerala has a population of about 30 million (less than 3% of the population of India) but has better health and social welfare infrastructure. The first case from Wuhan in India was identified in Kerala in March 2020. In the first few months of the pandemic, the state addressed the pandemic better than other parts of India. The reasons for this better response to contain the pandemic have been studied by many investigators. For example, Heller[11] identified four important characteristics of the Kerala response, namely: (i) a state response team; (ii) a broad and dense healthcare system; (iii) activation of an already highly mobilized civil society; and (iv) the capacity of state actors and civil society partners to coordinate their efforts at the level of panchayats, districts, and municipalities.

The state has managed the crisis by building on legacies of egalitarianism, social rights, and public trust. A state embedded in civil society—the women's empowerment Kudumbasree movement being a case in point—was in a good position to co-produce effective interventions, from organizing contact tracing to delivering 300,000meals a day through Kudumbasree community kitchens.

The author's understanding of the efforts in India, to date, is as follows. First, there is high awareness of the mental health impact of the COVID-19 pandemic in the general public and policymakers. Second, the current focus has been largely on the clinical dimensions and clinical care and not the larger public health approach. Third, the effort has been to reach people with help, rather than sharing of skills and empowerment of the population. There is recognition of the economic dimension of the pandemic and lockdown, but the bigger debate of the social dimensions (inequities, gender relations, welfare net, employment, tolerance, etc.) of the pandemic in terms of the origins of the pandemic, vulnerable groups, the inequalities in the society that contribute to mental health issues, and the need for working toward community resilience are yet to find voice in the professional and public spheres.[12]

The Pandemic and Social Psychiatry

Challenges

The current pandemic is not only a medical or economic challenge, but a social challenge. There are simultaneously needs around day-to-day survival, occupation, income, general healthcare, the infection-related issues, emotional reactions to the pandemic, disturbed relationships, fear of the future, and the limited health and welfare structures for care. There are larger challenges of the social issues relating inequities, social disadvantages, inadequacies in the education, health, social supports, and community trust and resilience. Equally importantly, there are opportunities for positive social changes.[13,14]

Opportunities

The emotional impact of the pandemic can be understood by a statement made, over 102 years back, during the Spanish flu, by the Father of the Nation, Sri. Mahatma Gandhi: "This protracted and first long illness in my life thus afforded me a unique opportunity to examine my principles and to test them."[1]

In the Indian situation, the following areas will need attention: Along with the number of reports of negative impact of the pandemic on the society, there are voices pointing to the possibility for positive outcomes. First, the pandemic provides social psychiatrists an opportunity to work toward a better society, a caring and equitable society for all the population. Second, the core of social psychiatry of recognition of the importance of historical, social, political, economic, and religious components of mental health has been brought to the forefront by the pandemic and offers the opportunity to develop decentralized local solutions. Third, the current experience reinforces the need for social psychiatrists to be not only clinicians but also social change agents, who work with the larger society for the common good. Fourth, there is need for caution to recognize the limitations of professional interventions, as mental health is dependent on so many other factors.

Action Points

The interventions can be at three time frames: immediate, short-term, and long term.

At the immediate level, of the coming weeks, the focus will have to be on the management of the distress and making psychiatric care both accessible, affordable, and acceptable to the population.

The bigger need is for the "non-clinical" population to work toward the prevention of mental disorders and the promotion of mental health. There are two components, namely strengthening of emotions by evidence-based activities like daily exercise, 8 hours of sleep, daily practice of yoga/meditation, eating fruits and vegetables, and spirituality as an essential part of life. All of these interventions, when they become a part of routine life, have the potential for better quality of life and decreased incidence of different forms of mental disorders.

In the short term, of the next year, the strengthening of the general medical services by training of the professionals and paraprofessionals in essentials of mental healthcare, along with making psychiatric care accessible through innovative measures like tele-psychiatry.

Another group that needs urgent addressing are the victims of domestic violence and substance abusers, and children traumatized by migration and other deprivations.

For the long-term actions, the most important psychiatric care would be professional services for the expected 30% with long-term effects like PTSD. Simultaneously, we should be addressing all the social factors that both predispose and perpetuate emotional health issues, and those with universal benefits are the following: inequalities in the society; health literacy; gender relationships; local governments and local leaderships; tolerance of differences; limiting childhood trauma; limited use of substance abuse; respect for elders; recognition of the vulnerability of the children in general and persons with disability in particular; social supports for migrants, lonely individuals; community spaces for interaction; greenery in the environment; and climate change.

Research should be an integral part of the above three levels of social psychiatry interventions for the purposes of understanding the needs, identifying vulnerable groups, simple assessment tools, identifying the strengths of the community, and the development of innovations and the evaluation of their effectiveness.

It is these two aspects of the disruption and construction of society that lie ahead.

Conclusion

The most fitting epitaph to the current American experience was written by Pope Francis, concluding in his November 2020 editorial:

> To come out of this crisis better, we have to recover the knowledge that as a people we have a shared destination. The pandemic has reminded us that no one is saved alone. What ties us to one another is what we commonly call solidarity. Solidarity is more than acts of generosity, important as they are; it is the call to embrace the reality that we are bound by bonds of reciprocity. On this solid foundation we can build a better, different, human future.

It is likely that the fight against the COVID pandemic will go well into 2022 and beyond. This is due to both the rapid development of virus mutation variants, with increasing virulence and transmissibility, as well as the sociocultural and political challenges of maintaining strong mitigation efforts. A case in point in recent months has been in India, where the excellent public health campaign it had mounted to control the pandemic was overwhelmed by pressures for political and cultural mass gatherings, which resulted in an explosion of cases to almost 30 million and close to 400,000 deaths. The promising development is a resurgence of international cooperation to support worldwide vaccination, attending to the needs of lower-income nations.

The values of solidarity and collective action, both within nations and internationally, need to be married to those of individual initiative/achievement and attainment and valuation of knowledge in order to address our current challenge of the COVID pandemic, but also the longer term and most dangerous existential threat faced by humanity, that of climate change. The recent return of the United States to the WHO and to international collaboration in general after the 2020 election may be a harbinger of positive efforts that will ultimately address the multiple challenges posed by this pandemic and other global existential threats. We do hope that mental health is considered as an important aspect of these responses, on a service level as well as a population/preventive level, with nations across the globe sharing and learning from each other's approaches.

References

A. UNITED STATES

1. Pope Francis. A crisis reveals what is in our hearts. *New York Times*, Editorial Section. November 16, 2020.
2. Bing COVID Tracker. https://www.bing.com/covid/local/unitedstates?form=C19ANS. 2021. Last accessed January 30, 2021.
3. Centers for Disease Control. COVID-19 vaccine: helps protect you from getting COVID-19. https://www.cdc.gov/coronavirus/2019-ncov/vaccines/index.html. 2022. Accessed January 30, 2021.
4. NBC News. Map: Coronavirus travel restrictions by state. https://www.nbcnews.com/news/us-news/map-coronavirus-travel-restrictions-inside-united-states-n1236157. 2020. Last accessed January 30, 2021.
5. Woodward R. *Rage*. New York: Simon & Schuster; 2020.
6. U.S. News and World Report. U.S. saw summer of Black Lives Matter protests demanding change. December 7, 2020. https://www.usnews.com/news/top-news/articles/2020-12-07/us-saw-summer-of-black-lives-matter-protests-demanding-change#:~:text=(Reuters)%20-%20The%20summer%20of%202020%20saw%20the,knelt%20on%20his%20neck%20for%20nearly%20nine%20minutes. Last accessed January 31, 2021.
7. Neiwert D. "White supremacists" arrested while trying to amplify protest violence, Richmond mayor says. *Daily Kylos*. July 27, 2020. https://www.dailykos.com/stories/2020/7/27/1964268/--White-supremacists-arrested-while-trying-to-amplify-protest-violence-Richmond-mayor-says. Last accessed January 31, 2021.
8. Willis C. The mental toll of COVID-19. *Scientific American*. December 2020;25.
9. Czeisler M, Lane R, Petrosky E, et al. Mental health, substance use, and suuicidal ideation during the COVID-19 pandemic: United States, June 24–30, 2020. *CDC MMWR*. 2020;69(32):1049–1057.
10. Lai J, Ma S, Wang Y, et al. Factors associated with mental health outcomes among health care workers exposed to coronavirus disease 2019. *JAMA Network Open*. 2020;3(3):e203976.
11. Armitage R, Nellums L. COVID-19 and the consequences of isolating the elderly. *Lancet Public Health*. 2020;5:e256.
12. Phelps C, Sperry L. Children and the COVID-19 pandemic. *Psychol Trauma*. 2020;12(S1):S73–S75.
13. Singha S, Royb D, Sinhac K, Parveenc S, Sharmac G, Joshic G. Impact of COVID-19 and lockdown on mental health of children and adolescents: A narrative review with recommendations. *Psychiatry Res*. 2020;293:113429.
14. Leeb R, Bitsko R, Radhakrishnan L, Martinez P, Njai R, Holland K. Mental health–related emergency department visits among children aged <18 years during the COVID-19 pandemic: United States, January 1–October 17, 2020. *CDC MMWR*. 2020;69(45):1675–1680.
15. Green AE, Price-Feeney M, Dorison SH. *Implications of COVID-19 for LGBTQ Youth Mental Health and Suicide Prevention*. New York: The Trevor Project; 2020. https://www.thetrevorproject.org/2020/04/03/implications-of-covid-19-for-lgbtq-youth-mental-health-and-suicide-prevention/. Last accessed on January 31, 2021.
16. Koonin L, Hoots B, Tsang C, et al. Trends in the use of telehealth during the emergence of the COVID-19 pandemic: United States, January–March 2020. *CDC MMWR*. 2020;69(43):1595–1599.

17. Arnold C. *Pandemic 1918: The Story of the Deadliest Influenza in History*. New York: St. Martin's Press, 2018.
18. Wikipedia. Spanish flu. https://en.wikipedia.org/wiki/Spanish_flu. Last accessed on January 31, 2021.

B. SCANDINAVIA

1. *WHO Policy Brief: COVID-19 and the Need for Action on Mental Health*. Geneva: WHO; May 13, 2020.
2. Danish Health Authority: Covid 19. https://www.sst.dk/en/English/Corona-eng. 2021. Last accessed February 3, 2021.
3. Government Offices of Sweden. April 2020. https://www.government.se/articles/2020/04/s-decisions-and-guidelines-in-the-ministry-of-health-and-social-affairs-policy-areas-to-limit-the-spread-of-the-covid-19-virusny-sida/. Last accessed February 3, 2021. Replaced by reference below.
4. Coronavirus: Sweden misjudged coronavirus resurgence. https://www.euronews.com/2020/12/15/coronavirus-sweden-s-health-officials-misjudged-covid-19-resurgence-says-pm-stefan-lofven. Last accessed February 3, 2021. Published on 12.15.2020.
5. Covid-19 epidemic in Norway. https://en.wikipedia.org/wiki/COVID-19_pandemic_in_Norway. Last accessed February 3, 2021.
6. The response of the Icelandic authorities. https://www.covid.is/sub-categories/icelands-response. Last accessed February 3, 2021.
7. Kristensen T. Søndergaard Danmark er ikke verdensmester i coronakamp [Denmark is not a world champion in fighting corona]. *Kronik (Column) Politiken*. July 4, 2020.
8. *WPA Position Paper on Psychiatry and the Covid 19 Pandemic*. https://3ba346de-fde6-473f-b1da-53649 8661f9c.filesusr.com/ugd/e172f3_0bec245159b946f287822b80e839b095.pdf. Last accessed February 3, 2021. Published on 09/15/2020.
9. Litteraturgennemgang ved Covid19 [A literature review of Covid 19]. 2020. https://www.legeforenin gen.no/contentassets/5181cf273d394c7fae314ea637d07e9d/litteraturgjennomgang-covid-19-pha-ous-4.4.2020.pdf. Last accessed February 3, 2021.
10. Svensk Psykiatrisk Forening: Covid19 och psykiatri. http://www.svenskpsykiatri.se/nyheter/2020/03/22/covid-19-och-psykiatri/. Accessed June 20, 2020. Published on 03/22/2020.
11. Questions and answers for patient in mental health services of Copenhagen about covid19. https://www.psykiatri-regionh.dk/undersoegelse-og-behandling/Sider/FAQ-m%C3%A5lrettet-patienter-under-COVID---19.aspx. Last accessed February 3, 2021.
12. Psychiatry and covid19. https://www.rm.dk/om-os/organisation/center-for-e-laering/kurser/hje mmedier-med-laringsindhold/covid19undervisningsmateriale/psykiatri-og-covid-19/. Last accessed February 3, 2021.
13. Information. Psykiatrien oplever fald i antal indlæggelser [There is a decline in the number of psychiatric admissions]. April 4, 2020. https://www.information.dk/indland/2020/04/psykiatrien-oplever-voldsomt-fald-indlaeggelser-coronakrisen. Last accessed February 3, 2021.
14. Monitoring the extent of covid19 in selected populations. https://www.psykiatri-regionh.dk/forskning/Udvalgte%20projekter/Forskningsprojekter-med-fokus-på-i-COVID-19-i-RHP/Sider/Monitorering-af-udbredelsen-af-COVID-19-i-udsatte-grupper-med-fokus-på-mennesker-med-psykisk-sygdom,-alkohol--og-stofmisbru.aspx?rhKeywords=covid19. Last accessed February 3, 2021.

C. INDIA

1. Spinney L. *Pale Rider: The Spanish Flu of 1918 and How It Changed the World*. London: Vintage; 2017.
2. Srinivasa Murthy R. Disaster mental health and social psychiatry: challenges and opportunities. *Indian J Soc Psychiatry*. 2018;34:323–327.
3. Lakshminarayana R, Srinivasa Murthy R, Diaz JOP. *Disaster Mental Health in India*. New Delhi: Indian Red Cross Society; 2004.
4. Srinivasa Murthy R. Conflict situations and mental health care in developing countries. In: Christodoulou GN, Mezzich JE, Christodoulou NG, et al., eds. *Disasters: Mental Health Context and Responses*. New Castle upon Tyne: Cambridge Scholars; 2016:153–172.
5. National Disaster Management Authority. *Guidelines on Psycho-Social Support and Mental Health Services (PSSMHS) in Disasters*. New Delhi: National Disaster Management Authority; 2009.

6. Vijayakumar L, Thara R. Because the mind matters. *The Hindu*. March 20, 2020.

7. Indian Psychiatric Society. *Position Statement*. New Delhi: Indian Psychiatric Society; 2020.

8. NIMHANS. *1. Mental Health in the times of COVID-19 Pandemic Guidance for General Medical and Specialised Mental Health Care Settings; 2. Telepsychiatry-Operational Guidelines; 3. Guidelines for Tele-Psychotherapy Services; 4. Resource Material: Online Training of Psychologists for Providing Brief and Basic Telephonic Psychological Support in the Context of COVID19*. Bangalore, India: NIMHANS; 2020.

9. Association for Psychiatric Social Work Professionals, Bengaluru, India. *Nurturing Children Through This Pandemic [A Family Guide]*. Bangalore: April 11, 2020.

10. Editorial: Kerala shows the way: decades of investment in public health is helping the state control Covid-19. *Times of India*. April 16, 2020.

11. Heller, P. A virus, social democracy and dividends for Kerala. *The Hindu*. April 18, 2020.

12. National Academy Press (NAM). *Developing a Framework for Measuring Community Resilience: Summary of a Workshop*. Washington, DC: NAM; 2015.

13 Orbach, S. Patterns of pain: what Covid-19 can teach us about how to be human. *The Guardian*, May 7, 2020.

14. Wright L. How pandemics wreak havoc—and open minds. *The New York*, July 20, 2020.

38

Mental Health Aspects of Information Technology

Impact on Behavior and on Treatment Applications

Kishan Nallapula and Andres J. Pumariega

Introduction

Information technology (IT) is defined by the *Oxford Dictionary of Physics* as "[t]he study or use of computers, telecommunication systems, and other devices for storing, retrieving, and transmitting information."[1] Information systems form the backbone of every single industry in the modern day. Information systems include but are not limited to telegraph, telephone, television, cellular phones, electronic mail, the World Wide Web, smartphones, digital media applications (apps), radio communication systems, global positioning systems (GPS), etc. The availability of these technologies has changed human communication and interaction patterns to the extent that it is nearly impossible to function in the society without the assistance of these technologies.

President Abraham Lincoln's inaugural address took 7 days and 17 hours to reach California in 1861.[2] Just 100 years later, the revolution of television meant that information could be transmitted within minutes or could be broadcast live for audiences living thousands of miles away. While interactions between like-minded individuals to spur innovation and scientific advancement took years or decades due to delays in information exchange, the advances in information technology have significantly decreased the time. In the year 1918, the United States Patent and Trademark Office issued 38,450 utility patents (inventions), while in 2018 the number was 307,760,[3] which is about an 8-fold increase in a matter of 100 years.

The *Merriam-Webster Dictionary* defines the internet as an electronic communications network that connects computer networks and organizational computer facilities around the world. What started as a network of computers has permeated into nearly almost every piece of equipment that we use currently with the proliferation of the Internet of Things (IoT). Consumer electronics, medical equipment, telephones, automobiles, small and large appliances, all are increasingly being made to connect to the network for ease of use and monitoring purposes. World economies, governmental enterprises, and private business all rely heavily on the internet as a platform to carry out their daily operations and broadcast information about their activities.

Information systems offer tremendous benefits to humans. In respect to communication, email has provided for secure, closed interpersonal sharing of information among individuals and groups in a matter of minutes to anyone located across the globe. This timely communication allows for increased work efficiency, better collaboration, and an improved quality of work.

There are also certain significant disadvantages with information technology use. It has changed human communication patterns: the younger generation are increasingly preferring to communicate electronically rather than in person. Attention to body language, which forms an important component of human interactions, is not present when a conversation is taking place via audio only, or via written messaging like email or instant messaging platforms.

The internet has also had a significant economic effect on certain industries, such as the demand for newsprint and paper products. The demand for printing and writing paper is significantly less in countries with widespread internet usage, while the demand for packaging paper and paperboard remains unchanged.[4] Due to the rise in e-commerce platforms, the United States has seen a record number of retail store closures from 2016 onward. This would naturally lead to a significant change in the drivers of local economies.

As mental health has a significant social component in the causation, maintenance, and treatment of mental illness, these rapid cultural changes due to the explosion of information technology are expected to have an effect.

IT Psychosocial Impact on Populations and Individuals

The standard of living across the globe has significantly changed in the latter half of the 20th century due to rapid dissemination of information and other advancements in sciences. As a result, information technology has had a significant impact on the daily lives of the overwhelming majority of the world population. The majority of that impact has been quite positive, but areas of negative impact and greater challenges do exist. Below we will outline the main areas of impact, both for the world's population as well as individuals.

Overall Impact on Society and Populations

Information technology has played a major role in the development of globalization of the world economy, including manufacturing, service industries, and finance. This has involved the worldwide distribution of services, global supply chains, and the provision of services across national boundaries and over long distances to minimize their expense. A family in the United States is just as likely to buy goods manufactured across a number of nations, and receive telephonic or online services from providers in different continents. Consumer goods and services have proliferated as a result of this high level of international and interregional commerce, with greater choices and rapid home delivery. The ability to communicate to the worldwide internet has been the major facilitator of these developments.[5]

Such global distribution of the economy has resulted in lower costs and greater efficiency, but has led to significant disruption in local employment and reduction in local goods and services except for niche products and services. There has also been significant dislocation of large brick and mortar stores and shopping malls, as well as small and large businesses. In addition to the impact on employment, this has also resulted in lower rates of public congregation around shopping, something that has been a key part of the human experience since the earliest bartering posts in early history.[5]

The impact on how education is delivered has also been revolutionized by information technology. The majority of higher educational institutions, and many web-based primary and secondary education entities, now provide completely online courses, including web-based and streaming lecture content, distance examinations and grades, discussion groups, and individualized online tutorial interaction with instructors. Such developments have greatly increased access to educational opportunities and have reduced geographic and time barriers, though cost reductions from the scalability of educational enterprises has yet to be realized. However, this revolution in education has had its negative aspects, with the reduction of interpersonal interaction, and barriers to customization of teaching techniques for individuals with learning and interpersonal challenges.[6,7]

Information technology has led to a revolution in interpersonal communication. It has led to more rapid and direct communication, first through electronic mail (email), then through telephonic text messages, and ultimately through distributed social media networks, ultimately leading to a convergence of interpersonal and mass communication. Social media networks are based on membership determined by group affiliations as diverse as friendships, organizational affiliation (political, religious, etc.) and even ideological beliefs. Communication across the internet facilitates distance interactions across geographic and national boundaries, and brings dispersed groups together.[8] However, it has had an adverse impact on time for more intimate one-on-one interaction, either via face to face or telephonic voice, leading to some degree of disconnection anlack of context through presumed anonymity.[9] More open communication has had a significant impact on political discourse and governance, with more open access to information and the ability to organize opinions and input. In some notable instances, it has allowed resistance to political oppression, in spite of efforts to suppress such resistance.[10,11] However, this has spawned backlash restrictions from oppressive regimes, as well as the use of misinformation to disrupt democratic processes.[12]

Another significant impact of the information technology revolution has been the increasing digital divides between the Global North (more developed and industrialized nations) and the Global South (developing and traditional nations). Though there is hope that these divides will be bridged as information technologies increasingly are adopted worldwide, in the meantime this divide exacerbates socioeconomic and cultural differences, to the point that many nations in Global South have experienced a backlash to outside influences, as well as barriers to economic and advancement opportunities for many people.[13]

Individual Impacts

As previously mentioned, electronic communication has greatly facilitated social connectedness across widely dispersed groups, including increased opportunities to connect with dispersed affinity groups, such as religious, social, political, or even illness support groups.[14] At the same time, it has contributed to less emphasis on live one-on-one communication, with some concerns that social skills are being lost in the process. The new formats of electronic communication have resulted in problems with appropriate boundaries and limits, with unfiltered communication outside of the context of nonverbal social cues from live interaction at times coming across as offensive or disruptive.[15-17] These effects are heightened by communication to social media, where negative feedback and negative group processes can escalate to the point that they become very distressing to the individual.[17] A well-known phenomenon around Facebook has been the distress experienced by some when they receive negative reaction to their posts or even an insufficient number of "likes."[16] Another phenomenon that has been described is that of "FOMO" (fear of missing out), experienced when attractive social events and activities are pictured on social media and individuals realize they were not invited or included.[18]

Electronic gaming has evolved from being an activity pursued individually or in small groups with a single console or terminal, involving simple graphics and simulations, to an interconnected experience that involves multiple players from around the globe and highly sophisticated images and graphics that are almost lifelike, with a high level of adventure. The games often have highly stimulating and engaging experiences driven by complex algorithms. These have led to widespread engagement of pre-adolescents and adolescents, particularly males, to the extent that they spend many hours per day or per week on gaming, to the detriment of both academic studies and interpersonal activities.[19,20] Unfortunately, some of the content of these games has skewed toward violent physical or even sexualized scenes, which then raises concerns about modeling disinhibition of impulsivity and aggression.[21] Such extent of virtual gaming has made it at times increasingly difficult for parents to set boundaries and limits with youth, setting up increasing parent-child conflict, especially for youth who already have difficulty with the need for novel stimuli and impulsivity.[22]

Another adverse aspect of the unrestricted and unfiltered nature and access of the internet is its use within the "dark web" for criminal activity and human trafficking. These applications have dangerous potential for many individuals, particularly those with poor impulse control, and of exposing youth to inappropriate content.[23]

Increasing research has focused on the impact of gaming and internet images and algorithms on the developing brain. Some studies have pointed to the development of shorter attention spans, reduced delay of gratification and patience, increased frustration, and increased impulsivity, resulting from exposure to the highly stimulating activities and images within the internet. Such results have even been found among adults as well as children and youth, to the extent that significant numbers of adults forgo an active interpersonal life for the sake of pursuing virtual electronic experiences.[24]

On the other hand, large segments of the population, particularly individuals who live in more traditional cultural settings or rural settings, with more limited socioeconomic status, and who may even be older in age, experience the opposite effect in the context of the intense activity of the internet. Being overwhelmed with the pace of electronic communication, information flow, and change is not unusual, especially for the older brain, which is less plastic and adaptable, while young brains have much more rapid cognitive assimilation/accommodation and more flexible and less ingrained neural circuits. These differences also contribute to an increased generational technological as well as cultural divide.[25]

Known Mental Health Impacts

Some studies have pointed to associations between time spent on internet activity and levels of depression, anxiety, and suicidality, especially among the youth. This is not only true for youth exposure to social media, but also for adults engaged in continual online communication that may even be work related.[26–28] Another adverse mental health phenomenon that has arisen is the increasing frequency of cyberbullying, the use of the internet to perpetrate aggression on others virtually through targeted negative and demeaning messages.[29] Other studies have also pointed to increasing problems with sleep disruption and/or disturbance resulting from after-hours internet activity. The adverse impact on the sleep cycle may be related to difficulty "winding down" from earlier activity, the engaging and nearly addictive quality of the activities themselves where the individual sacrifices sleep, and even the stimulation from back lighting emitted from devices, such as computer and smartphone screens.[30] Internet addiction (gaming, pornography, gambling) has also been found to be a significant mental health problem, sufficient to have been incorporated into psychiatric nomenclature and nosology.[20,31] The rapid and stimulating level of activity and images, the use of variable reinforcement approaches to maintain such activity, and the false sense of mastery that at times comes from engaging in such activity all contribute to these outcomes.[20]

IT Impact on the Delivery of Mental Health Services

Mental health service delivery traditionally involved in-person encounters. Individuals with serious mental illness have inherent deficiencies in information processing that limits them from utilizing their cognitive faculties to appropriately express themselves. Hence utilizing extant communication methods like postal mail, telephone, or telegraph were not appropriate for delivering mental health services.

Communication methods could be broadly classified into asynchronous and synchronous platforms. Asynchronous technologies include:

- Postal mail
- Telegraph
- Electronic mail (email)
- Short messaging service (SMS)/texting
- Instant messaging on the internet through various applications.

Synchronous technologies include:

- 2-way radio devices
- Telephone
- Audio-only internet applications
- Video conferencing or 2-way video calling applications.

Triaging the urgency of the information that needs to be exchanged is the key in selecting the appropriate modality to be used for a given situation. Below we briefly present when these different modalities may be utilized.

Postal mail: Needs paper, postage, and a trip to the nearest mailbox. Recipient usually receives the message in 2 to 3 days if there is no request for overnight mail. Mail is delivered to the address and the recipient will have to retrieve it at their convenience. May be utilized to send non-urgent messages or bills.

Telegraph: Transmission between 2 post offices is instantaneous; however, the message will have to be hand delivered to the recipient. Currently legacy technology with minimal usage across the globe.

Electronic mail: Requires access to internet. Written/typed messages can be transmitted instantaneously across the globe. Photographs and other documents could be attached if within specified size limits. The recipient should have a mechanism to be notified or check the mail at intervals to receive the message. Also provides for immediate responses. Used widely as the primary modality of information exchange among individuals and businesses alike. Could also be utilized to send non-urgent messages and bills. The limiting step is recipient dependent.

Short messaging service (SMS): Legacy SMS services allowed for text exchanges over the cellular network with a limit on the characters per message. These limitations are being phased out due to the advent of rich communication service (RCS). RCS also allows for other interactive messaging features like read receipts and whether the recipient is typing. This requires the sender and recipient to have cellular phone access and to be in a location with adequate coverage. This could be utilized for brief notification and to have a conversation that does not need a voice discussion. In health systems this is primarily utilized for appointment notification and confirmation.

Instant Messaging on the internet: This is akin to SMS but the information exchange occurs over the internet. This platform provides for a "conversation view." It has the easy ability to have group conversations, express emotions via "emoji," share pictures and videos. WhatsApp™ is the current worldwide leader in the instant messaging platforms.

Two-way radio devices: These wireless devices are primarily utilized by law enforcement, retail employees, taxi drivers, etc., which requires one message to be transmitted to a group of individuals and the recipient to have the ability to respond back to the group.

Telephone: Allows for real-time conversation between 2 individuals with variable ability to add others into a conference. This is the primary modality of voice communication currently. Provides some information about the patient's condition when doing a phone assessment. Visual stimuli are absent, which prevents certain assessments that require the patient to be seen.

Videoconferencing or 2-way video calling: This provides for audio and visual interaction in real time between parties. This is the closest to in-person conversations. Multiple video conferencing platforms exist with different levels of functionalities available to free and paid users. Many organizations enter into business associate agreements to utilize a product from a specific vendor. Mental health services can be adequately delivered through this platform if there is good internet connection and necessary hardware, which includes webcam, microphone, and speakers or a smartphone or a tablet with these capabilities.

Application of Some of These Technologies in Mental Health Service Delivery

Email: There is some usage of email as a means of delivering services.[32] However, this not widely practiced. It may be appropriate if the patient has difficulty or would like to express their feelings in writing.

Videoconferencing: As discussed above, videoconferencing mirrors the closest to in-person encounters. Mental health service delivery via 2-way audio-video communication platforms is growing exponentially worldwide. This improves access to care because of not needing to travel long distances to obtain care. This is particularly suited for increasing access to rural areas. In the urban setting this is beneficial, as this will significantly diminish tardy appointments due to traffic congestion. Major professional organizations like the American Psychiatric Association and others have standing committees that devote their time to promoting this platform and advocating its use in multiple avenues. Long-standing research and multiple review articles have shown that tele-mental health service is equivalent to in-person care. All the elements required for a comprehensive psychiatric interview and a mental status examination can be obtained by video calling. Studies have shown that acceptability across age groups is similar. The geriatric population prefer and accept this method of service delivery, similar to the younger generation.

Electronic Health Records(EHR)

The key to running a remote mental health service is the availability of electronic health records. A uniformed platform where information is shared among all members of the team involved in the service delivery is key. In the United States, EHR is an open market with multiple vendors and different levels of customization even with the same vendor. Although this model promotes competition and innovation in the field, sharing of information between the systems is not standardized, resulting in delays of information exchange and ultimately contributing to poor care. Major hospital systems like the Veterans Affairs administration hospitals have a unified system across the country. which helps care team members access patient information easily. Major EHR systems like Epic® have a system of linking the records at different institutions that subscribe to the same platform.

Having an EHR on most occasions provides the additional benefit of integrating the ability to prescribe medications including controlled substances. In countries where medication availability is strictly regulated, having the ability to e-prescribe is very important. In the United States, individual states have already mandated, or will mandate in the near future, that controlled substances with a potential for diversion be prescribed electronically directly by the physician to the pharmacy. This is a very important component in preventing and controlling substance use and drug trafficking.

EHR also allows for easy statistical analyses and the development of screening tools. Reviewing a large number of records can be accomplished by using a key word query method. Yuval Barak-Corren et al. did a longitudinal review of EHR from a large healthcare database spanning 15 years and found sensitive, specific, and early predictors of patients' future suicidal behavior.[33] Strongest predictors found were substance abuse, psychiatric disorder, injuries, and chronic conditions. EHR can also be utilized to administer screening tools like the Columbia Suicide Severity Rating Scale (CSSRS). Based on the scores of the screening tools, algorithms can be developed to find a disposition for the patient. Screening tools can be electronically provided to patients using patient portals that they may complete prior to their outpatient appointments.

EHRs allowing a patient portal integration is particularly beneficial for patients to track their appointments, receive and initiate secure communications to and from their providers, pay their bills, participate in telemedicine visits, upload pictures or other data, and complete rating scales, to name a few.

Utilizing Apps in the Delivery of Services

The ubiquity of smartphones worldwide has led to the proliferation of apps that address every single facet of life. Similarly, there are many apps that specialize in delivering mental health care. Talkspace is an asynchronous text-based psychotherapy service that has shown to have value in providing psychotherapy. A multitude of videoconferencing apps are available for the provision of tele-mental health services.[34,35] PTSD Coach, an app developed by the US Department of Veterans Affairs, helps patients with exposure therapy related to PTSD.[36] reSET is an FDA-approved app that requires a prescription, which is shown to have validity in the treatment of opioid addiction.[37]

In AVATAR therapy, therapists voice an online avatar which portrays the voices heard by schizophrenic clients. The clients converse with the avatar, with the avatar becoming less hostile as the dialogue progresses. In a randomized control trial, patients with schizophrenia or affective disorder who had enduring auditory verbal hallucinations were assigned to either AVATAR therapy or supportive counseling. "The reduction in PSYRATS–AH total score at 12 weeks was significantly greater for AVATAR therapy than for supportive counselling."[38]

Special Uses

Tele-mental health services are ideal to bridge disparity in the availability of services in rural and underserved areas. Expertise can be made available to where it is needed, easily and instantaneously, without needing to travel.[39,40] Tele-mental health services are being provided by hundreds of community agencies across the United States.

Tele-mental health services can be easily scaled and leveraged during the times of disasters when travel is restricted or not possible.[41] Natural disasters like inclement weather, earthquakes, and hurricanes prevent safe transportation. When power and communication lines are intact, tele-mental health services are ideal for continued care and also for emergency care needs. In pandemics like COVID-19, where international mobility is restricted, tele-mental health operations form a key piece in sustaining operations for clinics, hospitals, and community agencies.[42] In addition to providing care and treatment for patients, it also keeps the organizational revenue intact by minimizing cancellations.[42]

Regulations, Ethics, and Etiquette

Regulations around the practice of tele-psychiatry is highly variable. In the United States, the Health Insurance Portability and Accountability Act sets the standards for privacy, need for business associate agreements, etc. The individual states may have additional mandates for payment reimbursement, licensure requirements, and practice across state lines. The reader is referred to check with their local regulating agency on these matters.

The ethical considerations for the practice of tele-psychiatry remain the same as for an in-person encounter. It is imperative that consent is obtained for this form of care delivery, with a full discussion of alternative options. Ideally the patients are pre-screened for suitability in terms of acuity, technological availability (internet, audio-visual equipment, etc.), and proficiency. Clear protocols must be established by the individual provider or health systems regarding the need for disclosure of patient location and how emergencies in appointment would be handled. Having additional protocols for minors is needed, like a caregiver or adult to be present within immediate reach of the patient, and also a direct way for the provider to communicate with them. The provider must be aware of local emergency services where the patient is located and if the need arises, e.g., the patient disclosing suicidal ideations during the session, to contact them while engaging the patient.

Malpractice liability coverage is also carrier dependent and it may warrant discussion with the carrier while considering changes in practice delivery.

Etiquette

It is of paramount importance to maintain a professional etiquette while practicing tele-psychiatry. It is important to be mindful of lighting, background, acoustics, eye contact, multitasking, etc. Seeing the patients in their natural environment provides immense clinical information that helps in decision-making. However, technical issues on the patient's end may impede obtaining adequate mental status exam; it may necessitate the need for patience and also repeating oneself. The reader is referred to the American Psychiatric Association's Telepsychiatry Toolkit for further reading.[43]

Future Uses: Artificial Intelligence

Algorithms have been developed to mine EHR data. However, medical data are very complex and it is difficult to differentiate signal from noise. Data collection is asynchronous. The majority of clinical notes contain jargon that may be unique to specialty, locality, and culture. Also certain similar words, especially acronyms, are meant to mean different things in different contexts. The utilization of bots to screen social media posts for words like suicide is being investigated.

The ultimate question of whether artificial intelligence (AI) will replace physicians is a "no" at this point. Humans have an innate ability to defy algorithms at any given point, which is needed in unique patient situations. Although AI has the ability to incorporate new information, the ability to respond is as good as the algorithm, which is ultimately controlled by humans.

Conclusions

As it stands currently, technology and communication systems form an indispensable part of life in all domains. The ability to leverage these tools to enhance social activities, healthcare systems, and care delivery is very much necessary. Organizations and individuals will benefit if they use these technologies appropriately and efficiently in their lives.

References

1. Information Technology. https://www.oxfordreference.com/view/10.1093/oi/authority.20110803100003879.
2. Longfellow R. *Back in Time: Transportation in America's Postal System*. Washington, DC: U.S. Department of Transportation: Federal Highway Administration 2017. https://www.fhwa.dot.gov/infrastructure/back0304.cfm. Accessed on December 3, 2022.
3. *U.S. Patent Activity: Calendar Years 1790 to the Present*. U.S. Patent and Trademark Office. 2020. https://www.uspto.gov/web/offices/ac/ido/oeip/taf/h_counts.htm. Accessed on December 3, 2022.
4. Chiba T, Oka H, Kayo C. Socioeconomic factors influencing global paper and paperboard demand. *J Wood Science*. 2017;63:539–547.
5. Osland JS. Broadening the debate: the pros and cons of globalization. *J Management Inquiry*. 2003;12:137–154.
6. Raja R, Nagasubramani PC. Impact of modern technology in education. *J Appl Adv Res*. 2018;3:S33–S35.
7. Zhu X. The Integration of Media Technology and the Change of Education (IMTCE): a study of model of the impact of media technology on education. *Int J Inform Educ Technology*. 2018;8:422–427.
8. Flanagin AJ. Online social influence and the convergence of mass and interpersonal communication. *Human Comm Res*. 2017;43:450–463.

9. Subramanian KR. Influence of social media in interpersonal communication. *Int J Scien Progr Res.* 2017;38:70–75.

10. Koc-Michalska K, Lilleker D. Digital politics: mobilization, engagement, and participation. *Political Comm.* 2017;34:1–5.

11. Solo AMG, Bishop J. Network politics and the Arab Spring. In: Association IRM, ed. *Civic Engagement and Politics: Concepts, Methodologies, Tools, and Applications.* Hershey, PA: IGI Global; 2019:877–882.

12. Lakkysetty N, Deep P, Balamurugaan J. Social media and its impacts on politics. *Int J Adv Res, Ideas, and Innov Technology.* 2018;4(2):2108–2118.

13. Cruz-Jesus F, Oliveira T, Bacao F. The global digital divide: evidence and drivers *J Global Information Management.* 2018;26(2):1–26.

14. Conrad P, Bandini J, Vasquez A. Illness and the internet: from private to public experience. *Health.* 2016;20(1):22–32.

15. Khalil L. Identifying cyber hate: overview of online hate speech policies & finding possible measures to counter hate speech on internet. *J Media Studies.* 2016;31(1):61–73.

16. Reategui ASL, Palmer R. Unfiltered: the effect of media on body image dissatisfaction. *Int J Soc Sci Humanity.* 2017;7(6):367–372.

17. Schroeder R. Social theory after the internet: media, technology, and globalization. London: UCL Press; 2018:82–100. https://doi.org/10.2307/j.ctt20krxdr.

18. Wolniewicz CA, Tiamiyu MF, Weeks JW, Elhai JD. Problematic smartphone use and relations with negative affect, fear of missing out, and fear of negative and positive evaluation *Psychiatry Res.* 2018;262:618–623.

19. Martín-Perpiñá MM, Poch FV, Cerrato SM. Media multitasking impact in homework, executive function and academic performance in Spanish adolescents. *Psicothema.* 2019;31(1):81–87.

20. Muñoz-Miralles R, Ortega-González R, López-Morón MR, et al. The problematic use of Information and Communication Technologies (ICT) in adolescents by the cross sectional JOITIC study. *BMC Pediatrics.* 2016;16(1):1–11.

21. Lewis R. Literature review on children and young people demonstrating technology-assisted harmful sexual behavior. *Aggress Violent Behav.* 2018;40:1–11.

22. Symons K, Ponnet K, Walrave M, Heirman W. A qualitative study into parental mediation of adolescents' internet use *Computers Human Behav.* 2017;73:423–432.

23. Campbell C. Web of lives: how regulating the Dark Web can combat online human trafficking. *J Natl Assoc Admin Law Judiciary.* 2018;38(2):136–181.

24. Crone EA, Konijn EA. Media use and brain development during adolescence *Nature Communications.* 2018;9(1):1–10.

25. Cáceres RB, Chaparro AC. Age for learning, age for teaching: the role of inter-generational, intra- household learning in Internet use by older adults in Latin America *Inf Commun Soc.* 2019;22(2):250–266.

26. McCrae N, Gettings S, Purssell E. Social media and depressive symptoms in childhood and adolescence: a systematic review. *Adolesc Res Rev.* 2017;2:315–330.

27. Primack BA, Shensa A, Escobar-Viera CG, et al. Use of multiple social media platforms and symptoms of depression and anxiety: a nationally-representative study among U.S. young adults *Computers Human Behav.* 2017;69:1–9.

28. Notredame C-E, Morgiève M, Morel F, Berrouiguet S, Azé J, Vaiva G. Distress, suicidality, and affective disorders at the time of social networks. *Curr Psychiatry Rep.* 2019;21(10):

29. Savage MW, Tokunaga RS. Moving toward a theory: testing an integrated model of cyberbullying perpetration, aggression, social skills, and Internet self-efficacy *Computers Human Behav.* 2017;71:353–361.

30. Woods HC, Scott H. #Sleepyteens: social media use in adolescence is associated with poor sleep quality, anxiety, depression and low self-esteem. *J Adolescence.* 2016;51:41–49.

31. Giotakos O, Tsouvelas G, Spourdalaki E, Janikian M, Tsitsika A, Vakirtzis A. Internet gambling in relation to Internet addiction, substance use, online sexual engagement and suicidality in a Greek sample. *International Gambling Studies.* 2017;17(1):20-29.

32. Chechele PJ, Stofle G. Individual therapy online via email and Internet Relay Chat. In: Goss S, Anthony K, eds. *Technology in Counselling and Psychotherapy: A Practitioner's Guide.* London: Palgrave Macmillan; 2003:39–58.

33. Barak-Corren Y, Castro VM, Javitt S, et al. Predicting suicidal behavior from longitudinal electronic health records. *Am J Psychiatry*. 2017;174(2):154–162.

34. Marcelle E, Davis TS. BetterHelp members experience significant reduction in depression symptoms: viable alternative to traditional face-to-face counseling. *BetterHelp*. 2017. https://www.betterhelp.com/. Accessed December 3, 2022.

35. Hull TD, Mahan K. A Study of Asynchronous Mobile-Enabled SMS Text Psychotherapy. *Telemed J E Health*. 2017 Mar;23(3):240–247. doi: 10.1089/tmj.2016.0114. Epub 2016 Oct 31. PMID: 27797646.

36. Kuhn E, van der Meer C, Owen JE, Hoffman JE, Cash R, Carrese P, Olff M, Bakker A, Schellong J, Lorenz P, Schopp M, Rau H, Weidner K, Arnberg FK, Cernvall M, Iversen T. PTSD Coach around the world. *Mhealth*. 2018 May 25;4:15. doi: 10.21037/mhealth.2018.05.01. PMID: 29963560; PMCID: PMC5994444.

37. Chung J-Y. Digital therapeutics and clinical pharmacology. *Transl Clin Pharmacol*. 2019;27(1):6–11.

38. Craig TK, Rus-Calafell M, Ward T, et al. AVATAR therapy for auditory verbal hallucinations in people with psychosis: a single-blind, randomised controlled trial. *Lancet Psychiatry*. 2018;5(1):31–40, page 31.

39. Fortney JC, Pyne JM, Turner EE, et al. Telepsychiatry integration of mental health services into rural primary care settings. *Int Rev Psychiatry*. 2015;27(6):525–539.

40. David P. Paul I, Washington B, Robinson A, Tonnie M, Coustasse A. *Telepsychiatry: Access in Rural Areas*. Paper presented at: Northeast Business & Economics Association Forty-Fifth Annual Conference, 2018; Galloway, NJ.

41. *OCR Announces Notification of Enforcement Discretion for Telehealth Remote Communications During the COVID-19 Nationwide Public Health Emergency*. 2020. https://www.hhs.gov/about/news/2020/03/17/ocr-announces-notification-of-enforcement-discretion-for-telehealth-remote-communications-during-the-covid-19.html.

42. Reinhardt I, Gouzoulis-Mayfrank E, Zielasek J. Use of telepsychiatry in emergency and crisis intervention: current evidence. *Curr Psychiatry Rep*. 2019 Jul 1;21(8):63. doi: 10.1007/s11920-019-1054-8.

43. Telepsychiatry Toolkit. 2020. https://www.psychiatry.org/psychiatrists/practice/telepsychiatry/toolkit.

39

Social Psychiatry in Russia

Olga A. Karpenko and George P. Kostyuk

Social aspects of psychiatry have been acknowledged by the leading Russian psychiatrists since the 19th century; however, by the 21st century, a standardized definition of social psychiatry is still absent. Different experts have different views on social psychiatry and its place in medical science and practice. Some think that there is no need to define social psychiatry as a distinct branch of psychiatry, because psychiatry is "social" a priori. Others regard social psychiatry as a discipline located somewhere in between psychiatry and sociology. Some think that social psychiatry is a practical approach that includes rehabilitation and social support of patients and organization of mental healthcare; others consider it to be a special scientific discipline.

We would like to provide several definitions of social psychiatry as suggested by Russian psychiatrists. By the definition of T. B. Dmitrieva[1] and B. S. Polozhiy[2]: "Social psychiatry is an independent branch of psychiatry that studies the influence of environmental factors on the mental health, their relationship with the prevalence, incidence, clinical manifestations and course of the mental disorders, as well as the possibility of social therapy, rehabilitation and prevention of mental pathology. The subject of social psychiatry is a public mental health."[1]

According to the definition of Yu. A. Alexandrovskiy,[3] social psychiatry is "[a] branch of psychiatry that studies the influence of social factors on the mental health, the onset and

---

1. T. B. Dmitrieva (1951–2010), member of the Russian Academy of Science (RAS), psychiatrist, director of Serbskiy Institute of Social and Forensic Psychiatry (Serbskiy Institute) (1990–2010), minister of health of Russian Federation (1996–1998).

2. B. S. Polozhiy, professor of psychiatry, director of the department of ecological and social problems of mental health, Serbskiy Institute.

3. Yu. A. Alexandrovskiy, corresponding member of RAS, psychiatrist, head of the department of "Borderline mental disorders" in Serbskiy Institute.

course of mental illness. The mission of social psychiatry is also to develop social rehabilitation of mentally ill."[2]

From our point of view, social psychiatry is a branch of psychiatry that studies the mutual influence of social environmental factors and mental health of the person and society. It can be defined from several perspectives: clinical, organizational, and epidemiological. From the clinical perspective, social psychiatry deals with the social functioning of the patient and with factors that contribute to or influence the social functioning of the person. From the public health perspective, social psychiatry deals with the interaction between the person and the society and includes organization of care in the community, and social support depending on the level of maladjustment or disability of the patient. From the epidemiological perspective, social psychiatry studies social factors that can contribute to the mental health of the population, as well as the mental health of the person or a group of people.

Quite often "social" psychiatry is opposed to "biological" psychiatry, and the precise definition of social psychiatry remains to be a matter of reflection for specialists.[3]

In this chapter we provide a brief historical overview of the development of the social approach in Russian psychiatry from the end of 19th century until today.

The influence of social factors on mental health, to our knowledge, was first discussed in 1887 during the first Congress of Russian psychiatrists. The chair of the Congress, I. P. Merjeevskiy,[4] presented a plenary speech, "Environmental factors that predispose the development of mental diseases in Russia and means of their reduction,"[4] where he suggested that mental disorders in most cases are a consequence of abnormal social conditions like wars, economic crises, low education level, and alcohol consumption. This speech provoked a discussion about social etiology of mental disorders and the need of social preventive strategies.[5] At the end of the 19th century, the development of mental healthcare in Russia was under the influence of the humanistic ideas of S. S. Korsakov and his followers. The "no restraint" principle was introduced in mental hospitals, along with the development of family patronage for discharged patients. The topic of prevention of mental disorders by the modification of social factors was one of the most discussed at that time; Korsakov,[5] N. N. Bazhenov,[6] P. B. Gannushkin,[7] and V. P. Serbskiy[8] considered the social aspect to be a cornerstone of clinical psychiatry and organization of care for the mentally ill.

---

4. I. P. Merjeevskiy (1838–1908), psychiatrist, one of the founders of Russian psychiatry.

5. S. S. Korsakov (1854–1900), professor of psychiatry, head of the psychiatry department in Moscow University, founder of the "no restraint" principle in Russia, world renowned for the description of alcohol amnestic syndrome (Korsakov syndrome).

6. N. N. Bazhenov (1857–1923), professor of psychiatry, known for the development of the family patronage system in Russia.

7. P. B. Gannushkin (1875–1933), professor of psychiatry, follower of Korsakov, known for the systematization and description of personality types.

8. V. P. Serbskiy (1958–1917), professor of psychiatry, follower of Korsakov, the founder of forensic psychiatry in Russia and the law for the rights of the mentally ill.

Later, at the beginning of the 20th century, ideas of psycho-hygiene predisposed further development of mental care in Russia and then in the Soviet Union.[6] In 1919, under the supervision of Gannushkin, district psychiatry care was introduced in Moscow; later, since 1924, it was developed in the network of community-based mental health clinics (mental dispensaries).[7] Primary, secondary, and tertiary prevention of mental disorders was one of the goals of the mental dispensaries. One of the strategies was prevention at the workplace and mental checkup of various social groups. Therefore, psychiatrists collected mental characteristics of the population, and performed statistical analyses of psychopathology and calculation of the prevalence of "neuroses" in the population. On the basis of the obtained data, preventive strategies were developed, although the greater part of the efforts was focused on the prevention of alcohol consumption. In 1925 the first education program on social psychiatry was developed.[1]

Later, in Soviet Russia, studies of the influence of social factors on mental disorders of the population were somewhat unwelcome, as social factors were considered to be in a good state due to the efforts of the Soviet government. Nevertheless, medical system development was one of the priorities in the USSR, including mental care, and the system of community-based mental-health services continued to develop,[7] with day hospitals starting to function in 1933. Rehabilitation strategies focused mostly on labor rehabilitation. In this regard it is worth mentioning the input of D. E. Melekhov,[9] who developed a system of stepwise labor rehabilitation. According to this system, patients started to work in the special medical workplaces within mental-health facilities; then they began to work under the supervision of psychiatrists in real-life workplaces; and the final step was the ability to work independently. The aim of the rehabilitation strategy was the inclusion of patients with severe mental disorders in the working settings.

The system of mental dispensaries, on the one hand, guaranteed available and free-of-charge outpatient care for the mentally ill, but on the other hand, it led to various social limitations for people who applied for mental care;[8] this resulted in a fear of psychiatry in the population. The cases of political abuse of Soviet psychiatry, well promoted by mass media, added to the enhancement of the stigma of psychiatry in the society. One of the steps forward for human rights protection in psychiatry was the initiation of the Mental Health Law. Legislation for psychiatry was a part of the general healthcare law in the USSR; the independent Mental Health Law appeared first in 1988 and then was updated in 1992. All aspects of mental care provision since then are strictly regulated;[9] the rights of people who applied for mental healthcare cannot be limited due to the application for help. In 2021 the working group on the Mental Health Law update was created by the initiative of the Ministry of Health. The main purpose of the Law modification is to increase the availability of help for people with non-severe mental disorders.

In recent years the de-institutionalization of psychiatry and the development of the various types of day-care facilities became a tendency that can be regarded as a part of

9. D. E. Melekhov (1899–1979), professor of psychiatry, one of the founders of social psychiatry in Russia, director of Moscow Research Institute of Psychiatry (1951–1956), founder of the system of labor rehabilitation, author of a textbook on psychiatry for Orthodox priests.

social psychiatry.[7] Fighting the stigma of psychiatry is one of the tasks that can bring mental healthcare closer to potential consumers. We would like to mention two initiatives in the field of social psychiatry that appeared in Russia in the past 5 years.

The projects of the Moscow mental health service "To Say or Not to Say" aims to increase the awareness of the population about mental disorders, available help, and the state of modern mental healthcare. To achieve this goal, mental-health professionals perform public lectures and mental checkups at public facilities like libraries or popular art places in Moscow. This activity takes part monthly for the general public and became popular among young people and students.[10]

Another remarkable initiative that we would like to mention is the creation of the Mental Health Commission within the Russian Association for the Advancement of Science (RAAS) initiated by the prominent Russian physicist E. P. Velikhov[10] and chaired by G. P. Kostyuk. One of the missions of this Commission is to stimulate research projects in the field of mental health of the person and the society. As the result of these efforts, the comprehensive research program "Fundamental Research of the Mental Health of a Person and the Society" was initiated and sponsored by the Russian Foundation for Basic Research (RFBR). This interdisciplinary research program united specialists in medicine, biology, physics, psychology, sociology, and pedagogics who performed research in the field of the mental health during 2017–2020. It was the first time that mental health became the subject of research within RFBR grants. Annual conferences on the mental health of the person and society are organized in Moscow University as part of this initiative. These conferences unite professionals from various fields of science who speak on mental health issues as an interdisciplinary problem.

Thus, social issues of psychiatry historically were a very important part of Russian psychiatry, although they never have been an independent psychiatric discipline. Stigmatization of psychiatry still remains a problem in Russian society, but initiatives that are being undertaken by mental-health professionals, in collaboration with the interdisciplinary scientific community, aim to stress the attention of society, policymakers, and academia on the importance of mental health problems.

References

1. Дмитриева ТБ, Положий БС. Социальная психиатрия//Психиатрия: национальное руководство/под ред. ТБ Дмитриевой, ВН Краснова, НГ Незнанова, ВЯ Семке, АС Тиганова. М.: ГЭОТАР-Медиа, 2011. [Dmitrieva TB, Polozhiy BS. Social psychiatry. In: Dmitrieva TB, Krasnov VN, Neznanov NG, Semke VYa, Tiganov AS, eds. *Psychiatry: National Guidelines*. M.: Geotar-Media; 2011 (in Russian)].
2. Александровский ЮА. Краткий психиатрический словарь. М.: РЛС-2009, 2008. [Alexandrovskiy YuA. *Brief psychiatric glossary*. M.: RDG-2009, 2008 (in Russian)].

10. E. P. Velikhov, Soviet and Russian physicist, known for his works in nuclear science and in the field of education and basic science development, founder and president of the Russian Association for the Advancement of Science.

3. Priebe S. A social paradigm in psychiatry: themes and perspectives. *Epidemiol Psychiatr Sci.* 2016;25(6):521–527. doi: 10.1017/S2045796016000147.

4. Каннабих ЮВ. История психиатрии/ЮВ. Каннабих. Москва: Издательство Юрайт, 2019. [Kannabikh YuV. *History of Psychiatry.* Moscow: Urait Publishing House; 2019. (in Russian)].

5. Положий БС. Роль Центра им. В.П. Сербского в развитии социальной психиатрии // Российский психиатрический журнал. 2017. No. 1. C. 32–36. [Polozhiy BS. The role of the Serbskiy Center in the development of the social psychiatry. *Russian Journal of Psychiatry.* 2017;1:32–36 (in Russian)].

6. Kostyuk GP, ed. Outpatient mental health services in Moscow: history through today. M.: KDU; 2019. doi: 10.31453/kdu.ru.91304.0035.

7. Karpenko O, Kostyuk G. Community-based mental health services in Russia: past, present, and future. *Lancet Psychiatry.* 2018;5(10):778–780. doi: 10.1016/S2215-0366 (18) 30263-3.

8. Krasnov V, Gurovich I. History and current condition of Russian psychiatry. *Int Rev Psychiatry.* 2012;24(4):328–333. doi: 10.3109/09540261.2012.694857.

9. Kostyuk G, Karpenko O, Masyakin A, Burygina L. Mental health law in Russia. *Eur Psychiatry.* 2019;56:S157–S158.

10. Abramova LN, Shakhova EV. To say or not to say: medical and social project. *Consortium Psychiatricum.* 2020;1(2):72–76. doi: 10.17650/2712-7672-2020-1-2-72-76.

The Emergence and Development of Social Psychiatry in Romania

Alexandru Paziuc, Doina Cozman, and Mircea Lazarescu

Wolfgang Rutz wrote in Lancet in 2004:

> During this period of European transition, societal stress and loss of social cohesion and spiritual values directly affect patterns of morbidity and mortality. Life expectancy has dropped by 10 years in the space of a decade, cerebrovascular and cardiovascular mortality has increased four-fold, youth criminality five-fold, addiction four-fold, deaths from external causes seven-fold, and suicides eight-fold. In some countries, the very fabric of society and human togetherness is influenced by increasing rates of homicide and child manslaughter. A community syndrome can be identified consisting of depression, stress-related disorders, and death; of suicide, self-destructive behavior, violence, and aggression; of vascular morbidity and mortality; of alcoholism and addiction; of risk-taking behavior leading to accidents in the streets and workplaces; and even of the loss of moral and ethical values, leading to "moral insanity."[1]

Rutz recommends interventions to enhance control, empowering people in society and workplaces, supporting social connectedness, family cohesion, and spiritual values, and facilitating identity and dignity by increasing pluralism, tolerance, and democracy. Also, a new mental health approach, focusing on the psychosocial and existential determinants of mental and physical health—a holistically minded, public mental health approach.

For both contemporaneous commentators and historians, psychiatry within what was Communist Europe has largely been discussed through the prism of politics and ideology. Recently, scholars have begun to debate the extent to which psychiatric practices within post–World War II Eastern Europe were beholden to the ideological aspirations of the political elite. There is a difference between psychiatric practices that were socialist by design—where professional knowledge was theoretically guided by ideological considerations—and those that were socialist by default—where practices were shaped by the socialist context without being meaningfully inspired by ideology. This understanding makes it easier to connect Eastern Europe to the broader historiography of the twentieth century. In the current system of psychiatric care, dispensaries take a central position. Key issues of the discussion on mental healthcare include ways of coping with social stress disorders, strategies to redefine psychiatric rehabilitation in a changed socioeconomic context, and steps toward strengthening social support networks for people with mental illness.[2]

Psychiatry, while providing new insights into the experience of state-sponsored Communism.[3] Scholars debated the extent of psychiatric practices within post-WWII Eastern Europe were beholden to the ideological aspirations of the political the need and the need to differentiate between psychiatric practices that were socialist by design—where professional knowledge was theoretically guided by ideological considerations—and those that were socialist by default—where practices were shaped by the socialist context without being meaningfully inspired by ideology. By drawing a clearer distinction between "socialist by design" and "socialism by default," it became easier to reconnect Eastern Europe to the broader historiography of twentieth century psychiatry, while simultaneously providing new insights into the experience of state-sponsored Communism.

Professional knowledge is simultaneously shaped by a practitioner's own beliefs and social ambitions, as well as the legal, material, and political constraints of reality—themselves often consequences of the overarching ideological system. Psychiatry simply cannot be analyzed or understood independently from the social environment. The concept of "socialist by default" allows one to see how diagnostic and therapeutic practices could be impacted by ideology without necessarily being beholden to it, a notion worth considering because all forms of psychiatry occur within an ideological context of one sort or another.[3]

With these statements as the backdrop, this chapter aims to present the emergence and development of social psychiatry in Romania, the activity of the Association for Social Psychiatry of Romania, and models of good practice in the field of social and community psychiatry in Romania, as well as the future directions to take in this field.

Short History of Social Psychiatry in Romania

The history of Romanian psychiatry was marked by some significant sequences. Ever since the 19th century until the interwar period, some important psychiatric hospitals were established in Romania (for instance, Sibiu, Iași, Bucharest, Bălți, and Oradea) around which Romanian psychiatry developed. Most of the hospitals currently existing in Romania were founded during 1955–1965. A large part of them were in former barracks, mansions, schools, dorms, and even monasteries.[4] The decade that followed, 1965–1975, led to the establishment of most of the psychiatric wards of the unified hospitals in Romania. The third wave is the decade 1975–1985, when, in Romania, the services of community psychiatry were established: Laboratories for Mental Health (LMH) and the Day In-patient Units. The legal basis for them was a disposition from the Ministry of Health in 1974 stipulating the objectives and the way of functioning for these services, pleading also for the organization of occupational therapy. LMH were established in county capitals with the goals of active detection of the risk factors to prevent psychological disorders and treating them at an early stage. LMH aimed to organize and supervise research on the risk factors of psychological hygiene and psychological prophylaxis, promoting mental health based on the morbidity index.

The growing interest during the 1970s in Romania for mental health and the issues of social psychiatry saw an increase in the publication of books and scientific events and conferences on psychiatry: in Bucharest (1974) on the topic, "Recovery and Social Work in Psychological Disorders"; in Timisoara (1976) on "Issues of Social Psychiatry"; and the Third Conference of Social Psychiatry, in Timisoara (September 1978). National events on LMHs were organized at Pitești in 1979, 1984, and 1989, and the Fourth Conference of Social Psychiatry, in Timisoara in 1986. In addition, services of paid polyclinic occupational therapy were established in centers like Timisoara, Bucharest, Iasi, and Sibiu, the trainers being hospital employees. Tailoring, carpentry, cardboard, crafts, and assembling workshops carried out their activities, attended by psychotic patients from the polyclinic who received 70% of the earnings. Renowned psychiatrists, such as Mircea Lazarescu in Timisoara, Petre Branzei in Iasi, and Aurel Romila in Bucharest, supported and developed these services at that time. The activity of occupational therapy introduced a methodical program in the lives of psychotic patients who lived at home, which was amplified by participating in LMH programs, joint meals on holidays, and annual trips. Thus, the atmosphere of a genuine therapeutic community was created. During this period of 1975–1985, the psychiatric therapeutic system benefited from the support of many external collaborators, such as psychological, social, and art therapy, as "psychiatrists' friends."

The Establishment of the Association of Social Psychiatry of Romania (APSRO)

In 2005, an initiative group led by Alexandru Paziuc established at Campulung Moldovenesc the Association of Social Psychiatry of Romania in order to prepare, promote, and implement at all levels projects to support community psychiatric care for persons with mental disorders, aiming to support and encourage their social inclusion.[3] In recent years the association was promoting its purpose and goals, namely to change society's vision of the concept of mental disorder, of stimulating reintegration into society and family, psychological recovery and help for persons with mental health issues, and integrating the community with APSRO.

In Romania, the care delivered for mental disorders concentrates mostly in the psychiatric hospitals and is of a biological model. Over 75% of the experts in mental health (psychiatrists, psychologists, social workers) are employed or trained in academic centers. The rural areas are well under-represented in the workforce. Treatments remain psychopharmacological, with very limited psychosocial rehabilitation, multidisciplinary therapeutic team, and case management strategies. The persistence in the public opinion of a negative image of psychological disorders and stigma of illness, treatments, psychological recovery, and rehabilitation of psychological disorders resists necessary reforms in mental health in Romania.

The trend to institutionalize patients with mental disorders, the orientation more to biological therapies, and the lack of some (enough and efficient) services for social reinsertion and support also have caused an increase of frequent relapses, the psychiatric disorders turning chronic, and an increase of the hospitalization costs with the concomitant reduction of the quality and efficiency of psychiatric services. All these further contribute to the deepening of the stigmatization, marginalization, and isolation of persons with psychiatric problems. From the Association of Social Psychiatry of Romania perspective, we cannot talk of health in general without mental health. Mental health is part of the policies for public health, and psychological disorder must be considered and treated without discrimination, as any other somatic condition. The psychological disorder is not only an individual, family, and psychiatric services issue, it is also an issue of the community where the respective person lives and, by its costs and socioeconomic implications, and it is a national matter. Therefore, the association promotes the orientation of the psychiatric care from the hospital to the community and the complex multidisciplinary approach of the mental health and social support issues in the context of an appropriate motivating and stimulating legal framework.

APSRO promotes the issuing of a new policy in mental health, with a new vision, respectively to deliver accessible quality services, based on the existing needs, in as less restrictive as possible environment, especially at the community level, and the increase of the efficiency of the programs for promotion, prevention, and education to improve the population's state of mental health. The fundamental value at the ground to perform this policy was and continues to be the respect for human rights and the observance of the human dignity.

The passage from the institutionalized traditional system of care to one putting the emphasis on the person's integration into the community implies the acceptance and implementation of a set of principles such as:[5]

- **Autonomy**, defined as personal freedom, allowed the newly developed services to have the capacity to preserve and promote independence by discovering and stimulating the positive and "healthy" aspects of each patient's behavior, thus reinforcing such person's capacity to decide and have independent options regardless of the presence of the disability and of express symptomatology.
- **Responsibility** refers to the set of expectancies, which the patients, their familie,s and general population have about the functioning of the mental health services. Thus, the trust

in a certain service is given by the measure of how the service corresponds or satisfies the individual needs if the experts treating such persons observe the norms of medical ethics and deontology.

- **Effectiveness, efficiency, and equity** in using the resources in an underfinanced health-care system allowed for the gradual development of services quality.
- **Continuity, accessibility, and community participation** in the decision-making and co-ordination of the integrated services of mental healthcare facilitated the implementation of some community programs, in fighting against stigma and in reducing the community resistance to the mental disorder, the patient, and his/her family.

The setting up of the multidisciplinary team, the teamwork, the case management, and the definition of its members' responsibilities highlighted the process of:

- **Psychosocial rehabilitation** with the prevention of relapses, the improvement of the remaining functional skills, and patients' social reintegration. This in part became possible by making use of medical, psychiatric care in an integrative, multidisciplinary approach (psychologist, social worker, priest, occupational therapy trainer). Thus, the individual work was replaced with teamwork, emphasizing the individual's existential, biological, psychological, social, and spiritual sides, promoting the individual's real psychosocial recovery, integration, and rehabilitation.

Thus, in 1983 at Campulung Moldovenesc, with the establishment of a new modern general hospital in the old pavilion-like building located in the center of the town, a psychiatric ward with 80 beds and assigned area imprinted the further development of the psychiatric services adjusted to the local needs, means, and mentalities. The achieved results encouraged the further conceptualization of a model of psychiatric care in the community, where the experts, the beneficiaries of the psychiatric services, their families, and volunteers worked together to overcome the obstacles and find the solutions required for change.

The moment triggered a reform in mental health in 1999, with the separation of the psychiatric ward from the general hospital. The Foundation Orizonturi and AREAS, by the Town Hall and the representatives of the Ministry of Health, and by experts' associations (Romania Association of Psychiatry and Psychotherapy, and the Association of Social Psychiatry of Romania), turned the time of separation into the beginning of a genuine reform in mental health.

Being a region with strong religious customs, we arranged a chapel and employed a missionary priest who carried out, in addition to the specific activities (religious service and pastoral counseling), social reintegration. Besides the patients, people outside the hospital attended these services. This enhanced the relationship with the community and decreased marginalization, isolation, or stigmatization from the society.

Today, the CMH of Campulung Moldovenesc has a multidisciplinary community team formed of psychiatrist, psychologists, social worker, occupational therapy trainer, and nurse, which allows the possibility to continue, at the community level, the services initiated in the hospital. To deal with community resistances, we organized anti-stigma campaigns, exhibits of occupational therapy in the community, and round tables at the level of the partner town halls.

The large area assigned to the psychiatric sector of Campulung Bucovina (4000 km²), predominantly rural, with villages being isolated by mountains and woods, challenged the team of the Mental Health Centre for the process of evaluation, monitoring, and delivering mental healthcare services as close as possible to the patient's life environment. Thus, the idea was born to create the multidisciplinary mobile team to move in the territory, a project which received European funding. During 2008–2009, the European Union financed the project "Community Alternatives of Psychiatric Care" by the Program "Support for the Development of the Mental Health Community Services and Deinstitutionalization of the Persons with Mental Health Issues," Component B–Development of the Centres for Mental Health. The project was developed and implemented by the Foundation Orizonturi of Campulung Moldovenesc and the Centre for Mental Health of the Psychiatric Hospital of Campulung Moldovenesc with the support of the 13 partners represented by a hospital (the Psychiatric Hospital of Campulung Moldovenesc), a nongovernmental organization (NGO) (Association Effes of Siret), and the town halls of Campulung Moldovenesc.

Indirect/final beneficiaries were: the Centre for Mental Health and the Psychiatric Hospital of Campulung Moldovenesc, local public authorities, NGOs, patients' families, and the proximal community. The services delivered at beneficiaries' homes were adjusted to the individual needs and comprised medical support (psychosocial interventions), development of independent life skills, spending the spare time, promoting health, and counseling on other issues, for instance, legal or administrative.

A mobile team formed of experts delivered the services. It was created in the Centre of Mental Health of the Psychiatric Hospital of Campulung Moldovenesc and had a multidisciplinary approach, involving various specializations: psychiatrist, psychologists, social worker, nurse, priest, and occupational therapist, The project's activities and objective were promoted through the site www.echipamobila.ro and information materials, which were published and disseminated in the information areas organized at the premises of the town hall for each local community. At the end of the project implementation, a guide on the development of the community services was published: "Practical Guide for the Development of the Community Care Services for the Persons with Mental Health Issues Living in Small Towns and Rural Areas."

APSRO and Civil Society: Partnership with the Foundation Orizonturi

Nevertheless, not all these positive results would have been possible if we did not conclude a partnership relying on trust, respect, and mutual support with the direct beneficiaries of these services: patients and their families.

Thus, we established an NGO, Foundation Orizonturi, which is a charity, nongovernmental, apolitical, and spiritual organization acting in the field of mental health since 1995. In the Foundation Orizonturi vision, there is a future world where stigma and discrimination due to mental health issues disappear, and the psychiatric services' beneficiaries are integrated into the community socially and economically.

The organization has the mission to improve the quality of life for the beneficiaries of psychiatric services. The Foundation Orizonturi aims to support persons with mental health issues to regain self-confidence and to acquire some skills and competencies, allowing them to have an independent and active life at the community level.

The objectives of the Foundation Orizonturi include the information and education of persons with mental disorders on the health issues they are facing; the development of permanent activities of occupational and work therapies for the beneficiaries of psychiatric services; the improvement of community relations in order to increase comprehension and acceptance of the persons with mental health issues as active persons at the community level; and the socio-professional reinsertion of the persons with mental health disorders.

The activities of the Foundation Orizonturi mainly rely on its members' volunteer services and, along with them, of other persons who understand the organization's mission and are willing to support its development. The persons benefiting from the organization's activities are beneficiaries, former beneficiaries of psychiatric services, their kin, and legal supporters.

Current activities of the organization include:

- Starting in 1995, magazine of Romania's informative instructive and cultural character is designed to facilitate the relation of beneficiaries and society.
- Establishing some workshops for activities of occupational and work therapies (traditional sewing, carpet weaving, wood and canvas painting, pottery, tailoring) for the organization members, persons with mental disorders.
- Organizing weekly meetings for the organization members where they discuss current social issues and personal matters.
- Organizing meetings with persons who use the psychiatric services for the first time to provide them with information on the organization's role and activities.
- Club activities and monthly celebration of the organization members' birthdays.
- Exchanges, cooperation, and partnerships with Romanian and foreign NGOs working either in the same field of activity or in related fields.
- Participation in round tables, seminars, and conferences on topics of interest for the performance of the organization's activity and for its development.

More important projects run by the Foundation Orizonturi:

- journal realized by the beneficiaries of psychiatric services.
- **New ways of life through work**: ceramic workshop where the beneficiaries of psychiatric services work.
- **Campaigns against the discrimination and for the support and observance of the rights for the persons with mental health issues.**
- **Ways to policies**: program bringing together the beneficiaries of psychiatric services and their organizations, experts in the field, representatives of the state institutions, local

authorities, civil society, and mass media so they initiate together proper policies for mental health at local and national levels.

- **Integration in work:** warranty for equal opportunities and increase in the quality of life for the persons with disabilities, in partnership with the Romanian League for Mental Health.
- **International Journal of Grassroots Public Action:** a joint project run by InterAction, Whitstable–Kent, Centre for Citizenship and Community Mental Health, the University of Bradford, and the Foundation Orizonturi.

The publishing of the journal "A FI–TO BE" was the first important activity that provided the possibility to involve the beneficiaries. Both journal editing and desktop publishing are accomplished by the beneficiaries. The journal represents their "voice" on their life experiences, issues, and talent.

The beneficiaries are permanently involved in issuing, implementing, monitoring, and developing various projects. Their opinions are respected and used in the project's development. The beneficiaries are involved in organizing various events and are responsible for the organization of the current activities.

A program run in partnership by the Foundation Orizonturi, the Psychiatric Hospital of Campulung, Hamlet Trust of London, and the Town Hall of Campulung during 2003–2005 is the program Ways to Policies. The program is a good example, as it gives the beneficiaries of psychiatric services the possibility to contribute in the development of alternatives and to have a word in the drafting of better mental health policies at local and national levels; it facilitates the partnerships at national and local levels; it facilitates the partnerships between the groups of psychiatric services beneficiaries, institutions, political, and business environments, mass media, and other persons or groups interested in the problematic of mental health, providing them with the role of important "players" in the process of policymaking and in fighting against stigmatization and discrimination. The members of the Forum for Local Policies are among the psychiatric services' beneficiaries (33.33%), experts in the field (psychiatrists, nurses, psychologists), and persons from various fields of activity (education, police, justice, religious convictions, social work, local authority, mass media) interested in the matter of mental health. During the meetings that took place in the Town Hall council room during 2003–2005, the local forum activity focused on local problems in mental health, and highlighted a consistent and responsible participation by the forum members, who organized actions to address the identified issues. The program also stipulated 4 meetings at the national level, organized at Campulung Moldovenesc, Iaşi, Braşov, and Bucharest, at which other nongovernmental beneficiaries' organizations, local public authorities' representatives, and state institutions (Ministry of Public Health) participated.

Putting together knowledge, experience, opinions, and ideas, and so removing barriers once considered insurmountable, the participants in local and national forums drafted a list of priorities in mental health, as seen not only by the experts in the field but also by the beneficiaries of psychiatric services, and also by other institutions, persons, and groups of persons who are interested in mental health issues, and may intervene one way or another in solving them.

There were among the priority issues identified by the forum members:

- Stigmatization and marginalization of the persons with mental disorders due to population's insufficient information and education on psychological disorders, on their prevention and treatment, on the psychiatric services and the alternatives to those, and on the possibilities to reintegrate socio-professionally the persons with mental disorders. The potentially identified solutions were concretely implementing the provisions of Article 4 of the Law on mental health and protection for persons with psychological disorders; campaigns in mass media, schools, social environments with low education level; "open gates" policy; capitalization of the remaining capacities; community involvement.
- The absence of a consultative forum on the mental health issues at the national level to take and submit local matters and to represent the voice of the psychiatric services' beneficiaries, for their kin, for the experts, for the social services, and for those in the support system (church, business, mass media, etc.). Possible solution: creating a forum with wider representation of all above-mentioned categories meant to evaluate the issues and to monitor the resources by cooperation with local and regional forums, to create a database and to mediatize the activity, to keep the connection between the state institutions–nongovernmental organizations of mental health–experts–community, to identify and approach partners to discuss the improvement of the legal framework.
- The legal framework is insufficient on the protection of employments, the retirement and social aid system, fiscal facilities, norming the experts, the ratio set by law between the population's number and the community services (day-care centers, home care, community assistance). Possible solution: the consultative forum for mental health issues to initiate and support legal draft laws.
- The lack of funds at national and local levels for funding the community psychiatric assistance services and some social enterprises. Possible solution: legal draft laws through the consultative forum for mental health issues (protected housing, protected employments, urban and rural crisis centers).
- The lack of legal framework to regulate both a viable system of community assistance in psychiatry and the beneficiaries', kin's, and volunteers' training if they are willing to work in the system, and the training for the experts in the field (e.g., courses of community psychiatry, healthcare, and social services in psychiatry). Possible solution: to create a national center for mental health to cooperate directly with the decision-making bodies of the Ministry of Health, Ministry of Education, Ministry of Justice, and Ministry of Finance.
- The lack of communication and, implicitly, of cohesion between the state institutions, the nongovernmental organizations of mental health, experts, and the community. Possible solution: to organize local and regional forums to deliver information at the territorial level (identified issues and propositions for solutions and concrete actions) to the consultative forum for mental health issues which, at its turn, to act to facilitate the communication and, implicitly, the cohesion between the state institutions, the nongovernmental organizations of mental health, the experts, and the community.

Due to these activities carried out by the Psychiatric Hospital, the Foundation Orizonturi, and APSRO, in 2014, the prestigious journal *The Economist Intelligence Unit* published a paper, "Mental Health and Integration Services to Support the Persons with Psychological Disorders: Comparative Survey of 30 European Countries"; even though Romania took place 29 (due to the delay in the mental health reform), it still emphasized positively the activity at Campulung Moldovenesc, which was considered an example to follow.

Among the Association's objectives, there is also professional training for the persons involved in community psychiatric assistance, and the organization of several scientific and professional events with specific topics of community psychiatric assistance.

Since its establishment until now, the association members have participated with papers in the WASP International Congresses at Kobe, Prague, Marrakesh, and Lisbon, and decided to host the 23rd World Congress of Social Psychiatry, in Bucharest, October 25–28, 2019. The World Congress was a grand success with 653 delegates from 66 countries participating. The largest delegations came from Romania (297), but there were also large numbers of participants from India, the United Kingdom, Japan, Thailand, France, Australia, the United States, Portugal, Italy, and Germany There were 441 scientific presentations, including 12 plenary sessions, 53 symposia, 19 workshops, 97 free papers, and 81 e-posters. Early Career Psychiatrists Fellowships were awarded to 21 young colleagues from all parts of the world.

Conclusions and Lessons from Romanian Social Psychiatry and APSRO

1. The history of Romanian psychiatry was marked by significant sequences starting with pre-socialistic, socialistic, post-socialistic, and current advances in psychiatric rehabilitation
2. Therapeutic practices could be impacted by ideology without necessarily being beholden to it.
3. During this period of European transition, societal stress and loss of social cohesion and spiritual values directly affect patterns of morbidity and mortality.
4. The growing interest and active participation of Romanian social psychiatry in the 1970s advanced mental health and the issues of social psychiatry, with an increase clinical services and publications and scientific events.
5. Active participation in WASP Congresses and hosting the Congress in 2019 advanced the professional identity and scientific aspects of Romanian psychiatry. We feel fortunate and grateful.

References

1. Wolfgang Rutz. A need to rethink social psychiatry in Europe. *The Lancet*. 2004;363:1652. www.thelancet.com

2. Lăzărescu M. Aspects historic ale psihiatriei socio comunitare din Banat, Al 7-lea Congres National de Psihiatrie al ARPP, Sibiu, 29 Please add)Mai–01 Iunie 2019.
3. Mat Savelli. Beyond ideological platitudes: socialism and psychiatry in Eastern Europe Palgrave Communications. McMaster University, Hamilton; 2018. doi:10.1057/s41599-018-0100-1.
4. Paziuc A., Paziuc P. Spitalul de Psihiatrie Câmpulung Moldovenesc trecut, prezent și viitor, CNSM, București, 3–4 octombrie 2009.
5. World Health Organization. Organization of Services for Mental Health (Mental Health Policy and Service Guidance Package). Geneva: WHO 2022.

Epilogue

Anthropology, Social Psychiatry, and Mental Health

Rachid Bennegadi

Introduction

Social psychiatry deals with social factors associated with psychiatric morbidity, social effects of mental illness, psychosocial disorders and social approaches to psychiatric care, as has been described beautifully in the previous chapters of this volume. A social perspective in psychiatry and psychiatric research encompasses the social nature of human life. Social psychiatry is concerned with the interaction of the sociocultural environment and the individual. While recognizing the contribution of the individual's neurobiological and psychological factors, it incorporates anthropological, social, familial, cultural, religious, and technological contributions to understand and provide solutions for one's individual and social enhancement.

The psychological assistance of a person requires a certain number of competences: psychiatric competences in order to comprehend neuropsychiatric disorders, psychotherapeutic competences to discern psychological disorders or psychological suffering, plus being able to take into account the social determinants.

My long clinical experience as a psychiatrist and anthropologist at the Françoise Minkowska Centre, a French institution where we receive migrants, addressing their challenges of migration and as refugees in an exile context, has allowed me to learn a number of primary facts. At the Minkowska Centre, I received patients from all over the world, primarily those who spoke French, English, or Arabic. The mastery of these three languages enabled an adequate level of communication, but I realized that plurilingualism does not guarantee a cultural competence.

My patients were mainly affected by their migration trajectories and the disarray of exile in a rather violent way; in addition they encountered socioeconomic and administrative problems. The interference of these social determinants led me to establish a suitable support scheme for this population by involving as many social workers as possible to team up with the psychotherapists. This cooperation allowed us to tackle the problem in its true complexity.

The social psychiatry point of view of this issue intrigued me as much as transcultural psychiatry. I also realized that this was not just a theoretical problem. I don't mean to minimize the problem and to say that it's enough to be trained to be an expert in the matter, but the most helpful measure we took was the training of our psychotherapists in the assistance of migrants and refugees. I also realized an important concept in social psychiatry: the resistance of mental health professionals to anthropological and social discourses. The therapeutical care of a population who are more or less lost in French society requires a well-codified therapeutic framework.

Intercultural Communication

We find two circumstances: either the patient and the therapist share a common language; or they don't share a common language, in which case it is essential to have a linguistic and cultural interpreter in order to complete the therapeutic framework. The presence of an interpreter is not a matter translation, but a comparison of explanatory models and cultural references that the interpreter must be able to metaphorize simultaneously for the therapist and for the patient. This requires training, and I often noted the difficulties of this three-way communication that often impedes a coherent clinical framework.

An essential step to ensure an intercultural communication is to discuss with the interpreter beforehand. Moreover, the notion of countertransference is essential in this case; the fact that the therapist and the patient share the same language does not mean that they share the same cultural references.

So what competences can we expect from therapists, psychiatrists, psychologists, or psychoanalysts?

There has been plenty of research literature on the matter; the World Psychiatric Association has a vast collection of transcultural psychiatry papers that bring to light the intricacies of the therapeutic framework. Furthermore, the work on social and cultural psychiatry of the University of Montreal done by Laurence Kirmayer shows that the social dimension cannot be divided from the cultural dimension; it is necessary to integrate both elements into the therapeutic framework. All ethno-psychiatric theoretical approaches have advanced the debate on "cultural specificity."

Due to globalization, we've seen an increase in psychotherapeutic demand also because the access to mental health care is increasingly encouraged for people in precarious situations. Arthur Kleinman from Harvard University proposes a theoretical approach with a particular interest: clinical medical anthropology.[1]

The Interest of Clinical Medical Anthropology in Social Psychiatry

By differentiating "sickness, illness, and disease" as individual concepts, this approach allows us to integrate the social determinants (sickness) that impact the personality by allowing the patients to express their psychological suffering and their psychological or psychiatric disorders by means of their own cultural references and his explanatory models (illness). This allows the therapeutic framework to come together. I would like to emphasize that the therapist must be able, whatever his/her theoretical approach, to conceive an idea of the disorders from which his/her patients suffer, along with establishing a diagnosis and an appropriate therapeutic indication (disease). The patient may encounter individual difficulties and not only culture- and social-related difficulties at each stage of this particular setting.

In order to avoid countertransference concerns, which unconsciously stigmatize or else overvalue the patient, we must train therapists on this eclectic approach. It allows them and the patient to develop a person-centered framework in the most rewarding way.[2]

The Practical Application and the Therapeutic Reality

How can social psychiatry integrate this person-centered approach without neglecting a therapy's neuroscientific, psychoanalytic, and psychiatric dimensions?

In today's context, with globalization and worldwide human migration, it is no longer possible to assess a person on a single cultural criterion. This universal approach of humanity is not only a humanistic theory, but a pragmatic humanism that respects the person and offers competent mental healthcare.

If the therapist and the patient speak the same language, it will effectively allow the therapist to establish an easier-to-manage communication scheme compared to the scenario where they don't share the same language, or where the patient or the therapist has not mastered the metaphorical competences of the language they are speaking during therapy, thus creating discomfort (transference and countertransference). Any therapist who has had the opportunity to receive a patient who does not really speak the same language knows what I am talking about. This is why, when arranging a linguistic and cultural interpretation, it is necessary to prepare before the first interview by explaining these different aspects. If not, the most frequent outcome is that the dialogue will become exclusive between the patient and the interpreter, leaving the therapist out of the discussion.

The Means That Society Has to Offer Quality Mental Healthcare

Without the financial support to enable the therapeutic framework described above, either from an association or private funds, it would be difficult to incorporate the "cultural competences" to the social, psychological, and anthropological dimensions. It is important to address this matter because it clearly states the therapist's training as one of the main elements of cultural competences.

This training should be included already in university programs or it should be a complementary apprenticeship financed by a given society. Nevertheless, it has become a Cornelian dilemma because of globalization and the current increase of demand in mental healthcare. We will have to endure with what is available, but at the same time it is impossible to deal with the high demand through online counseling. The social and transcultural psychiatry services will eventually become overwhelmed by a high demand, not because it is inadequate, but because it requires previous training to be able to put in place an online therapeutic framework.

As important aspects of interpersonal relationship, how should we manage the transference and the countertransference in this case? Where is the place for empathy?

Once again, we tend to neglect the access to information when receiving a patient via internet or social media. From one positive point of view, the acceleration of online communication is beneficial for online therapy, but it can also have a disturbing effect because of its pace. In the case of social psychiatry, engaging in regular webinars and virtual conferences in the interest of synthesizing all the social, anthropological, economic, and ethical determinants, it will have a federating effect while it refers to mental illness with a universal approach of humanity.

However, it seems that social psychiatry cannot accept this strategy regardless of its goodwill, getting unconsciously trapped by the risk of stigmatization or cultural complicity.

Psychoanalysis, originally founded by Sigmund Freud, is a very good example of an attempt to universalize a problem by using arguments in which all humans should recognize themselves. Even if Freudian concepts of the id, the ego, and the superego knew a true success, the oedipal problematic remains difficult for many theorists because the cultural references of Greek mythology are not necessarily shared by the rest of humanity. Furthermore, Freud's biggest success was to raise awareness about the psychological defense mechanisms of human beings. The Jungian approach and its theory of anima and animus remains very interesting, and the current research in Lacanian and post-Lacanian psychoanalysis remains relevant in the debate on the functional capability of the brain and the psyche.[3] Following psychoanalytic research on the link between neurobiology and psychoanalysis, one must conclude that psychoanalysis remains pertinent regarding the human's performance of either the brain, the psyche, or the personality.

In addition, Boris Cyrulnik's[4] enlightening work about the establishment of a secure attachment between mother and child on their earlier interactions must be taken into account when taking charge of the post-traumatic syndrome, because in case of trauma it will allow the person to adopt a resilient posture. The most important point of this approach is that it complements, in a relevant way, the mobilization of energy from a vital impetus and the structure of personality to restore the meaning of a human life.

All of the methods mentioned in this book, which seeks to promote social psychiatry as a human and social science, show that it is important to appreciate clinical practices and clinical research because they enlighten us on the complexity of the mind.

It is also important to remember the cybernetic dimension of social psychiatry, especially the concepts of "transhumanism" and "post-humanism."[5,6]

Conclusion

Finally, it is necessary to establish a relation between the appearance of the homo-cyberneticus and the anguish of death. These will be competences that will allow us to tell the fake news apart from scientific reality. We must not neglect the threat of digital addiction. Ultimately, the responsibilities of each discipline must be clearly defined. Social psychiatry should not disassociate the social dimension and the cultural dimension. It is therefore necessary to train all of the mental health professionals on this new epistemological dimension of social psychiatry by learning to master the changes caused by the new social and cultural paradigms.

To summarize the content of the ideas, projects, and observations, I would like to make a few statements.

We must ask ourselves if the proverb "show me your friends and I'll tell you who you are" is applicable for those who are permanently connected to social media, including Twitter, Facebook, Instagram, Telegram, Linkedin, and all of the upcoming platforms. The law of the market is the one that actually decides the employability of the new softwares without taking into consideration their impact on our "mindware" (a neologism that tries to reconcile neurosciences and algorithms).

"Will humans and robots appreciate each other or will one end up demonizing or subjugating the other?" In this day and age, the debate over the impact of cybernetics on mental health revolves around the advocacy of transhumanism (improving human beings and increasing their skills and emotions) and post-humanism (disappearance of human beings in favor of humanoid structures).

Anyway, as far as we are concerned, it is important in the area of mental health to anticipate the disruptions that digital addiction may cause in people's daily lives, in their psychological care, and in the process of psychotherapeutic care. Consciousness is built within every human being through love and protection of those who educate us—our parents, school, and society.

None of us is "programmed"; we all have our own rituals and we have room to create our psychic and social lives. This implies a "right to error" that qualifies human beings, as well as a constant search for "the truth" that qualifies the human being. Transhumanism or post-humanism, where are we heading to with these new creatures created from cybernetics and meant to improve human intelligence? The question may seem ahead of schedule, but the digital world is not moving at the same pace as the field of emotions.

Can we consider those who are not connected to social media as lonely? We have a million friends and at the same time we have no friends. We have forums without any expertise, and we have an unprecedented flood of hate. All of this is part of our everyday intellectual environment without anyone knowing the slightest solution to regulate social media. This matter seems to be out of our hands, and it reminds us of the mythology of the

Golem, a creature made by humans who takes over humanity. It is a collective fear as old as human beings, except that today it has become a reality.

Psychiatric services need maximum flexibility, responding to changing needs; they must be ready to be confronted, ready to cooperate, ready to take responsibility toward society, ready to make their work and problems transparent, but resisting all attempts of society to delegate all responsibility to psychiatry. Only then will the community be ready to participate in shaping an acceptable life for our patients in their midst.[7]

References

1. Kleinman A. *Patients and Healers in the Context of Culture: An Exploration of the Borderland Between Anthropology, Medicine, and Psychiatry.* Berkeley: University of California Press; 1980.
2. Mezzich JE, Botbol M, Christodoulou GN, Cloninger CR, Salloum IM. *Person Centered Psychiatry.* Cham: Springer International; 2018.
3. Naccache L, Naccache MK. Parlez-vous cerveau? *Odile Jacob 7 Mars*; 2018. Sciences & Techniques.
4. Cyrulnik B. What approach to take to improve the quality of childhood in the European Union? the University of Toulon, France. 12 November 2008. https://www.allianceforchildhood.eu/files/Improving_the_quality_of_Childhood_Vol1/Hoofdstuk%2015%20pagina%20152-163.pdf
5. Ferry L. *La révolution transhumaniste.* Ed Plon; 2016.
6. Harari YN. *Homo Deus: une brève histoire de l'avenir.* Ed. Albin Michel; 2017.
7. Uchtenhagen AA. Which future for social psychiatry? *Int Rev Psychiatry.* 2008 Dec;20(6):535–539. https://doi.org/10.1080/09540260802565471.

Index

For the benefit of digital users, indexed terms that span two pages (e.g., 52–53) may, on occasion, appear on only one of those pages.

Tables, figures, and boxes are indicated by *t*, *f*, and *b* following the page number